P9-CRX-787

SOLID ORGAN TRANSPLANT REJECTION

Mechanisms, Pathology, and Diagnosis

edited by

KIM SOLEZ
University of Alberta
Edmonton, Alberta, Canada

LORRAINE C. RACUSEN
Johns Hopkins University School of Medicine
Baltimore, Maryland

MARGARET E. BILLINGHAM
Stanford University School of Medicine
Stanford, California

Marcel Dekker, Inc. New York • Basel • Hong Kong

Library of Congress Cataloging-in-Publication Data

Solid organ transplant rejection : mechanisms, pathology, and
diagnosis / edited by Kim Solez, Lorraine C. Racusen, Margaret E.
Billingham.
p. cm.
Includes index.
ISBN 0-8247-9510-5 (hardcover : alk. paper)
1. Transplant immunology. 2. Graft rejection. I. Solez, Kim.
II. Racusen, Lorraine C. III. Billingham, Margaret E.
[DNLM: 1. Graft Rejection. WO 680 S686 1996]
QR188.8.S66 1996
617.9'5—dc20
DNLM/DLC
for Library of Congress 95-46369
CIP

The publisher offers discounts on this book when ordered in bulk quantities. For more information, write to Special Sales/Professional Marketing at the address below.

This book is printed on acid-free paper.

Marcel Dekker, Inc.
270 Madison Avenue, New York, New York 10016

Current printing (last digit):
10 9 8 7 6 5 4 3 2 1

PRINTED IN THE UNITED STATES OF AMERICA

Foreword

This book details contemporary experience in molecular biology, histopathology, and rejection diagnosis in solid-organ transplantation, and enlightens us on the prospects of improving clinical results by more focused and rationally designed antirejection drug therapy.

We are at a point of transition in clinical transplantation medicine. Extensive scientific investments toward the understanding of immunology and molecular biology of acute allograft rejection, together with the discovery of cyclosporine and development of combination drug therapy, have improved short-term graft survival to levels that we could not dream about some 15 years ago. New challenges are, however, ahead. Regardless of the improvement in short-term graft survival of virtually all allografts, the half-life of transplants and the long-term success after the first year have not significantly improved. Multiple antigen-dependent and antigen-independent parameters influence the long-term survival, and result in clinical, metabolical, and histological manifestations in the transplant that are collectively called "chronic rejection."

The ultimate goal of this book is general application of the methods of diagnosis and treatment of rejection and allied conditions in grafted solid organs. However, the text is more than a summary or a progress report. The information is balanced between basic biology and clinical discussions reaching from microscopic anatomy to genetics, immunology, pharmacology, chemistry, microbiology, and more. This is what transplantation medicine is about, and where it is heading.

The first section of this book illuminates the basic principles of mechanisms of rejection, both cell- and antibody-mediated, and the immunopathology of rejection. The second section is devoted to the morphological pathology of rejection of heart, lung, liver, kidney, intestine, and pancreas, as well as to the pathology of post-transplant lymphoproliferative disorders. The third section focuses on clinical diagnosis of rejection, both acute and chronic, and on modern visualization techniques in the diagnosis of rejection. The molecular biology approaches are also included. The final section of the text addresses some of the most exciting new advances in the field of immunosuppression, future antirejection molecules, and forthcoming drugs. It reviews the mechanism of action of cyclosporine, as well as most of the new antirejection agents already in clinical trials. Emphasis is also placed on side effects, as well as on logical combination of these agents.

Taken together, this is a fascinating story that both illuminates today's knowledge and allows a glimpse of the future in transplantation diagnostics and medicine.

Pekka Häyry, M.D., Ph.D.
University of Helsinki
Helsinki, Finland

Preface

Solid-organ transplantation is a growing field, and with a generally excellent short-term outcome for many patients. Allograft rejection, however, remains a problem, both early after transplantation and in the late post-transplant period, when it is often the cause of allograft loss. The majority of solid-organ allograft recipients have episodes of acute rejection, which can often be successfully treated with the armamentarium of antirejection therapies currently available. Chronic allograft changes, however, which are likely due at least in part to rejection-induced injury, are not so amenable to treatment and represent a major ongoing challenge in solid-organ transplantation.

This book focuses on solid organ transplant rejection, considering mechanisms and pathology, clinical diagnosis, and molecular biological approaches as well as complications of antirejection therapy. Both acute and chronic rejection in all types of solid-organ allografts are considered at length by an international group of experts in the field of transplantation medicine.

In the initial section of the book, the emphasis is on basic mechanisms of rejection. The first and second chapters are specific discussions of cell-mediated and antibody-mediated rejection, including insights gained from clinical investigations as well as experimental model systems, focusing on acute and hyperacute rejection. A description of the immunopathology of rejection reactions follows, with emphasis on the contribution of this approach to defining mechanisms of rejection and sharpening the accuracy of diagnosis. The final chapters in this section review mechanisms and the molecular biology of chronic transplant changes, such as accelerated atherosclerosis, which threaten graft survival.

The second and third sections are arranged largely by organ system. In the second set of chapters, the pathology of rejection and allied conditions in each major solid-organ allograft is described. These chapters include the recently developed standardized schema for rejection diagnosis in heart, lung, kidney, and liver allografts, as well as rejection-related changes in intestinal and pancreatic allografts. For the pathology of rejection, chapters are included on fine-needle aspiration cytology in liver, kidney, and pancreas allografts, and the pathology of post-transplant lymphoproliferative disorder. Chapters on clinical diagnosis include radiologic imaging and molecular biological approaches to rejection, as these are powerful ancillary tools in the clinical evaluation of rejection.

Antirejection protocols, while critical for the survival of solid-organ allografts, also have important systemic and organ-specific effects. In the final group of chapters, the mechanism of action and specific toxic effects of cyclosporine as well as the numerous new immunosuppressive agents currently in therapeutic trials are reviewed.

This comprehensive work provides a valuable overview for the wide range of professionals involved in the care of solid-organ allograft recipients. It should be generally useful for transplant surgeons, medical subspecialists, immunologists, pathologists, radiologists, and nursing and technical staffs in transplantation medicine. For many of these professionals who care for recipients of several different types of solid-organ allografts, the inclusion of all these types of allografts in a single volume should prove particularly useful.

This book can only represent the current state of the art. Advances in important areas such as new immunosuppressive protocols, induction of tolerance, and xenografting can only be glimpsed on the horizon. This volume discusses these briefly, and provides a general background and context into which these and other breakthroughs can be assimilated in the future.

The editors wish to thank Syntex/Roche Biosciences for their generous contribution in support of the color illustrations in this book.

Kim Solez
Lorraine C. Racusen
Margaret E. Billingham

Contents

Contributors

Elnari Aavik Transplantation Laboratory, University of Helsinki, Helsinki, Finland

Sointu Alatalo, M.D. Transplantation Laboratory, University of Helsinki, Helsinki, Finland

Sami Asfar, M.D., F.R.C.S. (Ed.), F.A.C.S. Transplant Surgeon, University Hospital, London, Ontario, Canada

Hugh Auchincloss, Jr., M.D. Associate Professor of Surgery, Harvard Medical School, and Director, Pancreas Transplantation, Massachusetts General Hospital, Boston, Massachusetts

William M. Baldwin, III, M.D., Ph.D. Associate Professor, Department of Pathology, Johns Hopkins University School of Medicine, Baltimore, Maryland

Barbara F. Banner, M.D. Professor, Department of Pathology, University of Massachusetts Medical Center, Worcester, Massachusetts

Kenneth L. Baughman, M.D. Professor of Medicine and Director, Division of Cardiology, Department of Medicine, Johns Hopkins University School of Medicine, Baltimore, Maryland

William A. Baumgartner, M.D. Professor of Surgery and Cardiac Surgeon-in-Charge, Division of Cardiac Surgery, Johns Hopkins Hospital, Baltimore, Maryland

Margaret E. Billingham, M.B., B.S., F.R.C.Path., F.A.C.C. Professor of Pathology Emerita, Department of Cardiothoracic Surgery, Stanford University School of Medicine, Stanford, California

Barry J. Byrne, M.D., Ph.D. Assistant Professor of Pediatrics and Pathology, Department of Pediatrics, Johns Hopkins University School of Medicine, Baltimore, Maryland

Patricia M. Campbell, M.B.Ch.B., M.R.C.P.(UK), F.R.C.P.(C) Assistant Professor, Department of Medicine, University of Alberta, Edmonton, Alberta, Canada

B. D. Car Faculty of Medicine, Institute of Toxicology of the ETH and University of Zürich, Schwerzenbach-Zürich, Switzerland

John D. Day Department of Pathology, Johns Hopkins University School of Medicine, Baltimore, Maryland

Hans-Pietro Eugster, Ph.D. Department of Structural Toxicology, Institute of Toxicology of the ETH and University of Zürich, Schwerzenbach-Zürich, Switzerland

Judith Ann Ferry, M.D. Assistant Professor, Department of Pathology, Massachusetts General Hospital, Boston, Massachusetts

M. Roy First, M.D. Professor of Medicine, Department of Internal Medicine, University of Cincinnati Medical Center, Cincinnati, Ohio

David R. Grant, M.D., F.R.C.S.C. Professor, Department of Surgery, University of Western Ontario, London, Ontario, Canada

Rainer W. G. Gruessner, M.D., Ph.D. Associate Professor, Department of Surgery, University of Minnesota Medical School, Minneapolis, Minnesota

Fernando R. Gutierrez, M.D. Associate Professor, Department of Radiology, Mallinckrodt Institute of Radiology, Washington University School of Medicine, St. Louis, Missouri

Philip F. Halloran, M.D., Ph.D., F.R.C.P.(C) Professor, Departments of Medicine and Immunology, University of Alberta, Edmonton, Alberta, Canada

Ulrike M. Hamper, M.D. Associate Professor of Radiology, Division of Ultrasound, Department of Radiology and Radiological Science, Johns Hopkins University School of Medicine, Baltimore, Maryland

Nancy Lee Harris, M.D. Director of Anatomic Pathology, Department of Pathology, Massachusetts General Hospital, Boston, Massachusetts

Pekka Häyry, M.D., Ph.D. Professor of Transplantation Surgery and Immunology, Transplantation Laboratory, University of Helsinki, Helsinki, Finland

Ralph H. Hruban, M.D. Associate Professor, Department of Pathology, Johns Hopkins University School of Medicine, Baltimore, Maryland

Grover M. Hutchins, M.D. Professor, Department of Pathology, Johns Hopkins University School of Medicine, Baltimore, Maryland

Helena Isoniemi, M.D., Ph.D. Division of Transplantation, IV Department of Surgery, Helsinki University Central Hospital, Helsinki, Finland

Erkki Kallio, M.D. Transplantation Laboratory, University of Helsinki, Helsinki, Finland

Edward K. Kasper, M.D., F.A.C.C. Assistant Professor of Medicine and Director, Cardiomyopathy and Heart Transplant Service, Department of Medicine, Johns Hopkins University School of Medicine, Baltimore, Maryland

Dilip S. Kittur, M.D., Sc.D. Associate Professor, Department of Surgery, Johns Hopkins University School of Medicine, Baltimore, Maryland

Petri Koskinen, M.D. Transplantation Laboratory, University of Helsinki, Helsinki, Finland

Leena Krogerus, M.D. Transplantation Laboratory, University of Helsinki, Helsinki, Finland

Irmeli Lautenschlager, M.D., Ph.D. Assistant Professor of Transplantation Immunology, Transplantation Laboratory, Helsinki University Central Hospital, Helsinki, Finland

Karl Lemström, M.D. Transplantation Laboratory, University of Helsinki, Helsinki, Finland

L. Santiago Medina, M.D. Pediatric Radiology Fellow, Department of Radiology, Children's Hospital and Harvard Medical School, Boston, Massachusetts

Ari Mennander, M.D., Ph.D. Transplantation Laboratory, University of Helsinki, Helsinki, Finland

Michael Mihatsch Professor, Institut für Pathologie der Universität Basel, Basel, Switzerland

Marjukka Myllärniemi, M.B. Transplantation Laboratory, University of Helsinki, Helsinki, Finland

Joyce Nair-Menon Department of Cell Biology and Neurosciences, University of South Carolina School of Medicine, Columbia, South Carolina

Raouf E. Nakhleh, M.D. Director, Autopsy Pathology, and Senior Staff Pathologist, Division of Surgical Pathology, Department of Pathology, Henry Ford Hospital, Detroit, Michigan

N. Paul Ohori, M.D. Assistant Professor, Department of Pathology, University of Pittsburgh Medical Center, Pittsburgh, Pennsylvania

Steen Olsen, M.D. Professor of Pathology, University Institute of Pathology, Municipal Hospital, Århus, Denmark

Timo Paavonen, M.D., Ph.D. Department of Pathology, Transplantation Laboratory, University of Helsinki, Helsinki, Finland

Leendert C. Paul, M.D., Ph.D. Director, Division of Nephrology, Department of Medicine, St. Michael's Hospital, and Keenan Professor of Medicine, University of Toronto, Toronto, Ontario, Canada

Lorraine C. Racusen, M.D. Associate Professor, Department of Pathology, Johns Hopkins University School of Medicine, Baltimore, Maryland

Anne Räisänen-Sokolowski, M.D. Transplantation Laboratory, University of Helsinki, Helsinki, Finland

Lloyd E. Ratner, M.D. Assistant Professor, Department of Surgery, Johns Hopkins University School of Medicine, Baltimore, Maryland

Robert C. Robbins, M.D. Assistant Professor of Surgery, Department of Cardiothoracic Surgery, Stanford University School of Medicine, Stanford, California

Bernhard Ryffel, M.D., F.M.H.Path.* Professor, Faculty of Medicine, Institute of Toxicology of the ETH and University of Zürich, Schwerzenbach-Zürich, Switzerland

Marc S. Sabatine, M.D. Clinical Fellow in Medicine, Harvard Medical School, and Massachusetts General Hospital, Boston, Massachusetts

Fred Sanfilippo, M.D., Ph.D. Baxley Professor and Director, Department of Pathology, Johns Hopkins University School of Medicine, Baltimore, Maryland

**Present affiliation*: Institute of Pathology, Basel. Switzerland.

Sheila Sheth, M.D. Assistant Professor of Radiology, Department of Radiology and Radiological Science, Johns Hopkins University School of Medicine, Baltimore, Maryland

Marilyn J. Siegel, M.D. Professor, Department of Radiology, Mallinckrodt Institute of Radiology, Washington University School of Medicine, St. Louis, Missouri

Dale Craig Snover, M.D. Professor and Director, Anatomic Pathology, Laboratory Medicine and Pathology, University of Minnesota Medical School, Minneapolis, Minnesota

Kim Solez, M.D. Professor of Pathology, Department of Laboratory Medicine and Pathology, University of Alberta, Edmonton, Alberta, Canada

Qinjxiang Su, Ph.D. Faculty of Medicine, Institute of Toxicology of the ETH and University of Zürich, Schwerzenbach-Zürich, Switzerland

David E.R. Sutherland, M.D., Ph.D. Professor, Department of Surgery, University of Minnesota Medical School, Minneapolis, Minnesota

Eero Taskinen, M.D., Ph.D. Senior Pathologist, Transplantation Laboratory, University of Helsinki, Helsinki, Finland

James Theodore, M.D. Associate Professor, Division of Pulmonary and Critical Care Medicine, Department of Medicine, Stanford University School of Medicine, Stanford, California

Vincent G. Valentine, M.D. Medical Director, Lung Transplantation, Ochsner Transplant Center, and Assistant Professor of Medicine, Division of Pulmonary and Critical Care Medicine, Louisiana State University School of Medicine, New Orleans, Louisiana

Russell H. Wiesner, M.D. Professor of Medicine, Mayo Medical School, and Medical Director, Liver Transplantation, Mayo Clinic and Mayo Foundation, Rochester, Minnesota

Eeva von Willebrand, M.D., Ph.D. Docent in Clinical Immunology and Senior Consultant (Lecturer), Transplantation Laboratory, Helsinki University Central Hospital, Helsinki, Finland

Richard Wood, M.D., F.R.C.S. Professor, Department of Surgery, Clinical Sciences Centre, University of Sheffield, Sheffield, England

Serdar Yilmaz, M.D. Transplantation Laboratory, University of Helsinki, Helsinki, Finland

Samuel A. Yousem, M.D. Associate Professor, Department of Pathology, University of Pittsburgh Medical Center, Pittsburgh, Pennsylvania

Jeffrey S. Zaltzman, M.D., F.R.C.P.(C) Assistant Professor, Department of Medicine, St. Michael's Hospital and University of Toronto, Toronto, Ontario, Canada

1

Cell-Mediated Rejection

Marc S. Sabatine and Hugh Auchincloss, Jr.
Harvard Medical School and Massachusetts General Hospital, Boston, Massachusetts

I. INTRODUCTION

This chapter begins by briefly considering the three components central to any cell-mediated immune response: antigens, antigen-presenting cells (APCs), and T lymphocytes. Using these components, we then highlight the special features of alloreactivity that separate it from classic immunology. Next, we examine cell-mediated alloreactivity in detail, beginning with the potential responses of T cells to transplant antigens. We then review the various possible cognate interactions between transplant antigens and T cells, discuss the factors regulating those responses, and, finally, consider how T cells can bring about allograft rejection.

II. THE COMPONENTS: ANTIGENS, APCS, AND T LYMPHOCYTES

Cell-mediated immunity requires at least three components: foreign antigens, APCs, and T lymphocytes.

A. Transplantation Antigens

Research initiated in the early part of the 20th century on tumor and skin transplantation between inbred strains of mice revealed the genetic basis for allograft rejection (1–8). The proteins responsible for allograft rejection, called *histocompatibility antigens*, are the products of approximately 30 to 50 genetic loci that have codominant expression (9–12). These antigens can be divided into two categories: major and minor.

1. Major Histocompatibility Complex Antigens

Initially defined as the locus encoding the antigens responsible for rapid rejection of transplanted tissues, it was later realized that the major histocompatibility locus actually represents a complex containing several loci, each expressing highly polymorphic genes; hence, it is now called the major histocompatibility *complex* (MHC) (13). The MHC antigens actually have an important physiologic role in the immune system—that is, to present foreign antigens to responding T cells; their role as transplant antigens is accidental.

There are two classes of MHC molecules, and they differ in cellular distribution, types of antigens presented, and T cell subsets with which they interact.

a. Class I MHC Molecules. Class I MHC molecules, found on all nucleated cells, consist of an MHC-encoded α or heavy chain composed of three domains (α1 to α3) and a non-MHC-encoded β chain commonly known as β_2-microglobulin (13–16). The α1 and α2 segments form a peptide-binding region. Within this region, peptide fragments 8 or 9 amino acids in length, derived from endogenously synthesized proteins, are presented in a peptide-binding cleft. The cleft demonstrates a high degree of structural polymorphism which is caused by the allelic variation of the MHC genes found within a given species. The α3 segment of the molecule interacts with CD8 molecules on T cells, thereby explaining the observation that the T cells that recognize antigen presented in the context of class I MHC molecules are usually $CD8^+$ (17,18).

The β_2 microglobulin polypeptide is thought to be necessary for cell-surface stability of MHC I molecules; without it, expression of MHC I molecules is dramatically reduced (19–23). These observations led researchers to target the β_2-microglobulin gene for disruption via homologous recombination (24). The resulting β_2-microglobulin-deficient mice were found to have only rare distorted heavy chains on their cell surfaces (25).

b. Class II MHC Molecules. Class II MHC molecules are composed of two noncovalently associated polypeptide chains (13,26). The α and β chains are encoded by different MHC genes and both are polymorphic. The peptide-binding region is formed by the interaction between the α1 and β1 segments and presents peptides derived from exogenous proteins that have been taken up by the cell. The α2 and β2 segments combine to form a region that interacts with CD4 molecules on T cells, thus explaining why $CD4^+$ T cells almost always recognize antigen presented by class II MHC molecules. In contrast to class I MHC molecules, class II molecules constitutively appear on only a few cell types, including macrophages, Langerhans cells, dendritic cells, and B cells (27). Nonimmune cells express few to no class II molecules constitutively, but can be induced to do so by exposure to interferon gamma (IFN-γ) and potentially other cytokines, such as tumor necrosis factor (TNF) (28).

2. Minor Histocompatibility Antigens

a. Definition. Only a few histocompatibility loci encode major histocompatibility antigens. The rest, initiating slower rejection responses, encode minor histocompatibility antigens. This differentiation, however, based on the speed of graft rejection, does not hold up, because disparities of some class I antigens do not cause rapid rejection in the absence of class II differences, while the combination of some minor histocompatibility antigens does (29,30). Minor histocompatibility antigens are thus best defined as transplantation antigens capable of causing cell-mediated graft rejection but without the structural characteristics of MHC molecules (31).

b. Nature. Initially, it was thought that minor histocompatibility antigens were also cell surface glycoproteins similar to MHC molecules but simply incapable of generating as vigorous an immune response. Now it is clear that minor histocompatibility antigens are actually the peptides of self-proteins with allelic variations that are presented by MHC molecules. Between members of the species, these proteins are analogous to "nominal" foreign antigens (32–39). While some of the peptide determinants of minor histocompatibility antigens have been isolated, the nature of the proteins from which they are derived is still unknown (37–39).

c. The Immune Response to Minor Antigens. The idea that minor histocompatibility antigens are peptide fragments presented by self-MHC molecules is attractive, since it explains many of the observations regarding the immune response to these antigens (40,41). First, minor antigens do not stimulate a primary in vitro cell-mediated response (i.e., a mixed lymphocyte response (MLR) and a cell mediated lympholysis (CML), while major antigens do. This is in keeping with the observation that in vitro T-cell responses to nominal antigens require in vivo priming. Second, it has been difficult to detect humoral responses to minor histocompatibility antigens. We now realize that antibody production may, in fact, occur, but that without cell-surface expression of this protein, we have no way of detecting it. Third, secondary cell-mediated responses to minor histocompatibility antigens require that the minor antigens be presented in the context of the same MHC molecules they were exposed to during the primary exposure (33–35,42,43). Thus, the minor antigens demonstrate the phenomenon of MHC restriction.

3. Other Antigens Important in Transplantation

a. Tissue-Specific. There is evidence that some transplantation antigens presented by MHC molecules may be derived from proteins with limited tissue distribution (44–46). Perhaps the best example of a tissue-specific antigen is the Sk antigen found only in skin. Tissue-specific antigens need not display allelic variability. Rather, these antigens may generate a non-self determinant by being presented by donor MHC molecules on donor APCs. A recipient's T cells may be tolerant of "Self plus X_1" but not of "Allo plus X_1."

b. Hh Locus. The products of the hybrid histocompatibility (Hh) locus X are responsible for an unusual form of rejection of foreign tissue, which occurs even when the donor does not express novel histocompatibility antigens with respect to the recipient (5,6). Applicable only to grafts of hematopoietic origin, F_1 animals are resistant to the engraftment of parental-strain bone marrow cells unless very high doses are transferred. It seems that expression of Hh requires homozygosity at the particular loci and that the immune response to the Hh product by a recipient lacking that antigen is mediated by NK cells (47). To date, this phenomenon has not been shown to apply to grafts that are not of hematopoietic origin.

B. T Lymphocytes

1. Evidence for Role of T Cells

The importance of T cells in graft rejection has been demonstrated by many experimental observations. Both nude mice (which are athymic and therefore lack T cells) and neonatally thymectomized mice will accept allogenic and even xenogeneic skin grafts indefinitely (48). Moreover, reconstitution of these mice with purified T cells restores their ability to reject skin grafts (49–51). In humans, prolongation of graft survival relies upon immunosuppressive measures that are directed against T-cell activity (52).

2. Which T Cells Are Involved in Graft Rejection

Until fairly recently, however, it was unclear which subpopulations of T cells were involved in graft rejection. Much of the confusion arose from the erroneous assumption that cell surface markers on T cells corresponded perfectly with cell function (53).

T cells can be divided into two populations, based upon cell surface markers (abbreviated CD for cluster of differentiation): $CD4^+CD8^-$ and $CD4^-CD8^+$. As noted above, CD4 on T cells interacts with class II MHC molecules while CD8 interacts with class I MHC molecules. Thus, almost always, $CD4^+$ T cells recognize antigen presented by class II molecules while $CD8^+$ T cells recognize antigen presented by class I molecules.

With respect to function, T cells can be divided into two groups: helper T cells (T_h cells) and cytotoxic T lymphocytes (CTLs) (54–57). Helper T cells are lymphocytes which, when they recognize foreign antigen, secrete cytokines such as interleukins IL-2, IL-3, IL-4, and IL-5 and IFN-γ which cause other cells of the immune system to proliferate and differentiate. CTLs are lymphocytes which, when they recognize foreign antigen, bring about the destruction of the target cells bearing the foreign antigen by directly lysing the cell.

Although $CD4^+$ T cells tend to be helper cells and $CD8^+$ T cells tend to be CTLs, this distinction is far from absolute. $CD4^+$ T cells can have a cytotoxic function and $CD8^+$ T cells that make IL-2 have been identified. In addition, the CD4 and CD8 markers do not correspond perfectly with antigen specificity. CD8 cells specific for class II can be identified, although they are a minor population. However, because of the enormous strength of the alloresponse, even "minor" populations of T cells become important and may be able to bring about allograft rejection. Thus, the CD4 and CD8 distinction becomes much more complex.

C. Antigen-Presenting Cells

For T cells to be activated, they must have antigen presented to them by cells specialized for that function. These cells are called antigen-presenting cells (APCs). APCs are derived from the bone marrow and have the following properties (58–60):

1. Process Peptides and Present Antigen

Endogenously synthesized proteins tend to be cleaved in proteosomes and transported into the endoplasmic reticulum (ER), where their peptide fragments can bind to class I MHC molecules (61). The complex can then be transported to the cell surface. Alternatively, if a protein is exogenous, it tends to be internalized in endosomes and be subjected to partial proteolysis (58). These endosomes intersect vesicles transporting class II $\alpha\beta$ heterodimers, which are complexed with γ or invariant chains. The invariant chain is proteolytically cleaved, allowing the class II MHC molecules to bind to the peptide fragments. This complex can then be transported to the cell surface.

2. Transport

APCs have the ability to transport foreign antigens to lymph nodes. This transport function of APCs is useful, since naive T cells generally travel within the lymphoid circulation (62), whereas, after stimulation, T cells tend to express a different set of adhesion molecules that permit them to migrate into peripheral tissues (63,64).

3. Facilitate Adhesion Between T cell and APC

Binding of the TCR to the peptide/MHC complex by itself provides specificity but not sufficient stability to allow effective cell-cell communication. Thus, to facilitate binding, APCs express accessory adhesion molecules which serve as ligands for cell-surface molecules on T cells (65–71). Well-known APC–T cell combinations are listed in Table 1.

4. Costimulation

The fourth function of APCs is to provide the costimulatory or "second signals" to activate T cells. It is now well established that T-cell activation requires two signals (72–74). One of the best-characterized examples of cell surface costimulatory molecules is B7, a member of the immunoglobulin superfamily. This molecule binds to CD28 on T cells and engagement of CD28 by B7 enhances transcription of cytokine genes, especially the gene

Table 1 Adhesion Molecules

APC	T Cell	APC	T Cell
ICAM-1	LFA-1	CD72	CD5
ICAM-2		B7	CD28
ICAM-3		MHC II	CD4
LFA-3	CD2	MHC I	CD8

for IL-2 (75). Experimental evidence suggests that T cells become inactivated or anergized (i.e., unresponsive to an antigen when it is encountered again) if the first antigen encounter is without a costimulatory signal (73–76).

III. SPECIAL FEATURES IN TRANSPLANTATION

A. Alloreactivity Viewed in the Framework of Classic Immunology

If alloreactivity behaved like a classic immune response, we would use the following model to explain how allografts are rejected. A cell-mediated immune response would be triggered by any protein moieties expressed within a graft that do not exist in the recipient. Recipient APCs, such as macrophages, would infiltrate the graft and take up the alloantigens. These APCs would carry the alloantigens back to lymph nodes, where they would present processed peptide fragments. $CD4^+$ helper T cells would bind to the APCs via adhesion molecules and, while in contact, the T-cell receptors could recognize the foreign antigens presented on the APCs and become activated. Once fully activated, the helper T cells would proliferate and differentiate, secreting cytokines that would induce the proliferation and differentiation of other lymphocytes and nonspecific cells of the immune system. Foremost among the nonspecific effector cells are macrophages, which, when activated, would secrete cytokines that could stimulate inflammatory and cell-mediated immune responses, giving rise to the classic DTH response. Specific effector cells would also be activated and would include cytotoxic T lymphocytes which, when their TCRs recognize foreign antigens, could directly lyse target cells.

Cell-mediated allograft rejection is fundamentally different from classic immune responses, however, because allotransplantation involves two sets of APCs: those of the donor and those of the recipient. The recognition by T cells of MHC alloantigens on the donor APCs themselves has been called *direct recognition*, and this pathway activates several unusual T-cell responses (77–79). The recognition by T cells of alloantigens, MHC or otherwise, as peptide fragments presented by recipient APCs has been called *indirect recognition* (36,80–82). Despite the terminology, the "indirect" pathway is more like the process of classic immunology.

B. Donor APCs and Direct Recognition

Direct recognition is probably the most important feature that sets alloreactivity apart from classic immune responses. The recognition of MHC alloantigens on donor cells, without the requirement that these antigens be processed and presented by self MHC molecules, occurs because T cells that are specific for self MHC molecules plus foreign peptide cross-react with intact allogeneic MHC molecules.

1. Strength of the Direct Alloresponse

The exceptional strength of the immune response to MHC alloantigens is what first distinguished them from all other alloantigens and served as the basis for calling them "major" histocompatibility antigens. This strength is evident in several circumstances. First, one can generate a primary proliferative response to MHC alloantigens, whereas prior in vivo priming is required in attempting to generate a response to nominal antigens. Second, the precursor frequency of T cells reactive with allogeneic MHC antigens is roughly 100-fold greater than that for any nominal antigen (83,84). Third, MHC-disparate grafts are rejected with much greater speed than single minor antigen–disparate grafts.

There are two main theories to explain why the alloresponse is so powerful. The determinant density hypothesis is based on the notion that only a small fraction of the MHC molecules on an APC present the peptides of a given foreign antigen (78). Therefore, only TCRs with high affinity for these MHC-plus-peptide complexes will be activated. In the case of alloreactivity, however, *every* MHC molecule represents a foreign determinant; thus the density of foreign antigens on a single APC that can stimulate a single T cell is greatly increased. Therefore, even T cells with low affinity for the foreign determinants can be activated. Alternatively, the determinant frequency hypothesis is based on the idea that the TCR recognizes not just the allogeneic MHC molecules but also whatever peptide happens to be in the cleft of the allo-MHC molecule (79). As the MHC molecules on an allogeneic APC will present a large variety of different peptides in their clefts, each cell will have a high frequency of foreign determinants on its surface. Much recent experimental evidence favors determinant frequency as the cause of the strength of alloreactivity, but the two hypotheses are not mutually exclusive.

2. Unusual Cognate Interactions

Alloreactivity is so strong that atypical T-cell interactions, which are not of significance in classic immunology, are of great importance in transplantation immunology. For instance, most helper T cells are $CD4^+$ and most cytotoxic T cells are $CD8^+$, yet in alloreactivity, helper T cell function can be found in both $CD4^+$ and $CD8^+$ T cell subpopulations. Similarly, cytolytic functions have been demonstrated in both $CD4^+$ and $CD8^+$ cells (85). Moreover, in alloreactivity, the classic restrictions of $CD4^+$ and $CD8^+$ T cells can be broken on some occasions. Experimental findings suggest that some $CD8^+$ T cells can recognize allogeneic class II MHC molecules (86,87) and, likewise, some $CD4^+$ cells can recognize allogeneic class I MHC molecules (88,89).

C. Recipient APCs and Indirect Recognition

Indirect recognition is actually the normal means of antigenic presentation by the immune system: peptides of foreign proteins are usually presented by self MHC molecules on self (recipient) APCs. However, while the potential role of the indirect pathway in alloreactivity has been realized for some time, it has been difficult to demonstrate definitively its importance in the face of the enormous strength of the direct response. Recently, however, the advent of "knockout" mice, which lack MHC molecules, has made this possible (24,25, 90–93). Some features of the indirect pathway that seem likely to be important include the following:

1. Increasing Importance of the Indirect Pathway Over Time

Antigen-presenting cells are derived from the bone marrow. Therefore, in classic immunology, there is an inexhaustible supply of APCs. This is not necessarily the case in transplantation, where the supply of donor APCs may eventually be exhausted, to be replaced over time by recipient APCs. Therefore, the antigenic stimulus of an allograft, at least for naive T cells, is likely to rely progressively on the indirect pathway.

2. *The Indirect Pathway Sensitizes T Cells to the "Wrong " Determinant*

Helper T cells are sensitized by the indirect pathway to alloantigens presented in the context of self MHC molecules. These determinants, however, are not the ones expressed by the cells of the donor graft. Thus, the indirect pathway alone cannot sensitize T cells to antigens expressed in the donor graft.

3. *The Problem of Providing Help Generated by Indirect Sensitization to Cytotoxic Cells Sensitized Directly*

In classic immunology, the help provided by a $CD4^+$ T cell is thought to be limited in its availability to cells in very close proximity, because cytokines can only work over short distances. That proximity is achieved by the requirement that an APC present a helper determinant on its class II MHC molecule to a $CD4^+$ helper T cell and simultaneously, a cytotoxic determinant on its class I MHC molecule to a $CD8^+$ CTL. This is called *epitope linkage*. The use of the indirect pathway would seem to violate the requirement for epitope linkage (94), since the helper determinant, expressed on the recipient APC, would be on a different cell than the donor APC, which would have to express the relevant cytotoxic determinant. Evidence, however, does suggest that indirect recognition can bring about the activation of cytotoxic T cells directly reactive against allo-MHC molecules (95). The exact requirements and limitations of this interaction remain unknown, however.

IV. POTENTIAL T-CELL RESPONSES

Many different responses may occur when T cells encounter alloantigens.

A. Helper T-Cell Activation

Helper T-cell activation requires two signals. The first signal is provided by the TCR recognizing the peptide/MHC complex. The second signal can be either a cell surface molecule with a corresponding receptor on the T cell or a secreted cytokine. Reception of the two signals initiates a signal transduction cascade that activates the T cell. At the heart of T-cell activation is the transcriptional activation and expression of over seventy genes. These genes can be classified into immediate, early, and late, based on their time course of activation (96). In the immediate category are protooncogenes, such as c-*fos* and c-*myc*, and genes encoding transcription factors, such as NF-AT and NF-κB (97,98). In the early category are genes encoding cytokines and cytokine receptors, including IL-2, IL-4, IFN-γ, and the IL-2 receptor (99). The cytokines serve to activate nearby T cells, B cells, and macrophages, thereby magnifying the immune response. The upregulation of the IL-2 receptor, coupled with the T cell's secretion of increased amounts of IL-2, creates an autocrine growth pathway that plays a vital role in the proliferative response of the T cell to foreign antigen. Finally, in the late category are genes coding for cell-surface molecules such as CD2, CD45, class II MHC molecules, and the adhesion molecule VLA-1 (100). These changes in cell-surface molecules alter how the T cell interacts with the other cellular components of the immune system.

B. Helper T-Cell Subsets: T_H1 Versus T_H2

Activated helper T cells can be segregated into two distinct subsets, called T_H1 and T_H2, on the basis of the cytokines that they secrete (101–104). T_H1 cells tend to secrete IL-2, IFN-γ, and TNF_{β}, while T_H2 cells tend to secrete IL-4, IL-5, IL-6, and IL-10. Both subsets secrete IL-3, TNF_{α} and granulocyte-macrophage colony stimulating factor (GM-CSF). The different cytokine profiles suggest different functions, with T_H1 cells initiating a cellular immune response mediated by delayed-type hypersensitivity (DTH) and cytotoxic T lymphocyte (CTL) responses and T_H2 cells initiating a humoral immune response mediated by B cell proliferation and an antibody response (particularly IgG_1 and IgE).

C. Cytotoxic T Lymphocytes

CTLs are T lymphocytes that kill target cells bearing antigens to which the CTL's TCR can react. Just as in the activation of helper T cells, activation of CTLs from pre-CTLs requires two signals: first, antigen on a target cell presented by an MHC molecule, and, second, a cytokine such as IL-2, IL-4, or IFN-γ. Activation results in increased and then decreased levels of c-*fos* and c-*myc*, an increase in IL-2 production, and increased density of IL-2 receptor on the cell surface. Activated lymphocytes develop granules that contain a variety of cytotoxic molecules, including pore-forming proteins (e.g., perforins), serine esterases, and protein toxins (105). They also acquire the ability to secrete cytokines such as IFN-γ and lymphotoxin. Combined, these features allow CTLs to lyse target cells directly or to induce apoptosis (programmed cell death).

D. Tolerance and Anergy

In addition to activation, T-cell encounters with alloantigens can also produce downregulating responses (106,107). If T cells get deleted (108–111), are rendered nonresponsive (112–114), or are suppressed (115–118), the system becomes tolerant. It now appears that the nonresponsive state, called anergy, results from antigen receptor stimulation in the absence of the appropriate costimulatory signals (113,119,120). Functionally, anergic T cells are deficient in IL-2 secretion and remain nonresponsive even when restimulated with the appropriate antigens in the presence of costimulators (121).

E. Acquired Memory

Some T cells go on to become memory cells following their encounter with alloantigens (122). These cells respond more strongly and rapidly than naive T cells when they encounter antigen again. Several cell-surface markers appear to differentiate memory T cells from naive ones, including pgp-1, a low-molecular-weight isoform of CD45 known as CD45RO, and higher levels of CD2.

V. COGNATE INTERACTIONS IN ALLOREACTIVITY

Part of the control that determines the nature of a T cell's response to a foreign antigen includes the cognate interactions between the T-cell receptor and the MHC molecule-peptide complex. Although there is a relatively limited set of such interactions in classic immunology, additional interactions have been found to be important in transplantation.

A. $CD8^+$ Direct Response to Class I Alloantigens

In vitro, when purified $CD8^+$ responder cells are mixed with class I disparate stimulator cells, proliferation, IL-2 production, and cytotoxic responses are all generated (123–130).

Thus, CD8$^+$ T cells can demonstrate both helper and cytotoxic functions in response to class I alloantigens. In vivo, depletion studies demonstrate that the rejection of MHC class I disparate skin grafts depends on CD8$^+$ T cells, because anti-CD4 antibody often has no effect on allogeneic skin graft survival while anti-CD8 antibody greatly prolongs allograft survival (131–136). Similarly, adoptive transfer studies demonstrate that reconstituting recipient mice with CD8$^+$ T cells alone is sufficient to bring about the rejection of a class I disparate allograft, while mice reconstituted with CD4$^+$ T cells are unable to reject such allografts (49–51,137). Thus, CD8$^+$ T cells appear to be necessary and sufficient to bring about the rejection of class I disparate allografts.

B. CD8+ Direct Response to Class II Alloantigens

While a proliferative response by CD8$^+$ T cells against class II alloantigens has not been shown, a cytotoxic response has been demonstrated, both in bulk cultures and by analysis of individual T-cell clones (126). The anti-class II cytotoxic response can be blocked by the addition of an anti-Ia^b antibody, demonstrating that cytotoxic CD8$^+$ T cells directly recognize class II alloantigens and not peptide fragments presented on class I MHC molecules. Thus, apparently the direct pathway in alloreactivity is powerful enough to allow CD8$^+$ T cells to be activated by class II alloantigens despite the discordance between phenotype and classic MHC recognition specificity.

C. CD4+ Direct Response to Class II Alloantigens

In vivo, when CD4$^+$ responder cells are mixed with class II disparate stimulator cells, both proliferative and cytotoxic responses are generated (125,126,128). The response can be blocked by adding antibodies against the donor class II molecules, demonstrating that CD4$^+$ helper T cells can recognize class II MHC alloantigens directly. In vivo, matching donor and recipient class II antigens results in a survival advantage compared to grafts with no class II matching (138). Since CD4$^+$ responses to donor class II antigens via the indirect pathway would not be expected to be stronger than indirect responses to other antigens, the speed with which class II mismatched grafts are rejected suggests that CD4$^+$ cells are activated directly by class II alloantigens in vivo. Depletion studies show that survival of class II–only disparate grafts is prolonged when CD4$^+$ T cells are depleted (131–133, 136,139–141). Furthermore, adoptive transfer studies demonstrate that reconstituting recipient mice with CD4$^+$ T cells alone is sufficient to bring about the rejection of class II disparate allografts (49–51). Thus, CD4$^+$ T cells are both necessary and sufficient for the rejection of class II disparate allografts.

D. CD4+ Indirect Response to Alloantigens

In vitro, a proliferative response to class I alloantigens can be generated despite depletion of donor APCs and is only abolished completely upon depletion of recipient APCs as well (123–125). These findings suggest that CD4$^+$ helper T cells can be activated via the indirect recognition of allogeneic peptides presented on self class II MHC molecules by recipient APCs. In vivo, it is relatively easy to demonstrate that CD4$^+$ T cells can recognize alloantigens presented by recipient APCs but quite difficult to demonstrate that this response is responsible for graft rejection (142,143). This is both because CD4$^+$ T cells, stimulated via the powerful direct pathway, dominated the weaker indirect response whenever a class II antigen disparity is present, and because CD8$^+$ T cells provide help, even without CD4$^+$

Table 2 Cognate Pathways in Alloreactivity

	Direct		Indirect		Cytotoxic Pathways	
	Donor I	Donor II	Peptide + self I	Peptide + self II	Donor I	Donor II
CD4+	−	++++	−	+++	±	++
CD8+	++	−	±	−	++++	+

T cells, whenever there is a class I alloantigen disparity. However, opportunity to demonstrate the capacity of the CD4$^+$ indirect pathway has recently been afforded by the development of "knockout" mice lacking class II MHC molecules (144).

E. CD8$^+$ Indirect Response to Alloantigens

Activation of CD8$^+$ T cells via the indirect pathway has also been demonstrated by in vitro assays, giving rise to the phenomenon known as cross-priming. Since these CTLs are sensitized to determinants expressed by the recipient and not by the donor, it has again been unclear whether their activation is relevant to the process of rejection. A CD8$^+$ helper T-cell response to donor peptides presented by self class I probably is relatively weak but probably does exist.

F. The Response to Minor Antigen Disparate Allografts

As mentioned above, minor transplant antigens are peptide fragments from polymorphic proteins that are presented on MHC molecules. Therefore, these antigens can theoretically activate an alloresponse through either the direct or indirect pathways, depending on whether they are presented by donor or recipient APCs, respectively. As mentioned above, CD8$^+$ helper function against minor antigens appears to be relatively weak and CD4$^+$ T cells probably are the prime mediators of the helper response to minor histocompatibility antigens. Confirming the role of CD4$^+$ T cells, nude mice engrafted with multiple minor antigen-disparate allografts and then reconstituted with CD4$^+$ T cells are able to bring about the rejection of the allograft, while mice reconstituted with CD8$^+$ T cells are only inconsistently able to slowly reject the allograft (49,51,131–133,136,145). Mice reconstituted with both CD4$^+$ and CD8$^+$ T cells demonstrated the fastest rejection rates. This observed synergy is consistent with either the CD4$^+$ direct or the indirect pathways providing help and CD8$^+$ T cells providing effector functions.

G. Summary Correlating Phenotype, Specificity and Function

A summary of the different cognate interactions possible in alloreactivity is outlined in Table 2.

VI. FACTORS REGULATING T-CELL RESPONSES

With the multiple pathways of alloreactivity which can be called into play, it is clear that the immune response to allografts is extremely complex. Additional factors increase that complexity further by regulating the immune response to allografts.

A. Prior Sensitization: The Activation of Memory T Cells

Second-set graft rejection, mediated by memory T cells, is notable for its more rapid course and relative resistance to standard immunosuppressive therapy. Furthermore, once generated, the reactivation of $CD8^+$ CTLs from memory cells may occur independently of help from $CD4^+$ helper T cells (146–148). Thus, memory cell activation can have an important influence on the requirements for subsequent immune responsiveness.

B. Induction of Anergy

Sometimes, contact with donor cells does not stimulate T-cell activation but rather downregulation. Several features may decrease the tendency to activation.

1. APC Depletion

Nearly two decades ago, Lafferty et al. noted that the elimination of donor APCs prior to engraftment produced prolonged graft survival in murine thyroid allografts (149). While similar results have been obtained for a variety of types of organs in murine transplant models, investigators have not been able to succeed consistently in using APC depletion to prolong grafts in larger animals (119,150–153).

There are two problems with donor APC depletion. The first is that class II MHC molecule expression on donor cells can be upregulated, especially during an inflammatory process, and this increased antigen presentation may be able to offset the partial depletion of APCs. The other problem is that recipient APCs eventually infiltrate new grafts and therefore become available to present donor alloantigens to T cells via the indirect pathway. Yet if this is the case, why does APC depletion work at all? One important function of APCs is to bring antigens to lymph nodes for sampling by large numbers of naive T cells. Immediately after engraftment, donor APCs are better suited to carry out the transport of donor antigens than are recipient APCs. Thus, APC-depleted grafts may manifest prolonged graft survival because transport of alloantigens to lymph nodes is delayed.

2. Blocking the Secretion of Help

Therapy with anti-CD4 and sometimes with anti-CD8 monoclonal antibodies has been shown not only to be immunosuppressive but also to induce anergy and generate tolerance to allogeneic skin, islet, and heart grafts (154–159). The mechanism underlying this therapy may involve the temporary elimination of T cells and of IL-2 secretion, which are necessary for the generation of a cell-mediated immune response. Similarly, cyclosporine may help generate tolerance by blocking IL-2 production, for without the necessary IL-2, the T cells encountering antigens may become anergized.

3. APC Modification

Donor regulation of T cells may also occur when the costimulatory functions of APCs are blocked, so as to convert their antigen presentation into a tolerizing stimulus. In vitro, anergy is induced by exposing T_H1 $CD4^+$ T cell clones to antigen-MHC complexes in planar membranes or on chemically fixed APCs (113,120). Similar results have also been demonstrated in vitro using antigen presentation by non-APCs such as islet cells, keratinocytes, and T cells themselves. Immunoregulatory agents directed at B7, CTLA4, ICAM-1, LFA-1 and other costimulatory molecules may also promote T cell downregulation (160–164). One group has found that, in vitro, both B7 and ICAM-1 were equally potent costimulators of T-cell activation, but that only B7 costimulation prevented the induction of anergy (165). Correspondingly, both anti-B7 antibody and CTLA4-Ig (which blocks the B7-CD28 interaction) have been shown to induce anergy (166,167).

C. T_H1 Versus T_H2

Given that allograft rejection appears to be predominantly a cell-mediated immune response, it is possible that factors which shift the immune response from predominantly T_H1 to T_H2 might prolong graft survival. The ontogeny of helper T cells is thought to consist of the following stages (168–170). Naive T cells (or pre-T_H0 cells) secrete low levels of IL-2. Upon engagement of their T-cell receptor, they develop into T_H0 cells, which can secrete additional cytokines such as IL-3, IL-4, IL-5, and IFN-γ and perhaps all the cytokines helper T cells are capable of secreting. Upon full antigenic stimulation with the appropriate second signals, including cytokines and costimulatory molecules, T_H0 cells can then differentiate into T_H1 and T_H2 cells. The presence of IL-2, IFN-γ, and IL-12 and the absence of IL-4 and IL-10 favors the development of a T_H1 phenotype, while the presence of IL-4 and IL-10 and the absence of IFN-γ favors the development of a T_H2 phenotype. Therefore, cytokines secreted by one subset promote newly activated T cells to develop into that subset while inhibiting the development of the other subset. Thus, once one subset becomes predominant, it tends to maintain its dominance and direct the developing immune response along its lines.

Other factors also contribute to the tendency toward T_H1 versus T_H2. For example, macrophages as APCs seem to promote T_H1 cell development while B cells as APCs promote a T_H2 phenotype. The selective effect of different APCs is postulated to result from different cell-surface molecules that promote different costimulatory signals favoring the development of one subset over another. In addition, lower antigen doses favor T_H1 while higher antigen doses favor T_H2. Finally, the presence of activated $CD8^+$ CTLs favors T_H1 and inhibits T_H2.

Interestingly, while it has been easy to demonstrate anergy for T_H1 cells, it has been more difficult to do so for T_H2 cells, in part because their proliferative responses may not be as vigorous in the first place (171). Some researchers have noted that "anergized" T_H0 clones share many of the physiologic and morphologic characteristics of T_H2 cells (172). This suggests that stimulation in the absence of costimulatory molecules may not only inactivate T cells but may cause some of them to become activated as T_H2 cells. Others, however, have found that anergizing stimuli do not truly favor the T_H2 phenotype, because both IL-2 and IL-4 production is greatly reduced (173). Moreover, the fact that anergy and hence anergizing stimuli are often assessed on the basis of IL-2 production, such stimuli, by selectively decreasing IL-2 secretion, would naturally favor the development of a T_H2 phenotype. If, however, anergizing stimuli do favor a shift from T_H1 to T_H2, then the induction of anergy may prevent a cellular immune response only to promote a more vigorous humoral one.

D. Organ Transplantation as a Tolerogenic Stimulus?

By presenting a large numbers of alloantigens on non-APCs, such as parenchymal cells, which lack the appropriate costimulatory signals, organ transplantation itself may actually be downregulatory in certain cases. A manifestation of this clinically is that transplant recipients require less immunosuppression as time goes on. In murine models, certain organs have proven tolerogenic, some more than others, perhaps because of the relative density of APCs within the graft. The hierarchy favoring downregulation appears to be liver, kidney, heart, and then pancreatic islets. Skin grafts, on the other hand, are never tolerogenic on their own.

Other theories, however, besides anergy induction, have been invoked to explain an allograft's ability to induce tolerance. Some have suggested that an external suppressor mechanism is involved in the long-term survival of vascularized grafts. Others, using immunohistochemistry and polymerase chain reaction (PCR) analysis, have demonstrated the persistence of donor cells outside the transplanted organ in lymph nodes, skin, blood, and other tissues (174). This microchimerism may be responsible for tolerance induction or, alternatively, simply the result of long-term graft survival (175).

Regardless of the mechanism, the observation that certain organ grafts are themselves tolerogenic makes it challenging to ascertain precisely the effects of other so-called anergy-inducing strategies. If such strategies are only nonspecifically immunosuppressive, delay in graft rejection might allow sufficient time for the tolerance generated by the graft itself to come into play.

VII. GRAFT REJECTION

Despite the substantial evidence regarding the pathways of T-cell responses in alloreactivity, it is still not clear what effector mechanisms are responsible for allograft rejection.

A. Possible Cellular Effector Mechanisms

Several cellular effector mechanisms have been suggested as possible mechanisms of graft destruction, although the mere existence of these mechanisms, especially when measured by in vitro assays, does not prove that they are involved in the mechanism of graft destruction.

1. Delayed-Type Hypersensitivity (DTH)

In DTH, antigen-activated helper T cells secrete several different cytokines that recruit nonspecific effector cells of the immune system, the most prominent of which is the macrophage, and these cells eliminate the antigen (176). Although the activation of the helper T cells requires cognate interaction between antigen and TCR, the effector mechanism, albeit localized because of the local paracrine effects of cytokines, is nonetheless nonspecific because no antigen-receptor interaction is mandated.

The helper T cells can secrete cytokines such as TNF_{β} (also known as lymphotoxin or LT) and IFN-γ that "activate" vascular endothelium. Activation consists of at least three changes. First, the cell-surface expression of molecules such as ELAM-1 and ICAM-1 is upregulated. These molecules serve as ligands for the integrin family of molecules on the surface of leukocytes (e.g., LFA-1 and VLA-4), and increases in their levels make the endothelium more adhesive for leukocytes. Second, the endothelial cells secrete low-molecular-weight cytokines such as IL-8 and monocyte chemotactic protein-1 (MCP-1). These molecules increase the mobility of leukocytes. Third, the endothelial cells undergo morphologic changes that favor extravasation. Combined, these changes allow the endothelium to play a vital role in recruiting leukocytes to mount an inflammatory response.

Once recruited, blood monocytes differentiate into activated macrophages under the influence of IFN-γ. Activated macrophages effect the elimination of foreign antigen through several different means. First, they can directly eliminate foreign antigen through phagocytosis. Second, they can recruit additional nonspecific inflammatory cells, such as neutrophils, by secreting short-lived inflammatory mediators like PAF, prostaglandins, leukotrienes, and lipids. Third, they can become more efficient APCs, mainly via upregulation of class II MHC molecule expression. Fourth and finally, they can secrete cytokines such as TNF_{α} and IL-1, which augment the cellular immune response, and cytokines such as transforming growth factor beta (TGF-β) and PDGF, which stimulate fibrosis.

2. *Cytotoxic T Lymphocytes*

Cytotoxic T lymphocytes (CTLs) may play a role as effector cells in graft rejection, using their TCR to achieve antigen specificity (177). CTLs may be able to enter allografts after transplantation as small lymphocytes and subsequently be sensitized. More often, it appears that sensitization can occur in lymph nodes with activated CTLs then infiltrating the grafts (178–181).

Once CTLs are activated, they have at least two different ways in which they can eliminate target cells: pore formation and induction of apoptosis. Pore formation and lysis can be mediated by either granules or secreted proteins. The granules contain perforins, hydrolytic lysosomal enzymes, serine proteases, and proteoglycans (105,182). Perforin, the best-characterized of the granule components, is related to the ninth component of complement (182,183). Upon polymerization, perforins form tubular structures that, like the membrane attack complex (MAC) of the complement cascade, can span the membrane of target cells and initiate osmotic lysis (182). Among the secreted proteins are TNF_{β} (i.e., lymphotoxin) and ATP. TNF_{β} can lyse certain types of cells and ATP can induce increased membrane permeability (184–186).

Apoptosis or programmed cell death is essentially the internal disintegration of cells. If pore formation and osmotic lysis is necrosis or homicide, then apoptosis is suicide. Microscopically, apoptosis is characterized by chromatin condensation and DNA fragmentation and is associated with the activation of endogenous endonucleases (187,188). The signal transduction pathways by which CTLs induce apoptosis in their targets is still unknown.

3. *Natural Killer Cells*

Natural killer (NK) cells can be viewed as primitive CTLs that lack a TCR and are not MHC-restricted (189,190). NK cells have been shown to lyse virally infected cells and certain tumor cells. NK cells express the IL-2 receptor on their surface and, when stimulated by IL-2, become LAK (lymphokine-activated killer) cells, which demonstrate increased killing capabilities. Finally, NK cells have IgG Fc receptors (CD16) on their surface, allowing them to target cells coated with IgG. This form of lysis is called antibody-dependent cell-mediated cytotoxicity (ADCC) (191).

B. Examination of Grafts

Given the multiple possibilities for the effector cells responsible for graft rejection, investigators attempted to ascertain which cells were the primary mediators by examining the cellular subpopulations infiltrating rejecting allografts. Immunohistochemical staining, however, has generally revealed the presence of all the different cell types, including $CD4^{+}$ T cells, $CD8^{+}$ cells, NK cells, and macrophages (192–200). Further studies have attempted to identify more subtle histologic changes associated with rejection. For example, Sanfilippo et al. compared cellular infiltrates from rejecting grafts with infiltrates from functioning grafts (201). They found that the intensity of the T cell infiltrate could not be used to predict graft rejection, but a statistically significant increase in $CD8^{+}$ T cells could be identified in rejecting kidneys.

C. Correlating in Vivo Rejection with Demonstrable in Vitro Effector Functions: Support for the Cytotoxicity Model

1. Correlating the Responses to Alloantigens

Cytotoxic T-cell function is readily measurable in vitro using a standard CML assay. While the argument is indirect, if in vivo allograft rejection always correlated with in vitro cytotoxicity, it would suggest that CTLs are involved in rejection. Conversely, if cytotoxic activity in vitro was unrelated to in vivo graft rejection, then it would be harder to accept CTLs as the primary mediators of rejection.

Experiments looking at this correlation, using skin grafts with various antigenic disparities, have been performed by several laboratories. These experiments have compared the ability of T-cell subpopulations to reject the skin graft with the presence of helper and cytotoxic functions in vitro against the alloantigens. The results have generally shown that whenever a T cell subpopulation (e.g., $CD4^+$ T cells only, $CD8^+$ T cells only, or both) was able to reject a skin graft, that same T cell subpopulation demonstrated helper and cytotoxic functions against the alloantigens in vitro (49–51). Moreover T cell subpopulations that have helper but not cytotoxic capabilities against certain alloantigens are generally unable to mediate rejection (for example, $CD4^+$ T cells responding to class I or H-Y antigen disparities). These findings argue that cytotoxic T cells are necessary for graft rejection.

There have been, however, challenges to the strict correlation of cytotoxic activity and graft rejection. For example, the case of $CD4^+$ T cells attempting to reject a class I disparate graft has received additional scrutiny because several groups have reported that recipients depleted of $CD8^+$ T cells were able to reject class I disparate grafts despite the fact that cytotoxic $CD4^+$ T cells against class I alloantigens are very rare (49–51,131,134,135,198, 202). Rosenberg et al., however, were able to demonstrate that despite "$CD8^+$ T cell depletion" there still existed cytotoxic precursors of $CD8^+$ lineage in their animals (203). These residual cytotoxic cells required in vivo priming with $CD4^+$ helper T cells that were stimulated by other alloantigens. In addition, studies of the minor H-Y antigenic disparity have shown that not all cases of H-Y disparate graft rejection are associated with the subsequent demonstration of H-Y antigen cytotoxicity in vitro (204–206). These experiments, however, are technically difficult to carry out and the results are still controversial.

2. Both Helper and Effector Functions Are Required for Allograft Rejection

To further test the need for both helper and cytotoxic functions in graft rejection, Rosenberg et al. used a system for which it was known that the helper and cytotoxic functions were mediated by phenotypically distinct T-cell populations (49). The generation of an in vitro cytotoxic response to the male-specific H-Y antigen required $CD4^+$ helper T cells, which would recognize an H-Y helper epitope, to stimulate the proliferation and differentiation of $CD8^+$ cytotoxic T cells, which would recognize an H-Y cytotoxic epitope and lyse cells bearing that determinant. Rosenberg et al. grafted male $H\text{-}2^b$ skin onto female $H\text{-}2^b$ nude mice. Neither reconstitution with $CD4^+$ nor with $CD8^+$ T cells alone was sufficient to bring about the rejection of the single minor antigen disparate male skin. Only mice reconstituted with both cell types were able to reject the H-Y skin. Thus, skin allograft rejection required the presence of both helper and cytotoxic T cells.

3. CTL Cloning from Rejecting Allografts

Researchers have been able to clone cytotoxic T cells reactive against alloantigens (201,207–216). The experiments have been of two sorts. First, CTL clones have been generated in vitro which, when administered in vivo, can eliminate susceptible tumor cell grafts and cause local tissue necrosis in mice expressing skin-specific alloantigens recognized by the CTLs. Second, T lymphocytes found infiltrating allografts have been cultured in vitro and assessed for their cytotoxic abilities. $CD8^+$ T cells harvested from human renal allografts were found to possess cytotoxic activity against donor alloantigens. Furthermore, in a rat renal allograft model, T cells harvested from rejecting grafts showed higher alloantigen specific target lysis than cells from functioning grafts. These findings indicate that CTLs are generated in the rejection process and that their cytolytic activity may directly contribute to allograft rejection.

D. Antigen Specificity: Further Argument for the Cytotoxicity Model

One difference between a CTL-mediated and a DTH-mediated effector mechanism is the greater degree of antigen specificity associated with CTL activity. Thus, experiments have been performed testing the degree of antigenic specificity during allograft destruction.

1. Tumors

Murine tumor lines, being derived from inbred mouse strains, can serve as a model for allotransplantation when injected into a nonsyngeneic mouse strain. If the tumors are injected as a single-cell suspension, two different tumors can easily be mixed together. Lymphoid cells preimmunized to only one of the tumors can then be injected intraperitoneally along with the mixed tumor cells into irradiated mice. Only the tumor cells bearing the target alloantigens to which the lymphoid cells had been sensitized have been rejected in these experiments (217).

2. Tetraparental Grafts

Conceptually similar experiments have been performed with tissue transplants using tetraparental mice (218). These mice are created by fusing two different eight-cell-stage embryos, which then develop into genetic mosaics. This can be identified in some cases by mixed hair colors, reflecting the mosaicism of the parental melanocytes.

Rosenberg and Singer grafted trunk skin from B6↔A/J tetraparental mice onto immunoincompetent $H\text{-}2^b$ nude mice and allowed the grafts to heal. One month later, the nude recipients were reconstituted with unfractionated $H\text{-}2^b$ T cells, which were reactive against the white skin components but not the black ones. A nonspecific inflammatory rejection response ensued and resulted in complete hair loss and scab formation but no graft shrinkage. The tetraparental skin grafts survived this initial inflammation and regrew hair that was predominantly black. This demonstrated the selective survival of B6 melanocytes and hair follicles and suggested that the effector mechanism was highly antigen specific.

3. Rejection of Class II Disparate Grafts

Rosenberg and Singer went on to examine the rejection of MHC class II disparate skin (219). The rejection of such skin grafts was troubling to proponents of an antigen-specific cytotoxic effector phase because the alloantigens in these grafts was only present constitutively on Langerhans cells, which constitute less than 3% of skin cells. If the alloantigens were only on relatively few cells, how was the entire graft destroyed? They found that administration of anti-IFN-γ monoclonal antibody blocked the rejection of class II disparate grafts but not of class I disparate grafts (220). As discussed above, among IFN-γ's many roles is its ability to induce expression of class II MHC molecules and to activate macrophages. As the anti-IFN-γ prolonged class II disparate but not class I disparate graft survival, it suggests that it was the induction of class II MHC expression that was important in initiating graft rejection, confirming that graft rejection is antigen-specific and explaining how, under such a model, all elements of a class II disparate graft can be rejected in an antigen-specific manner.

E. Rejection of Skin from Bone-Marrow Chimeras: The DTH Counterargument

Although the specificity of allograft destruction provided a powerful argument for an antigen-directed, CTL-mediated effector arm, there were still certain unanswered questions posed by proponents of a DTH-mediated model. For example, in the tetraparental experiments, although the complete destruction of the allogeneic cells was easily documented, there was no way to quantify the amount of destruction of syngeneic or, in essence, bystander cells. In fact, the large inflammatory response suggests that significant bystander cell destruction did occur.

Rosenberg and Singer did a bone-marrow chimera experiment to test the ability of a nonspecific effector mechanism to bring about the destruction of an entire allograft (219). As the Langerhans cells (skin APCs) are of bone marrow origin while the keratinocytes are not, one can graft skin from an a→b bone marrow chimera onto a "b" animal and the only allogeneic elements in the graft will be the Langerhans cells. They found that the skin grafts were not rejected. Doody et al., however, performed similar experiments using skin from an a→b chimera grafted onto a "b" animal (221). The skin graft was rejected, albeit under somewhat different experimental conditions. This rejection process was confined sharply to the graft border and thus was highly selective, despite the fact that nonspecific effector mechanisms must have mediated the destruction of the majority of the cellular elements of the graft. The investigators postulated that a highly localized DTH response, triggered by the allogeneic Langerhans cells, caused the release of vasoactive and thrombogenic factors that disrupted the microvasculature in the immediate vicinity, leading to the selective necrosis of the skin graft.

F. Effector Mechanisms May Involve Both CTLs and DTH Mechanisms

Most of the data regarding the effector mechanisms of graft rejection can be reconciled by assuming that both CTL and DTH mechanisms are involved together. Work by Ando et al. using a transgenic mouse model of fulminant hepatitis to study a class I restricted response to foreign antigens has suggested the combination of effector mechanisms (222,223). Injection of a HBsAg-specific CTL clone into transgenic mice whose liver cells express the HBsAg protein resulted in an acute necroinflammatory response that had three components. First, Brd-U labeled injected CTLs came into direct contact with and brought about the apoptotic death of hepatocytes. Then, nonspecific and specific host inflammatory cells, including lymphocytes and neutrophils, were recruited and necroinflammatory foci appeared. Finally, concomitant with an abundant macrophage infiltrate, widespread hepatocellular necrosis ensued.

Administration of anti-IFN-γ antibody blocked both hepatocellular necrosis and the generation of necroinflammatory foci but did not inhibit the apoptosis induced by the CTLs. In addition, carrageenan (a macrophage inhibitor) blocked hepatocellular necrosis but had no effect on apoptosis or necroinflammatory development.

These results suggest that CTLs, reacting with their specific target antigens, can bring about apoptosis of their target cells, but that they can also secrete IFN-γ, which recruits other inflammatory cells that produce DTH-mediated tissue destruction.

VIII. SUMMARY

Besides summarizing the current state of knowledge regarding the basis of cell-mediated graft rejection, we hope that this review has amply illustrated one of the most interesting issues in transplantation today. That is, despite the power of alloreactivity, a recipient's immune system may eventually tolerate the foreign antigens and require no immunosuppression at all. As we come to a better understanding of the routes of antigen presentation, the regulation of T cell activation, and the mechanisms behind graft rejection, we come closer to being able to manipulate and regulate the immune system and thus closer to achieving our clinical goal of graft acceptance.

ACKNOWLEDGMENTS

M.S.S. is a 1993–1994 Howard Hughes Medical Institute Medical Student Research Training Fellow. H.A., Jr. is supported in part by USPHS grant HC-36372 and HC-18646.

REFERENCES

1. Little CC, Typper EE. Further experimental studies on the inheritance of susceptibility to a transplantable tumor, carcinoma (J.W.A.) of the Japanese waltzing mouse. J Med Res 1916: 33: 393–453.
2. Little CC. The Genetics of Tumor Transplantation. 1st ed. New York: Dover Publications, 1941.
3. Snell GD, Stimpfling JH. Genetics of Tissue Transplantation. 2d ed. New York: McGraw-Hill, 1966.
4. Winn HJ. Laws of Transplantation. 1st ed. New York: Marcel Dekker, 1988.
5. Cudkowicz G, Stimpfling JH. Hybrid resistance to parental marrow graft: association with the K region of H-2. Science 1964; 144:1339–1340.
6. Cudkowicz G, Nakamura I. Genetics of the murine hemopoietic-histocompatibility system: An overview. Trans Proc 1983; 15:2058–2063.
7. Little CC. A possible Mendelian explanation for a type of inheritance apparently non-Mendelian in nature. Science 1914; 40:904–906.
8. Little CC. The genetics of tissue transplantation in mammals. Cancer Res 1914; 8:75–95.
9. Barnes AD, Krohn PL. Estimation of number of histocompatibility genes controlling successful transplantation of normal skin in mice. Proc R Soc Lond, B 1957; 146:505–526.
10. Billingham RE, Hodge BA, Silvers WK. Estimate of number of histocompatibility loci in rat. PNAS 1962; 48:422–433.
11. Bailey DW. Four approaches to estimating number of histocompatibility loci. Transplant Proc 1970; 2:32–38.
12. Graff RJ, Brown DH. Estimates of histocompatibility differences between inbred mouse strains. Immunogenetics 1978; 7:367–373.
13. Hansen TH, Carreno BM, Sachs DH. The major histocompatibility complex. In: Paul WE ed. Fundamental Immunology. 3d ed. New York: Raven Press, 1993:577–628.
14. Caughman SW, Sharrow SO, Shimand S, et al. Ia+ murine epidermal Langerhans cells are deficient in surface expression of class I MHC. PNAS 1986; 83:7438–7442.
15. Harris HW, Gill TJ. Expression of class I transplantation antigens. Transplantation 1986; 42: 109–117.

16. Robinson PJ, Graf L, Sege K. Two allelic forms of mouse beta-2-microglobulin. Proc Natl Acad Sci USA 1981; 78:1167–1170.
17. Connolly JM, Potter TA, Wormstall EM, Hansen TH. The Lyt-2 molecule recognizes residues in the α3 domain in CTL responses. J Exp Med 1988; 168:325–341.
18. Salter RD, Norment AM, Chen BP, et al. Nature 1989; 338:345–347.
19. Hyman R, Stallings V. Characterization of a TL variant of a homozygous TL+ mouse lymphoma. Immunogenetics 1976; 3:75–84.
20. Krangel MS, Orr HT, Strominger JL. Assembly and maturation of HLA-A and HLA-B antigens in vivo. Cell 1979; 18:979–991.
21. Rock KL, Rothstein LE, Gambel SR, Benacerraf B. Reassociation with β_2-microglobulin is necessary for Kb class I major histocompatibility complex binding of exogenous peptides. Proc Natl Acad Sci USA 1990; 87:7517–7521.
22. Vitiello A, Potter TA, Sherman LA. The role of β_2-microglobulin in peptide binding by class I molecules. Science 1990: 250:1423–1426.
23. Kozlowski S, Takeshita T, Boehncke W-H, et al. Excess β_2 microglobulin promoting functional peptide association with purified soluble class I MHC molecules. Nature 1991; 349: 74–77.
24. Zijlstra M, Li E, Sajjadi F, Subramani S, Jaenisch R. Germ-line transmission of a disrupted B2-microglobulin gene produced by homologous recombination in embryonic stem cells. Nature 1989; 342:435–438.
25. Zijlstra M, Bix M, Simister NE, et al. β2-microglobulin deficient mice lack CD4-8+ cytolytic T cells. Nature 1990; 344:742–746.
26. Kaufman JF, Auffray C, Korman AJ, et al. The class II molecules of the human and murine major histocompatibility complex. Cell 1984; 36:1–13.
27. Daar AS, Fuggle SV, Fabre JW, et al. The detailed distribution of MHC Class II antigens in normal human organs. Transplantation 1984; 38:293–298.
28. Glimcher LH, Kara CJ. Sequences and factors: a guide to MHC class-II transcription. Ann Rev Immunol 1992; 10:13–49.
29. Graff RJ, Bailey DW. The non-H-2 histocompatibility loci and their antigens. Transplant Rev 1973; 15:26–49.
30. Loveland B, Simpson E. The non-MHC transplantation antigens: neither weak nor minor. Immunol Today 1986; 7:223–229.
31. Simpson E. Non-H-2 histocompatibility antigens: can they be retroviral products? Immunol Today 1987; 8:176–177.
32. Roopenian DC, Widmer MB, Orosz CG, Bach FH. Helper cell-independent cytolytic T lymphocytes specific for a minor histocompatibility antigen. J Immunol 1983; 130:542–545.
33. Roopenian DC, Orosz CG, Bach FH. Responses against single histocompatibility antigens: II. Analysis of cloned helper T cells. J Immunol 1984; 132:1080–1084.
34. Tekolf WA, Shaw S. Primary in vitro generation of cytotoxic cells specific for human minor histocompatibility antigens between HLA-identical siblings. J Immunol 1984; 132:1756–1760.
35. Czitrom AA, Gascoigne NR, Edwards S, Waterfield DJ. Induction of minor alloantigen-specific T cell subsets in vivo: Recognition of processed antigen by helper but not by cytotoxic T cell precursors. J Immunol 1984: 133:33–39.
36. Bevan MJ. Cross-priming for a secondary cytotoxic response to minor H antigens with H-2 congenic cells which do not cross-react in the cytotoxic assay. J Exp Med 1976; 143:1283–1288.
37. Wallny H-J, Rammensee H-G. Identification of classical minor histocompatibility antigen as cell-derived peptide. Nature 1990; 343:275–278.
38. Elliott T, Townsend A, Cerundolo V. Naturally processed peptides. Nature 1990; 348:195–197.
39. Falk K, Rotzschke O, Rammensee H-G. Cellular peptide composition governed by major histocompatibility complex class I molecules. Nature 1990; 348:248–251.

40. Lai PK, Waterfield JD, Gascoigne NR, et al. T-cell responses to minor histocompatibility antigens. Immunology 1982; 47:371–381.
41. Roopenian DC. What are minor histocompatibility loci? A new look at an old question. Immunol Today 1992; 13:7–10.
42. Roopenian DC, Widmer MB, Orosz CG, Bach FH. Response against single minor histocompatibility antigens: I. Functional immunogenetic analysis of cloned cytolytic T cells. J Immunol 1983: 131:2135–2140.
43. Bevan MJ. Minor antigens introduced on H-2 different stimulating cells cross-react at the cytotoxic T cell level during in vivo priming. J Immunol 1976; 117:2233–2238.
44. Steinmuller D, Wachtel SS. Transplantation biology and immunogenetics of murine skin-specific (Sk) alloantigens. Trans Proc 1980; 12:100–106.
45. Rosengard BR, Kortz EO, Ojikutu CA, et al. The failure of skin grafting to break tolerance to class I-disparate renal allografts in miniature swine despite inducing marked antidonor cellular immunity. Transplantation 1991; 52:1044–1052.
46. Lorenz R, Allen PM. Processing and presentation of self proteins. Immunol Rev 1988; 106:115–127.
47. Cudkowicz G. Genetic control of resistance to allogeneic and xenogeneic bone-marrow grafts in mice. Trans Proc 1975; 7:155–159.
48. Manning DD, Reed ND, Shaffer CF. Maintenance of skin xenografts of widely divergent phylogenetic origin on congenitally athymic (nude) mice. J Exp Med 1973; 138:488–494.
49. Rosenberg AS, Mizuochi T, Sharrow SO, Singer A. Phenotype, specificity, and function of T cell subsets and T cell interactions involved in skin allograft rejection. J Exp Med 1987; 165:1296–1315.
50. Sprent J, Schaefer M, Lo D, Korngold R. Properties of purified T cell subsets: II. In vivo responses to class I vs. class II H-2 differences. J Exp Med 1986; 163:998–1011.
51. Rosenberg A, Mizuochi T, Singer A. Analysis of T-cell subsets in rejection of Kb mutant skin allografts differing at class I MHC. Nature 1986; 322:829–831.
52. Cosimi AB, Burton RC, Colvin RB, et al. Treatment of acute renal allograft rejection with OKT3 monoclonal antibody. Transplantation 1981; 32:535–539.
53. Cantor H, Boyse EA. Functional subclasses of T lymphocytes bearing different Ly antigens: II. Cooperation between subclasses of Ly+ cells in the generation of killer activity. J Exp Med 1975; 141:1390–1399.
54. Reinherz EL, Schlossman SF. The differentiation and function of human T lymphocytes. Cell 1980; 19:821–827.
55. Swain SL. Significance of Lyt phenotypes: Lyt2 antibodies block activities of T cells that recognize class I MHC antigens regardless of their function. PNAS 1981; 78:7101–7105.
56. Swain SL. T cell subsets and the recognition of MHC class. Immunol Rev 1983; 74:129–142.
57. Swain SL, Bakke A, English M, Dutton RW. Ly phenotypes and MHC recognition: the alloheper that recognizes K or D is a mature Ly123 cell. J Immunol 1979; 123:2716–2724.
58. Neefjes JJ, Pleogh HL. Intracellular transport of MHC class II molecules. Immunol Today 1992; 13:179–183.
59. Germain RN, Margulies DH. The biochemistry and cell biology of antigen processing and presentation. Annu Rev Immunol 1993; 11:403–450.
60. Germain RN. Antigen processing and presentation. In: Paul WE ed. Fundamental Immunology. 3d ed. New York: Raven Press, 1993:629–676.
61. Monaco JJ. A molecular model of MHC class-I-restricted antigen processing. Immunol Today 1992; 13:173–178.
62. Kraal G, Breel M, Janse M, Bruin G. Langerhans cells, veiled cells, and interdigitating cells in the mouse recognized by a monoclonal antibody. J Exp Med 1986; 163:981–997.
63. Dustin ML, Springer TA. Role of lymphocyte adhesion receptors in transient interactions and cell locomotion. Annu Rev Immunol 1991; 9:27–66.
64. Springer TA. Adhesion receptors of the immune system. Nature 1990; 346:425–434.

65. Springer TA, Dustin ML, Kishimoto TK, Marlin SD. The lymphocyte function-associated LFA-1, CD2, and LFA-3 molecules: Cell adhesion receptors of the immune system. Annu Rev Immunol 1987; 5:223–252.
66. Hahn WC, Menu E, Bothwell A, et al. Overlapping but nonidentical binding sites on CD2 for CD58 and a second ligand CD59. Science 1992; 256:1805–1807.
67. Van de Velde H, von Hoegen I, Luo W, et al. The B-cell surface protein CD72/Lyb-2 is the ligand for CD5. Nature 1991; 351:662–665.
68. Parnes JR. Molecular biology and function of CD4 and CD8. Adv Immunol 1989; 44: 265–311.
69. Shimizu Y, Newman W, Tanaka Y, Shaw S. Lymphocyte interaction with endothelial cells. Immunol Today 1992; 13:106–111.
70. Butcher EC. Leukocyte-endothelial cell recognition: Three (or more) steps to specificity and diversity. Cell 1991; 67:1033–1036.
71. Hynes RO. Integrins: versatility, modulation, and signaling in cell adhesion. Cell 1992; 69: 11–25.
72. Mueller DL, Jenkins MK, Schwartz RH. Clonal expansion vs functional inactivation. Annu Rev Immunol 1989; 7:445–480.
73. Harding FA, McArthur JG, Gross JA, et al. CD28-mediated signalling co-stimulates murine T cells and prevents induction of anergy in T-cell clones. Nature 1992; 356:607–609.
74. Schwartz RH. Costimulation of T lymphocytes: The role of CD28, CTLA-4, and B7/BB1 in interleukin-2 production and immunotherapy. Cell 1992; 71:1065–1068.
75. June CH, Ledbetter JA, Linsley PS, Thompson CB. Role of the CD28 receptor in T-cell activation. Immunol Today 1990; 11:211–216.
76. Linsley PS, Ledbetter JA. The role of the CD28 receptor during T cell responses to antigen. Annu Rev Immunol 1993; 11:191–212.
77. Jerne NK. The somatic generation of immune recognition. Eur J Immunol 1971; 1:1–9.
78. Bevan MJ. High determinant density may explain the phenomenon of alloreactivity. Immunol Today 1984; 5:128–130.
79. Matzinger P, Bevan MJ. Hypothesis: why do so many lymphocytes respond to major histocompatibility complex antigens? Cell Immunol 1977; 29:1–5.
80. La Rosa FG, Talmage DW. Synergism between minor and major histocompatibility antigens in the rejection of cultured allografts. Transplantation 1985; 39:480–485.
81. Parker KE, Dalchau R, Fowler VJ, et al. Stimulation of CD4+ T lymphocytes by allogenic MHC peptides presented on autologous antigen-presenting cells. Transplantation 1992; 53: 918–924.
82. La Rosa FG, Talmage DW. The failure of a major histocompatibility antigen to stimulate a thyroid allograft reaction after culture in oxygen. J Exp Med 1983; 157:898–906.
83. Fischer Lindahl K, Wilson DB. Histocompatibility antigen-activated cytotoxic T lymphocytes: II. Estimates of frequency and specificity of precursors. J Exp Med 1977; 145:508–522.
84. Teh HS, Harley E, Phillips RA, Miller RG. Quantitative studies on the precursors of cytotoxic lymphocytes: I. Characterization of a clonal assay and determination of the size of clones derived from single precursors. J Immunol 1977; 118:1049–1056.
85. Lancki DW, Hsieh C-S, Fitch FW. Mechanisms of lysis by cytotoxic T lymphocyte clones: lytic activity and gene expression in cloned antigen-specific $CD4^+$ and $CD8^+$ lymphocytes. J Immunol 1991; 146:3242–3249.
86. Salgame P, Convit J, Bloom BR. Immunologic suppression by human $CD8^+$ T cells is receptor dependent and HLA-DQ restricted. Proc Natl Acad Sci USA 1991; 88:2598–2602.
87. Shinohara N, Bluestone JA, Sachs DH. Cloned cytotoxic T lymphocytes that recognize an I-A region product in the context of a class I antigen. J Exp Med 1986; 163:972–980.
88. Strassman G, Bach FH, $OKT4^+$ cytotoxic T cells can lyse targets via class I molecules and can be blocked by monoclonal antibody against T4 molecules. J Immunol 1984; 133:1705–1709.
89. McKisic MD, Sant AJ, Fitch FW. Some cloned murine $CD4^+$ T cells recognize H-2Ld class I

MHC determinants directly; other cloned CD4+ T cells recognize H-2Ld class I determinants in the context of class II MHC molecules. J Immunol 1991; 147:2868–2874.
90. Zijlstra M, Auchincloss HJ, Loring JM, et al. Skin graft rejection by beta$_2$-microglobulin-deficient mice. J Exp Med 1992; 175:885–893.
91. Grusby MJ, Johnson RS, Papaioannou VE, Glimcher LH. Depletion of CD4+ T cells in major histocompatibility complex class II-deficient mice. Science 1991; 253:1417–1420.
92. Grusby MJ, Auchincloss HJ, Lee R, et al. Mike lacking major histocompatibility complex class I and class II molecules. Proc Natl Acad Sci 1993; 90:3919.
93. Cosgrove D, Gray D, Dierich A, et al. Mice lacking MHC class II molecules. Cell 1991; 66:1051.
94. Mitchison NA, O'Malley C. Three-cell-type clusters of T cells with antigen-presenting cells best explain the epitope linkage and noncognate requirements of the in vivo cytolytic response. Eur J Immunol 1987; 17:1579–1583.
95. Lee RS, Grusby MJ, Glimcher LH, et al. Indirect recognition by helper cells can induce donor-specific cytotoxic T lymphocytes in vivo. J Exp. Med. 1994; 179:865–872.
96. Crabtree G. Contingent genetic regulatory events in T lymphocyte activation. Science 1989; 243:355–361.
97. Curran T, Bravo R, Muller R. Transient induction of c-fos and c-myc is an immediate consequence of growth factor stimulation. Cancer Surv 1985; 4:655–681.
98. Lewin B. Oncogenic conversion by regulatory changes in transcription factors. Cell 1991; 64:303–312.
99. Weiss A, Imboden JB. Cell surface molecules and early events involved in human T lymphocyte activation. Adv Immunol 1987; 41:1–38.
100. Hemler ME, Jacobson JG, Strominger JL. Biochemical characterization of VLA-1 and VLA-2 cell surface heterodimers in activated cells. J Biol Chem 1985; 260:15246–15252.
101. Mosmann TR, Cherwinski H, Bond MW, et al. Two types of murine helper T cell clones: I. Definition according to profiles of lymphokine activities and secreted proteins. J Immunol 1986; 136:2348–2357.
102. Cher DJ, Mosmann TR. Two types of murine helper T cell clones: II. Delayed-type hypersensitivity is mediated by Th1 clones. J Immunol 1987; 138:3688–3694.
103. Cherwinski HM, Schumacher JH, Brown KD, Mosmann TR. Two types of mouse helper T cell clones: III. Further differences in lymphokine synthesis between Th1 and Th2 clones revealed by RNA hybridization, functionally monospecific bioassays, and monoclonal antibodies. J Exp Med 1987; 166:1229–1244.
104. Mosmann TR, Coffman RL. Th1 and Th2 cells: Different patterns of lymphokine secretion lead to different functional properties. Annu Rev Immunol 1989; 7:145–173.
105. Henkart P, Henkart M, Millard P, et al. The role of cytoplasmic granules in cytotoxicity by large granular lymphocytes and cytotoxic lymphocytes. In: Henkart P, Martz E, eds. Mechanisms of Cell-Mediated Cytotoxicity II. Vol. 184. New York: Plenum Press, 1984:121–138.
106. Schwartz RH. Immunologic Tolerance. In: Paul WE ed. Fundamental Immunology. 3d ed. New York: Raven Press, 1993:677–731.
107. Charlton B, Auchincloss H, Fathman CG. Mechanisms of transplantation tolerance. Annu Rev Immunol 1994; 12:707–734.
108. Burnet FM. The Clonal Selection Theory of Acquired Immunity. New York: Cambridge University Press, 1959.
109. Kappler JW, Roehm N, Marrack P. T cell tolerance by clonal elimination in the thymus. Cell 1987; 4:273–280.
110. Fry AM, Matis LA. Self-tolerance alters T-cell receptor expression in an antigen-specific MHC restricted immune response. Nature 1988; 335:830–832.
111. Sha WC, Nelson CA, Newberry RD, et al. Positive and negative selection of an antigen receptor on T cells in transgenic mice. Nature 1988; 336:73–76.
112. Lamb JR, Skidmore BJ, Green N, et al. Induction of tolerance in influenza virus-immune T

lymphocyte clones with synthetic peptides of influenza hemagglutinin. J Exp Med 1983; 157:1434–1447.
113. Quill H, Schwartz RH. Stimulation of normal inducer T cell clones with antigen presented by purified Ia molecules in planar lipid membranes: Specific induction of a long-lived state of proliferative nonresponsiveness. J Immunol 1987; 138:3704–3712.
114. Roberts JL, Sharrow SO, Singer A. Clonal deletion and clonal anergy in the thymus induced by cellular elements with different radiation sensitivities. J Exp Med 1990; 171:935–940.
115. Tutschka RJ, Ki PF, Beschorner WE, et al. Suppressor cells in transplantation tolerance: II. Maturation of suppressor cells in the bone marrow chimera. Transplantation 1981; 32: 321–325.
116. Lancaster F, Chui YL, Batchelor JR. Anti-idiotypic T cells suppress rejection of renal allografts in rats. Nature 1985; 315:336–337.
117. Roser BJ. Cellular mechanisms in neonatal and adult tolerance. Immunol Rev 1989; 107: 179–202.
118. Maki T, Gottschalk R, Wood ML, Monaco AP. Specific unresponsiveness to skin allografts in anti-lympohcyte serum-treated, marrow-injected mice: Participation of donor marrow-derived suppressor T cells. J Immunol 1981; 127:1433–1437.
119. Lafferty K, Prowse S, Simeonovic C, Warren HS. Immunobiology of tissue transplantation: A return to the passenger leucocyte concept. Annu Rev Immunol 1983; 143–173.
120. Jenkins MK, Schwartz RH. Antigen presentation by chemically modified splenocytes induces antigen-specific T cell unresponsiveness in vitro and in vivo. J Exp Med 1987; 165.302–319.
121. Kang S-M, Beverly B, Tran A-C, et al. Transactivation by AP-1 is a molecular target of T cell clonal anergy. Science 1992; 257:1134–1138.
122. Gray D. Immunological memory. Annu Rev Immunol 1993; 11:49–77.
123. Mizuochi T, Golding H, Rosenberg AS, et al. Both L3T4+ and Lyt-2+ helper T cells initiate cytotoxic T lymphocyte responses against allogeneic major histocompatibility antigens but not against trinitrophenyl-modified self. J Exp Med 1985; 162:427–443.
124. Mizuochi T, Munitz TI, McCarthy S, et al. Differential helper and effector responses of Lyt-2 T cells to H-2Kb mutant (Kbm) determinants and the appearance of thymic influence on anti-Kbm CTL responsiveness. J Immunol 1986; 137:2740–2747.
125. Mizuochi T, Ono S, Malek TR, Singer A. Characterization of two distinct primary T cell populations that secrete interleukin 2 upon recognition of class I or class II major histocompatibility antigens. J Exp Med 1986; 163:603–619.
126. Golding H, Mizuochi T, McCarthy SA, et al. Relationship among function, phenotype, and specificity in primary allospecific T cell populations: Identification of phenotypically identical but functionally distinct primary T cell subsets that differ in their recognition of MHC class I and class II allodeterminants. J Immunol 1987; 138:10–17.
127. Singer A, Munitz TI, Golding H, et al. Recognition requirements for the activation, differentiation, and function of T-helper cells specific for class I MHC alloantigens. Immunol Rev 1987; 98:143–170.
128. Sprent J, Schaefer M, Properties of purified T cell subsets: I. In vitro responses to class I and class II H-2 alloantigens. J Exp Med 1985; 162:2068–2088.
129. McCarthy SA, Singer A. Recognition of MHC class I allodeterminants regulates the generation of MHC class II-specific CTL. J Immunol 1986; 137:3087–3092.
130. Mizuochi T, Hugin AW, Morse HC, et al. Role of lymphokine-secreting CD8+ T cells in cytotoxic T lymphocyte responses against vaccinia virus. J Immunol 1989; 142:270–273.
131. Wheelahan J, McKenzie IFC. The role of T4+ and Ly-2+ cells in skin graft rejection in the mouse. Transplantation 1987; 44:273–280.
132. Cobbold SP, Jayasuriya A, Nash A, et al. Therapy with monoclonal antibodies by elimination of T cell subsets in vivo. Nature 1984; 312:548–551.
133. Cobbold S, Waldmann H. Skin allograft rejection by L3T4+ and Lyt-2+ T cell subsets. Transplantation 1986; 41:634–639.

134. Smith DM, Stuart FP, Wemhoff GA, et al. Cellular pathways for rejection of class-I-MHC-disparate skin and tumor allografts. Transplantation 1988; 45:168–175.
135. Ichikawa T, Nakayama E, Uenaka A, et al. Effector cells in allelic H-2 class I-incompatible skin graft rejection. J Exp Med 1987; 166:982–990.
136. Auchincloss HJ, Mayer T, Ghobrial R, Winn HJ. T cell subsets, bm mutants, and the mechanism of allogenic skin graft rejection. Immunol Res 189; 8:149–164.
137. Rosenberg AS, Mizuochi T. A. S. Evidence for involvement of dual-function T cells in rejection of MHC class I disparate skin grafts: Assessment of MHC class I alloantigens as in vivo helper determinants. J Exp Med 1988; 168:33–45.
138. Pescovitz MD, Thistlethwait JRJ, Auchincloss HJ, et al. Effect of class II antigen matching of renal allograft survival in miniature swine. J Exp Med 1984; 160:1495–1508.
139. Woodcock J, Wofsy D, Eriksson E, et al. Rejection of skin grafts and generation of cytotoxic T cells by mice depleted of L3T4+ cells. Transplantation 1986; 42:636–642.
140. Madsen JC, Peugh WN, Wood KJ, Morris PJ. The effect of anti-L3T4 monoclonal antibody treatment on first-set rejection of murine cardiac allografts. Transplantation 1987; 44: 849–852.
141. Mottram PL, Wheelahan J, McKenzie IFC, Clunie GJA. Murine cardiac allograft survival following treatment of recipients with monoclonal anti-L3T4 or Ly-2 antibodies. Trans Proc 1987; 19:2898–2901.
142. Bradley JA, Mowat AM, Bolton EM. Processed MHC class I alloantigen as the stimulus for CD4+ T-cell dependent antibody-mediated graft rejection. Immunol Today 1992; 13: 434–438.
143. Kobayashi E, Kawai K, Ikarashi Y, Fujiwara M. Mechanism of the rejection of major histocompatibility complex class I-disparate murine skin grafts: Rejection can be mediated by CD4+ cells activated by allo-class I + II antigen in CD8+ cell-depleted hosts. J Exp Med 1992; 176:617–621.
144. Auchincloss HJ, Lee R, Shea S, et al. The role of "indirect" recognition in initiating rejection of skin grafts from major histocompatibility complex class II-deficient mice. Proc Natl Acad Sci USA 1993; 90:3373–3377.
145. Korngold R, Sprent J. Variable capacity of L3T4+ T cells to cause lethal graft-versus-host disease across histocompatibility barriers in mice. J Exp Med 1987; 165:1552–1564.
146. Andersson LC, Hayry P. Clonal isolation of alloantigen-reactive T cells and characterization of their memory functions. Transplant Rev 1975; 25:121–162.
147. Gurley KE, Hall BM, Dorsch SE. The factor of immunization in allograft rejection: Carried by cytotoxic T cells, not helper-induced T cells. Transplant Proc 1986; 18:307–309.
148. MacDonald HR, Sordat B, Cerottini J-C, Brunner KT. Generation of cytotoxic T lymphocytes in vitro: IV. Functional activation of memory cells in the absence of DNA synthesis. J Exp Med 1975; 142:622–636.
149. Lafferty KJ, Bootes A, Dart G, Talmage DW. Effect of organ culture on the survival of thyroid allografts in mice. Transplantation 1976; 22:138–149.
150. Bowen KM, Andrus L, Lafferty KJ. Survival of pancreatic islet allografts. Lancet 1979; 2:585–586.
151. Sollinger HW, Burkholder PM, Rasmus WR, Bach FH. Prolonged survival of xenografts after organ culture. Surgery 1977; 81:74–79.
152. Lechler RI, Batchelor JR. Restoration of immunogenicity to passenger cell-depleted kidney allografts by the addition of donor strain dendritic cells. J Exp Med 1982; 155:31–41.
153. Faustman D, Hauptfeld V, Lacy P, Davie J. Prolongation of murine islet allograft survival by pretreatment of islets with antibody directed to Ia determinants. PNAS 1981; 78:5156–5159.
154. Qin SX, Wise M, Cobbold SP, et al. Induction of tolerance in peripheral T cells with monoclonal antibodies. Eur J Immunol 1990; 20:2737–2745.
155. Cobbold SP, Martin G, Waldmann H. The induction of skin graft tolerance in major histocompatibility complex mismatched or primed recipients: Primed T cells can be tolerized in the periphery with anti-CD4 and anti-CD8 antibodies. Eur J Immunol 1990; 20:2747–2755.

156. Chen Z, Cobbold S, Metcalfe S, Waldmann H. Tolerance in the mouse to major histocompatibility complex-mismatched heart allografts, and to rat heart xenografts, using monoclonal antibodies to CD4 and CD8. Eur J Immunol 1992; 23:805–810.
157. Shizuru JA, Gregory AK, Chao CT, Fathman CG. Islet allograft survival after a single course of treatment of recipient with antibody to L3T4. Science 1987; 237:278–280.
158. Shizuru J, Seydel KB, Flavin TF, et al. Induction of donor-specific unresponsiveness to cardiac allografts in rats by pretransplant anti-CD4 monoclonal antibody therapy. Transplantation 1990; 50:366–373.
159. Alters SE, Shizuru JA, Ackerman J, et al. Anti-CD4 mediates clonal anergy during transplantation tolerance induction. J Exp Med 1991; 173:491–494.
160. Cosimi AB, Conti D, Delmonico FL, et al. In vivo effects of monoclonal antibody to ICAM-1 (CD54) in nonhuman primates with renal allografts. J Immunol 1990; 144:4604–4612.
161. Harding CV, Unanue ER. Modulation of antigen presentation and peptide-MHC-specific, LFA-1-dependent T cell-macrophage adhesion. J Immunol 1991; 147:767–773.
162. Wee SL, Cosimi AB, Preffer FI, et al. Functional consequences of anti-ICAM-1 (CD54) in cynomolgus monkeys. Transplant Proc 1991; 23:279–280.
163. Isobe M, Yagita H, Okumura K, Ihara A. Specific acceptance of cardiac allograft after treatment with antibodies to ICAM-1 and LFA-1. Science 1992; 255:1125–1127.
164. Tan P, Anasetti C, Hansen JA, et al. Induction of alloantigen-specific hyporesponsiveness in human T lymphocytes by blocking interaction of CD28 with its natural ligand B7/BB1. J Exp Med 1993; 177:165–173.
165. Boussiotis VA, Freeman GJ, Gray G, et al. B7 but not intracellular adhesion molecule-1 costimulation prevents the induction of human alloantigen-specific tolerance. J Exp Med 1993; 178:1753–1763.
166. Lenschow DJ, Zeng Y, Thistlethwaite JR, et al. Long-term survival of xenogeneic pancreatic islet grafts induced by CTLA4Ig. Science 1992; 257:789–792.
167. Seder RA, Germain RN, Linsley PS, Paul WE. CD28-mediated costimulation of interleukin 2 (IL-2) production plays a critical role in T cell priming for IL-4 and interferon γ production. J Exp Med 1994; 179:299–304.
168. Gajewski TF, Fitch FW. Differential activation of murine TH1 and TH2 clones. Res Immunol 1991; 142:19–23.
169. Fitch FW, McKisic MD, Lancki DW, Gajewski TF. Differential regulation of murine T lymphocyte subsets. Annu Rev Immunol 1993; 11:29–48.
170. Fitch FW, Lancki DW, Gajewski TF. T-cell-mediated immune regulation. In: Paul WE ed. Fundamental Immunology. 3d ed. New York: Raven Press, 1993:733–761.
171. Gilbert KM, Hobbs MV, Ernst D, Weigle DO. Heterogeneity in the ability of different antigen presenting cells to tolerize TH1 and TH2 clones. FASEB J 1991; A1688.
172. Gajewski TF, Lancki DW, Stack R, Fitch FW. "Anergy" of T_H0 helper T lymphocytes induces downregulation of T_H1 characteristics and a transition to a T_H2-like phenotype. J Exp Med 1994; 179:481–491.
173. Abehsira-Amar O, Gilbert M, Jolly M, et al. IL-4 plays a dominant role in the differential development of Th0 into Th1 and Th2 cells. J Immunol 1992; 148:3820–3829.
174. Starzl TE, Demetris AJ, Trucco M, et al. Systemic chimerism in human female recipients of male livers. Lancet 1992; 340:876–877.
175. Starzl TE, Demetris AJ, Murase N, et al. Cell migration, chimerism, and graft acceptance. Lancet 1992; 339:1579–1582.
176. Adams DO, Hamilton TA. The cell biology of macrophage activation. Annu Rev Immunol 1984; 2:283–313.
177. Berke G. The functions and mechanisms of action of cytolytic lymphocytes. In: Paul WE ed. Fundamental Immunology. 3d ed. New York: Raven Press, 1993: 965–1014.
178. Berke G, Sullivan KA, Amos DB. Rejection of ascites tumor allografts: I. Isolation, characterization and in vitro reactivity of peritoneal lymphoid effector cells from BALB/c mice immune to EL4 leukosis. J Exp Med 1972; 135:1334–1350.

179. Berke G, Rosen D, Ronen D. Mechanism of lymphocyte-mediated cytolysis: Functional cytolytic T cells lacking perforin and granzymes. Immunology 1993; 78:105–112.
180. Mason DW, Morris PJ. Effector mechanisms in allograft rejection. Annu Rev Immunol 1986; 4:119–145.
181. Roberts PH, Hayry P. Effector mechanism in allograft rejection: II. Density, electrophoresis and size fractionation of allograft-infiltrating cells demonstrating several classes of killer cells. Cell Immunol 1977; 30:236–253.
182. Podack ER. Molecular mechanisms of cytolysis by complement and by cytolytic lymphocytes. J Cell Biochem 1986; 3:129–157.
183. Young J-E, Cohn ZA, Podack ER. The ninth component of complement and the pore-forming protein (perforin) from cytotoxic T cells: Structural, immunological and functional similarities. Science 1986; 233:184–190.
184. Aggarwal BB, Eessalu TE. Human tumor necrosis factor and lymphotoxin: Their structural and functional similarities. In: Bonavida B, Coller RI, ed. Membrane-Mediated Cytotoxicity. Vol. 45. New York: Liss, 1987:297–301.
185. Ruddle NH, McGrath K, James T, Schmid DS. Purified lymphotoxin (LT) from class I restricted CTLs and class II restricted cytolytic helpers induce target cell DNA fragmentation. In: Bonavida B, Coller RJ, eds. Membrane-Mediated Cytotoxicity. Vol. 45. New York: Liss, 1987:379.
186. Zanovello P, Bronte V, Rosato A, et al. Responses of mouse lymphocytes to extracellular ATP: II. Extracellular ATP causes cell type-dependent lysis and DNA fragmentation. J Immunol 1990; 145:1545–1550.
187. Russel JH. Internal disintegration model of cytotoxic lymphocyte-induced target damage. Immunol Rev 1983; 72:97–118.
188. Tian Q, Streuli M, Saito H, et al. A polydenylate binding protein localized to the granules of cytolytic lymphocytes induces DNA fragmentation in target cells. Cell 1991; 67:629–639.
189. Ortaldo JR, Herberman RB. Heterogeneity of natural killer cells. Annu Rev Immunol 1984; 2: 359–394.
190. Nemlander A, Saksela E, Hayry P. Are "natural killer" cells involved in allograft rejection? Eur J Immunol 1983; 13:348–350.
191. Lovchik JC, Hong R. Antibody-dependent cell-mediated cytolysis (ADCC): Analyses and projections. Prog Allergy 1977; 22:1–44.
192. Roberts PJ, Hayry P. Sponge matrix allografts: A model for analysis of killer cells infiltrating mouse allografts. Transplantation 1976; 21:437–445.
193. Strom TB, Tilney NL, Paradyez J, et al. Cellular components of allograft rejection: Identity, specificity, and cytotoxic function of cells infiltrating acutely rejecting allografts. J Immunol 1977; 118:2020–2026.
194. Hall B, Dorsch S. Cells mediating allograft rejection. Immunol Rev 1984; 77:31–59.
195. Ascher NL, Hoffman R, Hanto D, Simmons R. Cellular basis of allograft rejection. Immunol Rev 1984; 77:217–232.
196. Hall B, Bishop G, Farnsworth A, et al. Identification of the cellular subpopulations infiltrating rejecting cadaver renal allografts: Preponderance of the T4 subset of T cells. Transplantation 1984; 37:564–570.
197. Hayry P, von Willebrand E, Parthenais E, et al. The inflammatory mechanisms of allograft rejection. Immunol Rev 1984; 77:85–142.
198. Bradley AJ, Bolton EM. The T-cell requirements for allograft rejection. Transplant Rev 1992; 6:115–129.
199. Preffer FI, Colvin RB, Leary CP, et al. Two color flow cytometry and functional analysis of lymphocytes cultured from human renal allografts: Identification of a Leu 2+3+ subpopulation. J Immunol 1986; 137:2823–2830.
200. Tilney NL, Strom TB, MacPherson SG, Carpenter CB. Surface properties and functional characteristics of infiltrating cells harvested from acutely rejecting cardiac allografts in inbred rats. Transplantation 1975; 20:323–330.

201. Sanfilippo F, Kilbeck PC, Vaughn WK, Bollinger RR. Renal allograft cell infiltrates associated with irreversible rejection. Transplantation 1985; 40:679–685.
202. Macphail S, Stutman O. L3T4+ cytotoxic T lymphocytes specific for class I H-2 antigens are activated in primary mixed lymphocyte reactions. J Immunol 1987; 139:4007–4015.
203. McCarthy SA, Kaldjian E, Singer A. Induction of anti-CD8 resistant cytotoxic T lymphocytes by anti-CD8 antibodies: Functional evidence for T cell signaling induced by multivalent cross-linking of CD8 on precursor cells. J Immunol 1988; 141:3737–3746.
204. Hurme M, Hetherington CM, Simpson E. Cytotoxic T-cell responses to H-Y: Correlation with the rejection of syngeneic male skin grafts. J Exp Med 1978; 147:768–775.
205. McKenzie IFC, Henning MM, Michaelides M. Skin graft rejection and delayed-type hypersensitivity responses to H-Y in an I-Ab mutant. Immunogenetics 1984; 20:475–480.
206. Gordon RD, Mathieson BJ, Samelson LE, et al. The effect of allogeneic presensitization on H-Y graft survival and in vitro cell-mediated responses to H-Y antigen. J Exp Med 1976; 144:810–820.
207. Kim B, Rosenstein M, Weiland D, et al. Clonal analysis of the lymphoid cells mediating skin allograft rejection. Transplantation 1983; 36:525–532.
208. Kilbeck PC, Miceli C, Finn OJ, et al. Relationships among renal allograft biopsy infiltrates, growth of T cell lines, and irreversible rejection. Transplant Proc 1988; 20:303–305.
209. Kilbeck PC, Tatum AH, Sanfillipo F. Relationships among the histologic pattern, intensity, and phenotypes of T cells infiltrating renal allografts. Transplantation 1984; 38:709–713.
210. Knechtle SJ, Wolfe JA, Burchette J, et al. Infiltrating cell phenotypes and patterns associated with hepatic allograft rejection or acceptance. Transplantation 1987; 43:169–172.
211. Wolfe JA, Knechtle SJ, Burchette J, et al. Phenotype and patterns of inflammatory cell infiltration associated with rejection or acceptance of rat liver allografts. Transplant Proc 1987; 19:364–368.
212. Straznickas J, Howell D, Ruiz P, Sanfillipo F. Phenotype and function of T cells propagated from donor-specific blood transfusion enhanced and autologous blood transfused rejecting rat renal allografts. Transplant Proc 1988; 20:276–280.
213. Miceli MC, Finn OJ. T cell receptor beta-chain selection in human allograft rejection. J Immunol 1989, 142:81–86.
214. Moreau JF, Peyrat MA, Vie H, et al. T cell colony-forming frequency of mononucleated cells extracted from rejected human kidney transplants. Transplantation 1985; 39:649–656.
215. Bonneville M, Moreau JF, Blokland E, et al. T lymphocyte cloning from rejected human kidney allograft: Recognition repertoire of alloreactive T cell clones. J Immunol 1988; 141:4187–4195.
216. Miceli MC, Barry TS, Finn OJ. Human renal allograft infiltrating T cells: Phenotype-function correlation and clonal heterogeneity. Transplant Proc 1988; 20:199–201.
217. Freedman LR, Cerottini J-C, Brunner KT. In vivo studies of the role of cytotoxic T cells in tumor allograft immunity. J Immunol 1972; 109:1371.
218. Rosenberg AS, Singer A. Evidence that the effector mechanism of skin allograft rejection is antigen-specific. PNAS 1988; 85:7739–7742.
219. Rosenberg AS, Katz SI, Singer A. Rejection of skin allografts by CD4+ T cells is antigen-specific and requires expression of target alloantigen on Ia- epidermal cells. J Immunol 1989; 143:2452–2456.
220. Rosenberg AS, Finbloom DS, Maniero TG, et al. Specific prolongation of MHC class II disparate skin allografts by in vivo administration of anti-IFN-gamma monoclonal antibody. J Immunol 1990; 144:4648–4650.
221. Doody DP, Stenger KS, Winn HJ. Immunologically nonspecific mechanisms of tissue destruction in the rejection of skin grafts. J Exp Med 1994; 179:1645–1652.
222. Ando K, Moriyama T, Guidotti LG, et al. Mechanisms of class I restricted immunopathology: A transgenic mouse model of fulminant hepatitis. J Exp Med 1993; 178:1541–1554.
223. Ando K, Guidotti LG, Wirth S, et al. Class I-restricted cytotoxic T lymphocytes are directly cytopathic for their target cells in vivo. J Immunol 1994; 152:3245–3253.

2

Antibody-Mediated Rejection

Patricia M. Campbell and Philip F. Halloran
University of Alberta, Edmonton, Alberta, Canada

I. HISTORICAL REFLECTIONS

Alloantibody is an inherent component of the immune response to alloantigens, and its role in rejection may be greater than previously appreciated. The tendency to downplay the role of antibody may have arisen because early studies in rodents showed that rejection was cell-mediated, not antibody-mediated. Early investigators found that acute rejection could not be induced by transferring serum (1–3) but could be induced by transferring cells. Yet it soon became clear that antibodies were able to mediate rejection of grafts under some circumstances, the most dramatic example being the description of hyperacute rejection (HAR) in renal transplant recipients who were ABO-incompatible or highly sensitized against class I human leukocyte antigens (HLA) (4–10).

Initially, it was believed that if typical acute rejection is mediated by T cells, presumably cytotoxic T cells, then alloantibody was a red herring. Recently we have come to realize that most acute rejection is T cell–mediated, but that mixed antibody and T-cell reactions and pure antibody-mediated rejection probably occur in clinical situations. In short, the fact that most acute rejection is T cell–mediated does not preclude the ability of alloantibody to also injure the graft in some situations.

A confusing feature of the antibody response is its lack of predictability in producing graft damage. Antibody can often mediate injury if a high concentration of antibody rapidly meets a graft that has not previously been exposed to the antibody and the antigen density is high. But if the antibody concentration is reduced or if prior exposure to antibody has reduced antigen density, the outcome becomes less predictable. These observations indicate "the need for an explosive response for extensive damage to occur" (3) as well as the capacity of the tissue to "accommodate" to antibody under some circumstances.

The purpose of this chapter is to reassess the role of the alloantibody response and to propose that alloantibody is an important player in some clinical rejection syndromes.

II. THE RANGE OF ANTIGENS THAT MAY EVOKE ALLOANTIBODY RESPONSES IN TRANSPLANTATION

Antibodies against a variety of antigens have been implicated in causing rejection. These include anti-class I, anti-class II, antiendothelial, and ABO antibodies. Many of these antibodies have been isolated in patients who rejected their allografts, but the relationship of the majority of these antibodies to the rejection is difficult to establish definitively, as discussed below. However, the role of anti-class I antibody in mediating rejection is well established, and this chapter focuses on anti-class I.

The antibodies most strongly associated with rejection are directed against antigens on endothelial cells. These include ABO system antigens, class I and class II HLA, and antibody against the ill-defined endothelial-monocyte (EM) alloantigens (11). This association suggests that the site of injury by antibody in an allograft is the resistance arteries and the microcirculation rather than the parenchyma.

III. CELLULAR EVENTS IN THE ALLOANTIBODY RESPONSE AGAINST MHC ANTIGENS

A. The Primary B-Cell Response

The B cell response against membrane antigens begins with antigen binding to the Ig receptor of the B cell. The antigen may be encountered as a membrane protein on the donor cell or as a soluble protein released from the donor cell and may be recognized within the graft or in the secondary lymphoid organs of the host (lymph nodes, spleen). The antigenic protein must be in its native conformation (as opposed to being denatured) because, to be an effective antigen, it must trigger B cells to make an antibody against the native protein on donor cells.

B. Antigenic Processing and Triggering in B Cells

As shown in Figure 1, the binding of the antigen to the Ig receptor partially triggers the B cell and the B cell internalizes the antigen. B-cell triggering involves antigen-receptor associated molecules (Igα and Igβ), tyrosine kinases, and intracellular signaling pathways such as the Ras-MAP kinase pathway and the IP_3-calcium pathway. Thus B-cell triggering is highly analogous to T-cell triggering. The triggering leads to an effective antibody response only in the presence of T-cell help.

Internalization of the Ig receptor introduces the antigen into the endosomal pathway, where it is broken down into peptides and permitted to occupy the groove of the recipient MHC class II and is expressed as such on the B cell membrane. It is then in a position to recruit CD4 T cells. Probably the CD4 T cells have already been primed by the antigenic peptides in the groove of other antigen presenting cells (APC) (e.g., dendritic cells of the host). Whether the donor APCs could present the donor peptide in the donor class II groove and recruit effective T-cell help for the antibody response is not clear. Alternatively, the antibody response requires host APCs to prime the CD4 T cells.

C. Recruiting "Helper" $CD4^+$ T Cells and T-B Cooperation

Primed CD4 T cells express gp39 (CD40 ligand) and now engage the B cell through its surface markers, particularly CD40. The induction of gp39 on T cells is inhibited by cyclosporine (CyA) (12). Other ligand pairs binding B cells to T cells include LFA-2

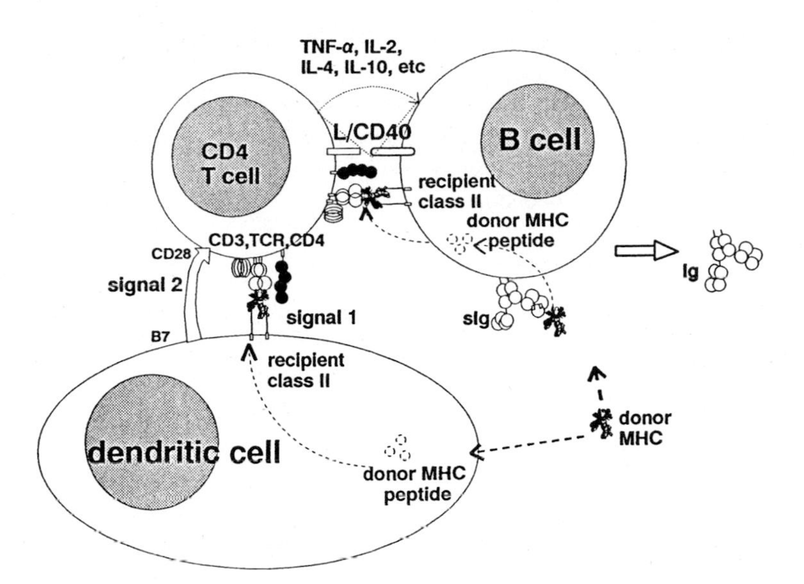

Figure 1 The donor MHC antigen is recognized by the host dendritic cell, internalized, and processed and presented in the class II groove to host CD4 cell. The antigen (signal 1) requires the presence of costimulatory molecules (signal 2) for effective activation. The identity of these costimulatory molecules has not been identified, but CD28 and B7/BB1 (B7) are the favored candidates. These events prime the T cell to express CD40 ligand (L) and secrete cytokines, TNF-α, IL-2, IL-4, and IL-10. Donor MHC is also recognized by the specific surface immunoglobulin (sig), internalized and presented to the CD4+ T cell, now primed to respond to donor peptide. The interaction of CD40 and its ligand stimulates the B cell to become sensitive to the cytokines produced by the T cell. The B cell now undergoes clonal expansion and proliferation and produces antibody for secretion.

(CD2)-LFA-3 (CD58); ICAM-1 (CD54)-LFA-1 (CD11a/CD18). Expression of B7 is induced on the surface of B cells, and this interacts with CD28 or CTLA-4 on T cells. Interaction between gp39 and CD40 stimulates the B cell directly, so that it becomes sensitive to cytokine production by the T cell (TNF-α, IL-4, IL-5, IL-2 and IFN-γ). Activation of B cells is dependent upon the CD40 ligand; if this is absent, an ineffective antibody response occurs (13).

Activated B cells divide rapidly. There is subsequent blast transformation, clonal expansion and differentiation occur, and antibody is produced for export. The first antibody is usually IgM, followed by "class switching" to IgG. The affinity of the antibody response matures over time by generating new somatic mutants, which bind antigen better than the original B-cell clone. Thus, as the antigen level decreases following the initial encounter, only cells expressing a high-affinity receptor will continue to proliferate. These events are dependent upon T-cell signals.

Antibody produced during the initial response returns to the germinal center complexed with antigen and opsonins, C3b and C3dg. CR2 receptor on the follicular dendritic cell binds the antigen to its cell surface, where it is recognized by B cells that now have receptors of high affinity. These cells, in turn, present antigen to T cells through gp39-CD40 interaction. This interaction induces expression of Bcl-2 on B cells, and programmed death by apoptosis is prevented. In the presence of costimulatory signals such as IL-2, IL-1α, or CD3, these cells differentiate to become plasma cells. Plasma cells produce large quantities of antibody and then die.

But in many cases the antibody response will persist for long periods of time. The persistence of the antibody response may reflect persistence of donor antigen or even of donor cells in the host. Whether circulating antibody persists or not, the antibody response can display memory when the antigen is encountered again.

D. The Secondary B-Cell Response

On reexposure to antigen, memory B cells bind antigen. Due to their high-affinity receptors, much lower levels of antigen are necessary to activate the B cells. These B cells are very efficient APCs; CD4 help is recruited, and these cells rapidly undergo clonal expansion and antibody production. A different class of antibody is produced, depending on its cytokine environment. Thus the secondary immune response is stronger, more rapid, and more specific, and it contains more IgG and less IgM.

IV. EFFECTOR MECHANISMS OF ALLOANTIBODY

A. The Role of Complement

The activation of the complement cascade is responsible for much of the tissue injury and inflammation in antibody-mediated rejection. The binding of C1 to IgG1, IGg2, IgG3, or IgM activates Cls and Clr (Fig. 2). Cls can now cleave C4 and then C2, forming the membrane-bound C4b2a (C3 convertase). The C3 convertase can cleave C3 into C3a and C3b. C3b attaches to C3 convertase to form the C5 convertase. C5 binds with low affinity to C4b2a3b and is cleaved into soluble C5a and C5b, which binds C6. C7, a highly hydrophobic molecule, inserts into the cell membrane and complexes with C56. C8 can associate and, together with the binding of multiple C9 monomers, completes the membrane attack complex (MAC). This creates a pore in the cell membrane, allowing the influx of water, resulting in osmotic lysis (Fig. 2).

A C3b-like molecule is normally generated at a low level in the circulation by the spontaneous slow hydrolysis of the thioester group in C3. This form of C3, abbreviated C3 (H_2O), can bind factor B in the fluid phase, making it susceptible to activation by factor D. This produces the alternative pathway C3 convertase, C3 (H_2O)Bb, which cleaves C3 into C3a and C3b. C3b can bind covalently to the membrane. On normal host cell membranes, C3b is rapidly inactivated by factors H and I, whereas on activating surfaces (e.g., certain pathological organisms or xenogeneic cells), C3b is inaccessible to factor H. Membrane-bound C3b can form the alternative pathway C3 convertase by binding factor B, which is activated by factor D. The C3b generated during the classic pathway can also activate the alternative pathway, providing a mechanism for greatly amplifying the complement cascade. It is likely that both pathways are involved in tissue injury in patients with antibody-mediated rejection.

It is important to understand the factors involved in the regulation of the complement system. As discussed above, soluble factors H and I prevent the activation of the alternative pathway by degrading C3b. Endothelial cells express a host of membrane-bound complement inhibitors. These include the C3 convertase regulators DAF and MCP. CD59 and homologous restriction factor (HRF) are expressed on numerous cells. In vitro, they inhibit the formation of MAC on the cell membrane. There is some species restriction in the function of these regulators of complement. This is one reason that complement activation

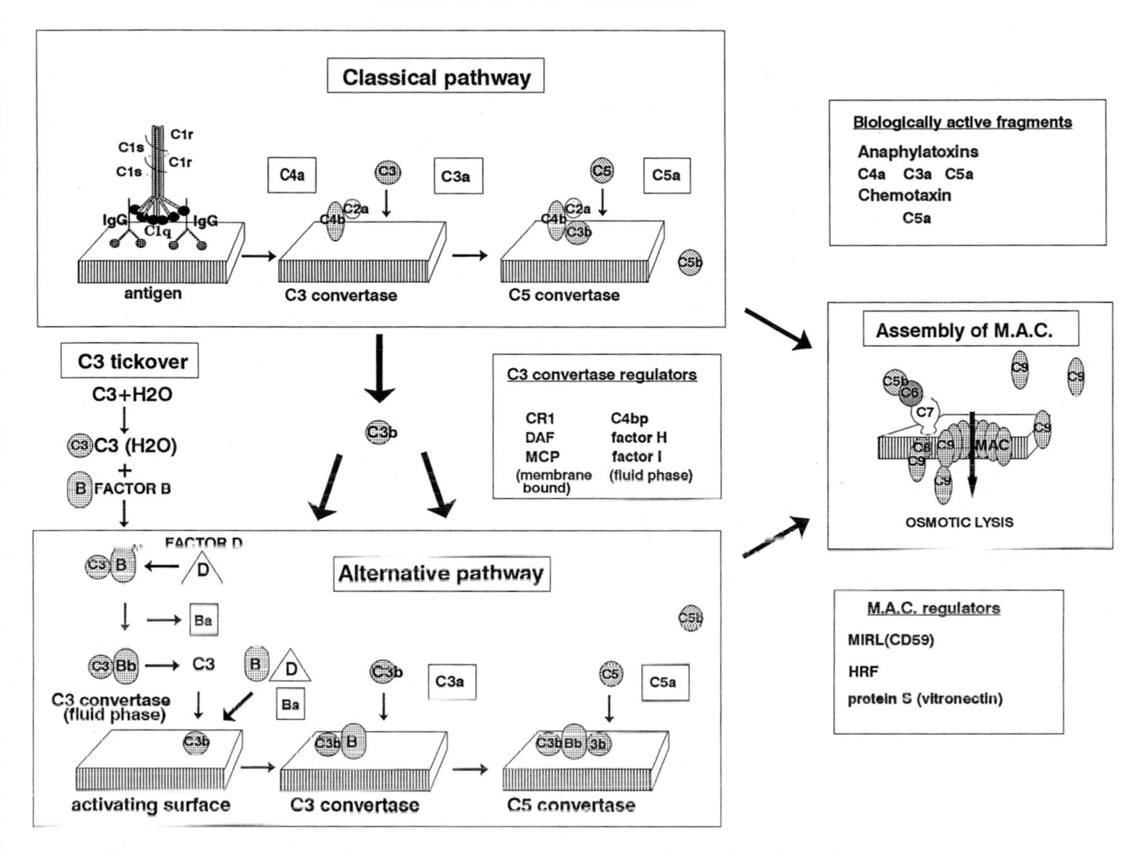

Figure 2 Activation of the classic pathway occurs following IgG binding to antigen. C3 convertase is formed and cleaves C3, producing C3b, which can either continue in the classic pathway or enter the alternative pathway. Both pathways result in formation of the membrane attack complex (MAC). The pathways are described in more detail in the text, and the function of the complement proteins are described in table 1. Key: △ = enzyme □ = soluble factor.

is a major problem in xenotransplantation. Other soluble proteins such as protein S (vitronectin) and Sp40,40 (clusterin) prevent the insertion of C5–9 into the membrane.

C3a and C4a, the soluble cleavage products of C3 and C4, bind to receptors expressed on mast cells, basophils, lymphocytes, and smooth muscle cells. They cause mast cells and basophils to release vasoactive substances (i.e., histamine, serotonin), which increase vascular permeability, and induce smooth muscle contraction. C5a has both anaphylactic and chemotactic properties, attracting monocytes and neutrophils to the site of injury, where they release cellular products such as proteases, oxidants, and growth factors, PAF and PDGF. Receptors for C5a are found on mast cells, basophils, neutrophils, macrophages, and endothelium. C5a is also a direct vasoconstrictor contributing to a reduced glomerular filtration rate (GFR). The effector functions of complement are summarized in Table 1. Cytokines released following T-cell activation (e.g., IFN-γ, IL-6) can induce synthesis of proteins involved in either the classic or alternative pathway or both.

Table 1 Effector Functions and Regulators of Complement

Complement protein	Receptor/ substrate	Receptor location/site of action	Function
Breakdown products of bound C3b			
C3b	CR1	All blood cells except platelets	Opsonisation, enhanced phagocytosis, B cell activation
C3dg	CR2	B cells, follicular dendritic cells (FDC)	Opsonisation, focuses antigen on surface of APC, B cell activation
C3bi	CR3/CR4	Monocytes, macrophages, FDC	Recognition by germinal B cell, production of antibody
Anaphylatoxins			
C3a	C3a R	Mast cells, basophils, lymphocytes, smooth muscle cells	Release of vasoactive substances (histamine, serotonins), vascular permeability, smooth muscle contraction
C4a	C4a R	Mast cells, basophils, lymphocytes, smooth muscle cells	Release of vasoactive substances (histamine, serotonins), vascular permeability, smooth muscle contraction
C5a	C5a R	Mast cells, basophils, neutrophils, monocytes, endothelial cells	Release of vasoactive substances, neutrophil lysosomes
Chemotaxins			
C5a	C5a R	Neutrophils and monocytes	Attracts monocytes and neutrophils to site of injury

Osmotic lysis			
MAC (C5–9)		Formed by binding of factors C5–9 on cell surface - cell membrane	Creates a hole in membrane, cell lysis
Regulators			
C1NH	C1r C1s	Soluble protein	Blocks activation of classic pathway
C4bp	C4b	Soluble protein	Accelerates decay of classic pathway
Factor H	C3b	Soluble protein	Accelerates decay of alternative pathway
Factor I	C3b	Soluble serine protease	In presence of C4bp, MCP or CR1 cleaves C4b and C3b
DAF (decay accelerating factor)	C4b2a C3bBb	Most blood cells, endothelium and epithelial cells	Accelerates decay of alternative and classic pathway
CR1	C4b, C4b2a, C3b, C3bBb	Erythrocytes and leukocytes	Accelerates decay of alternative and classic pathway
MCP (membrane cofactor protein)	C3b C4b	Most blood cells (not RBC), epithelial cells, endothelial cells, fibroblasts	Accelerates decay of alternative and classic pathway
Homologous restriction factor (HRF)	C8 C9	Red blood cells, lymphocytes, monocytes, neutrophils, platelets	Prevents MAC formation
CD59 (membrane inhibitor of reactive lysis)	C7 C8	Red blood cells, lymphocytes, monocytes, neutrophils, platelets ?endothelial cells, epithelial cells	Prevents MAC formation

Source: Ref. 82.

B. Antibody-Dependent Cell-Mediated Cytotoxicity (ADCC) and Killer (K) Cells

When circulating IgG binds to antigen on the target cell via the Fab region of the IgG molecule, the Fc portions can be recognized by Fcγ receptors. One class of Fc receptors (FcγRIII/CD16) is expressed on a population of lymphoid cells that include the effectors of ADCC (so-called "K" cells), which are in the same population of large granular lymphocytes as natural killer (NK) cells. Binding to the FcγRIII receptor activates the effector cell to secrete cytokines, including IFN-γ and TNF-α, and to release their granular proteins. These combined effects mediate cell lysis. The mechanism of lysis by the ADCC effector cells is likely to be similar to that of cytotoxic T lymphocytes, but the recruitment of the effector cells to the target is not due to T-cell receptors recognizing antigen but to Fc receptors recognizing the Fc portion of antibody.

C. Macrophages

Following upregulation of VCAM-1 on the vascular endothelium, chemokine-monocyte chemoattractant protein-1 (MCP-1) is released from leukocytes. MCP-1 changes the shape of the endothelial cells and increases permeability, and monocytes infiltrate the graft. There they differentiate into macrophages and, under the influence of IFN-γ, they are activated and mediate a number of effects through secretion of cytokines, tissue factors, antigen presentation, and phagocytosis. Macrophages also scavenge antibody-mediated material by virtue of their high-affinity Fcγ receptor, FcγRI. The role of the macrophage in antibody-mediated rejection is unknown.

D. IgE Mechanisms

It is puzzling that IgE responses are never encountered in clinical transplantation. This may reflect the tendency of the inflammatory cytokines (including the "TH1 cytokines" IL-2 and IFN-γ), to suppress the cytokines needed for the allergic response (IL-5).

V. EXPERIMENTAL MODELS OF ALLOANTIBODY-MEDIATED EFFECTS IN TRANSPLANTS

Animal models of skin grafts formed much of the early work on transplantation immunology (reviewed in Ref. 3). These experiments cannot be translated to transplantation of vascularized organs and therefore are not discussed.

The rapidity with which sensitized animals reject second-set transplants (14) and the histologic findings of fibrinoid necrosis in arterioles and glomerular capillaries suggested a role for antibody in mediating rejection of vascularized organ grafts. The ability to induce allograft rejection by the transfer of serum in some models provided further evidence for the role of antibody. Nevertheless, rodent models of vascularized organ grafts often lack alloantibody-mediated mechanisms such as HAR. However, a new transgenic model seems to have a prominent role for alloantibody. The ability of rats to reject $RTIA^a$ (MHC class I disparate) allografts depends on their (class I) haplotype (15); $RT1A^u$ rats readily reject a $Rt1A^a$ graft, whereas $RT1A^c$ rats do not. In the presence of monoclonal antibodies to CD8+ cells, $RTIA^a$ grafts are still rejected by $RT1A^u$, suggesting that CD8+ cells are not critical for rejection to occur. However, depletion of CD4+ cells prolonged graft survival. A strong antibody response correlates with the development of graft rejection, and passively transferred serum induces rejection in rats receiving RTIA[a] grafts and not third-party grafts, providing direct support for the role of antibody.

VI. DETERMINANTS OF THE DESTRUCTIVE POWER OF THE ALLOANTIBODY EFFECTOR MECHANISMS

Some alloantibody responses are more able to mediate destruction than others. There may be many factors determining the destructive power of the alloantibody response (Table 2). The characteristics of the antigen, the cell on which it is expressed, and in particular the level of expression could influence the destructive power. The quantity of alloantibody, especially alloantibody fixing in a short time, could be critical to achieving high density of immunoglobulin Fc portions per unit of endothelial area before accommodation and adaptation mechanisms reduce antigen density or increase endothelial resistance.

Antibody against broadly shared "public" determinants on MHC alleles could be more destructive than antibody against private determinants. ("Private" means confined to one MHC allele; "public" means expressed on many but not all MHC alleles, permitting some persons to make immune responses against these determinants.) Broadly reactive antibodies against a public determinant on all donor MHC alleles would be able to react to several times as many donor MHC molecules as would antibody against a single private specificity.

The existence of complement regulators and inhibitors (e.g., CD59) could be an important determinant of the effector function. By interrupting the assembly of C9 for the MAC, increased CD59 expression could make complement lysis less effective.

Table 2 Factors That Could Influence the Destructive Potential of an Alloantibody Response Against MHC Antigens

Antigen
1. Level of expression of antigen, especially in endothelium of small arteries and arterioles
2. "Public" versus "private" determinant: e.g., public would react with all class I antigens, private only with 25%
3. Class I versus class II

Antibody
1. Class and subclass
2. Affinity
3. Titer
4. Duration of the exposure: rapid deposition prevents accommodation

Effector mechanisms
1. Complement
2. Cellular effectors
3. Potential direct effect of antibody on endothelium

Adaptation
1. Time for accommodation to occur
2. Regulation of complement activity, inhibition of C1 in serum or on endothelium, e.g., CD59
3. Previous exposure (may induce accommodation)

A. Factors Affecting the Quantity, Specificity, and Class/Subclass and Duration of the Alloantibody Response

Antibody against donor MHC alleles is produced by some but not all transplant recipients and is sometimes induced by blood transfusions or pregnancies. Some of the factors affecting the response are as follows:

1. *Previous exposure (memory).* An anamnestic response is more rapid, more likely to involve IgG, less dependent on T-cell help, and higher-affinity.

2. *Antigenic determinants capable of engaging B cell Ig receptors.* The native MHC molecule must engage the antigen specific Ig receptor on a clone of B cells, triggering the internalization of the receptor MHC complex. Once internalized, the MHC is presented to peptides which can now occupy the groove of the recipient class I molecule being synthesized. Extensive MHC matching will result in few or no B-cell determinants, since the recipient will be extensively tolerized by its own MHC determinants.

3. *Antigenic determinants capable of recruiting T cell help.* CD4 T cells must be able to recognize determinants on the donor MHC molecule which the B cell has recognized. These determinants are presented to the T cell as peptides in the groove of the class II MHC molecule on the recipient B cell. Immunosuppression of alloantibody responses probably acts mainly on the CD4 T cell response, preventing help. MHC matching will reduce the MHC determinants available to recruit T-cell help.

4. *The cytokine environment affects the antibody class and subclasses produced.* CD4 cells can secrete two distinct phenotypic cytokine patterns: TH1 (IFN-γ, TNF, IL-2) and TH2 (IL-3, IL-4, IL-5, IL-10) (16). The phenotype expressed can be influenced by the cytokines present. IFN-γ promotes expression of TH1 phenotype and inhibits TH2 expression and IL-4 has the opposite effect. In turn, cytokine secretion determines the antibody produced: TH1 cytokines produce IgG2a and IgG3 while TH2 cytokines produce IgG1 and IgE. In general, the influence of TH1 cytokines seems to predominate in acute rejection, but a strong TH2 response is probably also present. This may explain why both cell-mediated and humoral immunity coexist. However, more work is needed on how the balance between TH1 and TH2 cytokines affects the alloantibody response.

5. *Graft injury may make a greater antigen load available to B cells, macrophages, and other APCs.* T cell responses produce IFN-γ, which increases the synthesis of MHC molecules.

6. *Some persons make high-titer, "broad" alloantibody responses.* One possible, reason is that the recipient cells with less common antigens or lacking broad public specificities are more likely to recognize a combination of T- and B-cell determinants and will make an antibody that reacts with sites on MHC alleles. There is little evidence that individuals preexist as "high antibody responders," but particular HLA phenotypes could be predisposed to make broad responses when challenged by particular HLA antigens.

7. *Anti-idiotypic antibodies.* The idiotype is the antigen-combining site of an antibody, and it can trigger an antibody response that neutralizes the original antibody (i.e., an anti-idiotype). The importance of anti-idiotypic antibodies in transplantation is controversial. It has been suggested that the development of antibodies to anti-HLA antibodies modifies the activity of anti-HLA antibodies. To study anti-idiotype antibodies, serum from patients who have anti-HLA antibody is incubated with donor cells and the test sample, either a second sample of serum from which the anti-HLA antibody has been absorbed or a later sample from which the anti-HLA activity has disappeared (17). Inhibition of cyto-

toxicity by the test serum suggests the presence of anti-idiotypic antibody. However, the assay is troublesome and cannot be demonstrated directly. The significance of anti-idiotypic anti-HLA antibodies is debated and the duration of the alloantibody response is highly variable.

8. *Persistence of donor cells (microchimerism).* It is possible that those persons who develop high sensitization for long periods of time and who are such a problem to transplant have persistence of some source of donor antigen. Persistence of donor cells has usually been evoked to explain hyporesponsiveness, but it could be a source of continued B-cell stimulation under some conditions.

VII. SUPPRESSIVE EFFECTS OF ALLOANTIBODY

A. Enhancement

One observation about alloantibody—which, in retrospect, may have misled investigators about the potential of alloantibody to injure the graft—was the phenomenon of enhancement in the rat. Immunological enhancement was described by Kaliss (18), Möller and Möller (19), and Batchelor (20) in the late '50s and mid-'60s. The term is defined as "enhanced graft survival induced by specific alloantibody against donor alloantigens." The initial studies involved inoculating mice with tumor homogenates prior to grafting allogeneic mouse tumors. The authors demonstrated that some tumor cells (i.e., dissociated lymphoid and myeloid cells) are readily lysed in vitro, whereas sarcomas or carcinomas are not. The ability to demonstrate enhancement depends on the combination of donor and tumor strains. Mice that do not show enhancement still produce antibody, as demonstrated by the ability to induce enhancement by injecting their sera into other animals prior to transplantation.

Early in vitro work has shown that the effect of antibody is dependent on the concentration, class, and affinity of the antibody, the density of antigen, and the ability of the antibody to fix complement. In vivo, dose of antibody, number of cells grafted, strain and species of animal, and complement activity determine whether the antibody response to the graft will be enhancement or rejection.

French and Batchelor (21) transplanted incompatible kidneys into rats that had received alloantibodies against the donor antigens. Prolonged graft survival was seen in the rats pretreated with antiserum, but the benefit was seen only in rats that were one haplotype mismatched. This may be explained by differences in the number of copies of the MHC class I antigens: the number of antigens limits the amount of antibody that can bind and activate complement. The rats used in these experiments were heterozygotes and thus had reduced antigenic density. Similar treatment of homozygous recipients showed less enhancement in graft survival and evidence of severe rejection. Rats treated with antibody did develop an antibody response, suggesting that the mechanism of enhancement cannot be explained by complete inhibition of the antibody response. As noted above, the rodent may have less potent effector systems than the human, and the lack of HAR may be a necessary precondition for enhancement. The complement-fixing ability of the antibody subclasses involved also determines enhancement, as do the characteristics of the antigen itself.

Experimental models of enhancement using skin allografts in mice showed that the antibody could not be absorbed by red blood cells. This implied that antibody responsible for enhancement was unlikely to be due to anti-class I but could be anti-class II (22). This led to the concept that anti-class II is enhancing because it damages the class II-positive interstitial dendritic cells (IDC), which are important immunogens.

A second theoretical mechanism of enhancement is that the antibody competes with cytotoxic lymphocytes (CTLs) for the antigens. This notion has been supported by the demonstration in vivo and in vitro that antigraft antibody can prevent CTLs from causing graft destruction. However, it fails to explain how antibody against one class of antigen (e.g., class II) could interfere with CTL recognition of another class of donor antigens (class I).

It is instructive to recall that passively administered antibody can suppress other immune responses. One example is the use of anti-D (Rh) antibody to suppress recognition of Rh incompatibilities in pregnancy. An Rh-ve mother can develop anti-D antibodies during pregnancy if the fetus is Rh+ve. Administration of anti-D immune globulin (23) during pregnancy binds the offending antigen and it is removed from the circulation, thus suppressing the development of an antibody response. Whether this mechanism has any relevance to the phenomenon of enhancement of graft survival by alloantibody is unknown.

B. Impact of Blood Transfusion on Graft Outcome

The potential benefit of transfusion on allograft survival was reported in 1973 (24) when Opelz et al. reviewed the outcome of renal transplant recipients and transfusion records of these patients. This finding was supported by reports of prolonged graft survival in animals that received fresh donor blood prior to transplantation. The ability of donor-specific blood transfusion to prevent rejection in the rat is influenced by the rat strain (25). In human studies (26), transfusion of three to four units of donor blood prior to living related transplantation resulted in 44% of recipients having an episode of rejection; 82% of recipients who did not receive donor-specific transfusion (DST) had a rejection episode. These patients were one haplotype mismatched and had a high MLC. The mechanism of the transfusion effect is still not understood; reduced levels of IL-2R and CD8 cells in the grafts have been reported, but their significance remains unexplained, and no difference in T cell function or NK cell activity has been demonstrated. Recently this minimal benefit is no longer seen, since the risk of evoking an antibody response to the potential donor remains significant.

C. Accommodation

Sometimes antibody can mediate injury that can be reversed, allowing graft survival to be maintained despite the persistence of the antibody response. Also, successful transplantation despite ABO incompatibility can be achieved by reducing pretransplant antibody levels by plasmapheresis or immunoadsorption (27). Post-transplant, the grafts survive despite the return of antibody to pretransplant titers. Some patients develop accelerated rejection, but this can be reversible and does not correlate with antibody levels. The ability of the grafts to function despite reexposure to antibody has been termed *accommodation*. This phenomenon has been demonstrated experimentally in xenotransplantation, where depletion of host natural antibodies prior to transplantation prolongs graft survival (28). The mechanism of accommodation is unknown. Modification in the antigen density or changes in the graft endothelial cell defenses against complement activation may occur. Thus on reexposure to antibody, the immune response is altered.

VIII. THE ANTIGENS AGAINST WHICH ANTIBODY-MEDIATED GRAFT INJURY IS DIRECTED

If there is a unifying feature in the list of antigens that mediate antibody-mediated rejection, it is that all are expressed on arterial endothelium, particularly the medium-sized and small arteries of the kidney.

A. ABO Blood Group Antigens

The potential of ABO antibodies to mediate rejection became apparent in the early days of renal transplantation (4). The A and B antigens are sugars, assembled by glycosyl transferases. Different glycosyl transferases are encoded by the alleles "A" and "B." These enzymes add sugars to the carbohydrate moiety *N*-acetyl-galactosidasamine (A) and galactose (B). The allele "O" product has no enzyme activity and therefore no antigen is expressed. Individuals, homozygous for "O" allele can therefore be universal donors. Expression of A or B allele, either homozygous or heterozygous, exposes antigens to a potential recipient. These antigens cross-react with many environmental antigens (i.e., pollen and membrane antigens on many of the normal bacteria found in the gut, milk and ovarian cyst fluid). Antibodies to these proteins "naturally" occur in most (but not all) members of the human population because of exposure to gut bacteria. Typically the antibodies are IgM, and they are directed against A1 and B but not A2.

The A and B antigens on renal vascular endothelium act as a target for anti-A or anti-B antibody. The binding of either anti-A or anti-B isoagglutinin to the endothelium is significant concentration activates complement and induces platelet and fibrin aggregation, resulting in microvascular occlusion. There is an associated infiltrate of neutrophils, monocytes, and endothelial cells, followed by rapid infarction of the graft.

There are two types of blood antigen A: A1 and A2. A1 antigens are thought to be the main antigen involved in anti-A responses, as the expression of A1 is both quantitatively (number of A determinants) and qualitatively (type of core saccharide antigen) higher than A2 (29). The A1 ag contains all four CHO chains, whereas A2 lacks type 4 and expresses 3 weakly. There have been reports of antibody-mediated rejection involving A2 antigens (30), and thus it appears safer to avoid transplanting across ABO incompatibility. Immunoadsorption of antibody by hemoperfusion and plasmapheresis has been successfully employed to reduce the antibody level to less than 1:16 (31) prior to transplantation.

The available columns for immunoadsorption have been claimed to be able to adsorb most of anti-A and anti-B antibody activity (32). Antibody that is not adsorbed has been identified as anti-A types 3 and 4 or anti-A types 2 and 6, implying that synthetic carbohydrates containing both the blood-group-specific terminal sugar sequence and part of the core carbohydrate chain would be necessary for immunoadsorption. Nevertheless, adsorption of some of the components may be sufficient if the requirement is only to reduce levels of antibody below a certain threshold amount.

B. Class I MHC Antigens

The ability of antibody against HLA class I to cause graft damage is well recognized in the context of HAR. In this phenomenon, the patient has developed preformed antibody prior to transplantation, most commonly anti-class I antibody, as a result of either transfusion, previous transplantation, or pregnancy. If the patient receives an allograft bearing the antigens to which he or she has been sensitized, the antibody will bind to the antigen expressed on the graft endothelium, activate complement, and attract polymorphs. HAR will ensue, manifested by rapid graft thrombosis and infarction. This typically does not respond to immunosuppressive therapies and almost invariably leads to graft loss. Fortunately, careful crossmatching has now largely eliminated this form of graft failure.

C. Class II MHC Antigens

Anti-class II antibody is able to cause graft injury, but infrequently. There have been several reports implicating a role for anti-class II antibody in HAR of renal allografts (33). The relative rarity of HAR due to anti-class II may be attributed to the low expression of class II on arterial endothelium in normal kidney (34) and may also explain the tendency toward few effects of anti-class II.

D. Non-HLA Antigens

The involvement of antibodies other than anti-HLA in allograft rejection is suggested by the occasional loss of HLA-identical allografts from apparent antibody-mediated rejection, which may be hyperacute or accelerated rejection (35). The antigens implicated include the endothelial/monocyte antigens (11,36,37) (see below).

E. Endothelial Cell Antigens

Cerilli et al. (38) and others (11) have reported the association of antibodies against antigens expressed on endothelial cells in patients undergoing acute allograft rejection. The antisera react with endothelial cells and monocytes but not T or B lymphocytes; thus they differ from HLA class I and II. Endothelial cell antigens also express a number of glycoproteins, including antigens shared with platelets, thrombin receptors, fibrinogen, and vWF (39). Despite many efforts, the particular antigen involved has not been identified and frequently anti-HLA antigens have been found to be responsible.

In xenotransplantation, IgM antibodies have been identified that react against glycoproteins that are found both on the endothelial cell and platelets, and it has been suggested that the EM antigen is a similar target (40). However, there is no evidence to support this.

Class I or II antigen expression may have a tissue-specific component and thus the EM antigen may be a tissue-specific modification of an MHC product, perhaps because of occupation of the MHC groove by a tissue-specific peptide. However, the peptides in MHC grooves to date are generally not tissue-specific.

F. Epithelial Cell Antigens

In the late 1980s a sudden increase in graft loss in pediatric renal transplant patients was reported in one center (41,42). These children rejected their grafts and were found to have IgM antibodies directed against epithelial cells (AEC). There was no evidence of anti-HLA antibodies. AEC antibodies were also demonstrated in adult patients, with a correlation between the presence of antibody and the development of rejection. These antibodies have since been found in dialysis patients awaiting transplantation; therefore their presence is unrelated to transplantation and may reflect exposure to antigen during dialysis. The significance of this isolated outbreak of rejection associated with AEC is unclear.

IX. THE ANTIBODY-MEDIATED REJECTION SYNDROMES IN CLINICAL TRANSPLANTATION

A. Hyperacute Rejection

The classic description of antibody-mediated rejection in renal transplantation is hyperacute rejection (HAR), now rare due to careful crossmatching practice. Classical HAR occurs rapidly, usually within minutes to hours of opening the vascular anastomosis. The hallmark is destruction of the renal endothelium and thrombosis of the renal vasculature. This phenomenon can be seen by the surgeon as soon as the anastomotic clamps are released. The reperfused kidney becomes pink and turgid, as expected, but then almost immediately turns mottled/blue and infarcts. Microscopically there is marked infiltrate of polymorphs. The pathogenesis of HAR is due to alloantibodies present in the recipient circulation that bind to the donor endothelium of the graft and activate complement. Complement activation recruits polymorphs and leads to endothelial injury, initiation of coagulation, and exposure of the subendothelial basement membrane proteins that activate platelets. It is not clear whether terminal complement (C) components (C 5–9) and assembly of the MAC are necessary for endothelial injury. The endothelial cells are stimulated to secrete von Willebrand's factor (vWf), which mediates platelet adhesion and aggregation. Activated platelets and other cells secrete platelet-activating factor (PAF), which stimulates the secretion of thromboxane and leukotrienes. Thromboxane, a potent vasoconstrictor, also induces platelet aggregation. Heparinase release by activated platelets degrades heparin sulfate, releasing cationic substances that alter the negative charges on the endothelial cell surface. The combined effect is a severe reduction of perfusion and infarction, too rapid to respond to immunosuppressive therapies.

The histologic changes seen on biopsy (43) are variable and not diagnostic. However, the most striking and consistent feature is infiltration of neutrophils. These are usually seen in the pertibular capillaries and glomeruli. Presumably the presence of neutrophils is in response to chemotactic substances C5a, IL-8 and the α chemokines, and others. The presence of platelet thrombi and fibrin deposition is well documented in HAR, and it may be difficult to differentiate from CyA-related hemolytic uremic syndrome (HUS). Immunofluorescence, which might be expected to show staining for IgG and complement, is usually negative. This is an important point, in that severe injury can be mediated by antibodies without sufficient accumulation of IgG to be detected in immunohistology. Electron microscopy may show widening of the subendothelial space.

The treatment of HAR is unsatisfactory. Severe systemic toxicity from necrotic renal tissue and mediators and consumption coagulopathy may develop. Graft nephrectomy is therefore recommended if the diagnosis of HAR with renal infarction can be confirmed. With current tissue-typing techniques, the classic form of HAR is rarely seen.

B. The Differential Diagnosis of Hyperacute Rejection

Hyperacute rejection must be distinguished from perfusion injury or thrombosis of the arterial anastomosis, which may present in a similar manner. A biopsy with frozen section is often helpful in this situation. HAR may not occur immediately but several hours after surgery and may be accompanied by the onset of fever, anuria, and graft tenderness. A fall in the platelet count or increase in fibrinogen degradation product support the diagnosis of HAR.

Another reported cause of early graft loss is the presence of red blood cell (RBC) cold agglutinins. These antibodies do not affect RBCs at normal body temperature, but the release of the anastomotic clamps, exposing the blood to the "cold" kidney, permits the antibodies to agglutinate the RBCs. After an initial period, of normal flow, blood flow rapidly deteriorates, and this typically results in graft loss (44,45). Histological findings include erythrocyte aggregates and fibrin deposits. Immunofluorescence reveals IgM staining in capillaries and arterioles. In contrast to HAR, neutrophils are rarely seen.

CyA-related HUS and spontaneous HUS may be difficult to differentiate from HAR. In these situations, blood should be drawn for a repeat donor-specific crossmatch and CyA should be discontinued. Treatment can be switched to OKT3 or antilymphocyte globulin to provide immunosuppression without CyA. Oral CyA may be reintroduced toward the end of therapy with OKT3 (46).

C. Antibody-Mediated Accelerated Acute Rejection of Kidney Transplants

We have recently demonstrated that anti-class I antibody against the donor can be found in some cases of acute rejection (47,48) and may be an important component of severe early acute rejection, particularly in presensitized patients. This typically occurs in the first week posttransplant and frequently occurs in patients whose kidneys are functioning well post-transplantation. Some of these patients have previously been sensitized against donor antigens, and the level of antibody may have subsequently fallen below detectable levels, giving a negative pretransplant crossmatch. This underlines the importance of identifying patients who have been highly sensitized and of crossmatching with historical sera as well as current sera prior to transplantation. Perhaps sensitive crossmatch techniques would have shown that these individuals had persistent antibody (see below).

Following transplantation, exposure to antigen may stimulate memory cells, resulting in an anamnestic response and rapid production of anti-class I antibody. Clinically this may be seen as a sudden severe deterioration of renal function. The patient develops oliguria, with or without systemic manifestations such as fever. Renal perfusion is compromised and the Doppler studies show increased resistance. The renal isotope scan often shows reduced perfusion and no function. Renal biopsy typically shows infiltration of polymorphs in the pertibular capillaries with or without fibrin thrombi. In some cases there is damage to the glomerular capillary endothelium, with widening of the subendothelial space. Often there is little of the lymphocytic infiltrate, tubulitis, or endothelialitis that is normally associated with acute cellular rejection. But some patients do display these features, suggesting that they may have both T cell–mediated rejection and antibody-mediated injury.

Typically these patients have detectable anti-class I antibody (47): the donor-specific T cell crossmatch becomes positive, the autologous crossmatch is negative, and the activity is platelet-absorbable. In our previous study, all patients who had detectable anti-class I–like antibody developed rejection, and the recovery of renal function was associated with loss of antibody. More recently, we have observed several patients in whom renal function recovered despite the persistence of anti-class I–like antibody for at least 6 months (see Table 3). Patient R.A. developed rejection 4 days after transplantation. Biopsy findings of arteritis—with endothelial swelling, foam cell change, and intimal thickening (Fig. 3)—suggested antibody involvement. There was no tubulitis, which is usually associated with cell-mediated rejection. Patient W.B., sensitized during rejection of a second kidney transplant, received a third cadaveric renal transplant. Initial renal function was good, but on day 7 oliguria developed, and a transplant biopsy showed solidification of the glomeruli

Table 3 Summary of Patients Demonstrating an Antibody Response Against Their Kidney Donor During the Course of Their Transplant

Name	Tx. No.	Peak PRA%	Xmatch at Tx.	DGF/ ATN	Day of Rej.	Xmatch at Rej.	Treatment	Loss of antibody	Outcome
RA	1	0	S−	No	4	S+	OKT3	71 days	Function
WB	3	54	T− B−	No	7	T+ B+	OKT3	+ve > 12 months	Function
AC	2	N/A	S−	No	5	S+	OKT3	245 days	Function
PK	3	4	T− B−	Yes	4	S+	OKT3	+ve > 12 months	Function
EP	2	23	S−	No	6	S+	OKT3 & ALG	Never	Nephrectomy

Xmatch results:
T, peripheral T cells
B, peripheral B cells
S, spleen
+, positive
−, negative
DGF, delayed graft function
ATN, acute tubular necrosis
Rej, rejection

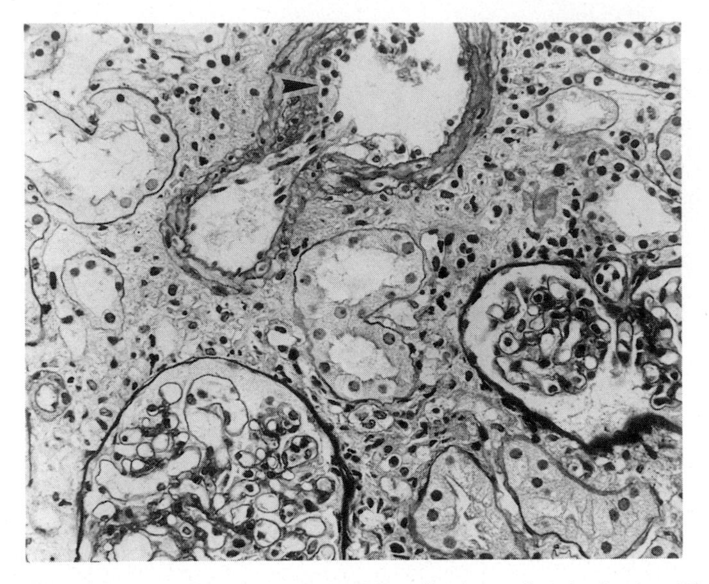

Figure 3 Arteritis in a patient with antibody-mediated rejection. There is swelling of endothelial cells (arrow) and intimal thickening. (PAS ×200.)

with neutrophil infiltration (Fig. 4). Neutrophils were also seen in the peritubular capillaries. These findings, together with a positive repeat donor-specific crossmatch, supported the diagnosis of antibody-mediated rejection.

Serum from all five donors demonstrated reactivity against their donor cells on repeating the donor-specific crossmatch. OKT3 treatment was used with good effect in all

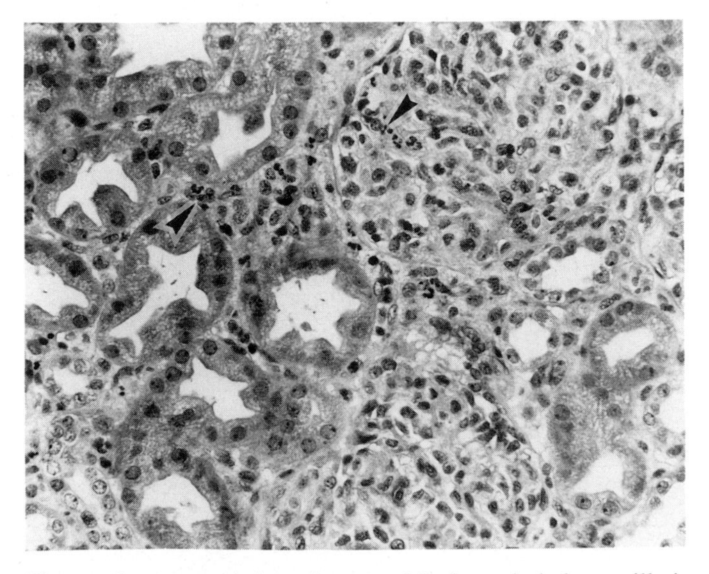

Figure 4 Accumulation of neutrophils in peritubular capillaries (left arrow) and in swollen glomeruli (right arrow). (H&E, ×200.)

except patient E.P. This patient rejected his first transplant and had received OKT3 when routine testing for antibodies to OKT3 was not done. Following OKT3 treatment this time, CD3 levels did not fall and therapy was switched to antilymphocytic globulin (MALG). Severe endothelialitis on biopsy and antidonor reactivity indicated the presence of both antibody and cell-mediated rejection, and the graft was lost to infarction. Three patients continued to demonstrate antidonor activity for more than 6 months after renal function had returned. Recovery of function despite the persistence of antibody is reminiscent of the phenomenon of accommodation and suggests that the endothelium can adapt to the presence of the antibody in some cases.

D. Mixed Antibody and T Cell–Mediated Acute Rejection

Cellular mechanisms have long been known to cause acute rejection, and most rejection episodes are probably T cell–mediated. The features of acute cellular rejection may coexist with the more subtle finding described in rejection associated with antibody, i.e., positive crossmatch, rapid loss of function, polymorphs. In this situation, anti-class I antibody may mediate the microvascular lesions. The presence of both may suggest severe injury, but, with aggressive treatment in the form of steroids and anti-lymphocytic therapy, these lesions may be reversible.

The introduction of the "Banff schema" (49) to provide a standardized working formulation for diagnosing and classifying rejection has helped to interpret and manage the various pathologies seen in the renal transplant biopsy appropriately. This morphological schema, however, does not fully reflect the immunologic and functional realities. Ultimately, additional immunologic and molecular techniques will be used to further refine this formulation.

X. CHRONIC REJECTION

An insidious deterioration in renal function associated with proteinuria and hypertension, after exclusion of other specific entities such as recurrent or de novo glomerulonephritis, strongly suggests the diagnosis of chronic rejection, dealt with in detail elsewhere in this volume. Biopsy characteristically shows intimal thickening due to arteriolar smooth muscle cell proliferation in the intima of small arteries, as well as tubular atrophy and interstitial fibrosis. Characteristic glomerular changes (transplant glomerulopathy) may be present, including thickening of the basement membrane, widening of the subendothelial space, and juxtaglomerular hyperplasia.

Controversy exists as to whether chronic rejection results from continued or repeated immune injury, mediated by cellular or humoral immune responses or both, or whether it is a later degenerative response to earlier events. Multiple episodes of acute T-cell–mediated rejection lead to graft injury along with induction of donor HLA antigens on the graft. Anti-HLA antibodies may contribute to the development of obliterative arterial lesions of chronic rejection in some cases (9). But there is no evidence at present to implicate a role for antibody in most cases of chronic rejection. It has been suggested that the reduced nephron mass following injury from rejection, nephrotoxicity, infection, or ATN may produce systemic and intraglomerular hyperfiltration and induce a variety of growth factors that have been implicated in the development of glomerular sclerosis in the failing kidney. However, the bulk of evidence suggests that chronic rejection is the late result of immunologic injury.

The concept that antibody mediates chronic rejection has also been considered in cardiac transplantation. Histologic findings in accelerated coronary artery disease (CAD) in heart transplants resemble the obliterative vascular changes described in chronic renal allograft rejection. Like other syndromes potentially mediated by alloantibody (HAR and accelerated acute rejection), the endothelium would be the prime target, with complement and neutrophils participating. Injury to the endothelium may initiate inflammatory response by altered expression of adhesion molecules and chemokines, thus attracting neutrophils, monocytes, lymphocytes, and lipids. Smooth muscle cells invade the intima and proliferate. The resultant intimal proliferation is usually uniform and distal, in contrast to the proximal focal lesions seen in CAD in the general population. However, there is little evidence correlating the presence of anti-HLA antibodies with the development of CAD in heart transplants (50).

The mechanisms responsible for chronic rejection are likely to be multifactorial and a number of risk factors have been identified, but at present the role of antibody remains speculative, and in most patients with chronic rejection, no alloantibody against the donor is demonstrable. There is no effective treatment for chronic rejection.

XI. MANAGEMENT ISSUES

A. Methods of Crossmatching

1. Complement-Dependent Cytotoxicity (CDC)

The standard method for crossmatching is the microlymphocytoxicity test. This is usually done with mononuclear cells (T cells, B cells, monocytes) that have been obtained either from the donor's peripheral blood or from spleen cells and separated by ficoll gradient and then by nylon wool or immunomagnetic beads. Recipient serum is incubated with donor cells for 30 min (T cells) or 60 min (B cells). Rabbit serum (as a source of complement) is then added with eosin and formaldehyde to fix the cells and prevent lysis. After 2 hr, complement-mediated injury is apparent in that the cells that have been damaged by complement have taken up eosin. Alternatively, immunofluorescence can be used to detect cell lysis. The use of donor spleen cells is preferable in the sensitized patient, as the cell preparation may be better than with peripheral blood, and low levels of reactivity may not be detected on the peripheral blood.

2. Flow Cytometry Crossmatching (FCXM)

The principle of flow cytometry involves the identification of cells according to some physical property: size, charge, light scatter, etc. This is achieved by focusing a beam of light (laser) on a stream of fluorescent labeled cells, arranged so that each cell passes through the light, fluoresces, and scatters the light. These emissions are converted to electronic signals. For crossmatching purposes, donor cells are incubated with recipient serum, and cells that have bound antibody are recognized by fluorescent-labeled anti-IgG. The green fluorescence scatter produced by these cells is compared to the pattern obtained with normal serum incubated with the donor cells. T and B cells can be further differentiated by the addition of a second monoclonal antibody labeled with phycoerythrin. As each cell is individually analyzed, even small amounts of antibody are detected.

Garovoy introduced the flow cytometry crossmatch test and demonstrated its increased sensitivity compared with the standard CDC (51). Other advantages offered by this method include its ability to distinguish between IgM and IgG antibodies and whether they are anti-T and anti-B (class I) or anti-B cell (class II) antibodies. The problem of poor cell viability is less. The system is very sensitive to antibody against lymphocytes, but it amplifies both true and false positives (e.g., autoantibodies and irrelevant reactions). One disadvantage is its requirement for a flow cytometry apparatus and a skilled technician on a 7-day-a-week basis.

3. *Antiglobulin Test*

The antihuman globulin (AHG) test is an alternative method, which is less expensive and is almost as sensitive as flow cytometry (52). In this method, recipient serum is incubated with donor cells, the cells are washed, and antihuman globulin (antihuman κ) is added. After 1 min at room temperature, rabbit complement is added. Eosin and formaldehyde are added and the degree of cell lysis is counted. The AHG increases the sensitivity of the system for complement lysis but amplifies both false positives and true positives, similar to FXCM flow cytometry.

B. Significance of the Positive T Cell Crossmatch

A positive CDC crossmatch is usually defined as cell lysis > 20% above background in CDC; similar criteria can be established for the FACS or antiglobulin tests. A positive CDC T cell crossmatch with current sera is a contraindication to proceed with transplantation (53). Whether a positive result with stored sera taken months or years earlier should be viewed in the same way is more controversial (54). In patients who have been identified as highly sensitized in the past, the stored sera may reveal the presence of donor-specific antibody that has the potential to recur following transplantation or which may still be present at subthreshold levels. A positive crossmatch with current sera in CDC does not always result in rejection and graft loss, but the graft survival curves are much lower in these recipients (55). With more sensitive methods, the predictive value of a positive crossmatch is less striking, due to "false positives." Three-month graft survival in retransplants was 64% in patients with a positive AHG versus 79% with a negative crossmatch. Recipients retransplanted across a positive FCXM had a 3-month graft survival of only 61%, compared with 81% in the negative group (56).

The introduction of flow cytometry in some centers has increased the number of positive crossmatches, both true positives and false positives. Whether the identification of such low levels of reactivity is significant and a contraindication to transplantation remains controversial. A higher incidence of early graft loss has been reported in recipients of a first cadaveric renal transplant who had a positive T cell FCXM compared with a negative result (57). A number of other centers have reported similar results with T-FCXM (58–61). The outcome of renal transplants performed on the basis of a negative CDC crossmatch was analyzed and a T and B FCXM was done on the same serum of these patients (62). In this report unsensitized recipients of a first cadaveric allograft did equally well if the CDC was negative, irrespective of the T-FCXM result, and these patients may be excluded from transplantation if T-FCXM is the only method used. Sensitized patients and retransplants have a higher incidence of a positive T cell FCXM. These patients have a poorer outcome compared to those with a negative T cell crossmatch (56). The T-FCXM should be regarded as significant in the sensitized patient, because a positive is very likely to be a true positive, not a false positive.

C. B Cell Crossmatch

The significance of a positive B-cell crossmatch with a negative T-cell crossmatch remains controversial for several reasons. Anti-B cell antibodies without T-cell reactivity can be anti-class II, weak anti-class I, or autoantibody; consequently they have a different impact on graft outcome. Autoantibodies (often but not always IgM), which react predominantly with B cells, are not a risk to successful transplantation but create serious confusion in the crossmatch process. The autocrossmatch, recipient serum crossmatched against the recipient's own cells, can identify circulating autoantibodies. Because autoantibodies can give rise to a positive crossmatch, they may obscure the presence of alloantibodies. In addition, xenoantibodies related to antilymphocytic antibody therapy (OKT3, antilymphocyte globulin) can give a positive crossmatch, and coexisting positive autocrossmatch helps to clarify this situation.

Weak anti-class I antibodies may be detected only against B cells, resulting in a positive B cell crossmatch and a negative T-cell crossmatch, because the B cell is more sensitive to anti-class I than is the T cell. These antibodies are obviously dangerous and their detection would mitigate against proceeding with transplantation. The key is demonstration of absorption by platelets, which will occur with anti-class I but not with anti-class II.

Cold and warm B-cell antibodies have been described (63), referring to the temperature at which activity is detected. Warm B-cell antibodies were reported to be detrimental, whereas cold antibodies were thought to be enhancing. However, more recent reviews suggest that the outcome associated with a positive B-cell crossmatch is not readily predicted by the temperature of the reaction.

D. Lymphocytic Antibodies in Systemic Lupus Erythematosus

Some patients with systemic lupus erythematosus (SLE) present a problem when they are screened prior to transplantation because of lymphocytotoxic autoantibodies against both T and B cells, giving high panel reaction antibody (PRA) and positive donor-specific and autocrossmatches. The problem is to determine whether donor-specific alloantibodies are also present and whether it is safe to proceed with transplantation.

A technique recently described by Terasaki et al. (64) to determine the presence of IgA antibodies may provide a means to detect anti-HLA antibody in these patients. This method is a modification of the monoclonal antibody–specific immobilization of leukocyte antigen (MAILA) test described by Mueller-Eckhardt et al. (65), in which a monoclonal antibody to HLA class I was used to isolate the anti-HLA antibody and antibodies to these complexes were then identified by an ELISA. Such assays may prove to be a useful general approach to solving difficult crossmatching problems.

At present, a positive B-cell crossmatch is not always a contraindication to transplantation unless it is likely to be a weak anti-class I. Further analysis is warranted to identify the antibody responsible for reactivity. An autocrossmatch will determine the presence of autoantibody, and a reducing agent, dithiothreitol (DTT), can be added to distinguish between IgM and IgG. Platelet absorption will remove anti-class I activity.

Sensitized or retransplanted patients should not be transplanted across positive IgG B-cell crossmatch, either CDC, antihuman globulin, or FACS. For the nonsensitized patient with a negative T-cell crossmatch and a positive B cell by CDC, where anti-class I activity has been excluded, transplantation can proceed. At present there is no evidence that these patients have a poorer outcome. But weak anti-class I or true anti-class II have been associated with HAR, and the advisability of proceeding across a positive B cell crossmatch must always be weighed against the risks.

E. Panel of Reactive Antibody

A traditional method for identifying patients at risk of antibody-mediated rejection is the panel of reactive antibody (PRA). This involves testing the potential recipient's serum against a selection of HLA-typed lymphocytes and calculating the percentage of positive reactions. This is a useful test because it can be done at any time before transplantation and can identify patients who may need particularly detailed crossmatching at the time of transplant (i.e., the use of spleen cells rather than peripheral blood lymphocytes). The PRA can also be followed in patients to determine the optimum time for transplantation (i.e., now that erythropoeitin is used routinely in the dialysis units, the number of patients becoming sensitized may diminish. However, it is still not clear that the number of transfusions is really decreased in the dialysis population in the era of erythropoeitin). The PRA in patients who have been sensitized and currently have a high PRA may decrease if transfusions are strictly curtailed. This also applies to patients who have become sensitized with previous transplantation. Perhaps all patients anticipating receiving renal transplants in the future should receive immunosuppression whenever they are transfused.

A high PRA in patients awaiting renal transplantation may alert their physician to the risk of antibody-mediated rejection with subsequent transplantation and allow time for further testing and identification of particular HLA antigens to be avoided in the future. PRA is not specific for anti-HLA antibodies: auto-antibodies can also give high PRA values. In patients with high PRA, further testing may be necessary, including an "auto-crossmatch" to screen for autoantibodies. A high PRA has been shown to correlate with increased risk of graft loss (55,66).

F. Should Previous Mismatches Be Repeated?

The issue of whether or not to repeat HLA mismatches remains controversial. Some centers have reported that this did not influence graft survival (67), whereas others have reported a poor outcome in patients who were retransplanted with repeat HLA DR mismatches (67,68). These studies cannot be directly compared. In most situations, repeating HLA mismatches appears to be safe (69), but in sensitized patients known to have antibody directed at a specific HLA antigen, the danger may be greater. In considering retransplants in patients with specific antibody, it is probably advisable to avoid reexposing patients known to have made antibodies against one HLA antigen to the same antigen.

XII. ISSUES IN PATIENT MANAGEMENT

A. Impact of Anti-HLA Antibodies on Graft Survival

The influence of donor-specific anti-HLA antibodies on long-term kidney graft survival is generally deleterious. The presence of such antibodies prior to transplantation will be detected by crossmatching, and thus the majority of antibody-mediated rejection situations will be avoided. The lower levels of antibody described earlier may escape detection and may proceed to cause accelerated rejection in the early posttransplant period. Sensitization carries a risk of rejection, and the peak PRAs rather than the PRA at the time of transplantation may more closely predict graft outcome (70). Antidonor antibody can be detected in some patients posttransplant (71), but in some cases these antibodies may be absorbed onto the graft endothelium and be undetectable.

The development of anti-HLA antibody reduces graft survival (71,72), and the incidence of chronic rejection may be higher in patients who had detectable anti-HLA antibodies. However, since the incidence of acute rejection increases the incidence of chronic rejection, it is unclear whether antibodies have an independent effect on chronic rejection.

B. Delayed Graft Function

Sensitization also carries a risk for delayed graft function (DGF) (55). The incidence of DGF in the sensitized patients rose from 20% in unsensitized recipients to 36% in primary transplants and 48% for regrafts. The nature of the association of DGF with sensitization is uncertain and potentially multifactorial. Preexisting antibody, especially detected in crossmatching, or early anamnestic responses against the donor could *cause* DGF. Alternatively, DGF could cause antibody responses to be more destructive by shedding antigen, inducing increased MHC expression, and by reducing renal blood flow, etc. Thus DGF could either be *caused by* or be *a cause of* antibody-mediated injury. If there is immediate graft function, the degree of sensitization has less influence on the outcome (55). However, in the presence of DGF, the sensitized recipient fares much worse than the unsensitized patient with DGF.

Consideration of the donor characteristics may therefore be important in evaluating a potential recipient. Any feature that may increase the chance of DGF should be avoided, if possible, in the sensitized individual.

C. Reducing the Risk of Sensitization

Avoiding sensitization must be viewed as the first goal in preventing antibody-mediated rejection. It is hoped that the routine administration of erythropoetin to dialysis patients will help.

Improved HLA matching could help to reduce sensitization. But the limited supply of organs makes this task difficult, and the present method of matching predicts the response of individual donor-recipient pairs very poorly. It is hoped that increasing molecular knowledge of the HLA antigens will generate options for predicting and avoiding uncontrolled responses. Matching "residues" may be a step toward this goal (73,74).

D. Detection of Antidonor Activity

Once the patient has been sensitized, the risk of antibody-mediated rejection can be minimized by detailed crossmatching at the time of transplant. This ideally would be by FACS analysis in the sensitized patient. The use of historical sera may be important, and increasing the emphasis on HLA matching and avoiding repeat mismatches should be considered.

The detection of a positive crossmatch with historical sera does not preclude transplantation, but the interval is important. The current practice is to avoid transplantation in patients who have had a positive crossmatch in the 6 months previously (75). But 6 months is arbitrary, and graft survival may be reduced in patients with a consistently positive crossmatch >6 months before transplant. The finding of an isolated antibody activity in only one of many sera may also reflect an intercurrent viral illness or transfusion and may not preclude a successful transplant.

Table 4 Possibilities for Prevention and Treatment for Antibody-Mediated Rejection

1. Prevention
   - Crossmatching
   - Prevent sensitization
2. Treatment
   - Antibody removal
     - Antigen absorption column (A, B blood groups)
     - IgG absorption column (protein A)
     - Plasmapheresis
   - Interruption of antibody synthesis
     - Suspend T cell help for B cells, e.g., OKT3
   - Interruption of complement cascade
   - Prevent recruitment of neutrophils
   - Anticoagulation

E. Strategies to Reduce the Immune Response

Once the decision to proceed had been made in the sensitized patient, several options are available (Table 4). A few centers have tried to reduce the level of circulating antibody by a variety of techniques. These include plasmapheresis and immunoadsorption of antibody (31,76) and the administration of intravenous immunoglobulin (IVIg) (77,78). At present we try to reduce the risk of reactivation of the antibody response by the use of induction therapy with intravenous OKT3. Some studies that suggest that this may offer some benefit in patients with DGF (79).

F. Reversal of Rejection

Recovery of renal function in patients with HAR is rare, but we and others have reported successful reversal of the acute antibody-mediated rejection with the use of OKT3 (80). In our report, the patients were all treated with methylprednisone (500 mg for 3 days IV) and OKT3 (5 mg/kg for 10 days). The recovery of renal function coincided with the donor-specific crossmatch becoming negative (in some, but others recovered despite persistence of antibody). Gannedahl et al. (81) also reported successful treatment of antibody-mediated rejection with intravenous methylprednisolone, plasmapheresis, and 15-deoxyspergualin, a new investigational immunosuppressive agent. Its mechanisms of action are not well established, but it has been reported to inhibit antigen B-cell proliferation in animal studies. It has not been shown to affect existing levels of antibody. The authors propose that it acts by preventing new antibody synthesis after the levels have been reduced with plasmapheresis. Since the new agents mycophenolate mofetil and brequinar act on B as well as T cells, they may have a role in reducing antibody formation.

XIII. CONCLUSIONS

Although HAR is rarely seen today, antibody still plays a major role in determining graft outcome. The degree of sensitization remains a strong factor in predicting risk of rejection and graft loss, particularly in the early posttransplant period. A burst of antibody against the class I antigens of the graft can be associated with severe deterioration in function.

Anti-HLA class I and II antibodies are both potentially injurious, and their presence should be viewed as a relative contraindication to transplantation. Repeating HLA DR mismatches in these patients should be avoided.

Standard crossmatching techniques (NIH CDC), both T and B, are adequate for the majority of recipients. However the high-risk patient (PRA >50%) and retransplants ideally should have FACS matching on current and historical sera. If FACS is not available, the CDC crossmatch should be done with donor spleen cells rather than peripheral blood, and a current, freshly drawn serum should be used for the final crossmatch.

There is a complex interaction between DGF and high PRA, which may reflect several mechanisms. Good initial function should be seen as important, particularly in the sensitized patient.

Early diagnosis of antibody-mediated rejection is important, as this is a potentially reversible situation. A repeat donor-specific crossmatch will help to confirm the diagnosis. If their grafts are successful, these patients do require close monitoring indefinitely, as they are still at risk of rejection, especially if they continue to demonstrate antidonor activity.

ACKNOWLEDGMENTS

We wish to thank Dr. D. Rayner (Department of Laboratory Medicine and Pathology, University of Alberta) for providing histologic material and advice, and Miss P. Publicover for her secretarial assistance. Dr. P. Campbell is supported by a Kidney Foundation of Canada Fellowship.

REFERENCES

1. Mitchison NA. Passive transfer of transplantation immunity. Proc R Soc Lond 1954; 142: 72–87.
2. Najarian JS, Feldman JD. Passive transfer of transplantation immunity: I. Tritiated lymphoid cells. II. Lymphoid cells in millipore chambers. J Exp Med 1962; 115:1083–1092.
3. Winn HJ. Antibody-mediated rejection. In: Burdick JF, Racusen LC, Solez K, Williams GM, eds. Kidney Transplant Rejection: Diagnosis and Treatment. 2d ed. New York: Marcel Dekker, 1992:319–329.
4. Starzl TE, Marchioro TL, Holmes JH, Waddell WR. The incidence, cause, and significance of immediate and delayed oliguria or anuria after human renal transplantation. Surg Gynecol Obstet 1964; 118:819–826.
5. Sheil AGR, Stewart JH, Tiller DJ, May J. ABO blood group incompatibility in renal transplantation. Transplantation 1969; 8:299–300.
6. Kissmeyer-Nielsen F, Olsen S, Peterson VP, Fjeldborg O. Hyperacute rejection of kidney allografts associated with pre-existing humoral antibodies against donor cells. Lancet 1966; 2: 662–665.
7. Williams GM, Lee HM, Weymouth RF, et al. Studies in hyperacute and chronic renal homograft rejection in man. Surgery 1967; 62:204–212.
8. Rolley RT, Williams GM, Lerner RA, et al. Homograft rejection. Transplant Proc 1969; 1: 275–278.
9. Jeannet M, Pinn VW, Flax MH, et al. Humoral antibodies in renal allotransplantation in man. N Engl J Med 1970; 282:111–117.

10. Williams GM, Hume DM, Hudson RP, et al. Hyperacute renal-homograft rejection in man. N Engl J Med 1968; 279:611–618.
11. Joyce S, Flye MW, Mohanakumar T. Characterization of kidney cell-specific, non-major histocompatibility complex alloantigen using antibodies eluted from rejected human renal allografts. Transplantation 1988; 46:362–369.
12. Fuleihan R, Ramesh N, Horner A, et al. Cyclosporin A inhibits CD40 ligand expression in T lymphocytes. J Clin Invest 1994; 93:1315–1320.
13. Gray D. Immunological memory. In: Paul WE, ed. Annual Review of Immunology. Palo Alto, CA: Annual Reviews, 1993:49–77.
14. Carpenter CB, d'Apice AJF, Abbas AK. The role of antibodies in the rejection and enhancement of organ allografts. In: Dixon FJ, Kunkel HG, eds. Advances in Immunology. Vol 22. 22d ed. New York: Academic Press, 1976:1–65.
15. Gracie JA, Bolton EM, Porteous C, Bradley JA. T cell requirements for the rejection of renal allografts bearing an isolated class I MHC disparity. J Exp Med 1990; 172:1547–1557.
16. Mosmann TR, Coffman RL. Th1 and Th2 cells: Different patterns of lymphokine secretion lead to different functional properties. Annu Rev Immunol 1989; 10:145–173.
17. Hardy MA, Suciu-Foca N, Reed E, et al. Immunodulation of kidney and heart transplants by anti idiotypic antibodies. Ann Surg 1991; 214:522–530.
18. Kaliss N. Immunological enhancement of tumor homografts in mice: A review. Cancer Res 1958; 18:992–1003.
19. Möller E, Möller G. Quantitative studies of the sensitivity of normal and neoplastic mouse cells to the cytotoxic action of isoantibodies. J Exp Med 1962; 115:527–553.
20. Batchelor JR. The use of enhancement of studying tumor antigens. Cancer Res 1968; 28: 1410–1414.
21. French ME, Batchelor JR. Immunological enhancement of rat kidney grafts. Lancet 1969; 2: 1103–1106.
22. Staines NA, Guy K, Davies DAL. The dominant role of Ia antibodies in the passive enhancement of H-2 incompatible skin grafts. J Immunol 1975; 5:782–789.
23. Clarke CA. Prophylaxis of rhesus iso-immunization. Br Med Bull 1964; 24:3–9.
24. Opelz G, Sengar DP, Mickey MR, Terasaki PI. Effect of blood transfusions on subsequent kidney transplants. Transplant Proc 1973; 5:253–259.
25. Wasowska B, Baldwin WM III, Howell DN, Sanfilippo F. The association of enhancement of renal allograft survival by donor-specific blood transfusion with host MHC-linked inhibition of IgG anti-donor class I alloantibody responses. Transplantation 1993; 56:672–680.
26. Salvatierra O Jr, Vincenti F, Amend W, et al. Deliberate donor-specific blood transfusions prior to living related renal transplantation: A new approach. Ann Surg 1980; 192:543–552.
27. Alexandre GPJ, Squifflet JP, De Bruyére M, et al. Present experiences in a series of 26 ABO-incompatible living donor renal allografts. Transplant Proc 1987; 19:4538–4542.
28. Bach FH, Platt JL, Xenotransplantation: A view of issues. Transplant Proc 1992; 24:S49–S52.
29. Breimer ME, Samuelsson BE. The specific distribution of glycolipid-based blood group A antigens in human kidney related to A_1/A_2 Lewis, and secretor status of single individuals: A possible molecular explanation for the successful transplantation of A_2 kidneys into O recipients. Transplantation 1986; 42:88–91.
30. Hanto DW, Brunt EM, Goss JA, Cole BR. Accelerated acute rejection of an A_2 renal allograft in an O recipient: Association with an increase in anti-A_2 antibodies. Transplantation 1993; 56: 1580–1583.
31. Palmer A, Taube D, Welsh K, et al. Removal of anti-HLA antibodies by extracorporeal immunoadsorption to enable renal transplantation. Lancet 1989; 1:10–12.
32. Mendez R, Sakhrani L, Aswad S, et al. Successful living-related ABO incompatible renal transplant using the Biosynsorb Immunoadsorption Column. Transplant Proc 1992; 24:1738–1740.

33. Scornik JC, Le For WM, Cicciarelli JC, et al. Hyperacute and acute kidney graft rejection due to antibodies against B cells. Transplantation 1992; 54:61–64.
34. Kaufman JF, Auffray C, Korman AJ, et al. The class II molecules of the human and murine major histocompatibility complex. Cell 1984; 36:1–13.
35. Kalil J, Guilherme L, Neumann J, et al. Humoral rejection in two HLA identical living related donor kidney transplants. Transplant Proc 1989; 21:711–713.
36. Mathew JM, Joyce S, Lawrence W, Mohanakumar T. Evidence that antibodies eluted from rejected kidneys of HLA-identical transplants define a non-MHC alloantigen expressed on human kidneys. Transplantation 1991; 52:559–562.
37. Jordan SC, Yap HK, Sakai RS, Alfonso P, Fitchman M. Hyperacute allograft rejection mediated by anti-vascular endothelial antibodies with a negative monocyte crossmatch. Transplantation 1988; 46:585–602.
38. Cerilli J, Brasile L, Galouzis T, et al. The vascular endothelial cell antigen system. Transplantation 1985; 49:286–289.
39. Cerilli J, Holliday JE, Fesperman DP, Folger MR. Antivascular endothelial cell antibody—Its role in transplantation. Surgery 1977; 81:132–138.
40. Yard B, Spruyt-Gerritse M, Claas F, et al. The clinical significance of allospecific antibodies against endothelial cells detected with an antibody-dependent cellular cytotoxicity assay for vascular rejection and graft loss after renal transplantation. Transplantation 1993; 55:1287–1293.
41. Harmer AW, Rigden SPA, Koffman CG, Welsh KI. Preliminary report: Dramatic rise in renal allograft failure rate. Lancet 1990; 335:1184–1185.
42. Martin S, Brenchley PE, Postlethwaite R, et al. Detection of anti-epithelial cell antibodies in association with pediatric renal transplant failure using a novel microcytotoxicity assay. Tissue Antigens 1991; 37:152–155.
43. Porter KA. Morphological aspects of renal homograft rejection. Br Med Bull 1965; 21: 171–175.
44. Lobo PI, Sturgill BC, Bolton WK. Cold-reactive alloantibodies and allograft malfunction occurring immediately post-transplant. Transplantation 1984; 37:76–81.
45. Schweizer RT, Bartus SA, Perkins HA, Belzer FO. Renal allograft failure and cold red blood cell autoagglutinins. Transplantation 1982; 33:77–79.
46. Buturovic J, Kandus A, Malovrh M, et al. Cyclosporine-associated hemolytic uremic syndrome in four renal allograft recipients: Resolution without specific therapy. Transplant Proc 1990; 22:1726–1727.
47. Halloran PF, Schlaut J, Solez K, Srinivasa NS. The significance of the anti-class I response: II. Clinical and pathologic features of renal transplants with anti-class I-like antibody. Transplantation 1992; 53:550–555.
48. Halloran PF, Wadgymar A, Ritchie S, et al. The significance of the anti-class I antibody response: I. Clinical and pathologic features of anti-class I mediated rejection. Transplantation 1990; 49:85–91.
49. Solez K, Alexlsen RA, Benediktsson H, et al. International standardization of criteria for the histologic diagnosis of renal allograft rejection: The Banff working classification of kidney transplant pathology. Kidney Int 1993; 44:411–422.
50. Rose ML. Antibody-mediated rejection following cardiac transplantation. Transplant Rev 1993; 7:140–152.
51. Garovoy MR, Rheinschmidt MA, Bigos M, et al. Flow cytometry analysis: A high technology crossmatch technique facilitating transplantation. Transplant Proc 1983; 15:1939–1943.
52. Kerman RH, Kimball PM, Van Buren CT, et al. AHG and DTE/AHG procedure identification of crossmatch-appropriate donor-recipient pairings that result in improved graft survival. Transplantation 1991; 51:316–320.
53. Scornik JC, Brunson ME, Howard RJ, Pfaff WW. Alloimmunization, memory, and the interpretation of crossmatch results for renal transplantation. Transplantation 1992; 54:389–394.

54. Cardella CJ, Falk JA, Nicholson MJ, et al. Successful renal transplantation in patients with T-cell reactivity to donor. Lancet 1982; 1:1240–1243.
55. Zhou YC, Cecka JM. Sensitization in renal transplantation. In: Terasaki P, ed. Clinical Transplants 1991. Los Angeles, California: UCLA Tissue Typing Laboratory, 1991; 313–323.
56. Ogura K, Cecka JM. Cadaver retransplants. In: Terasaki P, ed. Clinical Transplants. Los Angeles, CA: UCLA Tissue Typing Laboratory, 1990; 471–483.
57. Ogura K, Terasaki PI, Johnson C, et al. The significance of a positive flow cytometry crossmatch test in primary kidney transplantation. Transplantation 1993; 56:294–298.
58. Mahoney RJ, Ault KA, Given SR, et al. The flow cytometric crossmatch and early renal transplant loss. Transplantation 1990; 49:527–535.
59. Chapman JR, Deierhoi MH, Carter NP, et al. Analysis of flow cytometry and cytotoxicity crossmatches in renal transplantation. Transplant Proc 1985; 17:2480–2481.
60. Cinti P, Bachetoni A, Trovati A, et al. Clinical relevance of donor-specific IgG determination by FACS analysis in renal transplantation. Transplant Proc 1991; 23:1297–1299.
61. Talbot D, Cavanagh G, Coates E, et al. Improved graft outcome and reduced complications due to flow cytometric crossmatching and DR matching in renal transplantation. Transplantation 1992; 53:925–928.
62. Scornik JC, Brunson ME, Schaub B, et al. The crossmatch in renal transplantation: Evaluation of flow cytometry as a replacement for standard cytotoxicity. Transplantation 1994; 57: 621–625.
63. Ferguson RM, Rynasiewicz JJ, Sutherland DER, et al. Cyclosporine A in renal transplantation: A prospective randomized trial. Surgery 1982; 8:175–182.
64. Koka P, Chia D, Terasaki PI, et al. The role of IgA anti-HLA class I antibodies in kidney transplant survival. Transplantation 1993; 56:207–211.
65. Mueller-Eckhardt G, Kiefel V, Schmidt A, et al. Discrimination of antibodies against antigens of different MHC loci in human sera by monoclonal antibody-specific immobilization of leukocyte antigens. Hum Immunol 1989; 25:125–134.
66. Rankin GW, Jr., Wang X, Terasaki PI. Sensitization to kidney transplants. In: Terasaki PI, ed. Clinical Transplants 1990; Los Angeles, California: UCLA Tissue Typing Laboratory, 1991: 417–424.
67. Farney AC, Noreen HJ, Sutherland DER, et al. Effect of reexposure to mismatched major histocompatibility complex antigens on renal retransplant allograft survival. Transplant Proc 1993; 25:213–214.
68. Ting A, Morris PI. Development of donor-specific antibodies after renal transplantation. Transplantation 1979; 28:13–17.
69. Cecka JM, Terasaki PI. Repeating HLA antigen mismatches in renal retransplants—A second class mistake? Transplantation 1994; 57:515–519.
70. Ogura K. Sensitization. In: Terasaki PI, Cecka JM, eds. Clinical Transplants 1992: Los Angeles, CA: UCLA Tissue Typing Laboratory, 1992:357–369.
71. Suciu-Foca N, Reed E, D'Agati VD, et al. Soluble HLA antigens, anti-HLA antibodies, and antiidiotypic antibodies in the circulation of renal transplant recipients. Transplantation 1991; 51:593–601.
72. Barr ML, Cohen DJ, Benvenisty AI, et al. Effect of anti-HLA antibodies on the long-term survival of heart and kidney allografts. Transplant Proc 1993; 25:262–264.
73. Takemoto S, Gjertson DW, Terasaki PI. Increasing the proportion of matched kidney recipients by using HLA amino acid residues (abstr). 12th Annual ASTP Meeting 1993; May 17–19:56.
74. Takemoto S, Gjertson DW, Terasaki PI, HLA matching: Maximizing the number of compatible transplants. In: Terasaki PI, Cecka JM, eds. Clinical Transplants. Los Angeles, CA: UCLA Tissue Typing Laboratory, 1993:521–531.
75. Turka LA, Goguen JE, Gagne JE, Milford EL. Presensitization and the renal allograft recipient. Transplantation 1989; 47:234–239.

76. Hiesse C, Kriaa F, Rousseau P, et al. Immunoabsorption of anti-HLA antibodies for highly sensitized patients awaiting renal transplantation. Nephrol Dial Transplant 1992; 7:944–951.
77. Glotz D, Haymann JP, Sansonetti N, et al. Suppression of HAL-specific alloantibodies by high-dose intravenous immunoglobulins (IVIg): A potential tool for transplantation of immunized patients. Transplantation 1993; 56:335–337.
78. Tyan DB, Li VA, Czer L, et al. Intravenous immunoglobulin suppression of HLA alloantibody in highly sensitized transplant candidates and transplantation with a histoincompatible organ. Transplantation 1994; 57:553–562.
79. Cecka JM, Gjertson D, Terasaki PI. Do prophylactic antilymphocyte globulins (ALG ad OKT3) improve renal transplant survival in recipient and donor high-risk groups? Transplant Proc 1993; 25:548–549.
80. Gaber LW, Gaber AO, Vera SR, et al. Successful reversal of hyperacute renal allograft rejection with the anti-CD3 monoclonal OKT3. Transplantation 1992; 54:930–932.
81. Gannedahl G, Ohlman S, Persson U, et al. Rejection associated with early appearance of donor-reactive antibodies after kidney transplantation treated with plasmapheresis and administration of 15-deoxyspergualin: A report of two cases. Transplant Int 1992; 5:189–192.
82. Abbas KA, Lichman AH, Pober JS. Cellular and molecular immunology. Second Edition. Philadelphia: WB Saunders, 1994.

3

Immunopathology of Rejection

Ralph H. Hruban, William M. Baldwin, III, and Fred Sanfilippo
Johns Hopkins University School of Medicine, Baltimore, Maryland

I. INTRODUCTION

The mechanisms of cellular and antibody-mediated allograft rejection outlined in the previous two sections provide a basis for understanding the immunopathology of rejection and the techniques used to monitor transplant recipients for graft rejection. This chapter is intended to provide a bridge between the basic mechanisms and resultant pathological changes of rejection and a basis for understanding the techniques currently employed in evaluating the immunopathological changes associated with rejection. The chapter is divided into three sections. The first describes the categorization of rejection into relatively distinct clinical, temporal, and immunopathological groups, the second reviews how the manifestations of humoral mediated rejection can be used to monitor transplant recipients for rejection, and the third section does the same for the manifestations of cell-mediated rejection. While occasional organ-specific examples are given, more detailed organ-specific pathology is presented in later chapters.

II. CATEGORIZATION OF REJECTION

Rejection can be classified according to the rate at which it occurs, and this, in turn, reflects to some degree the underlying histology. *Hyperacute rejection* occurs within minutes to hours after circulation is reestablished to the graft and is due to antibody-mediated inflammation (1–3). It is characterized histologically by the presence of an acute inflammatory infiltrate with vascular injury, leading to necrosis and hemorrhage in the graft. *Acute rejection* develops over a span of days to weeks. Most acute rejection episodes occur within the first 3 months after transplantation, but episodes of acute rejection can occur much later and may be associated with changes in immunosuppression or with other causes of in situ inflammation, such as infections. Acute rejection can be caused by almost purely cellular or antibody-mediated events (4,5), but it is most often a mixture of the two immune responses. Histologically, acute rejection is characterized by the presence of a mononuclear cell infiltrate in the parenchyma of the graft and inflammatory vascular changes. *Chronic rejection* evolves gradually over months to years and may have its origins in damage incurred during earlier "reversible" episodes of acute rejection (6). The final stages of this lesion are characterized by fibrointimal proliferation in the vascular walls, interstitial fibrosis, and a relatively mild mononuclear cell infiltrate.

While these clinical classifications are useful for the general characterization of rejection reactions, increasingly sophisticated immunopathological studies of allografts have yielded a more complete appreciation of the multiple mechanisms involved in the rejection process. Some of the newer approaches to evaluating the immune responses to transplanted organs are discussed in this chapter.

III. MANIFESTATIONS OF HUMORALLY MEDIATED REJECTION

In hyperacute rejection, immunofluorescent stains can demonstrate antibody and complement components deposited on the vascular endothelium (1–3). When hyperacute rejection is due to ABO incompatibility, IgM isohemagglutinins are deposited on the vessels, whereas, when hyperacute rejection results from presensitization to HLA-A or B antigens (class I MHC antigens), the deposits are predominantly IgG (7). Preexisting antibodies to HLA-DR or DQ (class II MHC antigens) have been reported to cause hyperacute or accelerated acute rejection in a few renal allografts (8–11). In about half of these cases, IgM was deposited in the arterioles.

Antibodies are very efficient activators of complement to the extent that one IgM or two IgG molecules within 40 nm can activate complement. Microaggregates of IgG below the detection level of immunohistology can activate the complement cascade (12). As a result, staining for IgM or IgG in tissue sections can be expected to detect antibody deposition only in hyperacute rejection and in the more vigorous cases of antibody-mediated acute rejection. Staining for some of the secondary and tertiary effectors activated by antibody can provide a more sensitive indicator of antibody deposition than staining directly for IgM or IgG (see Table 1). For example, complement can be detected in some biopsies in the absence of demonstrable antibodies (5,8,13). This may represent activation of complement by antibodies deposited in quantities that are below the threshold of

Table 1 Histological Correlates for Antibody-Mediated Rejection

Staining	Correlation
IgM	Typical of isohemagglutinins to A or B blood group antigens, and some antibodies to class II MHC antigens
IgG	Typical of antibodies to MHC antigens, particularly HLA-A or -B
C4b or C4d	Classic pathway component, covalently bound to target in clusters
Bb	Alternative pathway component
C3b	Present in the highest concentration, covalently bound to tissue
MAC	MAC neoantigen only detectable after terminal C components are assembled
Platelets	Can be activated by FcR and C1qR on their surfaces
Neutrophils	Have receptors for IgG, C1q, C4b, C3b iC3b, and C5a
Monocytes	Have receptors for IgG, C1q, C4b, C3b iC3b, and C5a
FcR	On platelets, neutrophils, macrophages and NK cells
CD11b/CD18	Complement Receptor 3 (CR3) on neutrophils, macrophages, and NK cells
CD11c/CD18	Complement Receptor 4 (CR4) on neutrophils, macrophages, NK cells, and subsets of B and T cells

detection by immunohistology (4,5). Alternatively, it may be the result of direct activation of complement by injured tissues (14–21).

The remainder of this section emphasizes the complement-mediated events leading to reactions that can be detected by normal tissue stains or by immunohistology. Complement is a cascade of sequentially activated proteins that have multiple functions (14). The most important complement components in their order of activation are highlighted.

The first complement component to be activated by antibody deposited in a transplant is C1 (see Fig. 2 in Chap. 2). C1 is a complex composed of one large bifunctional binding protein (C1q) and two pairs of enzymes ($C1r_2$ and $C1s_2$). When C1q binds to antibody or directly to tissue constituents by its globular domains, it can interact through its exposed collagenlike tail region with cells bearing C1q receptors (C1qR). This mechanism accounts for some of the accumulation of platelets, neutrophils, and monocytes present in many biopsies from allografts with acute rejection. Platelet activation through C1qR results in increased procoagulant activity (22). C1qR on neutrophils and macrophages mediate increased oxidative metabolism and ADCC of antibody opsonized targets (23–25). Consequently, focal accumulations of platelets, neutrophils, or macrophages should suggest the possibility of antibody and complement deposition. Although intact platelets and granulocytes can be discerned on routinely stained tissue sections, degranulated cells are not easily appreciated. We have found that immunofluorescent stains with antibodies directed to platelet-specific antigens are particularly useful in evaluating the extent of intravascular platelet aggregation in experimental models of antibody-mediated graft rejection (26). Similarly, Ten and co-workers (27) have reported that immunofluorescent stains for granule contents can be used to evaluate the extent of granulocyte involvement in acute renal allograft rejection in humans.

C4, the second component to be activated in the classic pathway of complement, is cleaved into a small, soluble fragment (C4a) and a large fragment (C4b) that has a short-lived thioester binding site, which can bind covalently to cell surfaces or to the antibody itself. Staining for C4b (Fig. 1; see also color plate), or its further breakdown product C4d may be particularly informative for several reasons. Once C1 is activated by binding to antibody, it can cleave about 35 molecules of C4. The short half-life of the thioester binding site ensures that the C4b binds in clusters around the site of antibody deposition. This localized concentration of C4b covalently bound to target tissues increases the sensitivity of staining for C4b without distorting the distribution of the lesion. In addition, it indicates that the complement cascade has been activated through the classic pathway (Fig. 2). Staining for C4d may also be useful. Feucht and colleagues (28,29) have reported that capillary deposits of C4d in renal transplants were associated with circulating antibodies to class I MHC antigens and with early graft loss.

C2 binds to C4b and is cleaved by C1s into C2a and C2b. C2a remains attached to C4b to form the C3 convertase, C4b2a, of the classic pathway of complement. Factor B of the alternative complement pathway is structurally and functionally homologous to C2 of the classic pathway, and the $C3(H_2O)Bb$ complex is the C3 convertase of the alternative pathway of complement. A positive stain for Bb, therefore, indicates that complement has been activated through the alternative pathway. The Bb fragment of factor B is mitogenic for B lymphocytes. It has been calculated that conversion of as little as 1 to 5% of factor B to Bb at the site of inflammation would stimulate the local expansion of B lymphocytes (30). This mechanism could account for the nests of B lymphocytes that are observed in some acute rejection reactions (31).

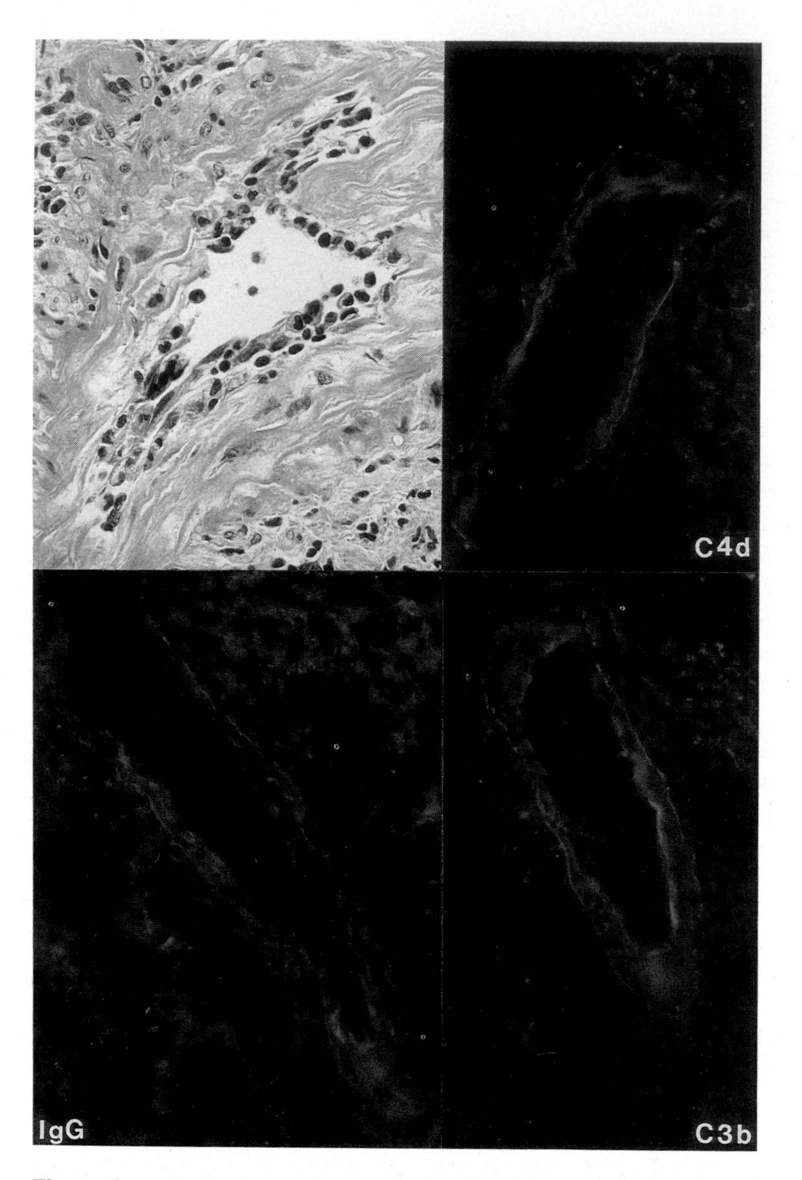

Figure 1 Kidney biopsy 9 days after transplantation. Routine hematoxylin and eosin staining (top left) of formalin-fixed tissue demonstrates marked endothelialitis of an artery, with lymphocytes, monocytes, and neutrophils disrupting the endothelium. Immunofluorescence stains on frozen sections from the same biopsy revealed little IgG but strong linear staining for C4d and C3b on the endothelium of an artery. (For optimal reproduction, see color plate.)

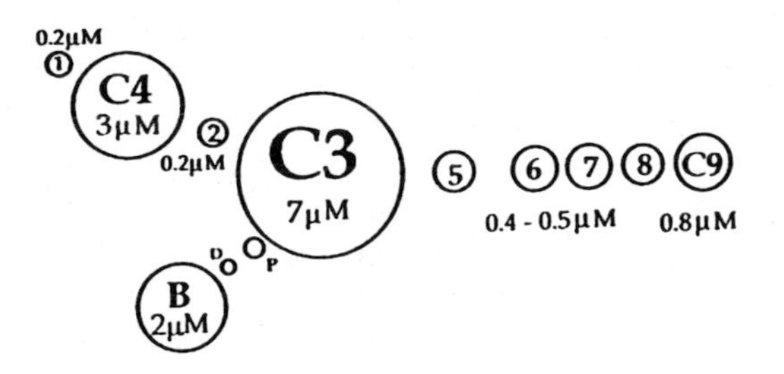

Figure 2 Relative serum concentrations of components of the classic and alternative pathways of complement. C3, which is activated by both pathways, circulates in the highest concentration. C4, which is specific for the classic pathway, and factor B, which is specific for the alternative pathway, are also present in high concentrations.

Activation of the complement cascade by either the classic or alternative pathway results in the cleavage of C3 and then of C5 into their active fragments. The smaller cleavage products (C3a and C5a) are extremely potent proinflammatory mediators. C5a is about 10- to 1000-fold more active than C3a on a molar basis (32,33), but C3 is present in about 20-fold greater concentrations in the plasma (1.4 mg/mL vs. 0.07 mg/mL in humans). Both C3a and C5a cause histamine release from mast cells and basophils, contraction of smooth muscle, and increased permeability of vessels. C5a also activates endothelial cells (34). Activated endothelial cells release heparan sulfate (35) and synthesize tissue factor (36), making their cell membrane more thrombogenic. In addition, C5a is a powerful chemoattractant for granulocytes (eosinophils and basophils as well as neutrophils) and monocytes. Activation through the C5a receptor (C5aR) causes enzyme release by granulocytes (37), cytokine (interleukins-1, -6, and -8 and tumor necrosis factor–alpha (IL-1, IL-6, and IL-8 and TNF-α)) production by monocytes (38,39), and upregulation of complement receptors CR1 and CR3 (40,41). These mechanisms may lead to the neutrophil activation that has been correlated with acute rejection episodes in hepatic transplants (42).

The larger cleavage product of C3, namely C3b, can bind via a thioester group to cell membranes. Each C3 convertase can cleave several hundred C3 molecules and about 10% of the C3b fragments bind to the adjacent cell membranes. Membrane-bound C3b and its further breakdown product, iC3b, serve as accessory adhesion molecules, strengthening the contact between the target cell and effector cells, expressing CR1 and CR3 respectively (25). CR3 (also known as Mac-1, Mo-1 or CD11b/CD18) is a member of the leukocyte integrin family and has binding affinity for fibrinogen, factor X, and beta-glucan as well as iC3b (43,44). C5a activation of neutrophils and monocytes not only enhances CR1 and CR3 attachment to fixed C3b and iC3b but also exposes a binding site in CR3 for ICAM-1 (45), which is upregulated in renal, cardiac, and hepatic transplants during rejection (46–52) and infection (53). CR4 (p150,95 or CD11c/CD18) and LFA-1 (CD11a/CD18), two other members of the leukocyte adhesion molecule family that bind to iC3b and ICAM-1, 2, and 3, respectively, are also upregulated by C5a. Through these adhesion receptors, C5a promotes adherence of monocytes and neutrophils to endothelial cells and their extravascular migration.

Monocytes, macrophages neutrophils, platelets, and some lymphocytes coexpress receptors for iC3b, C3b, or C1q with Fc receptors (FcR). All three well-defined FcRs for IgG (the high-affinity FcRI and the two low-affinity FcRII and III receptors) preferentially bind the complement-activating IgG1 and IgG3 subclasses (54). When suboptimal concentrations of antibody are bound to antigen, binding of iC3b, C3b, or Clq can induce dose-dependent target-cell killing through FcR-bearing cells (23–25,55). In this way, concentrations of antibodies and complement that are not histologically detectable have the potential to cause injury through platelets, neutrophils, and macrophages. Several groups have demonstrated cells with FcR by immunohistology in rejecting allografts (56–58). Similarly, the presence of C3 deposits and infiltrates containing large amounts of macrophages has been correlated with severe rejection episodes in clinical biopsies (9).

C5b-C9, the membrane attack complex (MAC), is the terminal effector phase of complement activation. The importance of MAC in acute and hyperacute rejection has been demonstrated in rodent models using recipients with a profound deficiency of C6 (26,59). C5b, C6, C7, C8, and C9 assemble as a polymeric complex to form a channel through the plasma membrane that can cause cell lysis. After the separate components are assembled, the MAC complex can be detected on cell surfaces with reagents specific for the neo-epitopes of the MAC complex (59). If only low densities of MAC are assembled on the surface of a metabolically active cell, lysis is prevented by exocytosis or endocytosis of the injured membrane. This transient insertion of MAC through the cell membrane releases calcium from intracellular stores and initiates signaling (60). The insertion of MAC into endothelial cells causes an array of changes in membrane characteristics and the release of mediators that are of direct relevance to acute and chronic rejection. Platelet-derived growth factor (PDGF) and basic fibroblast growth factor (bFGF) are released by endothelial cells following insertion of MAC (61). These potent mitogens for mesangial cells together with direct MAC-induced proliferation of fibroblasts (62) could contribute to chronic proliferative changes observed in vascular walls and the interstitium of transplanted organs. Insertion of MAC causes a rapid fusion of cytoplasmic granules with the endothelial cell membrane exposing P-selectin (GMP-140) to interact with platelets, neutrophils, and monocytes in the circulation (63). In addition, vesiculation of the plasma membrane exposes a catalytic surface on vascular endothelial cells for the prothrombinase enzyme complex (64), which could contribute to fibrin deposition associated with acute rejection episodes.

Thus, an understanding of the interaction of antibodies, complement, and inflammatory cells is helpful in selecting and interpreting immunohistological stains of transplant biopsies. In particular, stains for C4 and C3 are more sensitive than stains for immunoglobulin (Ig). In addition, deposition of C4 in a lesion indicates activation of the classic pathway of complement, whereas the presence of factor B suggests that the alternative pathway has been activated. In the future, MAC may be correlated with the endothelial cell activation that is thought to initiate chronic rejection.

IV. MANIFESTATIONS OF CELL-MEDIATED REJECTION

As outlined in the previous chapter, cell-mediated immunity can be initiated by one of two mechanisms. Recipient antigen presenting cells (APC) can process foreign antigens and then present these processed antigens on their surface in conjunction with self class II major histocompatibility complex molecules. Antigen-specific recipient T-helper lymphocytes can then be activated when their T-cell receptor binds to this foreign peptide-recipient class II complex. Alternatively, donor class II antigens expressed on the surface of donor APCs can directly stimulate recipient T-helper lymphocytes. This mode of direct alloantigen presentation generally provides a much greater stimulus for rejection and is more difficult to reverse with standard immunosuppressive therapy (65,66). Regardless of the stimulus, once activated, these lymphocytes produce a variety of cytokines that in turn activate additional leukocytes, including cytotoxic T lymphocytes and macrophages, resulting in graft rejection. While further details of cell-mediated rejection (CMR) are given in the earlier chapter by Drs. Sabatine and Auchincloss, each of the basic components of CMR outlined above provides a basis for understanding the manifestations of rejection in the peripheral blood and in the graft as well as the usefulness and limitations of these manifestations in monitoring transplant recipients for rejection.

The morphological changes associated with lymphocyte activation are probably the simplest manifestations of cell-mediated rejection (67). These changes can be detected in the peripheral blood by light microscopic examination of peripheral blood smears. The technique of "cytoimmunologic monitoring," or CIM, refers to the monitoring of transplant recipients for rejection based on the percentage of lymphoblasts (number of lymphoblasts/total number of lymphoid cells) in the peripheral blood (68–70). As one would expect, the percentage of lymphoblasts in the peripheral blood increases during allograft rejection (67–71). Unfortunately, there are two major limitations to CIM. First, it can be difficult to classify reproducibly the activation states of lymphocytes based solely on their morphology (69). Second, activation of peripheral lymphocytes caused by infection cannot be distinguished from activation of lymphocytes due to rejection (68,72–74).

It was hoped that the identification of a number of the molecular mediators of cell-mediated rejection would overcome the first problem listed above, that is, the difficulty in reproducibly classifying the activation status of immune cells. For example, it has been demonstrated that both the release of interleukin-2 (IL-2) and the expression of specific membrane receptors for IL-2 accompany the activation of T-lymphocytes (75). These receptors, designated IL-2R, are also released into extracellular fluids (76). The expression of these receptors is induced within a few hours of activation, and they are a potentially more specific marker of lymphocyte activation than is morphology. Indeed, the number of lymphocytes expressing IL-2R has been shown to increase in the peripheral blood of heart transplant recipients with rejection (77–78), and the levels of soluble IL-2R have been shown to increase during acute rejection in heart, lung, kidney, and liver transplant recipients (79–85). While the expression of the IL-2R does appear to be a good marker of lymphocyte activation, the usefulness of IL-2R expression is limited because the activation of peripheral blood lymphocytes caused by rejection cannot be distinguished from activation by infection (70,76,79,81,84).

The recognition that phenotypically identifiable T-lymphocyte subsets play distinct roles in cell-mediated rejection provides another avenue for monitoring peripheral blood lymphocytes after transplantation. As discussed in Chap. 1, $CD4^+$ lymphocytes exhibit class II antigen restriction, secrete IL-2, IL-4, IL-5, γ-interferon and TNF-β, and they usually function as T-helper cells. In contrast, $CD8^+$ lymphocytes exhibit class I antigen restriction, and they usually function as T-cytotoxic or T-suppressor cells. These two phenotypically identifiable T-cell subpopulations, $CD4^+$ and $CD8^+$, can be identified in the peripheral blood by flow cytometry, and a number of investigators have suggested that the ratio of $CD4^+$ to $CD8^+$ cells can be used to distinguish rejection from other reactions (78,85,86). For example, Molajoni et al. monitored the peripheral blood of 10 heart-transplant recipients for lymphocytes expressing CD3, CD4, CD8, Leu-7, CD16, or CD19 antigens and found that heart allograft rejection was associated with an increased prevalence of $CD3^+$ and $CD4^+$ cells in the peripheral blood (85). Unfortunately, as was true for IL-2R, rejection episodes cannot be consistently detected by monitoring the T-lymphocyte subsets in the peripheral blood, and episodes of infection can yield false-positive results (72,77,87,88).

An alternative approach to looking at the phenotype of the T-cell subsets is to examine the antigen specificity of the lymphocytes circulating in the peripheral blood (88–91). T lymphocytes employ clonotypic T-cell receptors (TCR), which recognize foreign antigen in association with class I or class II human leukocyte antigens. This antigen specificity of T-lymphocytes can be useful in determining whether or not activated lymphocytes in the peripheral blood are responding to donor antigens or to infections. For example, Debruyne et al. used "limiting dilution analysis" (LDA) to quantify the number of donor alloantigen-reactive helper T lymphocytes in the peripheral blood of 12 heart-transplant recipients (89). Cryopreserved cells obtained from the donor's spleen were used as a source of donor alloantigen stimulation, and the results of the LDA were compared to the findings in the patient's heart biopsies (89). They found that donor-*specific* T lymphocytes in the peripheral blood increased more than sixfold during episodes of rejection, and in some patients this increase occurred before a biopsy diagnosis was established (89). The advantage of this technique is that it is donor-antigen–specific and so it can be used to distinguish between infection and rejection; however, it is technically difficult to perform, and it may be positive even in mild cases of rejection (89).

It is disappointing that most of these peripheral blood monitoring techniques fail to establish clearly whether or not a graft is being rejected. However, it is to be expected if one remembers the basic mechanisms of cell-mediated rejection outlined earlier. As there is preferential homing and selective trapping of activated lymphocytes in the graft, the most important reactions are not necessarily manifested systemically (92–95). Indeed, Suitters et al. demonstrated that considerably higher frequencies of donor-specific cytotoxic lymphocytes are present in heart biopsies obtained from heart-transplant recipients than in the peripheral blood of the same patients (94). Clearly, the best way to determine with certainty what is going on within a graft is to examine the graft itself.

Biopsy of an allograft is the most direct way to monitor allografts for the presence of cell-mediated rejection. Currently, most allograft biopsies are evaluated at the light microscopic level by the examination of sections stained with hematoxylin and eosin. The changes assessed in each biopsy are organ-specific and are described in later chapters on organ-specific pathology. In general, however, the mere presence of lymphocytes in a biopsy is not sufficient to establish a diagnosis of rejection, because virtually all allografts are infiltrated to some degree by recipient lymphocytes. Thus, the evaluation of biopsies relies heavily on the expertise of the pathologist interpreting the slides. For example, in heart allografts, it can be difficult to determine whether an inflammatory reaction in a heart biopsy is due to prior biopsy site change or to rejection (96).

The hallmark of graft rejection is inflammation, and the leukocytes infiltrating a graft can be phenotyped just as those in the peripheral blood can be. In acute and chronic rejection, the majority of the lymphocytes infiltrating allografts are T lymphocytes (97–99). These T lymphocytes consist of a mixture of $CD4^+$ and $CD8^+$ cells, and a variety of investigators have examined the value of phenotyping for CD4 and CD8 in allograft biopsies (92,93,98,100–104). In general, these studies have demonstrated that mild early acute allograft rejection is associated with an increase in the number of $CD4^+$ cells (Fig. 3; see also color plate) and that later moderate rejection is associated with an increase in $CD8^+$ T lymphocytes (92,102). Leu-7–positive natural killer cells and macrophages have also been identified (58,93,98,102,105,106). de Blic et al. (98) stained 72 lung biopsies from 21 lung-transplant recipients with a panel of monoclonal antibodies that included antibodies to CD3, CD4, and CD8; they found that (a) regardless of grade, there were more $CD3^+$ cells in biopsies from transplant recipients than in biopsies from nontransplanted controls and (b)

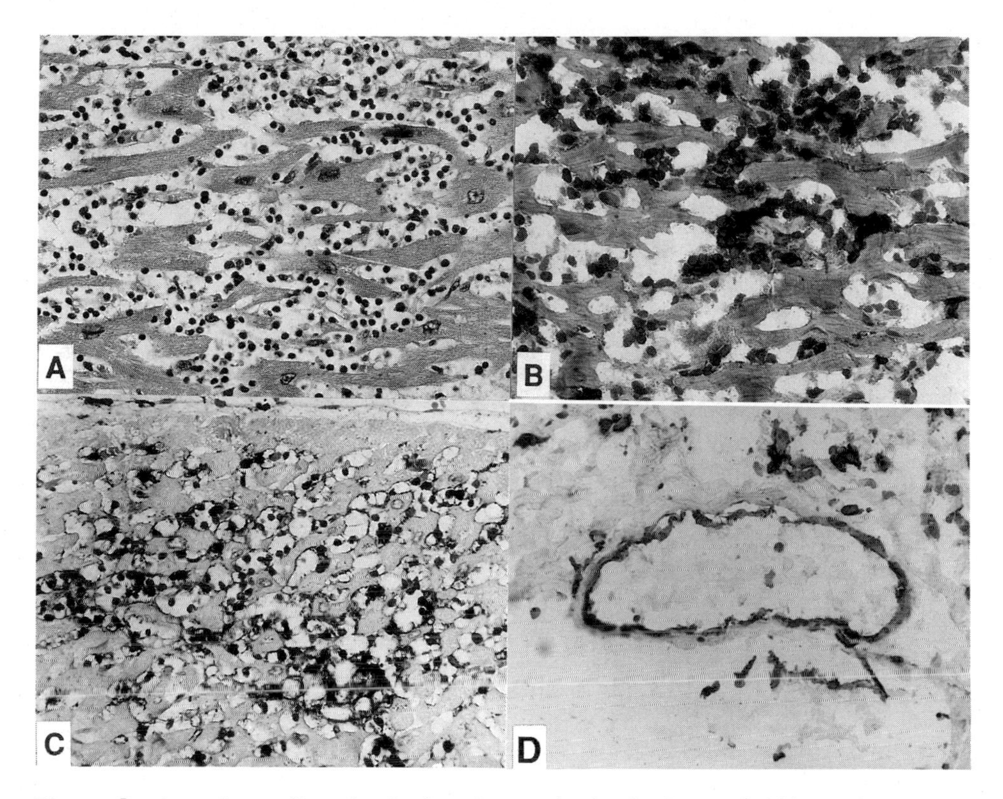

Figure 3 Acute heart allograft rejection. Acute rejection is characterized by an intense mononuclear cell infiltrate associated with myocyte necrosis (A). In this case, immunohistochemical staining demonstrated that the infiltrate was composed of a mixture of CD4 (B) and CD8-positive cells, most of which expressed CD45RO (C). The infiltrate was accompanied by the upregulation of class II antigen expression on endothelial cells (D). [A, hematoxylin and eosin; B–D, immunostaining for CD4 (B), CD45RO (C), and HLA-DR(D); all ×400.] (For optimal reproduction, see color plate.)

there is a correlation between the histological grade of rejection and the number of CD3$^+$, CD8$^+$, and CD25$^+$ (IL-2R) cells. The CD4/CD8 ratio did not, however, correlate with rejection (98). The predominance of CD8 vs. CD4 T cells in renal allografts can, however, suggest that rejection is more likely than other causes of renal dysfunction such as CSA toxicity (104).

The different subsets of T lymphocytes also express different isoforms of CD45, and the coexpression of these isoforms provides additional information about the status of the T lymphocytes (92). Cells expressing CD45RA are predominantly naive (inactivated) lymphocytes, while CD45RO–positive cells are believed to be memory T cells (92). Ibrahim et al. stained 33 endomyocardial biopsies from heart-transplant recipients using double labeling for CD4, CD8, CD45RA, and CD45RO. They found that mild rejection was associated primarily with CD4$^+$/CD45RA$^+$ lymphocytes, while moderate rejection was accompanied by an increase in CD8$^+$/CD45RO$^+$ lymphocytes (Fig. 3C) (92). Immunophenotyping studies such as these demonstrate that T lymphocytes are the predominant type of leukocyte seen during organ rejection, and suggest that phenotypic characterization of the lymphocytes infiltrating a graft might be helpful in distinguishing rejection from other reactions (92). Similar findings have also been reported for liver (107) and kidney allografts (108).

Recently, antibodies have been produced against a number of the activation markers associated with cell-mediated rejection, and the expression of these markers has been examined in allograft biopsies. The expression of IL-2 and IL-2R, perhaps the best-characterized of these activation markers (58,80,98,99,109–111), has not proven to be a reliable marker for allograft rejection (111). Lipman et al. analyzed 24 kidney biopsies for IL-1, IL-2, IL-2R, IL-6, and TNF-α, and found no significant change in any of the cytokines or IL-2R with rejection (111). Although the expression of IL-2 and IL-2R in biopsies is not a specific marker for allograft rejection, the identification of lymphocytes expressing IL-2 and IL-2R in rejecting allografts demonstrates that these lymphocytes can be the source of the soluble IL-2 and IL-2R found in the peripheral blood of transplant recipients (80).

The expression of class II human leukocyte antigens is another potential activation marker. As outlined in Chaps. 1 and 2, the class II antigens HLA-DR, HLA-DP and HLA-DQ are normally expressed only on monocytes, macrophages, dendritic cells, B lymphocytes, and some endothelial cells (112). Class II antigen expression can be induced, however, in other cell types by γ-interferon (112). Thus, the expression of class II antigens by parenchymal and endothelial cells is a potential marker of immune activation in a biopsy (Fig. 3D). We examined 10 sets of bronchial epithelial biopsies obtained from 6 heart-lung–transplant recipients for the presence of induced class II antigen expression on bronchial epithelial cells and found induced class II antigen expression in 6 of these 10 biopsies (113). However, this expression of class II antigen was neither a sensitive nor a specific marker of lung allograft rejection (113). This lack of specificity of class II antigen expression is not surprising, because any inflammatory stimulus that results in the production of γ-interferon could potentially induce class II antigen expression (98).

The mechanism by which cytolytic cells kill their targets has recently been characterized, and several of the mediators of this process are specific markers for the functional activation of lymphocytes in allograft biopsies (114–116). For example, perforin is a potent cytolytic pore-forming protein expressed in cytoplasmic granules of functionally active cytolytic T lymphocytes (114–117). Perforin is released by cytolytic cells into the intercellular space adjacent to the target cells by granule exocytosis, and it kills target cells by a mechanism similar to that seen with the terminal components of the complement cascade. Perforin inserts itself into the target cell membrane and polymerizes to form a transmembrane pore (117). This pore has been demonstrated in the cell membranes of myocytes injured in myocarditits, and the pore results in the osmotic lysis of the target cell (117). The expression of perforin is highly regulated (118). Although resting lymphocytes contain little or no perforin, perforin expression can be rapidly induced by IL-2 stimulation (118). Perforin is, therefore, a specific marker for functionally active cytolytic lymphocytes. Perforin expression has been examined in animal models of allograft rejection and in human heart, lung, and kidney transplants; in general, it has proven to be a sensitive and specific marker of rejection (119–126). Griffiths et al. examined 29 endomyocardial biopsies obtained from 17 heart-transplant recipients for perforin expression using in situ hybridization and found that all of the biopsies obtained from patients with rejection contained perforin-expressing lymphocytes (122). Remarkably, perforin gene expression could be used to identify rejection before histological damage occurred to the graft (122). Six of the ten patients whose biopsies had lymphocytes that expressed perforin but lacked histological evidence of rejection went on to develop rejection in subsequent biopsies (122).

Thus, perforin expression appears to be a useful and potentially early marker for acute allograft rejection.

In addition to perforin, the cytoplasmic granules of cytolytic lymphocytes also contain granzymes. The granzymes belong to the serine protease family and, like perforin, they are released into the intercellular space by granule exocytosis upon effector-target cell interaction (119). Granzyme mRNA expression has been shown to peak just prior to maximum killing activity in an in vitro system (122). Granzyme-A and granzyme-B expression have been examined in heart, lung and kidney grafts and, like perforin, the expression of these serine proteases has been shown to correlate with rejection (111,119–122,126,127). Indeed, in most grafts that have been examined, the expression of the granzymes tends to parallel that of perforin (119–122,126,127). Markers of the functional activation of lymphocytes, such as perforin and the granzymes, are potentially highly specific markers of allograft rejection.

While the presence of functionally active lymphocytes in a graft appears to be a good marker for allograft rejection, significant damage to the graft could be prevented if the diagnosis of rejection could be established *before* the lymphocytes injure their target cells. Lymphocytes must bind to adhesion molecules expressed on graft endothelial cells before they can migrate into a graft. The expression of adhesion molecules therefore occurs before significant numbers of lymphocytes have entered the graft. One potential approach to the early diagnosis of rejection would be to look for the expression of these adhesion molecules. While some adhesion molecules, such as intercellular adhesion molecule-1 (CD54, ICAM-1), are probably constitutively expressed (128), others, like vascular cell adhesion molecule-1 (VCAM-1), are not expressed on resting endothelial cells and are induced by the immune-mediated activation of endothelial cells by IL-1 and TNF-α (52,110,128–130). Indeed, the induced expression of VCAM-1 on endothelial cells has been shown to precede leukocyte accumulation in an animal model of heart-allograft rejection (130). Similarly, Ferran et al. have demonstrated VCAM-1 expression on capillaries and postcapillary venules just prior to the development of rejection in human heart-allograft recipients (50). Thus, the expression of adhesion molecules such as VCAM-1 on endothelial cells has the potential of being a very *early* marker of allograft rejection.

Clearly, recent advances in our understanding of the mechanisms underlying humoral and cell-mediated rejection have contributed to the development of techniques that can aid in the interpretation of graft biopsies. These techniques may even reveal "impending" graft rejection, so that patients can be given augmented immunosuppression tailored to the specific type of the immune response before significant graft injury takes place. Unfortunately, since the rejection process has proven to be remarkably graft-specific, most of these techniques must be applied directly to biopsy tissue in order to be useful. Moreover, because of the many different pathways of immune-mediated injury, it is likely that evaluation of multiple parameters such as activation and adhesion molecules, phenotypic markers of infiltrating cells, and presence of soluble mediators such as complement, cytokines, and other factors will be necessary for the consistent and accurate characterization of the presence and prognosis of rejection reactions.

ACKNOWLEDGMENTS

The authors would like to thank Jane Ann Day and Amanda Schlott Lietman for their assistance with this manuscript and Donna Suresch for preparing the immunofluorescent sections. W.M.B. and F.S. are supported in part by grant R01 HL53245-01.

REFERENCES

1. Kissmeyer-Nielsen F, Olsen S, Petersen VP, Fjeldborg O. Hyperacute rejection of kidney allografts associated with pre-existing humoral antibodies against donor cells. Lancet 1962; 2:662–665.
2. Patel R, Terasaki PI. Significance of the positive crossmatch test in kidney transplantation. N Engl J Med 1969; 280:735–739.
3. Williams GM, Hume DM, Hudson RP, et al. "Hyperacute" renal-homograft rejection in man. N Engl J Med 1968; 279:611–618.
4. Halloran PF, Wadgymar A, Ritchie S, et al. The significance of the anti-class I response: I. Clinical and pathological features of anti-class I-mediated rejection. Transplantation 1990; 49:85–91.
5. Halloran PF, Schlaut J, Solez K, Srinivasa NS. The significance of the anti-class I response: II. Clinical and pathological features of renal transplants with anti-class I-like antibody. Transplantation 1992; 53:550–555.
6. Almond PS, Matas A, Gillingham K, et al. Risk factors for chronic rejection in renal allograft recipients. Transplantation 1993; 55:752–756.
7. Busch GJ, Reynolds ES, Galvanek EG, et al. Human renal allografts: The role of vascular injury in early graft failure. Medicine 1971; 50:29–83.
8. Scornik JC, LeFor WM, Cicciarelli JC, et al. Hyperacute and acute kidney graft rejection due to antibodies against B cells. Transplantation 1992; 54:61–64.
9. Mohanakumar T, Rhodes C, Mendez-Picon G, et al. Renal allograft rejection associated with presensitization to HLA-DR antigens. Transplantation 1981; 31:93–95.
10. Ahern AT, Artruc SB, Della Pelle P, et al. Hyperacute rejection of HLA-A, B-identical renal allografts associated with B lymphocyte and endothelial reactive antibodies. Transplantation 1982; 33:103–106.
11. Baldwin WM III, Pruitt SK, Sanfilippo F, Alloantibodies: Basic and clinical concepts. Transplant Rev 1991; 5:100–119.
12. Steen HB. Characteristics of flow cytometers. In: Melamed MR, Lindmo T, Mendelsohn ML, ed. Flow Cytometry and Sorting. New York: Wiley-Liss, 1990:11–25.
13. Svalander C, Nyberg G, Blohme I, et al. Acute early allograft failure and the C3/macrophage phenomenon. Transplant Proc 1993; 25:903–904.
14. Baldwin WM III, Pruitt SK, Brauer RB, Daha MR, Sanfilippo F. Complement in organ transplantation: contributions to inflammation, injury and rejection. Transplantation 1995; 59:797–808.
15. Baker PJ, Adler S, Yang Y, Couser WG. Complement activation by heat-killed human kidney cells: Formation, activity, and stabilization of cell-bound C3 convertases. J Immunol 1984; 133:877–881.
16. Seifert PS, Catalfamo JL, Dodds J. Complement activation after aortic endothelial injury. Semin Thromb Hemost 1986; 12:280–283.
17. Maroko PR, Carpenter CD, Chiariello M, et al. Reduction by cobra venom factor of myocardial necrosis after coronary artery occlusion. J Clin Invest 1987; 61:661–670.
18. Weisman HF, Bartow T, Leppo MK, et al. Soluble human complement receptor type 1: In vivo inhibitor of complement suppressing post-ischemic myocardial inflammation and necrosis. Science 1990; 249:146–151.
19. Linas SL, Whittenburg D, Parsons PE, Repine JE. Mild renal ischemia activates primed neutrophils to cause acute renal failure. Kidney Int. 1992; 42:610–616.
20. Pemberton M, Anderson G, Vetvicka V, et al. Microvascular effects of complement blockade with soluble recombinant CR1 on ischemia/reperfusion injury of skeletal muscle. J Immunol 1993; 150:5104–5113.
21. Seekamp A, Mulligan MS, Till GO, Ward PA, Requirements for neutrophil products and L-arginine in ischemia-reperfusion injury. Am J Pathol 1993; 142:1217–1226.

22. Peerschke EI, Reid KB, Ghebrehiwet B. Platelet activation by C1q results in the induction of alpha IIb/beta 3 integrins (GPIIb-IIIa) and the expression of P-selectin and procoagulant activity. J Exp Med 1993; 178:579–587.
23. Eggleton P, Ghebrehiwet B, Coburn JP, Sastry KN, Zaner KS, Tauber AI. Characterization of the human neutrophil C1q receptor and functional effects of free ligand on activated neutrophils. Blood 1994; 84(5):1640–1649.
24. Leu RW, Kriet D, Zhou A, et al. Reconstitution of murine resident peritoneal macrophages for antibody dependent cellular cytotoxicity by homologous serum C1q. Cell Immunol 1989 122:48–61.
25. Wahlin B, Perlmann H, Perlmann P, et al. C3 receptors on human lymphocyte subsets and recruitment of ADCC effector cells by C3 fragments. J Immunol 1983; 130:2831–2836.
26. Brauer RB, Baldwin WM III, Daha MR, et al. The use of C6-deficient rats to evaluate the mechanism of hyperacute rejection of discordant cardiac xenografts. J Immunol 1993; 151:7240–7248.
27. Ten RM, Gleich GJ, Holley KE, et al. Eosinophil granule major basic protein in acute renal allograft rejection. Transplantation 1989; 47:959–963.
28. Feucht HE, Felber E, Gokel MJ, et al. Vascular deposition of complement-split products in kidney allografts with cell-mediated rejection. Clin Exp Immunol 1991; 86:464–470.
29. Feucht HE, Schneeberger H, Hillebrand G, et al. Capillary deposition of C4d complement fragment and early renal graft loss. Kidney Int 1993; 43:1333–1338.
30. Peters M, Ambrus JL Jr, Fauci A, Brown E. The Bb fragment of complement factor B acts as a B cell growth factor. J Exp Med 1988; 168:1225–1235.
31. Sun J, McCaughan GW, Matsumoto Y, et al. Tolerance to rat liver allografts: I. Differences between tolerance and rejection are more marked in the B cell compared with the T cell or cytokine response. Transplantation 1994; 57:1349–1357.
32. Bitter-Suermann D. The anaphylatoxins. In: Rother K, Till GO, ed. The Complement System. New York: Springer-Verlag, 1988:367–384.
33. Morgan BP. Complement: Clinical Aspects and Relevance to Disease. New York: Academic Press, 1990:36–56.
34. Murphy HS, Shayman JA, Till GO, et al. Superoxide responses of endothelial cells to C5a and TNF-alpha. Divergent signal transduction pathways. Am J Physiol 1992; 263:L51–59.
35. Platt JL, Dalmasso AP, Lindman BJ, et al. The role of C5a and antibody in the release of heparan sulfate from endothelial cells. Eur J Immunol 1991; 21:2887–2890.
36. Carson SD, Johnson DR. Consecutive enzyme cascades: Complement activation at the cell surface triggers increased tissue factor activity. Blood 1990; 76:361–367.
37. Gulbins E, Schlottmann K, Rauterberg EW, Steinhausen M. Effects of rC5a on the circulation of normal and split hydronephrotic rat kidneys. Am J Physiol 1993; 265:F96–103.
38. Barton PA, Warren JS. Complement component C5 modulates the systemic tumor necrosis factor response in murine endotoxic shock. Infect Immun 1993; 61:1474–1481.
39. Morgan EL, Ember JA, Sanderson SD, et al. Anti-C5a receptor antibodies: Characterization of neutralizing antibodies specific for a peptide, C5aR-(9-29), derived from the predicted amino-terminal sequence of the human C5a receptor. J Immunol 1993; 151:377–388.
40. Arnaout MA, Spits H, Terhorst C, et al. Deficiency of a leukocyte surface glycoprotein (LFA-1) in two patients with Mo1 deficiency: Effects of cell activation of Mo1/LFA-1 surface expression in normal and deficient leukocytes. J Clin Invest 1984; 74:1291–1300.
41. Fearon DT, Collins LA. Increased expression of C3b receptors on polymorphonuclear leukocytes induced by chemotactic factors and by purification procedures. J Immunol 1983; 130:370–375.
42. Adams DH, Wang LF, Burnett D, et al. Neutrophil activation—An important cause of tissue damage during liver allograft rejection? Transplantation 1990; 50:86–91.
43. Rosen H, Law SK. The leukocyte cell surface receptor(s) for the iC3b product of complement. Curr Top Microbiol Immunol 1990; 153:99–122.

44. Diamond MS, Garcia-Aguilar J, Bickford JK, et al. The I domain is a major recognition site on the leukocyte integrin Mac-1 (CD11b/CD18) for four distinct adhesion ligands. J Cell Biol 1993; 120:1031–1043.
45. Diamond MS, Staunton DE, Marlin SD, Springer TA. Binding of the integrin Mac-1 (CD11b/CD18) to the third immunoglobulin-like domain of ICAM-1 (CD54) and its regulation by glycosylation. Cell 1991; 65:961–971.
46. Bishop GA, Hall BM. Expression of leukocyte and lymphocyte adhesion molecules in the human kidney. Kidney Int 1989; 36:1078–1085.
47. Cosimi AB, Conti D, Delmonico FL, et al. In vivo effects of monoclonal antibody to ICAM-1 (CD54) in nonhuman primates with renal allografts. J Immunol 1990; 144:4604–4612.
48. Taylor PM, Rose ML, Yacoub MH, Pigott R. Induction of vascular adhesion molecules during rejection of human cardiac allografts. Transplantation 1992; 54:451–457.
49. Brockmeyer C, Ulbrecht M, Schendel DJ, et al. Distribution of cell adhesion molecules (ICAM-1, VCAM-1, ELAM-1) in renal tissue during allograft rejection. Transplantation 1993; 55:610–615.
50. Ferran C, Peuchmaur M, Desruennes M, et al. Implications of de novo ELAM-1 and VCAM-1 expression in human cardiac allograft rejection. Transplantation 1993; 55:605–609.
51. Fuggle SV, Sanderson JB, Gray DW, et al. Variation in expression of endothelial adhesion molecules in pretransplant and transplanted kidneys—Correlation with intragraft events. Transplantation 1993; 55:117–123.
52. Hancock WW, Whitley WD, Tullius SG, et al. Cytokines, adhesion molecules, and the pathogenesis of chronic rejection of rat renal allografts. Transplantation 1993; 56:643–650.
53. Koskinen PK. The association of the induction of vascular cell adhesion molecule-1 with cytomegalovirus antigenemia in human heart allografts. Transplantation 1993; 56:1103–1108.
54. van de Winkel JG, Capel PJ. Human IgGFc receptor heterogeneity: Molecular aspects and clinical implications. Immunol Today 1993; 14:215–221.
55. Symer DE, Paznekas WA, Shin HS. A requirement for membrane-associated phospholipase A2 in platelet cytotoxicity activated by receptors for immunoglobulin G and complement. J Exp Med 1993; 177:937–947.
56. Tilney NL, Kupiec-Weglinski JW, Heidecke CD, et al. Mechanisms of rejection and prolongation of vascularized organ allografts. Immunol Rev 1984; 77:185–216.
57. Häyry P, von Willebrand E, Parthenais E, et al. The inflammatory mechanisms of allograft rejection. Immunol Rev 1984; 77:85–142.
58. Wijngaard PLJ, Tuijnman WB, Meyling FHJG, et al. Endomyocardial biopsies after heart transplantation: The presence of markers indicative of activation. Transplantation 1993; 55:103–110.
59. Brauer RB, Baldwin WM III, Sanfilippo F. Evidence that terminal complement components contribute to acute allograft rejection. Transplantation 1995; 59:288–293.
60. Morgan BP. Effects of the membrane attack complex of complement on nucleated cells. Curr Top Microbiol Immunol 1992; 178:115–140.
61. Benzaquen LR, Nicholson-Weller A, Halperin JA. Terminal complement proteins C5b-9 release basic fibroblast growth factor and platelet-derived growth factor from endothelial cells. J Exp Med 1994; 179:985–992.
62. Halperin JA, Taratuska A, Nicholson-Weller A. Terminal complement complex C5b-9 stimulates mitogenesis in 3T3 cells. J Clin Invest 1993; 91:1974–1978.
63. Hattori R, Hamilton KK, McEver RP, Sims PJ. Complement proteins C5b-9 induce secretion of high molecular weight multimers of endothelial von Willebrand factor and translocation of granule membrane protein GMP-140 to the cell surface. J Biol Chem 1989; 264:9053–9060.
64. Hamilton KK, Hattori R, Esmon CT, Sims PJ. Complement proteins C5b-9 induce vesiculation of the endothelial plasma membrane and expose catalytic surface for assembly of the prothrombinase enzyme complex. J Biol Chem 1990; 265:3809–3814.
65. Schulick RD, Muluk SC, Clerici M, et al. Value of in vitro CD4+ T helper cell function test for predicting long-term loss of human renal allografts. Transplantation 1994; 57:480–482.

66. Muluk SC, Clerici M, Via CS, et al. Correlation of in vitro CD4+ T helper cell function with clinical graft status in immunosuppressed kidney transplant recipients. Transplantation 1991; 52:284–291.
67. Fieguth HG, Haverich A, Schaefers HJ, et al. Cytoimmunologic monitoring for the noninvasive diagnosis of cardiac rejection. Transplant Proc 1987; 19:2541–2542.
68. Wijngaard PLJ, van der Meulen A, Schuurman H-J, et al. Cytoimmunologic monitoring for the diagnosis of acute rejection after heart transplantation. Transplant Proc 1989; 21:2521–2522.
69. Schübel C, Caca K, Dirschedl P, et al. Reliability of cytoimmunological monitoring after heart transplantation by consensus measurement: A multicenter study. Transplant Proc 1990; 22:2317–2318.
70. Kemkes BM, Schütz A, Engelhardt M, et al. Noninvasive methods of rejection diagnosis after heart transplantation. J Heart Lung Transplant 1992; 11:S221–S231.
71. Hammer C, Klanke D, Lersch C, et al. Cytoimmunologic monitoring (CIM) for differentiation between cardiac rejection and viral, bacterial, or fungal infection: Its specificity and sensitivity. Transplant Proc 1989; 21:3631–3633.
72. Hammer C, Reichenspurner H, Klima G. Immunologic parameters for the diagnosis of graft rejection. Transplant Proc 1993; 25:26–29.
73. Jutte NHPM, Daane R, van den Bemd JMG, et al. Cytoimmunological monitoring to detect rejection after heart transplantation. Transplant Proc 1989; 21:2519–2520.
74. May RM, Cooper DKC, Du Toit ED, Reichart B. Cytoimmunologic monitoring after heart and heart-lung transplantation. J Heart Transplant 1990; 9:133–135.
75. Zucchelli GC, Clerico A, De Maria R, et al. Increased circulating concentrations of inter leukin-2 receptor during rejection episodes in heart- or kidney-transplant recipients. Clin Chem 1990; 36:2106–2109.
76. McNally CM, Luckhurst E, Penny R. Cell free serum interleukin-2 receptor levels after heart transplantation. J Heart Lung Transplant 1991; 10:769–774.
77. Coles M, Rose M, Yacoub M. Appearance of cells bearing the interleukin-2 receptor in peripheral blood of cardiac transplant patients and their correlation with rejection episodes. Transplant Proc 1987; 19:2546–2547.
78. Roodman ST, Miller LW, Tsai CC. Role of interleukin-2 receptors in immunologic monitoring following cardiac transplantation. Transplantation 1988; 45:1050–1056.
79. Jordan SC, Marchevski A, Ross D, et al. Serum interleukin-2 levels in lung transplant recipients: correlation with findings on transbronchial biopsy. J Heart Lung Transplant 1992; 11:1001–1004.
80. Simpson MA, Madras PN, Cornaby AJ, et al. Sequential determinations of urinary cytology and plasma and urinary lymphokines in the management of renal allograft recipients. Transplantation 1989; 47:218–223.
81. Simpson MA, Madras PN, Cornaby AJ, et al. Origin of elevated IL-2 and IL-2R in the urine of rejecting renal allograft recipients. Transplant Proc 1989; 21:299–300.
82. Young JB, Lloyd KS, Windsor NT, et al. Elevated soluble interleukin-2 receptor levels early after heart transplantation and long-term survival and development of coronary arteriopathy. J Heart Lung Transplant 1991; 10:243–250.
83. Perkins JD, Nelson DL, Rakela J, et al. Soluble interleukin-2 receptor level as an indicator of liver allograft rejection. Transplantation 1989; 47:77–81.
84. De Maria R, Zucchelli GC, Masini S, et al. Nonspecific increase of interleukin-2 receptor serum levels during immune events in heart transplantation. Transplant Proc 1989; 21: 440–441.
85. Molajoni ER, Bachetoni A, Cinti P, et al. Relevance of immunological parameters to detect allograft rejection in heart transplant recipients. Transplant Proc 1989; 21:2534–2536.
86. Holzinger C, Zuckermann A, Laczkovics A, et al. Monitoring of mononuclear cell subsets isolated from the coronary sinus and the right atrium in patients after heart allograft transplantation. J Thorac Cardiovasc Surg 1991; 102:215–223.

87. Eidelman FJ, Guttmann RD. Serial monitoring of peripheral blood lymphocyte subsets in cardiac allograft rejection in the rat. Transplantation 1989; 47:1079–1081.
88. Reader JA, Burke MM, Counihan P, et al. Noninvasive monitoring of human cardiac allograft rejection. Transplantation 1990; 50:29–33.
89. DeBruyne LA, Ensley RD, Olsen SL, et al. Increased frequency of alloantigen-reactive helper T lymphocytes is associated with human cardiac allograft rejection. Transplantation 1993; 56:722–727.
90. Rabinowich H, Zeevi A, Paradis IL, et al. Proliferative responses of bronchoalveolar lavage lymphocytes from heart-lung transplant patients. Transplantation 1990; 49:115–121.
91. Reinsmoen NL, Bolman RM, Savik K, et al. Are multiple immunopathogenetic events occurring during the development of obliterative bronchiolitis and acute rejection? Transplantation 1993; 55:1040–1044.
92. Ibrahim S, Dawson DV, Van Trigt P, Sanfilippo F. Differential infiltration by CD45RO and CD45RA subsets of T cells associated with human heart allograft rejection. Am J Pathol 1993; 142:1794–1803.
93. Malinowski K, Waltzer WC, Jao S, et al. Homing of CD8CD57 T lymphocytes into acutely rejected renal allografts. Transplantation 1992; 54:1013–1017.
94. Suitters AJ, Rose ML, Dominguez MJ, Yacoub MH. Selection for donor-specific cytotoxic T lymphocytes within the allografted human heart. Transplantation 1990; 49:1105–1109.
95. Vaessen LMB, Baan CC, Ouwehand AJ, et al. Acute rejection in heart transplant patients is associated with the presence of committed donor-specific cytotoxic lymphocytes in the graft but not in the blood. Clin Exp Immunol 1992; 88:213–219.
96. Tazelaar HD, Edwards WD. Pathology of cardiac transplantation: Recipient hearts (chronic heart failure) and donor hearts (acute and chronic rejection). Mayo Clin Proc 1992; 67: 685–696.
97. Bishop DK, Shelby J, Eichwald EJ. Mobilization of T lymphocytes following cardiac transplantation. Transplantation 1992; 53:849–857.
98. de Blic J, Peuchmaur M, Carnot F, et al. Rejection in lung transplantation—An immunohistochemical study of transbronchial biopsies. Transplantation 1992; 54:639–644.
99. Brousse N, Canioni D, Rambaud C, et al. Intestinal transplantation in children: Contribution of immunohistochemistry. Transplant Proc 1990; 22:2495–2496.
100. deLourdes Higuchi M, de Assis RVC, Sambiase NV, et al. Usefulness of T-cell phenotype characterization in endomyocardial biopsy fragments from human cardiac allografts. J Heart Lung Transplant 1991; 10:235–242.
101. Trentin L, Zambello R, Faggian G, et al. Phenotypic and functional characterization of cytotoxic cells derived from endomyocardial biopsies in human cardiac allografts. Cell Immunol 1992; 141:332–341.
102. Hoshinaga K, Mohanakumar T, Goldman MH, et al. Clinical significance of in situ detection of T lymphocyte subsets and monocyte/macrophage lineages in heart allografts. Transplantation 1984; 38:634–637.
103. Platt JL, LeBien TW, Michael AF. Interstitial mononuclear cell population in renal graft rejection: Identification by monoclonal antibodies in tissue sections. J Exp Med 1982; 155: 17–30.
104. Sanfilippo F, Kolbeck PC, Vaughn WK, Bollinger RR. Renal allograft cell infiltrates associated with irreversible rejection. Transplantation 1985; 40:679–685.
105. Hruban RH, Beschorner WE, Baumgartner WA, et al. Diagnosis of lung allograft rejection by bronchial intraepithelial Leu-7 positive T lymphocytes. J Thorac Cardiovasc Surg 1988; 96: 939–946.
106. Beschorner WE, Burdick JF, Williams GM, Solez K. The presence of Leu 7 reactive lymphocytes in renal allograft undergoing acute rejection. Transplant Proc 1985; 17:618–622.
107. Ibrahim S, Dawson DV, Killenberg PG, Sanfilippo F. The pattern and phenotype of T-cell infiltration associated with human liver allograft rejection. Hum Pathol 1993; 24:1365–1370.

108. Ibrahim S, Dawson DV, Sanfilippo, F. Predominant infiltration of rejecting human renal allografts with T cells expressing CD8 and CD45RO. Transplantation 1995; 59:724–728.
109. Noronha IL, Eberlein-Gonska M, Hartley B, et al. In situ expression of tumor necrosis factor-α, interferon-γ, and interleukin-2 receptors in renal allograft biopsies. Transplantation 1992; 54:1017–1024.
110. Ruan X-M, Qiao J-H, Trento A, et al. Cytokine expression and endothelial cell and lymphocyte activation in human cardiac allograft rejection: an immunohistochemical study of endomyocardial biopsy samples. J Heart Lung Transplant 1992; 11:1110–1116.
111. Lipman ML, Stevens AC, Bleackley RC, et al. The strong correlation of cytotoxic T lymphocyte-specific serine protease gene transcripts with renal allograft rejection. Transplantation 1992; 53:73–79.
112. Chandler C, Passaro E Jr. Transplant rejection: Mechanisms and treatment. Arch Surg 1993; 128:279–283.
113. Hruban RH, Beschorner WE, Baumgartner WA, et al. Evidence that the expression of class II MHC antigens is not diagnostic of lung allograft rejection. Transplantation 1989; 48:529–530.
114. Fox WM III, Hruban RH, Hameed A, Hutchins GM. Perforin. CorNotes 1992; 7:10.
115. Fox WM III, Hameed A, Hutchins GM, et al. Perforin expression localizing cytotoxic lymphocytes in the intimas of coronary arteries with transplant-related accelerated arteriosclerosis. Hum Pathol 1993; 24:477–482.
116. Hameed A, Olsen KJ, Cheng L, et al. Immunohistochemical identification of cytotoxic lymphocytes using human perforin monoclonal antibody. Am J Pathol 1992; 140:1025–1030.
117. Young LHY, Joag SV, Zheng LM, et al. Perforin-mediated myocardial damage in acute myocarditis. Lancet 1990; 336:1019–1021.
118. Smyth MJ, Ortaldo JR, Shinkai Y-I, et al. Interleukin-2 induction of pore-forming protein gene expression in human peripheral blood CD8+ T cells. J Exp Med 1990; 171:1269–1281.
119. Clément MV, Haddad P, Soulié A, et al. Perforin and granzyme B as markers for acute rejection in heart transplantation. Int Immunol 1991; 3:1175–1181.
120. Clément MV, Soulié A, Legros-Maida S, et al. Perforin and granzyme B: Predictive markers for acute GVHD or cardiac rejection after bone marrow or heart transplantation. Nouv Rev Fr Hematol 1991; 33:463–470.
121. Clément MV, Maïda SL, Israël-Biet D, et al. Perforin and granzyme B expression is associated with severe acute rejection. Transplantation 1994; 57:322–326.
122. Griffiths GM, Namikawa R, Mueller C, et al. Granzyme A and perforin as markers for rejection in cardiac transplantation. Eur J Immunol 1991; 21:687–692.
123. Kataoka K, Naomoto Y, Shiozaki S, et al. Infiltration of perforin-positive mononuclear cells into the rejected kidney allograft. Transplantation 1992; 53:240–242.
124. Matsuno T, Sakagami K, Saito S, et al. Does perforin mediate the direct injury of renal allograft in acute rejection? Transplant Proc 1993; 25:879–880.
125. Matsuno T, Sakagami K, Saito S, et al. Expression of intercellular adhesion molecule-1 and perforin in kidney allograft rejection. Transplant Proc 1992; 24:1306–1307.
126. Mueller C, Shao Y, Altermatt HJ, et al. The effect of cyclosporine treatment on the expression of genes encoding granzyme A and perforin in the infiltrate of mouse heart transplants. Transplantation 1993; 55:139–145.
127. Mueller C, Shelby J, Weissman IL, et al. Expression of the protease gene HF as a marker in rejecting allogenic murine heart transplants. Transplantation 1991; 51:514–517.
128. Carlos T, Gordon D, Fishbein D, et al. Vascular cell adhesion molecule-1 is induced on endothelium during acute rejection in human cardiac allografts. J Heart Lung Transpl 1992; 11:1103–1109.
129. Pelletier RP, Morgan CJ, Sedmak DD, et al. Analysis of inflammatory endothelial changes, including VCAM-1 expression, in murine cardiac grafts. Transplantation 1993; 55:315–320.
130. Tanaka H, Sukhova GK, Swanson SJ, et al. Endothelial and smooth muscle cells express leukocyte adhesion molecules heterogeneously during acute rejection of rabbit cardiac allografts. Am J Pathol 1994; 144:938–951.

4

Molecular Biology of Chronic Rejection and Predictive Value of Biopsies

Pekka Häyry, Serdar Yilmaz, Karl Lemström, Petri Koskinen, Anne Räisänen-Sokolowski, Ari Mennander, Leena Krogerus, Eero Taskinen, Timo Paavonen, Marjukka Myllärniemi, Erkki Kallio, Elnari Aavik, and Sointu Alatalo
University of Helsinki, Helsinki, Finland

Helena Isoniemi
Helsinki University Central Hospital, Helsinki, Finland

I. INTRODUCTION

Regardless of the dramatic progress in short-term results of organ transplantation, the half-life of the transplants after the first year has not improved (1). This is illustrated in Fig. 1, which is based on the results of the Batelle-Seattle Research Center National Cooperative Transplant Study, 1991 (2).

The half-life of the first cadaveric kidney transplants in the United States has been approximately 7.5 years since 1977, and it was not altered after the introduction of cyclosporine. Although the short-term results in genetically more homogeneous populations, such as that of Finland, are approximately 10% units higher than the U.S. average, the half-life is only marginally better: 8.5 years.

Another interesting feature deriving from Fig. 1 is that the short half-life after the first year is predominantly a problem in kidney transplants; in heart transplants, the half-life is approximately 11 years; in adult liver transplants, it is even longer, 17 years. The longest half-life to our knowledge is in pediatric liver transplants: more than 30 years.

II. INCIDENCE, MANIFESTATIONS, AND RISK FACTORS FOR CHRONIC REJECTION

A. Incidence of Chronic Rejection in Organ Transplants

Several lines of evidence indicate that chronic allograft rejection is a prime contributing factor to less satisfactory long-term allograft survival and the largest single reason for late graft loss. A recent prospective study in Helsinki, employing protocol core biopsies,

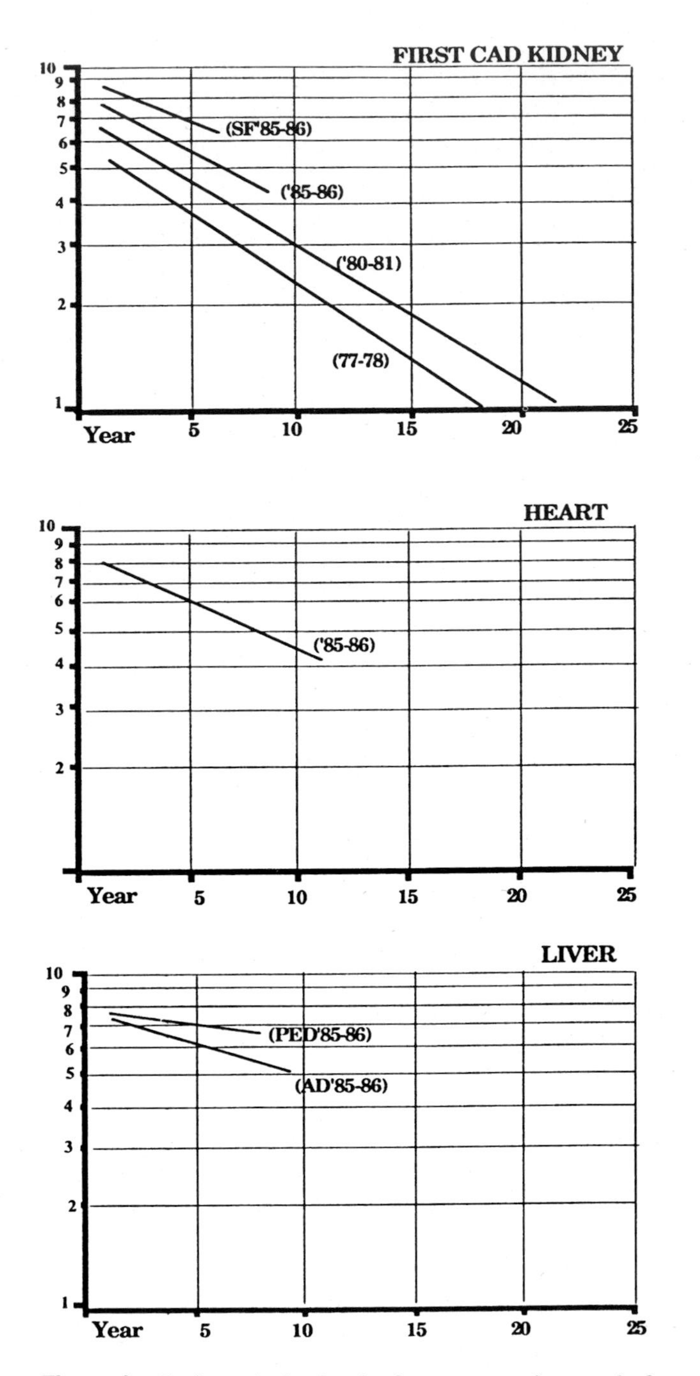

Figure 1 Graft survivals after the first postoperative year in first cadaveric kidney, heart, and liver allografts. Years in parentheses indicate the time period when the transplants were performed. SF's 85–86 indicates first cadaveric kidney allografts in Finland performed during 1985–86; the remainder of the graphic is based on the Seattle Batelle Transplant Study (2).

demonstrated incipient (though mostly mild) histological changes of chronic rejection in approximately 50% of cadaveric renal transplants at 2 years (3,4). Also, transplants with normal or near-normal function displayed such changes (3,4). A second study, performed independently in Uppsala, demonstrated similar chronic histopathological alterations in 40% of kidney allografts by 6 months after transplantation (5).

Cardiac allograft arteriosclerosis is the main cause of death after the first posttransplant year. On coronary angiography, the incidence of coronary arteriosclerosis is 6 to 18% at 1 year, 23% at 2 years and up to 50% at 5 years (6,7). Moreover, comparisons between autopsy histopathology and angiographic studies indicate that there is an underestimation of this disorder in angiography (8).

Liver is evidently the least sensitive organ to chronic rejection: slowly declining liver transplant function, associated in biopsy with the "vanishing bile duct" syndrome, affects only 10% of all liver transplants (9–11). On the other hand, chronic rejection is a major indication for liver retransplantation.

As the half-life of these organs has not changed since the introduction of cyclosporine, it appears that the current therapeutic modalities are not sufficient to prevent chronic rejection. Therefore, major emphasis is on several lines of research to develop drugs and procedures that will prevent and/or stop the progression of this disorder.

B. Common and Organ-Specific Features in Morphological Pathology of Acute and Chronic Rejection

The conspicious histological feature of acute rejection in all organs is the infiltration by mononuclear leukocytes together with evidence of tissue destruction.

The Banff classification (12) of human renal allograft rejection grades acute rejection as "mild" if only focal or moderate tubulitis is present, "moderate" is there is significant interstitial infiltration with several foci of inflammation and/or severe tubulitis and/or mild or moderate intimal arteritis, and "severe" if severe intimal arteritis and/or transmural arteritis with fibrinoid damage and necrosis of medial smooth muscle cells is present.

The ISHLT classification (13) for acute heart allograft rejection classifies rejection "mild" if focal or diffuse perivascular or interstitial infiltrates are present without evidence of myocyte necrosis, "moderate" if the infiltration is more aggressive and focal myocyte damage is present, and "severe" if the infiltrate consists also of polymorphs and there is evidence of edema, hemorrhage, vasculitis, and widespread myocyte necrosis.

Three grading systems for acute liver allograft rejection (14)—the National Institute of Diabetes and Digestive and Kidney Disease (NIDDK), Minnesota, and "European" systems—consider rejection "mild" if inflammatory infiltrate is present in some but not all of the triads and is confined within portal spaces; "moderate" if the infiltrate involves all of the triads with or without spillover into the lobule but without evidence of centrilobular hepatocyte necrosis, ballooning, or drop-out; and "severe" when the inflammatory infiltrate is present in all of the triads and there is evidence of arteritis, paucity of bile ducts, or central hepatocellular ballooning with confluent dropout of hepatocytes.

Thus the intensity of inflammation, the extent of tissue damage, and, particularly, the extent of vascular involvement indicate increasing severity of the acute episode.

The histopathology of chronic rejection is entirely different (15–17). As in acute rejection, the different organs share common features and display organ-specific manifestations.

The common denominator for chronic rejection in all organs (Table 1) is persistent focal, often perivascular inflammation that is associated with focal myocyte necrosis in the

Table 1 Histopathology of Chronic Rejection in Different Organs

Heart	Kidney	Liver
Inflammation	Inflammation	Inflammation
Arteriosclerosis	Arteriosclerosis	Arteriosclerosis
Fibrosis	Glomerular basal membrane thickening and sclerosis	Hepatocellular ballooning
		Vanishing bile ducts
	Tubular atrophy	Giant cell transformation
	Fibrosis	Fibrosis

Sources: Refs. 15–17

media; occasional breaks in internal elastic lamina; and concentric, generalized intimal thickening (18) or "allograft arteriosclerosis" (19).

The most conspicious organ-specific feature in the heart is widespread fibrosis between the myocytes. The kidney displays glomerular mesangial cell proliferation, glomerular sclerosis, tubular atrophy, and fibrosis. In the liver, the organ-specific features are vanishing bile ducts, hepatocellular ballooning, giant cell transformation, and fibrosis.

Thus, whereas in acute rejection the histopathology is "lytic," the overall picture in chronic rejection is "proliferative."

C. Risk Factors for Chronic Rejection

Considering the common manifestations of chronic rejection in all organs, persistent focal perivascular inflammation (often with a fairly low activation level of lymphoid cells) and concentric, generalized intimal thickening (18), a hypothesis has been put forward that these changes result from continuous low-level trauma to the vascular endothelium which, in turn, responds by synthesis of growth factors, leading to smooth muscle cell replication and intimal thickening (19,20).

Several lines of clinical evidence support this hypothesis (Table 2).

The initiating event in allograft arteriosclerosis is most likely immunological, as both histoincompatibility (21,22) and—by far the most important—the frequency of acute rejection episodes (23–27) are prime risk factors for development of chronic rejection. The impact of acute rejection is more clear in genetically heterogeneous populations (e.g., that of the United States) (24–29) than in genetically homogeneous populations (e.g., that of Finland) (28). In addition, other peri- and postoperative damage may contribute to endothelial trauma. Long cold ischemia time (29) and high and low donor-recipient age (30) are risk factors for chronic rejection. Long ischemia time may contribute via increased reperfusion injury. On the other hand, in transplants deriving from elderly donors, some of these manifestations may already be present. Cytomegalovirus (CMV) infection is a known risk factor in heart and liver transplants (31,32), and the vascular wall seems to be a target for CMV infection. Hyperlipidemia has been reported as a risk factor for chronic allograft rejection (28); hyperlipidemia is also a risk factor in common atherosclerosis.

Once the trauma has been initiated, it may become independent of the immune response and other contributing factors, and a vicious circle is induced. Retransplantation

Table 2 Risk Factors for Chronic Rejection

Risk factor	References
Frequency and intensity of acute rejection episodes	23–27
Histoincompatibility	21, 22
Long cold ischemia time	29
Low and high donor-recipient age	30
Hyperlipidemia	28
Cytomegalovirus infection (heart, liver)	31, 32
Hypertension?	35
Diabetes mellitus?	28
Inadequate immunosuppression—noncompliance	24, 26
Contributing Factors	
Decrease of renal mass and intraglomerular hemodynamic factors	34

of a rat kidney allograft back to donor strain, if it is performed prior to the appearance of the arteriosclerotic manifestations, prevents the development of chronic vascular rejection (33). On the other hand, if the transplantation is performed after the arteriosclerotic manifestations have appeared, the disorder seems to progress (33).

Also other factors, such as transplant hemodynamics, contribute. Once the initial trauma has occurred, there is a gradual decrease of renal mass and increase in intraglomerular pressure, both of which contribute to glomerular pathology (34). This may also be the reason why the kidneys of very young donors do less well than adult kidneys (30).

III. EXPERIMENTAL EVIDENCE FOR ACUTE REJECTION LEADING TO CHRONIC REJECTION

Numerical quantitation of rejection episodes, upon which the current clinical evidence is based, does not take into account the intensity and length of the episodes, both of which may contribute to the severity of chronic rejection. We have recently proposed a single numerical parameter for the frequency, intensity, and length of acute rejections, the area under the serum creatinine versus time curve (AUC_{cre}), and tested the validity of this parameter in an experimental study with renal transplants between inbred rat strains.

Renal transplants were performed from DA (Ag-B4, $RT1^a$) to WF (Ag-B2, $RT1^v$) strains. The rats were immunosuppressed subcutaneously with 5 mg/kg body weight of cyclosporine A (CyA) for 1, 2, 3, and 12 weeks, resulting in different numbers (0 to 4) of biopsy-confirmed acute rejections with different intensities (s-cre: 100 μmol/L to 448 μmol/L) and length (3 to 24 days), all of which were reversible with additional CyA treatment. The intensity of chronic changes in graft histology was quantitated as a chronic allograft damage index (CADI) (see below), and the endpoint of transplant function as the level of serum creatinine at sacrifice.

AUC_{cre} from 1 to 3 weeks (AUC_{cre} 1–3), describing the recovery period from the operation with no rejections, did not correlate to CADI ($r = 0.230$, $p = 0.249$; Fig. 2). All

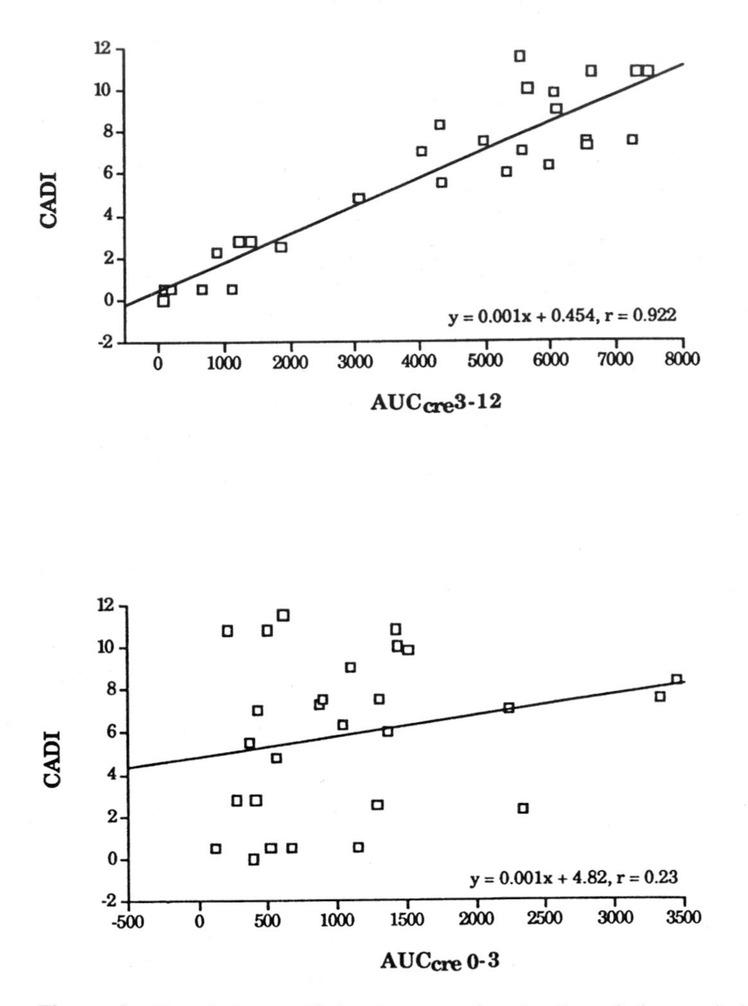

Figure 2 Correlation coefficient between chronic allograft damage index (CADI) and area under the curve of serum creatinine (AUC_{cre}) at 0 to 3 weeks and 3 to 12 weeks posttransplantation of DA kidneys to WF recipients. See text for details.

AUC_{cre} from the third week onward correlated with CADI. The best correlation to CADI was obtained with AUC_{cre} from 3 to 12 weeks (AUC_{cre} 3–12; $r = 0.922$, $p = 0.0001$), which covered the time period of all acute rejection episodes. AUC_{cre} 3–12 correlated equally well to endpoint transplant function ($r = 0.89$, $p = 0.0001$). The correlations of AUC_{cre} 3–12 to CADI and to endpoint transplant function were better than correlations of the number of acute rejections to CADI ($r = 0.876$, $p = 0.0001$) and to endpoint transplant function ($r = 0.811$, $p = 0.0001$), indicating that AUC_{cre} 3–12 is a more sensitive parameter than the number of acute rejections to predict chronic rejection (Table 3). Thus the results also indicate that there is, indeed, a causal relationship between acute and chronic rejection and that not only the frequency but also the intensity and length of acute rejections contribute to chronic rejection. Indirectly, these results suggest that acute trauma leading to chronic rejection may be reduced by aggressive treatment of acute rejection.

Table 3 Correlations Between AUC_{cre} 3–12 and the Number of Rejections to CADI and to Endpoint Serum Creatinine

	Correlation coefficient		
	r	r^2	p value
AUC_{cre} 3–12 vs. CADI	0.922	0.851	0.0001
No. of rejection episodes vs. CADI	0.876	0.767	0.0001
AUC_{cre} 3–12 vs. endpoint serum creatinine	0.89	0.793	0.0001
No. of rejection episodes vs. endpoint serum creatinine	0.811	0.657	0.0001

IV. BIOLOGY OF VASCULAR SMOOTH MUSCLE CELLS IN ALLOGRAFT ARTERIOSCLEROSIS (CHRONIC REJECTION)

A. Vascular Smooth Muscle Cell Biology in Classic Atherosclerosis and in Transplant Arteriosclerosis

Assuming that the initiating event for allograft arteriosclerosis (chronic rejection) is peri- and postoperative trauma and the driving force persistent perivascular inflammation, the following question arises: How do these events regulate smooth muscle cell replication in the vascular wall?

For reasons linked with classic athreosclerosis and because of issues such as coronary artery ballooning reinjury, the subject of smooth muscle cell biology has been under intensive investigation for more than a decade. This information has been summarized in recent reviews by Ross (36,37) and Thyberg et al. (38) and may be abbreviated as follows:

Smooth muscle cells exist in two phenotypes, the "synthetic" phenotype prevalent in embryonic and young, growing organisms and the "contractile" phenotype, prevalent in adult arterial wall. During atherogenesis, there is a phenotypic change from contractile to synthetic. Only the synthetic phenotype of smooth muscle cell is able to replicate.

A whole number of factors, induced by initial endothelial trauma, have been linked with proliferative behavior of smooth muscle cells in classic atherosclerosis. These have recently been reviewed by Ross (36). Some of these are products of the endothelial cells, like platelet-derived growth factor (PDGF), basic fibroblast growth factor (bFGF), transforming growth factor–beta (TGF-β), insulinlike growth factor 1 (IGF-1) as well as interleukin-1 (IL-1), prostaglandin (PGI_2), nitric oxide, and oxidized low-density lipoproteins (oxLDL). Some of these factors derive from inflammatory T cells, especially if they are in an activated state, like gamma interferon (IFN-γ), TGF-β, and tumor necrosis factor-alpha (TNF-α). Platelets deposited along the vascular wall contribute by producing PDGF, epidermal growth factor/transforming growth factor alpha (EGF/TGF-α), TGF-β, IGF-1 and thromboxane-A_2 (TX-A_2). A whole wealth of these factors derive from inflammatory macrophages, which are often closely associated anatomically with the replicating smooth muscle cells. Activated macrophages produce particularly PDGF, bFGF, EGF/TGF-α, TGF-β, TNF-α, IL-1, PGI_2, Tx-A_2 and oxLDL. In addition, smooth muscle cells themselves can produce many of these factors—such as bFGF, IGF-1, IL-1, TGF-β, and EGF/TNF-α—and are able to stimulate themselves via autocrine or paracrine pathways. In addition, they produce myeloid colony stimulating factor (M-CSF), monocyte chemotactic protein-1 (MCP-1), and granulocyte-monocyte colony-stimulating factor (GM-CSF). They also induce the synthesis of collagen, elastic fibers, and proteoglycans, which are proproliferative.

It is a general belief, although not always formally documented, that similar molecular cascades as in classic atherosclerosis, operate also in allograft arteriosclerosis. In the allograft, the situation is, however, more complex, as the initial trauma may be more complex in nature than simple mechanical stress associated with lipid deposits, and as the inflammatory cells in adventitia provide additional molecules, such as IL-2 and IFN-γ, which stimulate inflammatory leukocytes and induce the expression of adhesion molecules on microvascular endothelium.

Thus, taken together, three molecular cascades are most likely operational in allograft arteriosclerosis: (a) cytokines deriving from the inflammatory leukocytes and/or occasionally from the parenchymal cells themselves; (b) lipid mediators of inflammation (eicosanoids and platelet activating factor) deriving particularly from inflammatory macrophages but also from parenchymal cells; and (c) the peptide "growth factors" deriving from the endothelium, from the inflammatory leukocytes, and occasionally also from the vascular smooth muscle cells themselves.

Thus one may ask: Which of these factors are relevant in the process and how can this be experimentally documented?

B. Aortic Allograft as a Model for Allograft Arteriosclerosis

Considering that the problem in chronic rejection focuses on smooth muscle cell replication in the vascular wall and that the remainder of the organ-specific manifestations can be explained either as consequences of allograft arteriosclerosis (i.e., ischemic events) or parallel biological responses (e.g., mesangial proliferation in kidney), the question arises how these inflammatory cascades may be quantitated at the molecular level. Use of ordinary organ allografts—such as kidney, heart, or liver allografts—would be difficult, as this would require the dissection of the vascular tree apart from the tissue parenchyma. We therefore decided to transplant only the vascular wall and use the largest available vessel, the aorta, as an allograft.

The basic layout of this experimental setup in aorta allografts has been described and amply reviewed (19,20,39). Therefore, it is considered here only briefly.

Aortic allografts are transplanted from DA to WF rat strains across the major and minor histocompatability barriers. For control, DA-to-DA transplants are done, and, as an additional control, normal aortas are used. When the transplants are done without immunosuppression, the allografts undergo a short, spontaneously reversible episode of acute rejection, peaking at 1 to 2 months posttransplantation, that subsides spontaneously (39). This is very prominent in allograft adventitia but is largely lacking in the syngeneic transplants. Concomitantly with the increase in the inflammatory infiltrate in allograft adventitia, a high-level expression of IL-2 receptor in the activated lymphoid cells is recorded. Shortly thereafter, a gradual necrosis of media begins and medial nuclei disappear. In the intima, there is a gradual increase in the number of intimal nuclei and intimal thickness up to 1 year posttransplantation, after which the situation stabilizes (Figs. 3 and 4).

Immunocytochemical studies demonstrate heavy infiltration of T-helper cells in the allograft adventitia, which is largely lacking in syngeneic transplants, as well as the presence of monocytes and macrophages at different stages of maturation. The excess of T cytotoxic and NK cells in the allograft compared with the syngeneic graft is less impres-

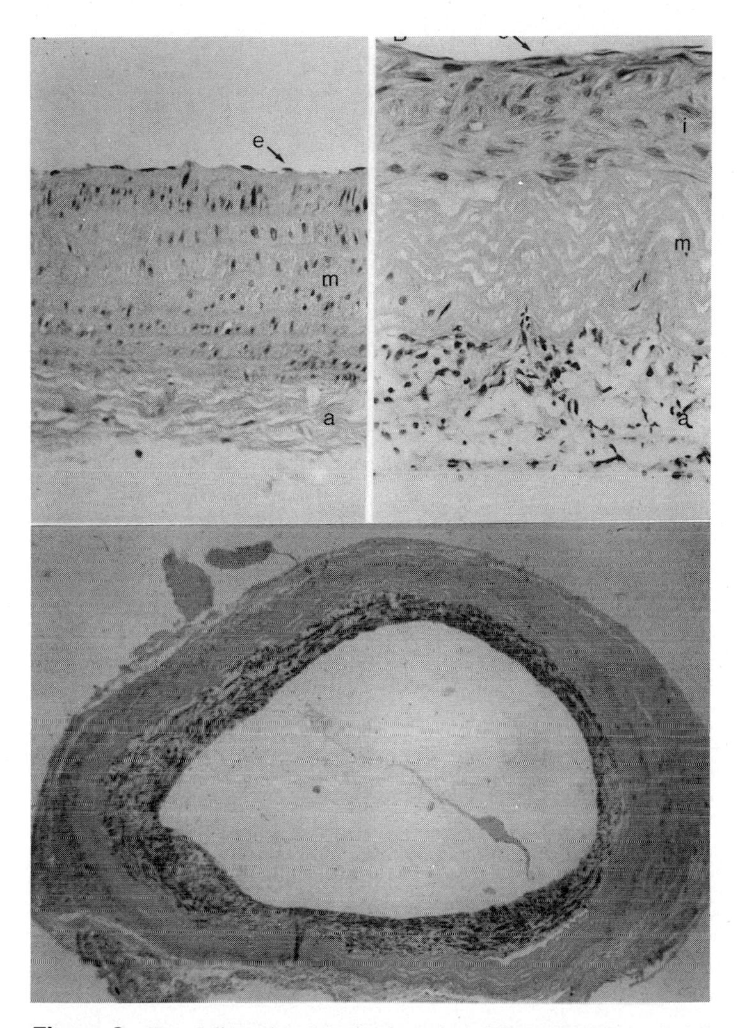

Figure 3 Top: Microphotograph of a DA-to-WF syngeneic transplant (to the left) and an allograft (to the right) approximately 2 months posttransplantation. Hematoxylin and eosin, ~×400. The endothelium is facing up. Note the intimal thickening, media necrosis, and adventitial inflammation in the allograft lacking in the syngeneic transplant. Abbreviations: a = adventitia, m = media, i = intima. Bottom: Low-power microphotograph of the whole aortic cross section, stained for smooth muscle cell alpha-actin. Note complete media necrosis and accumulation of the SMC in the intima.

sive. The level of IL-2 receptor expression during the acute stage in the inflammatory population is 200- to 300-fold greater in the allograft compared to the syngeneic graft, and the level of class II expression is approximately fivefold greater. Thereafter the expression of IL-2 receptor subsides. More ICAM-1 and its ligand LFA-1-α are also expressed in the allograft compared to the syngeneic transplants (Fig. 5). The high level of class II expression is also seen in the aortic endothelium as well as in the intramural capillaries of the allograft, and staining for immunoglobulin G and complement demonstrates extensive deposits in the allograft compared to syngeneic transplants (40).

Taken together, the alterations in the aortic allograft closely mimick the vascular wall

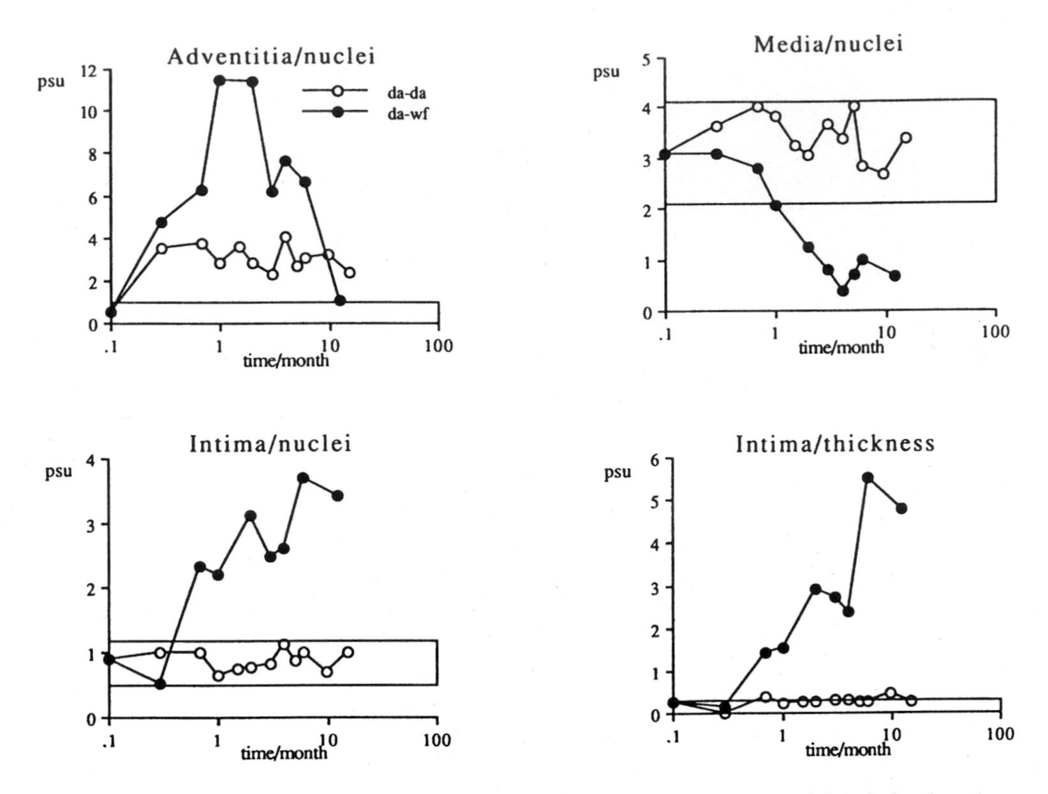

Figure 4 Adventitial inflammation (top left), media nuclear contents (top right), intimal nuclear contents (bottom left) and intimal thickness (bottom right) in DA-to-WF aortic allografts (closed circles) and in DA-to-DA syngeneic grafts (open circles) up to 12 months posttransplantation. The scale is given in "point score units," psu (39). Note logarithmic time axis. The box indicates corresponding control area ±2 × SD in normal aorta.

alterations in human chronic allograft rejection. There is first an acute and later a chronic inflammation in allograft adventitia, deposits of Ig and complement in the vascular wall, a proliferative response of smooth muscle cells and a gradual loss of their nuclei from the media, breaks in internal elastic lamina, appearance of proliferating smooth muscle cells in the intima (intermixed with some T cells and macrophages) and a concentric intimal thickening plus a gradual occlusion of the graft. The only difference from the constellation of findings in the human is a more extensive medial necrosis in the experimental animals than in man, where only occasional necrotic nuclei are observed.

Currently the aorta allograft model for allograft arteriosclerosis is widely used in several laboratories with highly concordant results (41,42,43) and/or femoral artery transplants are used instead (44).

The more extensive media necrosis under experimental conditions is explained by a higher lymphoid activation level in the allograft adventitia. If the recipient rats are immunosuppressed with CyA (45), the drug profoundly suppresses the immune response towards the allograft and practically eliminates the adventitial inflammation and lymphoid activation. Consequently there is no medial necrosis although, due to the pro-atherosclerotic features of CyA, there is intensive intimal thickening (45). On the other hand, if the

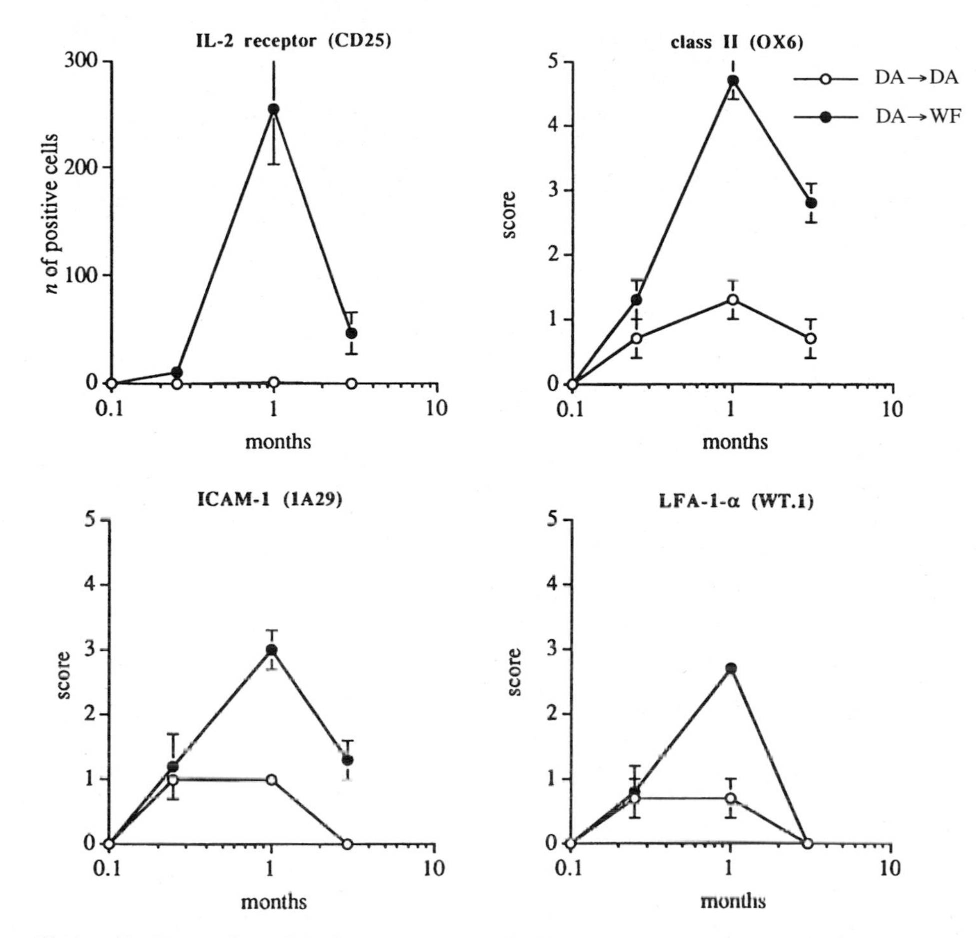

Figure 5 Expression of IL-2 receptor, class II, ICAM-1, and LFA-1 alpha in the adventitia of DA-to-WF aortic allografts (solid circles) and in DA-to-DA syngeneic transplants (open circles) up to 3 months posttransplantation. See text for details.

adventitial inflammation is induced by starch particles, this results in granuloma formation in the adventitia consisting mainly of activated macrophages with no or only minimal level of lymphoid activation. Consequently, there is strong intimal thickening at the site of the granulomas but no medial necrosis occurs (46).

C. Is Allograft Arteriosclerosis a Self-Limiting Process?

If the recipient rats are injected with tritiated thymidine (3H-TdR) or bromodesoxyuridine (BUDR) prior to sacrifice and the reaction product is visualized, the frequency of labeled nuclei gives the actual replication rate of the cells in the three different layers of the vascular wall. As seen in Fig. 6, there is a high level proliferative response of the cell population in allograft adventitia, peaking 1 month posttransplantation and subsiding gradually thereafter. There is practically no proliferation of adventitial cells in syngeneic transplants. Double labeling with leukocyte common antigen (47) demonstrates that most of the replicating cells in the adventitia are leukocytes.

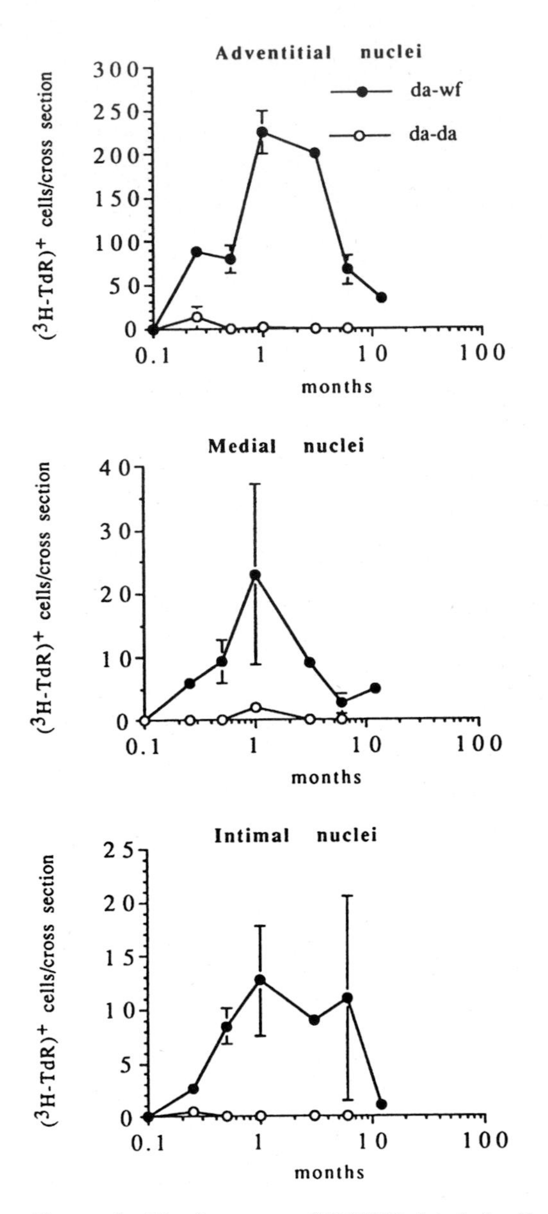

Figure 6 The frequency of 3H-TdR–labeled cells per aortic cross section in the aortic adventia, media, and intima of DA-to-WF aortic allografts (closed circles) and DA-to-DA syngeneic transplants (open circles). The rats were pulse-labeled with 250 uCi of 3H-TdR at −3 hr before sacrifice, and the autoradiograms were performed from formalin-fixed specimens. (Ilford L.4; IIIford, Mobberley, Cheshire, UK.)

In the media and the intima, a strong proliferative response is also recorded, although on this occasion the proliferating cells are practically all alpha-actin–positive smooth muscle cells. No proliferation is observed in syngeneic transplants. It is noteworthy that, in the media and the intima, the proliferation also gradually subsides, in the media by 9 months and in the intima by 12 months after transplantation.

This observation—together with the observation of plateauing of the intimal thickening—indicates that the process of allograft arteriosclerosis is self-limiting. There are two possible explanations for this. One is that, after the immune response (and active inflammation in the adventitia) is "burned out," the triggering force disappears. The other possibility is based on the observation by Ross (48) when he performed smooth muscle cell cultures either from atherosclerotic human plaques or from underlying intima. He demonstrated that whereas the smooth muscle cells obtained from the plaques replicated for only a few cycles, the smooth muscle cells obtained from media replicated for some 50 cycles, as is customary for human diploid cells (49).

D. Synthesis of Smooth Muscle Cell Regulatory Molecules in the Vascular Wall

As the regulatory molecules described in the preceding section most likely operate at a close range, using autocrine, paracrine or even intracrine interactions, we found it important to investigate the presence of these molecules in the vascular wall itself. For controls, we again used either syngeneic grafts of the same age or normal aortas.

To quantitate the various molecules in the allograft vascular wall, three technical approaches were used. First, we used immunohistochemistry to assess most of the lymphokines as well as the expression of IL-2 receptor (IL-2r), class II antigens (46), and adhesion molecules and their ligands (47). Second, the vascular wall was minced, the molecules were extracted from the transplant by acid extraction, and commercially available RIA assays for IL-1, TX-B_2, prostacyclin (6-keto-$PGF_1\alpha$), LT-B4, EGF, IGF-1, PDGF-beta chain, and endothelin were used (47). Third, we prepared the primers and probes for the following growth factors—PDGF-BB, IGF1, EGF, TGF-β, aFGF, and bFGF—and used semiquantitative reverse transcriptase–polymerase chain reaction (RT-PCR) with built in GAP-dehydrogenase standard for the quantitation (unpublished). Generally similar results were obtained with all these techniques when the same molecule was assessed with two different methods.

Table 4 demonstrates the presence of certain cytokines, eicosanoids, and growth factors in the rejecting vascular wall 2 to 5 months after aortic transplantation. As can be seen in the table, more IL-1, IFN-γ, TX-B_2, EGF, IGF-1 and PDGF-BB was extracted from the allograft than from syngeneic transplants or normal control aorta. The expression of IL-2r was increased severalfold. There was no difference in the level of 6-keto-PGF1-α or LTB-4, and to our astonishment, the expression of endothelin (type 3) was not altered either.

The aortic neointima is relatively loosely attached to the internal elastic lamina during the "cellular" stage of intimal thickening and can be detached along this line up to 2 to 3 months posttransplantation. This makes it possible to investigate separately the expression of these growth factors in the intima as opposed to the remaining of the vascular wall—i.e., in the media plus adventitia, where media is already mostly acellular. This information is also included in Table 4. Il-1 was equally present in adventitia and intima, IL-2r, IFN-γ and TX-B_2 were mainly present in the adventitia, whereas 6-keto-$PGF_1\alpha$, EGF, IGF-1 and PDGF-BB, were mostly present in the intima.

Table 5 demonstrates the expression of the mRNA for several growth factors in aorta vascular wall in 3-month-old aortic allografts compared to syngeneic transplants and normal control aortas. As can be seen in the table, the level of PDGF-BB, IGF-1, and TGF-β messages was increased severalfold compared to syngeneic or normal aortas; the

Table 4 Synthesis of Cytokines and Eicosanoids in the Vascular Wall 2 to 5 Months After Aortic Transplantation

	Normal aorta	DA→DA	DA→WF	Adventitia/intima ratio in allograft
IL-1, pg/mg	0.6	0.8	1.6	1.2
IL-2R, psu	0.0	0.4	2.5	6.6
IFN-gamma, pso	0.0	0.1	2.3	23
6k-PGF-1-alpha, ng/mg	16.3	16.8	13.9	0.5
T×B2, ng/mg	0.2	2.3	5.5	5.7
LTB4, ng/mg	0.0	<2	<2	ND
EGF, pg/mg	80	165	594	0.8
IGF-1, pg/mg	460	1492	4811	0.7
PDGF-BB, pg/mg	65	50	460	0.5
Endothelin, pg/mg	14	9.1	11.6	ND

IL-1, interleukin 1; IL-2R, interleukin 2 receptor; IFN-gamma, interferon gamma; 6k-PGF-1-alpha, 6-ketoprostaglandin Fl-alpha(α); TxB2, thromboxane B2; LTB4, leukotriene B4; EGF, epidermal growth factor; IGF-1, insulin-like growth factor 1; PDGF-BB, platelet derived growth factor BB-chain; psu, point score units; DA, rat strain Dark Agouti (AG-B4, RT1[a]); WF, rat strain Wistar Furth (AG-B2, RT1[u]). *Source*: Modified from Ref. 47.

level of bFGF message was marginally increased; and there was no enhanced expression of EGF or acidic fibroblast growth factor (aFGF) in the allograft in this assay.

Our results thus indicate that multiple molecular cascades operate in the induction of smooth muscle cell replication in rejecting transplants. Comparable results have ben obtained by several other investigators. These studies are summarized briefly in Table 6. As can be seen, TGF-β is amply expressed by immunohistochemistry and by Northern blot analysis in rejecting human and rat kidney and rat liver tissue (44,50–53). Enhanced expression of EGF has been observed in rat heart and rat kidney transplants (51,54); basic FGF in human heart and rat femoral artery (44,55); and acidic FGF in human heart (56). Several investigators have demonstrated the presence of PDGF, either by in situ hybridiza-

Table 5 Expression of Growth Factor mRNA in Aorta Vascular Wall of 3-Month-Old Aortic Allografts[a]

Growth factors	Allogeneic	Syngeneic	Normal aorta
PDGF-BB	2481	454	634
IGF-1	3105	330	251
EGF	675	481	1140
TFG-β	2299	304	270
aFGF	2734	1073	1883
bFGF	1283	543	473

[a]Semiquantitated from RNA isolated from the graft vascular wall using RT-PCR and GAPDH as standard. PDGF-BB, platelet derived growth factor BB-chain; IGF-1, insulin-like growth factor 1; EGF, epidermal growth factor; TGF-β, transforming growth factor β; aFGF, acidic fibroblast growth factor; bFGF, basic fibroblast growth factor; RT-PCR, reverse transcriptase polymerase chain reaction; GAPDH, glyceraldehyde-3-phosphate dehydrogenase.

Table 6 Expression of Growth Factors and Their Receptors in Chronically Rejecting Transplants

Molecule[a]	Type	Localization	Species and organ	Method of demonstration	Reference
TGF	β3	Endothelium inflammatory cells, fibrosis	Human kidney	Immunohistochemistry	50
	β	Vessels, interstitium	Rat kidney	Immunohistochemistry	51
	β	NA[b]	Rat liver	Northern blot analysis	52
	β	NA[b]	Rat heart	Northern blot analysis Immunohistochemistry	53
	β	Intima	Rat femoral artery	In situ hybridization	44
EGF		Media, myocytes	Rat heart	Immunohistochemistry	54
		Vessels, interstitium	Rat kidney	Immunohistochemistry	51
FGF	Basic	Intima	Human heart	Immunohistochemistry	55
	Basic	Intima	Rat femoral artery	In situ hybridization	44
	Acidic	NA[b]	Human heart	Quantitative PCR In situ hybridization Immunohistochemistry	56
PDGF	AA	Intima	Rat femoral artery	In situ hybridization	44
	AA	Intima	Baboon femoral graft	In situ hybridization	57
	BB	Intima endothelium	Baboon femoral graft	In situ hybridization	57
	AB/BB	Intima, glomeruli, endothelium	Human kidney	Immunohistochemistry	50
PDGF receptor	β	Vascular myocytes	Rat heart	Immunohistochemistry	54
	β	Intima, glomeruli, endothelium	Human kidney	Immunohistochemistry	50
	β	Intima, glomeruli	Human kidney	Immunohistochemistry	59
	β	Vessels	Human kidney	Immunohistochemistry	60
	β	Interstitium, vessels, glomeruli	Human kidney	Immunohistochemistry	58

[a]TGF, transforming growth factor; EGF, epidermal growth factor; FGF, fibroblast growth factor; PDGF, platelet-derived growth factor.
[b]NA, information not available.
For abbreviations see Table 5.

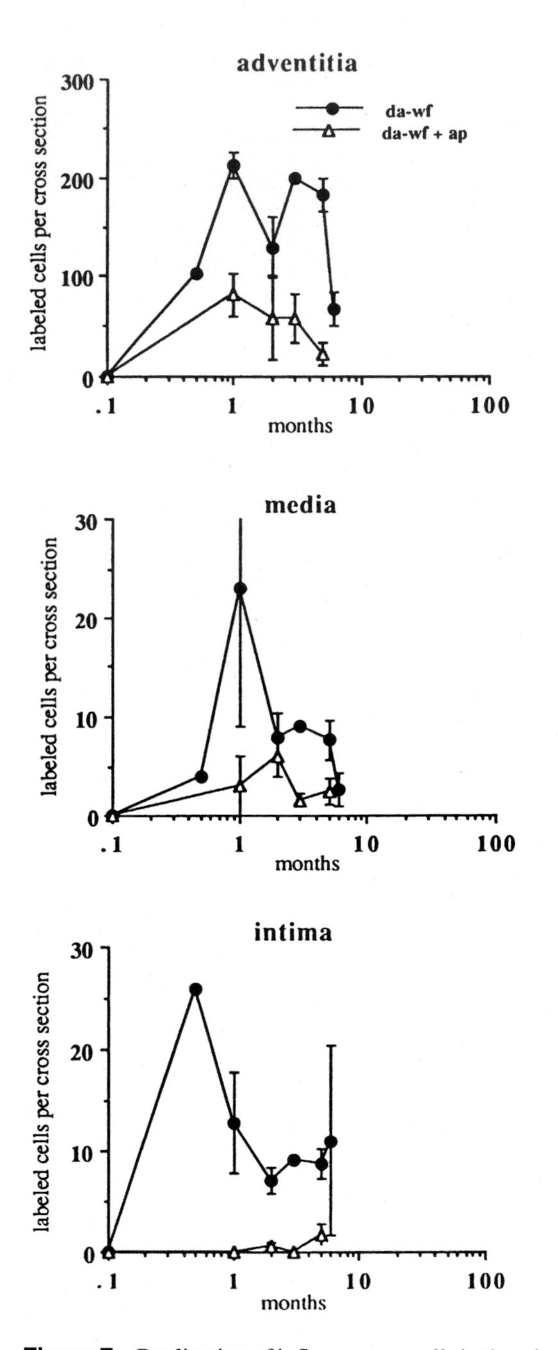

Figure 7 Replication of inflammatory cells in the adventitia, media, and intima of DA-to-WF aortic allografts (closed circles) and in allografts of recipients infused with 80 μg/mL/kg/day of angiopeptin (AP). Note that the replication rate of adventitial inflammatory cells was reduced to approximately 50% of the nontreated control, the media cells to 20%, and the intimal cells to 10%. (Modified from ref. 67.) See text for details.

Table 7 Inhibition of Cytokine, Eicosanoid, and Growth Factor Synthesis by BIM23014 in the Allograft Vascular Wall

	Allograft	Allograft + BIM23014	Nontreated (%)
IL-1, pg/mg	1.6	1.9	118%
T×B2, ng/mg	5.5	5.4	100%
6k-PGF1α, ng/mg	13.9	16.5	123%
EGF, ng/mg	594	376	68%
IGF-1, ng/mg	4811	3625	75%
PDGF-BB, ng/mg	460	160	35%

For abbreviations see Table 4.
Source: Modified from Ref. 47.

tion or by immunohistochemistry, in chronically rejecting rat femoral artery, baboon femoral graft, or human kidney (44,50,57). Subsequently, the PDGF-β receptor has been reported in rat heart and human kidney by several individual investigators (50,54,58–60).

F. Relevance of Growth Factors as Regulatory Molecules in Chronic Rejection

The presence of a given molecule does not indicate, however, that it is functional in the process of allograft arteriosclerosis or how relevant it is in this process. We have approached this question by using a new investigative molecule, BIM-23014 (Angiopeptin). BIM-23014 is an analogue of somatostatin, the antihormone for somatotropin (growth hormone). Somatostatin and its analogue lanreotides (like Angiopeptin) and octreotides (like Sandostatin (61,62) have been shown to antagonize angiogenesis and smooth muscle cell replication after endothelial injury (63–66). We therefore investigated the effect of Angiopeptin on intimal thickening and correlated the inhibitory effect to the expression of the different growth factors in the vascular wall.

Administration of 80 μg/kg/day of Angiopeptin with continuous Alzet infusion minipumps, dramatically reduced the replication of smooth muscle cells in the allograft media and intima and moderately also that of the inflammatory cells in the adventitia (Fig. 7). Concomitantly, Angiopeptin reduced the expression of three major growth factors—EGF, IGF-1 and PDGF-BB—by nearly 50% in the vascular wall (Table 7). Finally it reduced the intimal thickening by approximately 50 percent (47,67). These observations strongly suggest that the growth factors present in the vascular wall are relevant to intimal thickening.

V. MOLECULAR BIOLOGY OF CHRONIC REJECTION

An outline of the cellular and molecular cascades in chronic rejection is given in Fig. 8. During chronic rejection, there is continuous low-level inflammation in the transplant parenchyma, particularly in the vicinity of the intragraft arteries and arterioli, and low-level activation of lymphoid cells. This is facilitated by continuous low-level expression of endothelial adhesion ligands, bringing the inflammatory cells into the parenchyma. They exit through the lymphatics. The prominent effector molecules regulating class II expres-

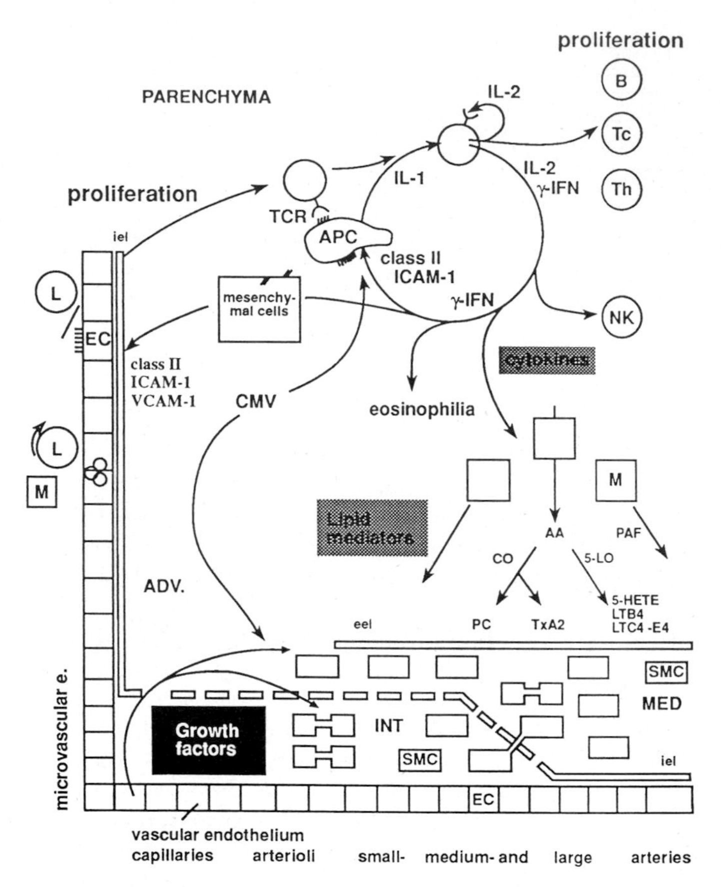

Figure 8 Summary of the main cellular and molecular events in chronic allograft vasculopathy. There is an influx of inflammatory cells through the graft microvascular endothelium (to the left). This is facilitated by the expression of the adhesion ligands (class II, ICAM-1, VCAM-1, and others). The contact of the antigen-responsive lymphocytes to the antigen-presenting cells (of either donor or recipient type) expressing the donor antigens on their surface carries on the antiallograft immune response. In chronic rejection, the level of lymphoid activation is far lower than in acute rejection, but it is still detectable. As a consequence of this interaction, cytokines are released from inflammatory lymphoid cells, which facilitates the maturation of B cells (B), cytotoxic cells (Tc), and helper cells (Th) in situ. The same mechanism also brings in immunologically nonspecific lymphocytes, NK effector cells, monocytes, and macrophages until the noncommitted cells dominate over the immunologically committed cells at a ratio of >99 to <1%. The cytokines and lipid mediators of inflammation (eicosanoids and PAF), released by the inflammatory leukocytes in the allograft adventitia and also in the neointima, induce continuous low-level damage to the graft vascular endothelium. This induces the endothelial cells to defend themselves via secretion of peptide growth factors such as IGF1, PDGF-BB, etc., also released by other parenchymal cells and by the inflammatory cells. These growth factors together with cytokines (e.g., IL-1) induce the media smooth muscle cells to replication and to migrate through the breaks in the internal elastic lamina (eel) into the neointima. Abbreviations: L = lymphocyte; M = monocyte/macrophage; NK = natural killer cell; B = B cell; Tc = T cytotoxic cell; Th = T helper cell; APC = antigen-presenting cell; SMC = smooth muscle cell; EC = endothelial cell; TCR = T-cell receptor; AA = arachinodic acid; CO = cyclooxygenase; 5-LO = 5-lipoxygenase; PC = prostacyclin; 5-HETE = hydroxyeicosatetraenoic acid; LT = leukotriene; iel = internal elastic lamina; eel = external elastic lamina, ADV = adventitia, MED = media, INT = intima.

sion and the expression of binding ligands are the cytokines secreted by the immunocompetent lymphocytes, particularly IFN-γ.

In addition to the donor-specific B cells, T-cytotoxic and T-helper cells, most of the inflammation during episodes of acute rejection (68) consist of immunologically noncommited lymphoid cells (69–72). NK-effector cells (73), and monocytes in various degrees of maturation toward macrophages. This is most likely also the case in chronic rejection. These cells, particularly the macrophages at higher maturation levels, bring in the lipid mediators, eicosanoids, and PAF, molecules which are known to induce tissue damage and may also act as growth-regulatory molecules for smooth muscle cells.

The inflammatory response in the allograft adventitia, the presence of inflammatory leukocytes in the subendothelium and in the intima, and the cytokines and lipid mediators released by them induce continuous low-level endothelial damage, though this is not always visible by endothelial morphology. Endothelial cells release growth factors in response to injury, and these growth factors, as shown, are potent mitogens for smooth muscle cells. Thus the molecular pathology of allograft arteriosclerosis consists of the following components: chronic low-level inflammation, release of cytokines and lipid mediators of inflammation, injury to vascular endothelium, secretion of growth factors, and induction of smooth muscle cell replication.

VI. PREDICTIVE VALUE OF BIOPSIES IN CHRONIC RENAL ALLOGRAFT REJECTION

A. Quantitation of Renal Allograft Pathology

Once the experimental cascades of chronic rejection were roughly outlined under experimental conditions, we wanted to follow these alterations closely in human transplants also. In order to generate quantitative data, we developed a numerical scoring system for chronic allograft pathology. Due to limitations of space, we deal here only with renal allografts.

The Banff classification of renal allograft pathology (12) deals primarily with acute rejection and its differential diagnosis. Chronic rejection in the Banff classification is considered under three different categories—mild, moderate, and severe transplant nephropathy—and the grading is based on the intensity of interstitial fibrosis and tubular atrophy and loss.

In order to identify and quantitate the histopathological features relevant to chronic rejection, we first performed rat renal transplants from DA to WF strains and immunosuppressed these animals for 2 or 3 weeks to induce long-term survivors (74). For controls, syngeneic transplants were done, and to rule out the CyA effect, these recipients were equally immunosuppressed. At the end of the observation period, 3 months posttransplantation, when the transplant function was significantly compromised, the animals were sacrificed, paraffin sections were done for transplant histopathology, and 30 different histological variables (Table 8) were scored blindly by two observers. Eight parameters appeared significantly higher in the allograft compared to syngeneic transplants: interstitial inflammation and fibrosis, interstitial pyroninophilia, glomerular mesangial matrix increase, basement membrane thickening and sclerosis, and vascular intimal proliferation and obliteration. The intensity of tubular epithelial vacuolation and atrophy, though higher in the allograft than in the syngeneic graft, did not reach statistical significance (Table 9).

In addition, 89 consecutive protocol core biopsies were performed in human renal transplant recipients, representing patients with entirely normal, slightly compromised, and

Table 8 Parameters Evaluated in the Histological Specimens of Renal Grafts

Interstitium[a]	*Glomeruli*
Inflammation	Number of glomeruli
Lymphocytes	Mesangial cell proliferation
Neutrophils	Mesangial matrix increase
Macrophages	CBM[d] thickening
Eosinophils	CBM duplication
Pyroninophilic cells	Capillary thrombosis
Edema	Bowman's capsule thickening
Hemorrhage	Glomerular inflammation
Fibrin deposits	Glomerular sclerosis
Fibrosis	Glomerular necrosis
Tubuli[b]	*Vessels*[c]
Epithelial swelling	Endothelial swelling
Epithelial vacuolation; isometric	Endothelial proliferation
Epithelial vacuolation; anisometric	Intimal proliferation
Epithelial atrophy	Inflammation
Necrosis	Sclerosis
Casts	Obliteration
Inflammation	
Dilatation	
Basement membrane thicking	

Scored separately for [a]diffuse and focal changes; [b]proximal and distal tubuli; [c]arteries, arterioles and veins; [d]capillary basal membrane. The histopathological changes were scored from 0 to 3 (0 = none, 1 = mild, 2 = moderate, 3 = severe).

severely compromised transplant function (Table 10). The biopsy histology (Table 8) was again quantitated by the same pathologists and scored blindly and independently. Eight of these variables correlated significantly with the impairment of kidney function as measured by the level of serum creatinine: interstitial inflammation, pyroninophilia and fibrosis, glomerular mesangial matrix increase and sclerosis, vascular intimal proliferation, and tubular dilation and atrophy (Table 10). Thus the changes observed in human kidneys during chronic rejection were virtually identical to those seen in chronically rejecting rat kidneys and nearly the same as those suggested by Hume et al. (16) 40 years ago!

As we wanted to quantitate the pathology with plain histology, without additional staining or use of monoclonal antibodies, we excluded pyroninophilia from the scoring. Thus the chronic allograft damage index (CADI) in biopsy histology became equivalent to the sum score of interstitial inflammation and fibrosis, glomerular mesangial matrix increase and sclerosis, vascular intimal proliferation, and tubular atrophy. When each one of these parameters is scored from 0 to 3, the minimum CADI index is 0 and the theoretical maximum 18.

B. Predictive Value of Renal Allograft CADI Index for Chronic Allograft Rejection

As mild histological changes compatible with chronic rejection were also seen in well-functioning transplants 2 years posttransplantation (4), we wanted to investigate the impact of these alterations on subsequent clinical chronic rejection.

Table 9 Correlations Between Late (3-month) Transplant Function and Histopathology in DA to WF Rat Renal Allografts and in DA-to-DA Syngeneic Grafts

	Cyclosporine dose (mg/kg/d)[a]	
	Allograft	Syngeneic graft
Number of rats	5	5
Mean s-creat.(μmol/L)	437[b]	105
Interstitium		
Inflammation	1.80[c]	0.50
Pyroninophilic cells (%)	28.0[b]	2.60
Fibrosis	1.40[b]	0.70
Glomeruli		
Mesangial matrix increase	2.10[c]	1.00
CBM[d] thickening	1.40[c]	0.40
Sclerosis	1.00[c]	0.00
Vessels		
Intimal proliferation	2.20[b]	0.20
Obliteration	1.60[c]	0.00
Tubuli		
Epithelial vacuolation	1.10	0.80
Epithelial atrophy	0.70	0.40
Basement membrane thickening	0.60	0.20

[a]Allogeneic rats received cyclosporine 15 mg/kg/day SC for 2 weeks; syngeneic rats for 3 weeks.
[b]$p < 0.01$ (significance in Mann-Whitney U test).
[c]$p < 0.05$.
[d]Capillary basal membrane.
Source: Modified from Ref. 74.

We first correlated the CADI index at 2 years to transplant function during the subsequent years of follow-up. The correlation of the 2-year CADI index to the recipient serum creatinine level at 6 years posttransplantation is given in Fig. 9. As can be seen in the figure, the correlation coefficient (r value) between CADI index at 2 years and graft function at 6 years posttransplantation was 0.717 and was highly significant ($p = 0.0001$).

In the second analysis, three groups of patients were formed on the basis of their CADI index and graft function at 2 years and correlated to clinical graft outcome at 6 years (Table 11). Of the grafts with a low CADI index and stable graft function at 2 years (group I), 3/43 (7%) were in chronic rejection at 6 years after transplantation. Of the grafts with high CADI index and stable graft function at 2 years (group II), 13/31 (42%) were in chronic rejection at 6 years. All patients in groups I and II who had died had good and stable graft function at the time of death. Of the grafts with high CADI index and deteriorated graft function at 2 years (group III), 13/14 (93%) were in chronic rejection at 6 years. All deceased patients in this group had deteriorated graft function at the time of death. The 6-year graft survival in groups I, II, and III was 91, 77, and 29% ($p = 0.001$), and the median serum creatinine was 106, 181, and 303 μmol/L ($p = 0.001$) respectively.

Thus, taken together, our results support our previous findings (4) that the presence of incipient histological changes of chronic rejection, even in well-functioning grafts, is a significant risk factor for subsequent chronic rejection, and that the CADI index obtained at

Table 10 Intensity of Late Histopathological Findings in Human Renal Allografts According to Graft Function

	Creatinine			
	Normal (<115 μmol/L)	Slightly increased (116–200 μmol/L)	Increased (>200 μmol/L)	p[a]
Number of patients with biopsy	37	32	20	
Mean number of glomeruli	7.2	7.8	7.3	NS
Interstitium				
Diffuse inflammation	0.2	0.4	0.7	0.0050
Pyroninophilic cells	0.1	0.2	0.4	0.0410
Diffuse fibrosis	0.1	0.7	1.5	0.0002
Glomeruli				
Mesangial matrix increase	0.1	0.5	0.7	0.0015
Bowman's capsule thickening	0.2	0.3	0.3	NS
Glomerular sclerosis	0.2	0.8	0.7	0.0019
Vessels				
Intimal proliferation	0.2	0.4	0.6	0.0483
Obliteration and sclerosis	0.2	0.4	0.4	NS
Tubuli				
Epithelial swelling	0.3	0.4	0.3	NS
Isometric vacuolation	0.1	0.2	0.1	NS
Anisometric vaculolation	0.4	0.3	0.4	NS
Tubular atrophy	0.4	0.8	1.3	0.0001
Basement membrane thickening	0.2	0.2	0.5	NS
Tubular dilatation	0.0	0.2	0.4	0.0065

[a]Spearman rank correlation coefficient used for statistics.
Source: Modified from Ref. 4.

2 years posttransplantation accurately predicts transplant function at 6 years (unpublished). These results also emphasize the importance of protocol core biopsy in long-term follow-up of renal transplant recipients. This emphasis is further supported by an independent study deriving from Uppsala (5). In this study, 104 protocol core biopsies were performed at 6 months after transplantation and the chronic graft damage (CGD) index was calculated as the CADI index. Patients with a high histopathology score had significantly higher graft loss rates 2 years later than those with a low score ($p = 0.037$).

C. Quantitation of Heart Allograft Histology and Correlation with Angiography

Also in heart allografts, the prime manifestation of chronic rejection is a generalized, concentric intimal thickening (allograft arteriosclerosis) together with a mild inflammatory infiltrate of the vascular wall and periphery of the vessels (75–77). Endothelial dysfunction, recorded as an impaired response to the endothelium-dependent vasodilator acetylcholine, is also a common early finding in coronary angiograms of heart-transplant recipients (78).

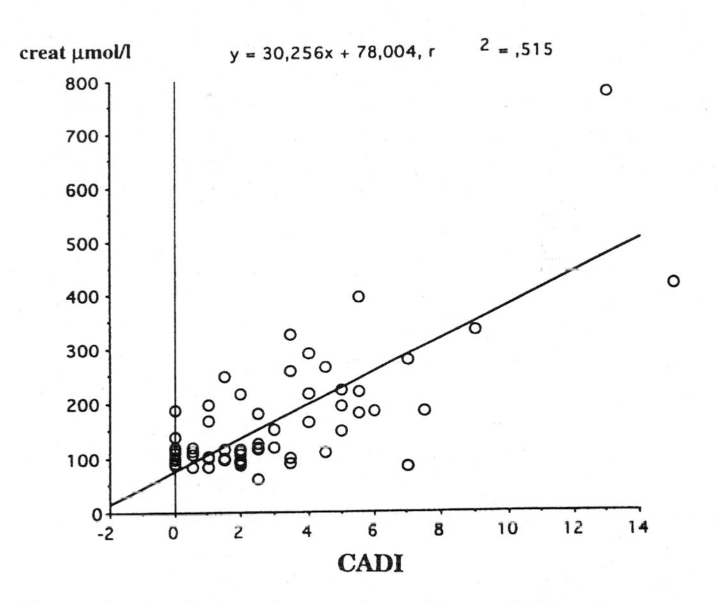

Figure 9 Correlation of protocol core biopsy CADI at 2 years posttransplantation to endpoint transplant function at 6 years. See text for details.

Radiological imaging methods are widely considered the only reliable method to monitor heart allograft arteriosclerosis (6). In coronary angiography, the lesions are usually either proximal focal lesions with asymmetrical plaques similar to those seen in non-transplant atherosclerosis or diffuse concentric luminal narrowing of the vessel affecting the entire length of the vessel wall, including the smallest branches (6). However, a new imaging technique, intravascular ultrasonography, applicable only to large vessels, has

Table 11 The 6-Year Outcome of Grafts in the Three Patient Groups Formed at 2 Years on the Basis of the CADI Index and Recipient Clinical Status[a]

	Group I: CADI ≤2 and stable graft function	Group II: CADI >2 and stable graft function	Group III: CADI >2 deteriorated graft function	
	(n = 43)	(n = 31)	(n = 14)	
Clinical chronic rejection (deteriorated graft function or on dialysis)	3 (7%)	13 (42%)	13 (93%)	p = 0.0001
Patient died with a functioning graft	2	3	2	NS
Number of functioning grafts	38	24	4	p = 0.005
Graft survival (%)	91%	77%	29%	
S-creat. mean ± SD (µmol/L)	115 ± 37	198 ± 141	288 ± 102	p = 0.001
S-creat. median (µmol/L)	106	181	303	

[a]CADI = chronic allograft damage index calculated from renal allograft biopsy.

become available to detect early intimal changes in large coronary arteries of heart-transplant patients (79). Autopsy findings have demonstrated that almost every heart-transplant patient surviving for more than 1 year has vascular changes (8). In explanted allografts, the basic histological lesion of cardiac allograft arteriosclerosis is concentric intimal thickening and a low-level perivasculitis affecting intramyocardial branches of the coronary arteries (76,80).

There is relatively broad agreement that histological features of endomyocardial biopsy (EMB) relating to chronic rejection are nonexistent. However, we believe that this may not be the case. Along the lines of the results obtained in our renal transplants, we constructed a prospective study of heart-transplant patients. We quantitated blindly the histological changes in endomyocardial biopsies from 0 (no change) to 3 (severe changes) with respect to the 12 independent histological parameters given in Table 12. We then correlated these histological changes to angiographic results obtained from the very same patients (81). The following histological alterations in biopsies significantly correlated with narrowing of coronary arteries in annual angiograms: endothelial cell proliferation and intimal thickening characterized by accumulation of acellular matrix beneath the endothelium of small intramyocardial arteries (Table 13).

The frequency of vascular changes in EMB specimens was significantly higher than in angiograms during the first 3 postoperative years (Fig. 10). The most common type of early vascular changes in EMB specimens, to which cardiac allograft vasculopathy in angiography could be attributed, was endothelial cell proliferation, which was observed in most biopsy specimens studied. Later on, intimal thickening was also observed. However, the intensity of vascular changes in EMB was usually mild, so it is difficult to decide whether these histological findings of the vascular wall reflect the true state of allograft arteriosclerosis in the same way as seen in coronary angiography.

VII. CONCLUDING REMARKS

The hallmarks of chronic rejection (also called chronic vascular rejection) are persistent perivascular inflammation, often with low-level of lymphoid activation, and a concentric generalized intimal thickening of all intragraft intramural arteries to the level of arterioli. The high similarity of these changes in different types of allografts suggest that "allograft

Table 12 Parameters Evaluated in the Histological Specimens of Heart Allografts[a]

Inflammation	Arterioles/Capillaries
Vascular wall	Endothelial nuclear enlargement
Perivascular space	Endothelial cell proliferation
Mononuclear cells	Intimal thickening
Polymorphonuclear cells	Fibrosis
Pyroninophilic cells	Endocardial
Myocyte morphology	Interstitial
Nuclei	Patchy
Vacuolar degeneration	Diffuse
Hypertrophy	

[a]Histopathological changes were scored semiquantitatively from 0 to 3 (0 = none, 1 = mild, 2 = moderate, and 3 = severe).

Table 13 Correlation of Histological Scores with Normal and Abnormal Coronary Angiography at 1 Year Postoperatively

Histologic parameter in EMBs	Coronary angiography without CAV[a]	Coronary angiography with CAV	p Value[b]
Capillary endothelial cell proliferation	0.79	1.5	<0.02
Arteriolar endothelial cell proliferation	0.33	0.79	<0.05
Arteriolar intimal thickness	0.45	1.43	<0.005

[a]CAV, cardiac allograft vasculopathy.
[b]Significance values were obtained by the Mann-Whitney U test.
Source: Modified from Ref. 81.

arteriosclerosis" is a key manifestation of chronic rejection and that other "organ-specific" changes may be explained either on the basis of this manifestation (e.g., anoxia) or of parallel biological events (glomerular sclerosis in kidneys).

The peri- and postoperative trauma, particularly earlier episodes of acute rejection, seems to be the key initial trigger for chronic rejection. Once the cascade of events leading to smooth muscle cell replication in vascular wall is initiated, the process seems to become independent of the trigger.

Studies employing vascular wall transplants have demonstrated an excess of certain cytokines (IL-1, IL-2, IFN-γ) and their receptors (IL-2r), certain lipid mediators of inflammation (TX-B_2), and an abundance of growth factors (IGF-1, PGDG-BB, TGF-β, and bFGF) in the allograft vascular wall during the development of allograft arteriosclerosis. As peptides downregulating the growth factor expression, such as angiopeptin, are also

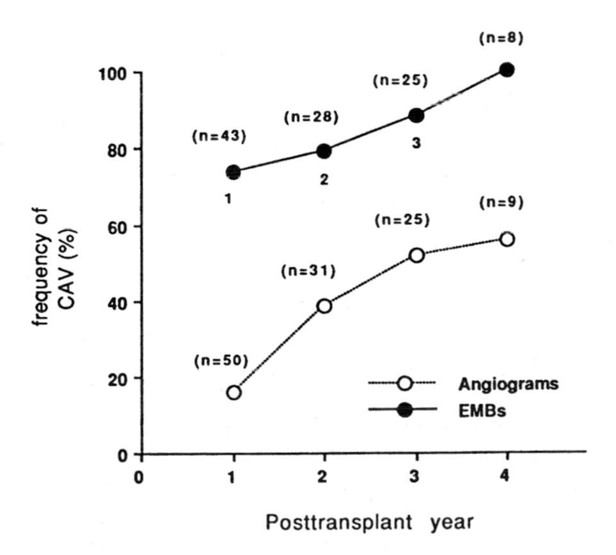

Figure 10 Frequency of chronic vascular disease (CAV) independently estimated from endomyocardial biopsy and from simultaneously performed coronary angiography at 1 to 4 years posttransplantation. Numbers indicate the number of patients at each time point. (Modified from Ref. 81).

strongly inhibitory to vascular smooth muscle cell replication in vivo, it is likely that they are important regulatory molecules in this process.

In order to monitor chronic vascular rejection in human transplants, it is necessary to quantitate the histological changes and express these in numerical figures. We have therefore created the chronic allograft damage index (CADI) equivalent to the sum score of interstitial inflammation and fibrosis, glomerular mesangial matrix increase and sclerosis, vascular intimal proliferation, and tubular atrophy in allograft biopsy. As each one of these parameters is scored from 0 to 3, the minimum CADI index is 0 and the theoretical maximum 18.

We have also demonstrated, based on sequential protocol core biopsies, that the histological CADI index at 2 years is an early predictor for chronic allograft rejection. The 2-year CADI index correlated in linear regression analysis to the transplant function at 6 years posttransplantation ($p = 0.0001$). When the same patients were categorized at 2 years in three different groups—those with CADI index ≤ 2 and stable graft function, those with CADI index >2 and stable graft function, and those with CADI index >2 and deteriorated graft function—the frequency of clinical chronic rejection at 6 years posttransplantation was 7, 42, and 93% respectively ($p = 0.0001$).

The incipient histological findings quantitated as the CADI index is, to our knowledge, the earliest predictor of chronic allograft rejection. Thus, a protocol core biopsy and the CADI index may be used as an (ad interim) endpoint in clinical studies for chronic rejection, before the necessary 5- to 10-year follow-up is completed.

REFERENCES

1. Cho YW, Terasaki PI. Long-Term Survival. In: Terasaki PI, ed. Clinical Transplants 1988. Los Angeles: UCLA Tissue Typing Laboratory, 1988:277–282.
2. Evans RW. Executive Summary: The National Cooperative Transplantation Study. Seattle, WA: Battelle-Seattle Research Center, June 1991 (BHARC-100-91-020).
3. Isoniemi H, Krogerus L, von Willebrand E, et al. Renal immunosuppression: VI. Triple drug therapy versus immunosuppressive double drug combinations: Histopathological findings in renal allografts. Transplant Int 1991; 4:151–156.
4. Isoniemi HM, Krogerus L, von Willebrand E, et al. Histopathological findings in well-functioning, long-term renal allografts. Kidney Int 1992; 41:155–160.
5. Dimény E, Wahlberg J, Larsson E, Fellström B. Can histopathological findings in early renal allograft biopsies identify patients at risk for chronic vascular rejection? Clin Transplantation 1995; 9:79–84.
6. Gao SZ, Alderman EL, Schroeder JS, et al. Accelerated coronary vascular disease in the heart transplant patient: Coronary arteriographic findings. J Am Coll Cardiol 1988; 12:334–340.
7. Olivari MT, Homans DC, Wilson RF, et al. Coronary artery disease in cardiac transplant patients receiving triple-drug immunosuppressive therapy. Circulation 1989; 80(suppl III):111–115.
8. Johnson DE, Alderman EL, Schroeder JS, et al. Transplant coronary artery disease: Histopathologic correlations with angiographic morphology. J Am Coll Cardiol 1991; 17:449–457.
9. Freese DK, Snover DC, Sharp HL, et al. Chronic rejection after liver transplantation: A study of clinical, histopathological and immunological features. Hepatology 1991; 13:882–891.
10. Klintmalm GB, Nery JR, Husberg BS, et al. Rejection in liver transplantation. Hepatology 1989; 10:978–985.
11. Quiroga J, Colina I, Demetris AJ, et al. Cause and timing of first allograft failure in orthotopic liver transplantation: A study of 177 consecutive patients. Hepatology 1991; 14:1054–1062.
12. Solez K, Axelsen RA, Benediktsson H, et al. International standardization of criteria for the

histologic diagnosis of renal allograft rejection: The Banff working classification of kidney transplant pathology. Kidney Int 1993: 44:411–422.
13. Billingham ME, Nathaniel RB, Cary NRB, et al. A working formulation for the standardization of nomenclature in the diagnosis of heart and lung rejection: Heart rejection study group. J Heart Transplant 1990; 9:587–593.
14. International Working Party (Chair of Panel on Hepatic Allograft Rejection: Demetris AJ). Terminology for hepatic allograft rejection. 1995.
15. Rose AG, Uys CJ. Pathology of graft atherosclerosis (chronic rejection). In: Cooper DKC, Novitzky D, ed. The Transplantation and Replacement of Thoracic Organs. Dordrecht: Kluwer, 1990:161–167.
16. Hume DM, Merrill JP, Miller BF, Thorn GW. Experiences with renal homotransplantation in the human: Report of nine cases. J Clin Invest 1955; 34:327–382.
17. Oguma S, Belle S, Starzl TE, Demetris AJ. A histometric analysis of chronically rejected human liver allografts: Insights into the mechanisms of bile duct loss: Direct immunologic and ischemic factors. Hepatology 1989; 9:204–209.
18. Demetris AJ, Zerbe T, Banner B. Morphology of solid organ allograft arteriopathy: Identification of proliferating intimal cell populations. Transplant Proc 1989; 21:3667–3669.
19. Hayry P, Mennander A, Raisanen SA, et al. Pathophysiology of vascular wall changes in chronic allograft rejection. Transplant Rev 1993; 7:1–20.
20. Hayry P, Isoniemi H, Yilmaz S, et al. Chronic allograft rejection. Immunol Rev 1993; 134: 33–81.
21. Opelz G, for the Collaborative Transplant Study. Strength of HLA-A, HLA-AB, and HLA DR mismatches in relation to short- and long-term kidney graft survival. Transplant Int 1992; 5 (suppl 1):S621–S624.
22. Takemoto S, Terasaki PI, Cecka JM, et al. Survival of nationally shared, HLA-matched kidney transplants from cadaveric donors: The UNOS Scientific Renal Transplant Registry (see comments). N Engl J Med 1992; 327:834–839.
23. Abele R, Novick AC, Braun WE, et al. Long-term results of renal transplantation in recipients with a functioning graft for 2 years. Transplantation 1982; 34:264–267.
24. Almond PS, Matas A, Gillingham K, et al. Risk factors for chronic rejection in renal allograft recipients. Transplantation 1993; 55:752–756.
25. Basadonna GP, Matas AJ, Gillingham KJ, et al. Early versus late acute renal allograft rejection: Impact on chronic rejection. Transplantation 1993; 55:993–995.
26. Lindholm A, Ohlman S, Albrechtsen D, et al. The impact of acute rejection episodes on long-term graft function and outcome in 1347 primary renal transplants treated by 3 cyclosporine regimens. Transplantation 1993; 56:307–315.
27. Tesi RJ, Henry ML, Elkhammas EA, Ferguson RM. Predictors of long-term primary cadaveric renal transplant survival. Clin Transplant 1993; 7:343–352.
28. Isoniemi H, Nurminen M, Tikkanen MJ, et al. Risk factors predicting chronic rejection of renal allografts. Transplantation 1994; 57:68–72.
29. Lim EC, Terasaki PI. Early graft function. In: Terasaki PI, Cecka JM, eds. Clinical Transplants 1991. Los Angeles: UCLA Tissue Typing Laboratory, 1991:401–407.
30. Yuge J, Cecka JM. Sex and age effects in renal transplantation. In: Terasaki PI, Cecka JM, ed. Clinical Transplants 1991. Los Angeles: UCLA Tissue Typing Laboratory, 1991:257–267.
31. Grattan MT, Moreno-Cabral CE, Starnes VA, et al. Cytomegalovirus infection is associated with cardiac allograft rejection and atherosclerosis. JAMA 1989; 261:3561–3566.
32. O'Grady JG, Alexander GJM, Sutherland S, et al. Cytomegalovirus infection and donor/recipient HLA antigens: Interdependent co-factors in pathogenesis of vanishing bile duct syndrome after liver transplantation. Lancet 1988; 2:302–305.
33. Tullius SG, Heemann UW, Wagner K, Tilney NL. Changes of chronic kidney allograft rejection are reversible after retransplantation. Transplant Proc 1993; 25:906–907.

34. Kingma I, Chea R, Davidoff A, et al. Glomerular capillary pressures in long-surviving rat renal allografts. Transplantation 1993; 56:53–60.
35. Cheigh JS, Haschemeyer RH, Wang JC, et al. Hypertension in kidney transplant recipients: Effect on long-term renal allograft survival. Am J Hypertens 1989; 2:341–348.
36. Ross R. The pathogenesis of atherosclerosis: A perspective for the 1990s. Nature 1993; 362:801–809.
37. Ross R. Rous-Whipple Award Lecture. Atherosclerosis: a defense mechanism gone awry. Am J Pathol 1993; 143:987–1002.
38. Thyberg J, Hedin U, Sjölund M, et al. Regulation of differentiated properties and proliferation of arterial smooth muscle cells. Arteriosclerosis 1990; 10:966–990.
39. Mennander A, Tiisala S, Halttunen J, et al. Chronic rejection in rat aortic allografts: An experimental model for transplant arteriosclerosis. Arterioscler Thromb 1991; 11:671–680.
40. Hayry P, Mennander A, Yilmaz S, et al. Towards understanding the pathophysiology of chronic rejection. Clin Invest 1992; 70:780–790.
41. Plissonnier D, Amichot G, Lecagneux J, et al. Additive and synergistic effects of a low-molecular-weight, heparin-like molecule and low doses of cyclosporin in preventing arterial graft rejection in rats. Arterioscler Thromb 1993; 13:112–119.
42. Dumont CE, Plissonnier D, Guettier C, Michael JB. Effects of glutaraldehyde on experimental arterial iso- and allografts in rats. J Surg Res 1993; 54:61–69.
43. Steele DM, Hullett DA, Bechstein WO, et al. Effects of immunosuppressive therapy on the rat aortic allograft model. Transplant Proc 1993; 25:754–755.
44. Gregory CR, Huie P, Billingham ME, Morris RE. Rapamycin inhibits arterial intimal thickening caused by both alloimmune and mechanical injury: Its effect on cellular, growth factor, and cytokine response in injured vessels. Transplantation 1993; 55:1409–1418.
45. Mennander A, Tiisala S, Paavonen T, et al. Chronic rejection in rat aortic allografts: II. Administration of cyclosporine induces accelerated allograft arteriosclerosis. Transplant Int 1991; 4:173–179.
46. Mennander A, Paavonen T, Hayry P. Intimal thickening and medial necrosis in allograft arteriosclerosis (chronic rejection) are independently regulated. Arterioscler Thromb 1993; 13:1019–1025.
47. Hayry P, Raisanen A, Ustinov J, et al. Somatostatin analog lanreotide inhibits myocyte replication and several growth factors in allograft arteriosclerosis. FASEB J 1993; 7:1055–1060.
48. Ross R, Wight TN, Strandness E, Thiele B. Human atherosclerosis: I. Cell constitution and characteristics of advanced lesions of the superficial femoral artery. Am J Pathol 1984; 114: 79–93.
49. Hayflick L. The limited lifetime of human diploid cell strains. Exp Cell Res 1965; 37:614–636.
50. Noronha IL, Weis H, Hartley B, et al. Expression of cytokines, growth factors, and their receptors in renal allograft biopsies. Transplant Proc 1993; 25:917–918.
51. Hancock WH, Whitley WD, Tullius SG, et al. Cytokines, adhesion molecules, and the pathogenesis of chronic rejection of rat renal allografts. Transplantation 1993; 56:643–650.
52. Rao P, Sun H, Snyder J, et al. Effect of FK 506 on FK-binding protein and transforming growth factor beta gene expression. Transplant Proc 1991; 23:2873–2874.
53. Waltenberger J, Wanders A, Fellstrom B, et al. Induction of transforming growth factor-beta during cardiac allograft rejection. J Immunol 1993; 151:1147–1157.
54. Higgy NA, Davidoff AW, Grothman GT, et al. Expression of platelet-derived growth factor receptor in rat heart allografts. J Heart Lung Transplant 1991; 10:1012–1022.
55. Gordon D. Growth factors and cell proliferation in human transplant arteriosclerosis. J Heart Lung Transplant 1992; 11:S7.
56. Zhao XM, Frist W, Yeoh TK, et al. Role of acidic fibroblast growth factor (aFGF) and its receptor (FGFR-1) in pathogenesis of cardiac allograft vasculopathy (CAV). J Heart Lung Transplant 1994; 13(1(2)):S55.

57. Golden MA, Au YP, Kirkman TR, et al. Platelet-derived growth factor activity and mRNA expression in healing vascular grafts in baboons: Association in vivo of platelet-derived growth factor mRNA and protein with cellular proliferation. J Clin Invest 1991; 87:406–414.
58. Fellstrom B, Klareskog L, Larsson E, et al. Tissue distribution of macrophages, class II transplantation antigens, and receptors for platelet-derived growth factor in normal and rejected human kidneys. Transplant Proc 1987; 19:3625–3627.
59. Fellstrom B, Klareskog L, Heldin CH, et al. Platelet-derived growth factor receptors in the kidney—Upregulated expression in inflammation. Kidney Int 1989; 36:1099–1102.
60. Rubin K, Tingstrom A, Hansson GK, et al. Induction of B-type receptors for platelet-derived growth factor in vascular inflammation: Possible implications for development of vascular proliferative lesions. Lancet 1988; 1:1353–1356.
61. Brazeau P, Vale W, Burgus R. Hypothalamic polypeptide that inhibits the secretion of immunoreactive pituitary growth hormone. Science 1973; 179:77–79.
62. Fassler JE, Hughes JH, Titterington L. Somatostatin analog: An inhibitor of angiogenesis. Clin Res 1988; 36:869.
63. Conte JV, Foegh ML, Calcagno D, et al. Peptide inhibition of myointimal proliferation following angioplasty in rabbits. Transplant Proc 1989; 4:3686–3688.
64. Foegh ML, Khirabadi BS, Chambers E, et al. Inhibition of coronary artery transplant atherosclerosis in rabbits with angiopeptin, an octapeptide. Atherosclerosis 1989; 78:229–236.
65. Fellström B, Dimeny E, Foegh ML, et al. Accelerated atherosclerosis in heart transplants in the rat simulating chronic vascular rejection: Effects of prostacyclin and angiopeptin. Transplant Proc 1991; 23:525–528.
66. Lundergan C, Foegh ML, Vargas R, et al. Inhibition of myointimal proliferation of the rat carotid artery by peptides, angiopeptin and BIM 23034. Atherosclerosis 1989; 80:49–55.
67. Mennander A, Raisanen A, Paavonen T, Hayry P. Chronic rejection in the rat aortic allograft: V. Mechanism of the angiopeptin (BIM23014C) effect on the generation of allograft arteriosclerosis. Transplantation 1993; 55:124–128.
68. Hayry P, von Willebrand E, Parthenais E, et al. The inflammatory mechanisms of allograft rejection. Immunol Rev 1984; 77:83–142.
69. Doveren RFC, Buurman WA, van der Linden CJ, et al. Analysis of cytotoxic T-lymphocyte response in rejecting allografted canine kidneys. Transplantation 1986, 41:33–38.
70. Orosz CG, Zinn NE, Sirinek L, Ferguson RM. In vivo mechanisms of alloreactivity: I. Frequency of donor-reactive cytotoxic T-lymphocytes in sponge matrix allografts. Transplantation 1986; 41:71–83.
71. Manca F, Ferry B, Jaakkola M, et al. Frequency and functional characterization of specific T-helper cells infiltrating rat kidney allografts during acute rejection. Scand J Immunol 1987; 25:255–264.
72. Tiisala S, Leszczynski D, Halttunen J, et al. The frequency of B cells secreting antibodies against donor MHC antigens in rats rejecting renal allografts. Transplant Int 1990; 3:86–91.
73. Nemlander A, Saksela E, Hayry P. Are natural killer cells involved in allograft rejection? Eur J Immunol 1983; 13:348–350.
74. Yilmaz S, Taskinen E, Paavonen T, et al. Chronic rejection of rat renal allograft: I. Histological differentiation between chronic rejection and cyclosporin nephrotoxicity. Transplant Int 1992; 5:85–95.
75. Uys CJ, Rose AG. Pathologic findings in long-term cardiac transplants. Arch Pathol Lab Med 1984; 108:112–116.
76. Billingham ME. Cardiac transplant atherosclerosis. Transplant Proc 1987; 19:19–25.
77. Hruban RH, Beschorner WE, Baumgartner WA, et al. Accelerated arteriosclerosis in heart transplant recipients is associated with a T-lymphocyte-mediated endothelialitis. Am J Pathol 1990; 137:871–882.
78. Fish RD, Nabel EG, Selwyn AP, et al. Responses of coronary arteries of cardiac transplant patients to acetylcholine. J Clin Invest 1988; 81:21–31.

79. St.Goar FG, Pinto FJ, Alderman EL, et al. Intracoronary ultrasound in cardiac transplant recipients—In vivo evidence of "angiographically silent" intimal thickening. Circulation 1992; 85:979–987.
80. Billingham ME. Graft coronary disease: The lesions and the patients. Transplant Proc 1989; 21:3665–3666.
81. Koskinen PK, Nieminen MS, Krogerus LA, et al. Cytomegalovirus infection and accelerated cardiac allograft vasculopathy in human cardiac allografts. J Heart Lung Transplant 1993; 12:724–729.

5

Accelerated Arteriosclerosis in Heart Transplant Recipients: The Central Pathogenetic Role of Endothelial Cell Injury

John D. Day, Grover M. Hutchins, Barry J. Byrne, Kenneth L. Baughman, Edward K. Kasper, and Ralph H. Hruban
Johns Hopkins University School of Medicine, Baltimore, Maryland

William A. Baumgartner
Johns Hopkins Hospital, Baltimore, Maryland

I. INTRODUCTION

Since the first heart transplant was performed in 1967, cardiac transplantation has emerged as an effective therapy for otherwise fatal heart disease. Most heart transplant recipients return to productive and satisfying lives. With the introduction of cyclosporine-based immunosuppression and improvements in the treatment of acute infections, 1 year survival rates are now approaching 90% (1). However, with increased survival, accelerated arteriosclerosis has emerged as the major cause of morbidity and mortality in heart transplant recipients.

The characteristic progressive narrowing of the coronary arteries that develops in heart-transplant recipients has been reported under a variety of names, including accelerated atherosclerosis, graft vasculopathy, and graft coronary disease; however, we prefer the term *accelerated arteriosclerosis*. This name not only conveys the speed with which the lesion develops but also distinguishes the process from the more common natural atherosclerosis seen in the general population.

This chapter focuses on the cellular and molecular basis for the development of accelerated arteriosclerosis in heart transplant recipients. However, the process also occurs in kidney and lung allografts, and at least some of the observations made in heart allografts may apply to these other organs as well.

II. EPIDEMIOLOGY

Accelerated arteriosclerosis was first observed in human heart-transplant recipients by Thomson in 1969 (2). Now it is known to be a progressive and almost universal complication in long-term survivors (3,4). Accelerated arteriosclerosis can develop as early as 3 months posttransplantation (5); it occurs in the pediatric (6–8) as well as the adult population; its prevalence is not decreased by cyclosporine immunosuppression (9); and it is the leading cause of death in transplant recipients beyond the first year (5). While angiography can detect accelerated arteriosclerosis in as many as 40% of heart transplant recipients 3 to 5 years following transplantation (10,11), almost all patients have histological evidence of accelerated arteriosclerosis as early as 1 year after transplantation (12).

III. CLINICAL PRESENTATION

One of the most devastating aspects of accelerated arteriosclerosis is that it can strike without symptoms of myocardial ischemia, because the transplanted heart is denervated (10). Many of the transplant recipients with accelerated arteriosclerosis are completely without symptoms until they acutely develop a life-threatening arrhythmia, congestive heart failure, or sudden death. Thus, in the absence of reliable clinical signs, annual coronary angiography is the main diagnostic technique for establishing the presence of the disease. More recently, intracoronary ultrasound has also become a valuable tool (13).

IV. RISK FACTORS

The immunosuppressive therapy that heart transplant recipients receive often causes hypertension, hypercholesterolemia, hyperglycemia and obesity, but few of these "traditional" risk factors have been shown to contribute to the development of accelerated arteriosclerosis (14–19). As more sensitive means of recognizing accelerated arteriosclerosis become available (13), some of these risk factors may be found to be significant.

Of the numerous potential risk factors that have been studied, cytomegalovirus (CMV) infection has been the one most clearly linked with accelerated arteriosclerosis (20,21). Grattan et al. followed 321 heart transplant recipients and demonstrated that the death rate from accelerated arteriosclerosis was much higher in the 91 recipients who developed CMV infections than it was in the 230 recipients who did not (20). In their study, less than 10% of the CMV-negative patients developed severe coronary obstruction (defined as ≥70% stenosis by angiography) by the fifth year after transplantation, as compared with nearly 30% of the CMV-positive patients (20). Furthermore, Wu et al. have demonstrated CMV nucleic acids in vessels with accelerated arteriosclerosis (22).

Ischemic injury at the time of transplantation has also been associated with accelerated arteriosclerosis. We recently examined the first three endomyocardial biopsies of 50 heart transplant recipients for peritransplant ischemic injury and found that the presence of significant ischemic injury in these biopsies was the strongest predictor of the development of accelerated arteriosclerosis (23).

Additional factors, some more controversial than others, have been associated with accelerated arteriosclerosis. These include major and minor histocompatibility mismatches between donor and recipient (24–27), hyperlipidemia (10,28), major rejection episodes (11), advanced donor age (10,21), and therapy with cyclosporine (29).

V. PATHOLOGY

Although the clinical risk factors for the development of accelerated arteriosclerosis are not well defined, the gross and microscopic features of the process are certainly striking and characteristic. As illustrated in Fig. 1 (see also color plate), accelerated arteriosclerosis is

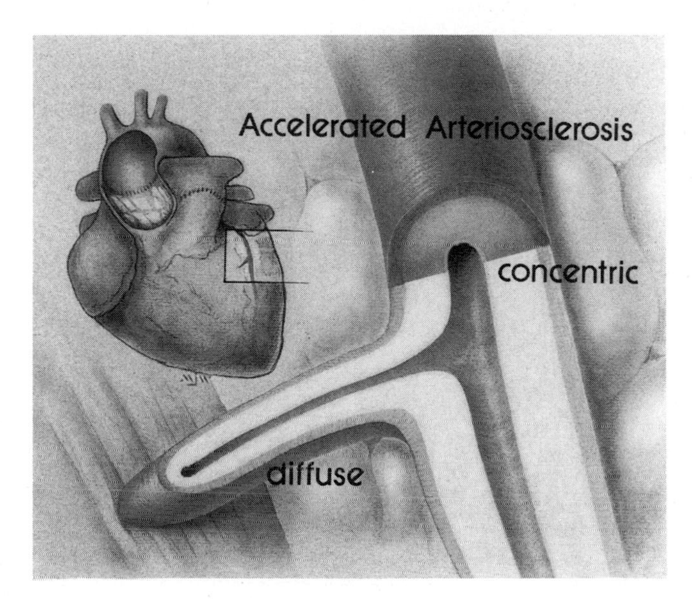

Figure 1 Schematic representation of transplant-related accelerated arteriosclerosis illustrating the diffuse and concentric luminal narrowing characteristic of this lesion. (From Ref. 33.) (For optimal reproduction, see color plate.)

characterized by a *concentric* narrowing of the coronary arteries. The process is *diffuse* and even extends into intramyocardial vessels (30). Because even the small vessels are involved, patients with accelerated arteriosclerosis are usually not candidates for bypass surgery. This gross appearance sharply contrasts with that of natural atherosclerosis, which is focal and eccentric. Interestingly, accelerated arteriosclerosis does not involve the recipient's vasculature but rather is localized to the allograft (31,32). These characteristic gross changes result in the angiographic finding of diffuse concentric luminal narrowing of the coronary arteries with pruning of the smaller distal vessels (Fig. 2 [see also color plate] and Fig. 3) (10). At the light microscopic level (Fig. 4), the external and internal elastic laminae are usually intact, and the intima is thickened by an accumulation of smooth muscle cells, lipid-laden macrophages, and lymphocytes (32). In particular, there is significant accumulation of lymphocytes and macrophages in the subendothelial space (32). Ultrastructurally, smooth muscle cells, macrophages, and two populations of lymphocytes are observed in the intima of affected vessels. The first population of lymphocytes has cytoplasmic granules and cell processes extending into injured endothelial cells, a phenotype suggestive of cytotoxic T lymphocytes. The second lacks cytoplasmic granules, is in contact with macrophages, is located slightly deeper in the intima, and is suggestive of helper T lymphocytes (33). Microthrombi and platelet adherence to the endothelium have also been observed (33).

VI. PATHOGENESIS

While a variety of mechanisms—including ischemia, CMV infection, humoral and cellular rejection, and cyclosporine therapy—have been proposed to account for the rapid development of arteriosclerosis in heart transplant recipients, no single factor accounts for its development. The etiology of accelerated arteriosclerosis is clearly multifactorial. Never-

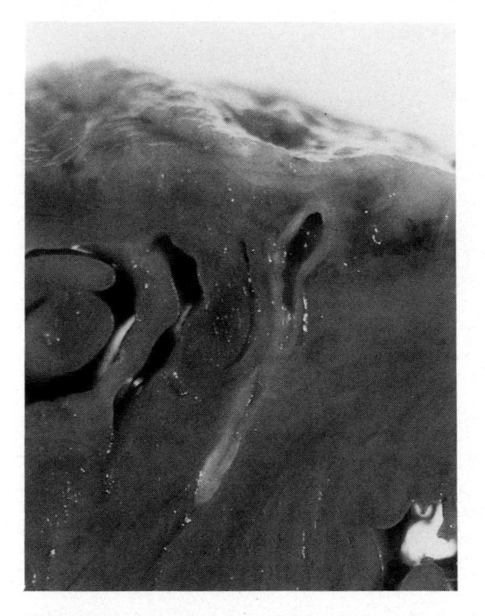

Figure 2 Gross photograph of a section of a coronary artery of the heart from a patient with accelerated arteriosclerosis. Note the concentric nature of the luminal narrowing and the diffuse involvement of both the larger epicardial and smaller perforating coronary arteries. (From Ref. 163.) (For optimal reproduction, see color plate.)

theless, many of the contributing factors have a common denominator: *endothelial injury*. This is not surprising considering the central role that the endothelium plays in the control of vascular tone, permeability, and coagulopathy and in the generation of and response to growth factors and cytokines. Below, we review the mechanisms by which the endothelium is injured after transplantation and the cellular and molecular mechanisms by which endothelial injury, in turn, promotes the development of accelerated arteriosclerosis.

A. Ischemia

As seen in Fig. 5, the heart may sustain significant ischemic injury at the time of transplantation (34). Based on posttransplant serum levels of myosin light chain, it has been reported that the heart transplant procedure can be associated with myocardial injury comparable to that seen in acute infarction (34). Similarly, at the ultrastructural level, ischemic injury to the endothelium can be significant. Billingham et al. examined 15 donor hearts for ultrastructural evidence of ischemic injury, comparing the 12 hearts obtained from distant locations to the 3 procured on site. They observed vascular changes consisting of moderate to severe capillary endothelial swelling and bleeding in all of the distantly procured hearts but not in any of the locally procured hearts (35).

This acute ischemic injury to the heart and to its endothelium can have long-term consequences (23). For example, in an animal model of renal transplantation, Yilmaz et al. have demonstrated that merely increasing the graft ischemic time from 30 to 60 min causes accelerated arteriosclerosis (36).

Furthermore, this relationship between ischemia and accelerated arteriosclerosis appears to be a causal one. Therapies that decrease ischemic injury at the time of transplantation also decrease the development of accelerated arteriosclerosis. In a prospective, ran-

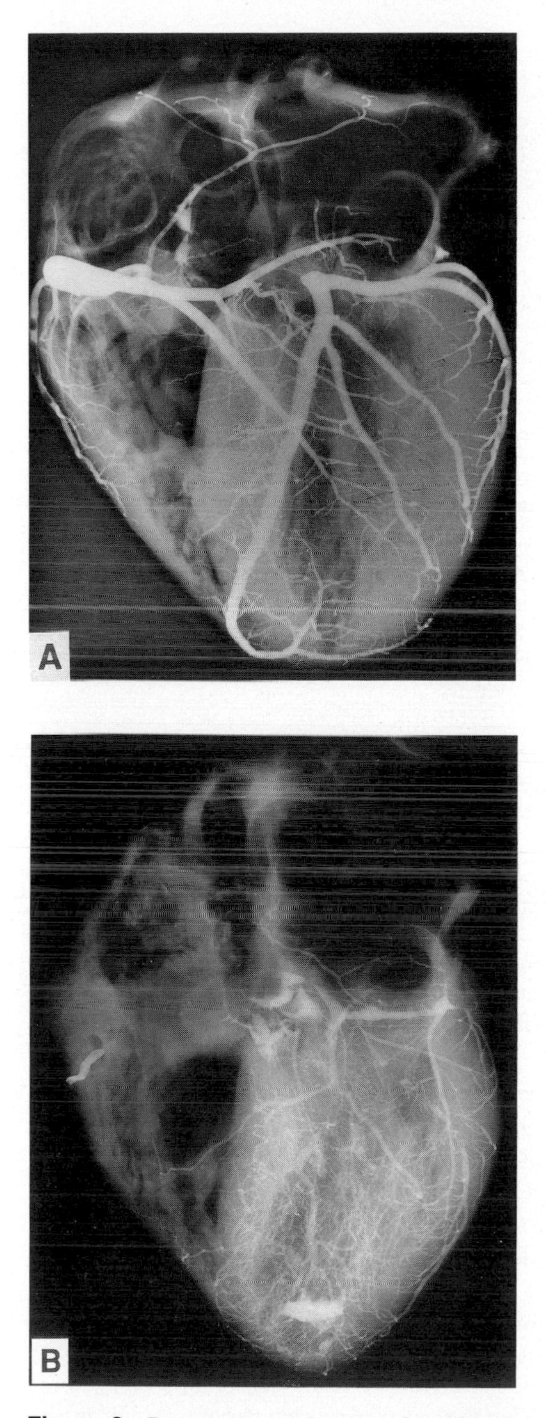

Figure 3 Postmortem angiogram of a normal heart (A) and of the heart from a patient with moderate accelerated arteriosclerosis (B). In contrast to the normal, note the diffuse nature of the involvement of the vessels in B. (B from Ref. 163.)

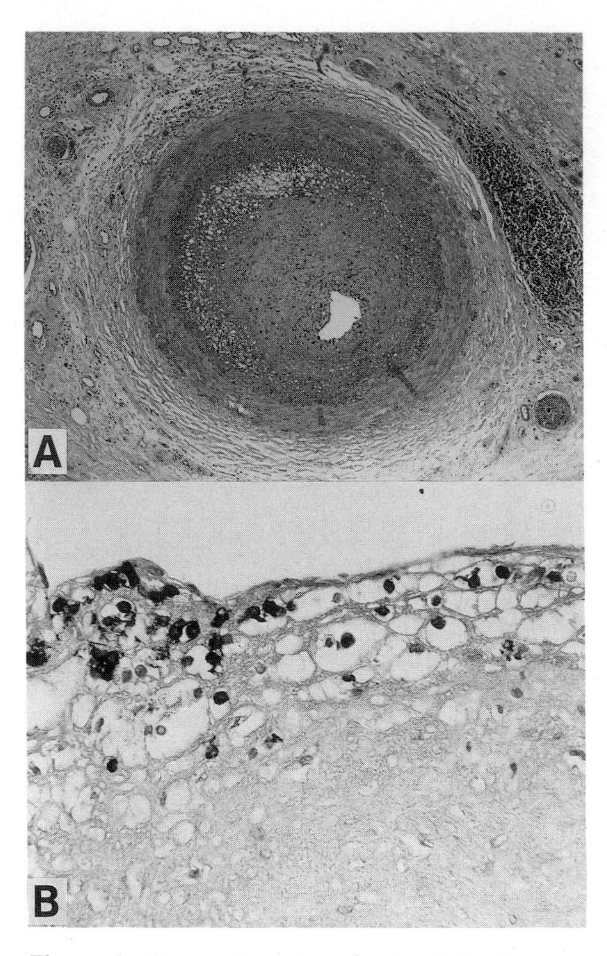

Figure 4 The accelerated arteriosclerosis in this case was characterized by a concentric luminal narrowing (A). The intimal thickening was associated with a T-lymphocyte endothelialitis (B). (From Ref. 32.) (A: hematoxylin and eosin, ×60; B: immunohistochemical staining for CD45RO, ×400.)

domized, double-blind, placebo-controlled trial of 177 cadaveric renal transplant recipients, Land et al. demonstrated that human recombinant superoxide dismutase (rh-SOD), given at the time of transplantation, significantly reduced acute and chronic rejection and increased 4-year graft survival by 22% (37). Superoxide dismutase mitigates free-radical–mediated reperfusion injury, supporting a causal role for ischemic injury in the development of accelerated arteriosclerosis.

As noted previously, a relationship between early ischemic injury and the development of accelerated arteriosclerosis is also seen in human heart-transplant recipients. When we examined the first three endomyocardial biopsies from 50 heart-transplant recipients for evidence of early ischemic injury, we found that the histological changes of ischemic injury (Fig. 5) were the strongest predictors of subsequent transplant-related accelerated arteriosclerosis (RR 2.6, 95% CI 1.2-5.8, p=0.02) (23).

There are a number of molecular and cellular mechanisms by which the ischemic injury that the heart sustains at the time of transplantation can promote the development of

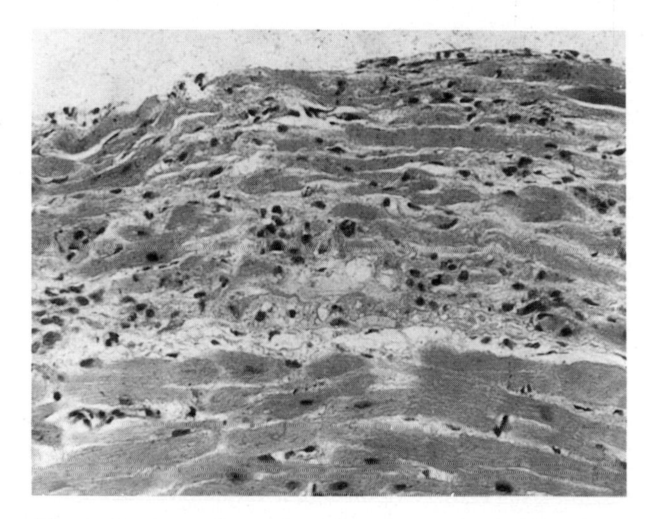

Figure 5 Large focus of myocyte necrosis with early macrophagic removal (top half of the figure). In contrast, the myocardium at the bottom of the figure appears viable. (From Ref. 23.)

accelerated arteriosclerosis (38). These include platelet activation and adherence, complement activation, the upregulation of adhesion molecules, the promotion of humoral rejection, the promotion of cellular rejection, and increased susceptibility to CMV infection. Each of these mechanisms is discussed in the following sections, as is the role of macrophages, cyclosporine, and the disregulation of vascular tone in the development of accelerated arteriosclerosis.

B. Platelet Activation

One of the most consistent and characteristic manifestations of endothelial damage is platelet aggregation and degranulation, with subsequent thrombus formation (2,33,39–41). Platelet adherence can be demonstrated in transplanted organs at the ultrastructural level (33) and immunohistochemically using antiplatelet antibodies (40). Once adherent to the endothelium, platelets promote the development of accelerated arteriosclerosis through a variety of mechanisms, including the release of growth factors that stimulate endothelial cells, smooth muscle cells, and fibroblasts.

Principal among the growth factors released by platelets is platelet derived growth factor (PDGF), which increases matrix deposition, lipid accumulation, directional cell migration, and, most importantly, smooth muscle cell proliferation (42,43). All of these effects of PDGF can contribute to the development of accelerated arteriosclerosis. Furthermore, increased PDGF receptor expression has been demonstrated in the smooth muscle cells and fibroblasts of coronary arteries with accelerated arteriosclerosis (44).

Platelet deposition may also contribute to the development of accelerated arteriosclerosis by the thickening of the intima caused by the organization of microthrombi. The demonstration that platelets play a role in the development of accelerated arteriosclerosis is important, because there are a variety of therapies that can be used to block platelet function, and these treatments have the potential for decreasing accelerated arteriosclerosis.

C. Complement

More subtle forms of ischemia-induced endothelial injury may also promote the development of accelerated arteriosclerosis. For example, endothelial cells injured by ischemia can activate complement (45). Weisman et al. (46) and Litt et al. (47) have shown that transient ischemia, with subsequent reperfusion, results in the deposition of C3, C5b–C9 (the membrane attack complex, or MAC) and leukocyte accumulation.

The insertion of MAC into the cell membrane of endothelial cells results in the release of PDGF and basic fibroblast growth factor (bFGF), and these growth factors can contribute to the subintimal thickening of the vasculature commonly seen in accelerated arteriosclerosis (48). Split products of complement can also enhance macrophage chemotaxis, adhesion, and phagocytosis. For example, C3a and C5a stimulate macrophages to synthesize and release cytokines, such as interleukin-1 (IL-1), which are mitogenic for smooth muscle cells (49).

MAC insertion into the endothelium also causes endothelial activation. The activation of endothelial cells increases their procoagulant activity, resulting in platelet deposition (50,51).

D. Upregulation of Adhesion Molecules and HLA Antigens

Ischemia also upregulates the expression of inflammatory cell adhesion molecules and human leukocyte antigens (HLA) on the vascular endothelium. Ischemia-induced reperfusion injury to the myocardium results in the production of oxygen free radicals by inflammatory cells (52). This local accumulation of inflammatory cells is made possible by the upregulation of inflammatory cell adhesion molecules—such as vascular cell adhesion molecule-1 (VCAM-1) and intercellular adhesion molecule-1 (ICAM-1)—on endothelial surfaces (53–55). The upregulation of adhesion molecules will lead to increased leukocyte binding which will result in cytokine release and ultimately in endothelial injury. The importance of this upregulation of adhesion molecules has recently been demonstrated by Isobe et al. They demonstrated that treatment with antibodies directed against ICAM-1 and its ligand, LFA-1, induces a donor-specific tolerance to heart grafts, resulting in indefinite survival in mice (56). Hence, the upregulation of adhesion molecules on endothelial cells can be caused by ischemia, and, in turn, this upregulation may play an important role in accelerated arteriosclerosis and graft rejection.

In addition to the upregulation of adhesion molecules, ischemic injury also results in increased expression of major histocompatibility complex antigen. Shoskes et al. demonstrated that 60-min unilateral vascular occlusion in the kidneys of mice resulted in 3- to 6-fold increase in class I HLA expression and in a 1.5- to 3-fold increase in HLA class II expression (57). This increased expression of HLA antigens secondary to ischemia may increase the immunogenicity of graft endothelial cells, thereby promoting both humoral and cellular rejection. As is discussed in the following two sections, humoral and cell-mediated rejection, in turn, promote the development of accelerated arteriosclerosis (58–60).

E. Antibody-Mediated Rejection

Ischemic injury at the time of transplantation may also result in the release of donor endothelial antigens, and this antigen release may, in turn, promote the development of a humoral (antibody-mediated) reaction against the graft (61). Indeed, antiendothelial antibodies have been demonstrated in the early posttransplant period and in long-term survivors with accelerated arteriosclerosis. Hammond et al. have identified a subgroup of heart transplant recipients in whom the deposition of immunoglobulins and complement can be demonstrated in endomyocardial biopsies taken shortly after transplantation (62,63). Similarly, antigraft antibodies can be demonstrated in long-term survivors, and these antibodies have been associated with the development of accelerated arteriosclerosis (58,64–66). In particular, Rose et al. demonstrated a 23% decrease in the 4-year survival rate for those patients whose panel reactive antibody levels were greater than 10% during the first 6 months after transplantation (59). Likewise, Dunn et al. found that antiendothelial antibodies were present in 71% of the patients with accelerated arteriosclerosis. Similar antibodies were found in only 5% of the patients who had not developed the disease (66).

The antibodies produced following transplantation may be directed at HLA class I and II antigens, endothelial cell-specific antigens, or tissue-specific antigens expressed on endothelial cells (59,66,67). Once host antibodies have bound to any of these graft antigens, the antigen-antibody complex is capable of stimulating proliferation of both helper and cytotoxic T lymphocytes, and with T-cell activation, lymphokines are released that further augment the secretion of antibodies by B lymphocytes (58). The complement component C1 is also activated by antibody deposited in a graft, and the binding of the C1q component of C1 to its receptor, C1qR, results in platelet activation and increased procoagulant activity (68). Furthermore, C5a activates endothelial cells, making their cell membranes more thrombogenic (50). Hence, initial ischemic injury may result in the production of antibodies specific for several different antigens on the endothelium of the graft. These antibodies can cause endothelial injury and the development of accelerated arteriosclerosis.

F. Cell-Mediated Immunity

Cell-mediated immunity has been shown to play a central role in the development of accelerated arteriosclerosis in both humans and experimental animals. Cardiac grafts between genetically identical animals do not develop vascular lesions, accelerated arteriosclerosis does develop across HLA barriers and can be enhanced by sensitization of the recipient to donor antigens, and the vascular lesions seen in the graft are not seen in the native vessels of transplant recipients (32). Furthermore, recipient lymphocytes have been demonstrated in contact with donor endothelial cells in vessels with accelerated arteriosclerosis (69). The presence of recipient lymphocytes infiltrating the donor coronary arteries was established using the technique of fluorescence in situ hybridization (FISH). We examined sections of coronary arteries from two heart-transplant recipients undergoing retransplantation because of accelerated arteriosclerosis by FISH for the presence of cells containing the Y chromosome (69). In both cases, the recipients were male and the original donor hearts were obtained from females. As shown in Fig. 6 (see also color plate), hybridization was detected in lymphocytes and macrophages closely associated with endothelial cells, establishing that these lymphocytes and macrophages in the donor hearts were of recipient origin. In contrast, hybridization was not detected in endothelial cells. Thus, recipient lymphocytes infiltrate vessels with accelerated arteriosclerosis (69).

While both $CD4^+$ and $CD8^+$ lymphocytes are present in approximately equal numbers within the subendothelium of vessels affected with accelerated arteriosclerosis (32), the relative contribution of helper and cytotoxic lymphocytes remains unclear. This section discusses the mechanisms whereby recipient helper lymphocytes and cytotoxic lymphocytes contribute to the development of accelerated arteriosclerosis.

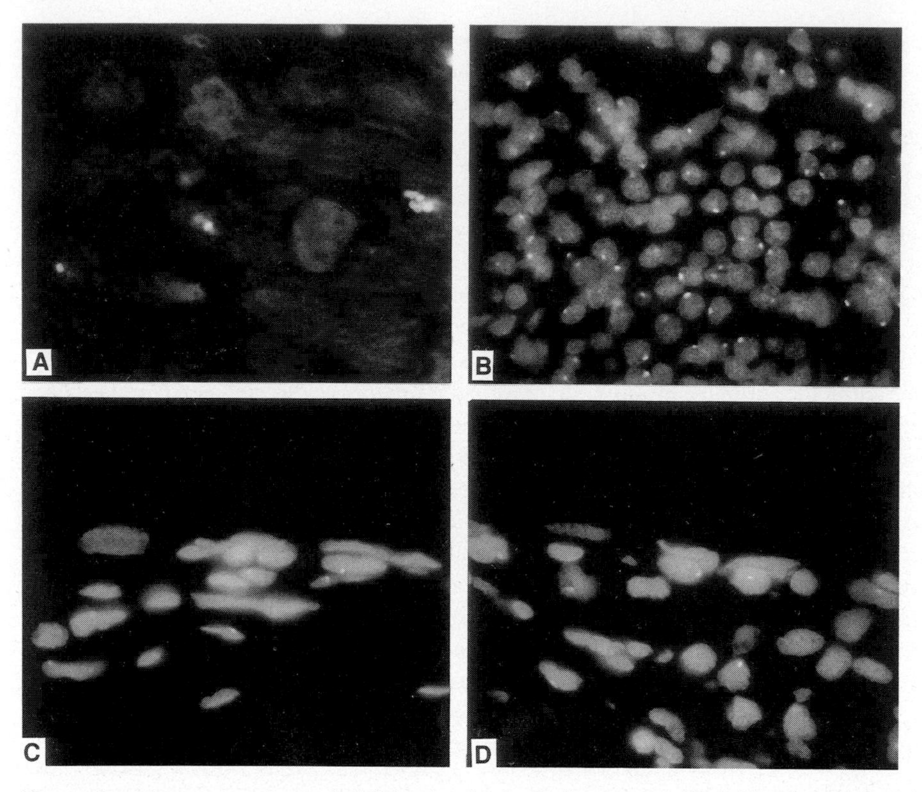

Figure 6 Fluorescence in situ hybridization for the Y chromosome. Hybridization was not detected in cardiac myocytes (A). In contrast, note the intense focal punctate yellow hybridization present in infiltrating lymphocytes (B) and in subendothelial lymphocytes and macrophages (C and D). C and D: The lumina of the vessels occupies the top third of the photograph, endothelial cells are identified as the single layer of flattened cells immediately lining these lumina, and the subendothelial lymphocytes and macrophages occupy the lower portion of the photograph. (From Ref. 69.) (For optimal reproduction, see color plate.)

T-helper lymphocytes are present in vessels with accelerated arteriosclerosis, they are functionally active, and they can promote accelerated arteriosclerosis in a variety of ways. The CD4 antigen is usually expressed on T-helper cells, and $CD4^+$ cells have been demonstrated in vessels with accelerated arteriosclerosis (32,70). Furthermore, these cells are morphologically consistent with helper T cells. At the ultrastructural level, we identified lymphocytes morphologically consistent with T-helper cells in contact with macrophages in coronary arteries with accelerated arteriosclerosis (33). T-helper cells are not only present but they are also functionally active. Salomon et al. demonstrated that the $CD4^+$ lymphocytes in vessels with accelerated arteriosclerosis proliferate and release interleukin-2 (IL-2), a known B- and T-lymphocyte stimulator, in response to activated foreign endothelial cells (70). Once activated, T-helper cells can promote accelerated arteriosclerosis by a delayed-type hypersensitivity reaction; T-helper cells are known to secrete a variety of lymphokines which activate macrophages, and activated macrophages have been shown to produce PDGF, which is a potent mitogen for smooth muscle cells.

In contrast to the indirect mechanism by which T-helper lymphocytes promote accelerated arteriosclerosis, cytotoxic lymphocytes may directly injure endothelial cells, which express foreign class I HLA antigens (71). As was true for T-helper cells, cytotoxic T lymphocytes have been identified in vessels with accelerated arteriosclerosis, they have been shown to be functionally active, and they are capable of promoting the development of accelerated arteriosclerosis through a number of mechanisms. Lymphocytes expressing CD8 have been demonstrated in vessels with accelerated arteriosclerosis (Fig. 7; see also color plate), and, ultrastructurally, some of the subintimal lymphocytes in these vessels have been shown to contain membrane-bound cytoplasmic granules within cellular processes (Fig. 8) (32,33). This morphology is consistent with a cytotoxic function for these lymphocytes, and they appear to be functionally active. Evidence of their functional activity comes from electron microscopy and immunohistochemical studies. Ultrastructurally, these lymphocytes are intimately associated with injured endothelial cells (33). Immunohistochemically, as shown in Fig. 9 (see also color plate), the lymphocytes have been shown to express perforin (71), a pore-forming protein that is expressed by functionally active cytotoxic lymphocytes (71–77). Therefore the expression of perforin by lymphocytes in vessels with accelerated arteriosclerosis suggests that these lymphocytes are functionally active cytotoxic T cells.

These ultrastructural and immunohistochemical studies have been combined to confirm that the lymphocytes seen at the ultrastructural level are the same ones that express perforin. We used an immunogold labeling technique to detect perforin at the ultrastructural level and found perforin expression in the granules of the lymphocytes in two coronary

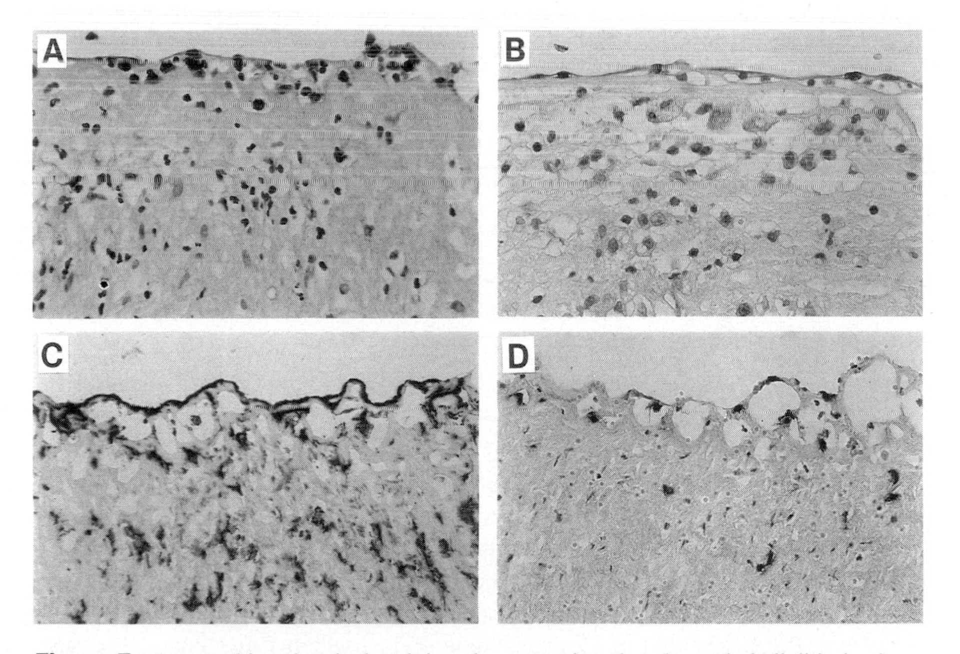

Figure 7 Immunohistochemical staining demonstrating that the endothelialitis in the coronary arteries of this explanted heart with accelerated arteriosclerosis is composed of macrophages (A) and T lymphocytes (B). The endothelialitis is associated with induced class II major histocompatibility antigen expression on endothelial cells (C), and the T lymphocytes stain as cytotoxic T lymphocytes (D). (From Ref. 32.) (A: Immunohistochemical staining, MAC-387, ×400; B: CD45RO, ×685; C: HLA-DR, ×575; D: CD8, ×575.) (For optimal reproduction, see color plate.)

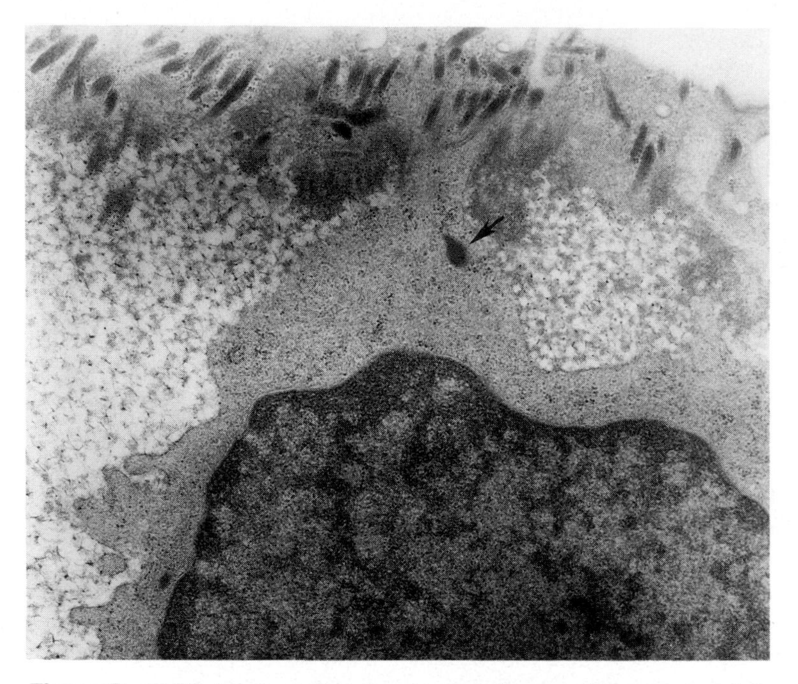

Figure 8 TEM showing a lymphocyte extending a cell process containing a single cytoplasmic granule (arrow) into an overlying endothelial cell. The endothelial cell shows evidence of injury, including cytoplasmic vacuoles and an increased number of Weibel-Palade bodies. (From Ref. 33.) (Magnification: ×26,500.)

arteries with transplant-related accelerated arteriosclerosis. This observation combines our previous findings of lymphocytes containing membrane-bound granules at the electron microscopic level (33) with the immunohistochemical staining for perforin by light microscopy (71). Hence, immunohistochemical and ultrastructural observations suggest that functionally active cytotoxic T lymphocytes reactive against the endothelium are present in grafts with accelerated arteriosclerosis. As is discussed in a later section, endothelial injury is, in turn, a major promoter of accelerated arteriosclerosis.

G. Macrophages

One of the earliest manifestations of accelerated arteriosclerosis is the appearance of large numbers of monocytes binding to the vascular endothelium (25,78). Once bound to the endothelium, these monocytes emigrate into the intima and transform into lipid-laden macrophages (79). Macrophages remain a constant feature of the vascular lesions, even in the later stages, when the inflammatory cells make up only a small portion of the actual arteriosclerotic lesion. Macrophages can promote the development of accelerated arteriosclerosis through the production of oxidized lipoproteins, which cause endothelial and smooth muscle cell injury, and by the promotion of foam-cell formation (80,81). Furthermore, macrophages play an integral role in the production and secretion of inflammatory mediators, such as PDGF and leukocyte chemotactic factors. These factors further contribute to the development of accelerated arteriosclerosis. Indeed, increased PDGF receptor expression is observed prominently on the smooth muscle cells and fibroblasts in areas of

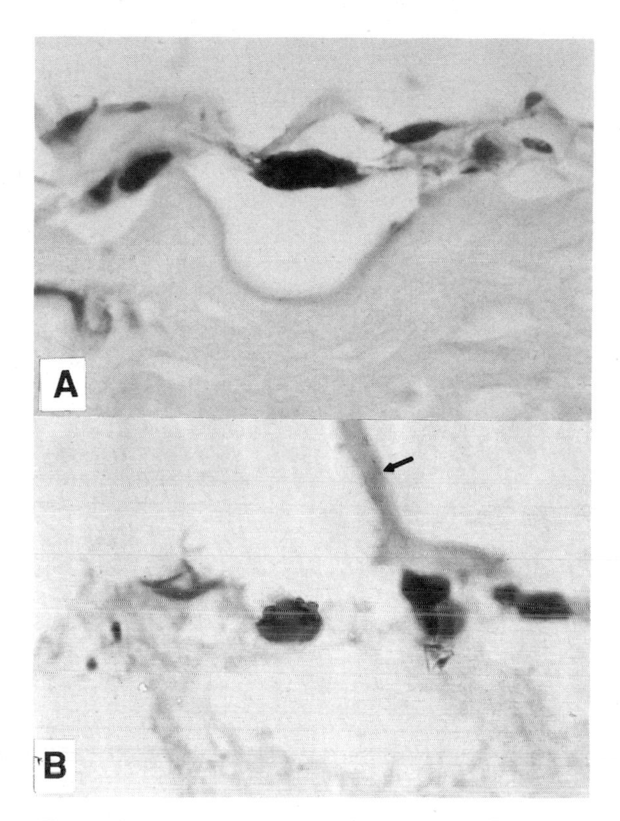

Figure 9 $CD8^+$ lymphocytes were identified in the subendothelial spaces of coronary arteries with transplant-related arteriosclerosis (A). In contrast to the diffuse staining seen with the anti-CD8 antibody, a granular cytoplasmic staining was seen when the same cells were stained for perforin (B). (From Ref. 71.) (A. immunohistochemical stain for CD8, ×960; B: immunohistochemical stain for perforin, ×900.) (For optimal reproduction, see color plate.)

the graft containing inflammatory cells (44). Macrophage involvement in the disease is not exclusively mediated by PDGF; other cytokines produced by macrophages, such as tumor necrosis factor-alpha (TNF-α), transforming growth factor-beta (TGF-β), and IL-1 (49), may cause further recruitment and proliferation of leukocytes into the vascular lesion. For example, TNF-α increases the expression of adhesion molecules on endothelial cells, increases cytokine production, promotes smooth muscle cell growth, increases endothelial prothrombotic activity, and increases HLA expression; TGF-β increases the production of extracellular proteins (82). Hence, macrophages play an active role in the direct formation of the lesion as well as synthesizing and secreting cytokines, which play a prominent role in the development of accelerated arteriosclerosis.

H. Cytomegalovirus

Ischemic injury can also promote accelerated arteriosclerosis by increasing the graft's susceptibility to cytomegalovirus (CMV). Cytomegalovirus infection, a common occurrence after cardiac transplantation, is one of the strongest risk factors for the development of accelerated arteriosclerosis studied to date. The infection typically occurs in the first 3 months after transplantation, and the link to vascular disease appears to be most significant in patients with viremia of more than 4 months' duration (83,84). The source of infection in transplant recipients can be infected donor grafts or a reactivation of a latent CMV infection in the host (85). In addition to the development of accelerated arteriosclerosis, CMV infection has been linked to increased graft rejection (20), myocarditis (83), and atherosclerosis in the nonimmunosuppressed population (86).

Although the association of CMV with accelerated arteriosclerosis has been well studied, the mechanism whereby the virus promotes arteriosclerosis is not entirely clear. Cytomegalovirus nucleic acids have been detected in endothelial cells, smooth muscle cells, and lymphocytes in coronary arteries with accelerated arteriosclerosis (Fig. 10) (22). Thus, it is quite possible that CMV infection may induce accelerated arteriosclerosis by any or all of the following mechanisms: (a) direct viral injury to endothelial cells (87),

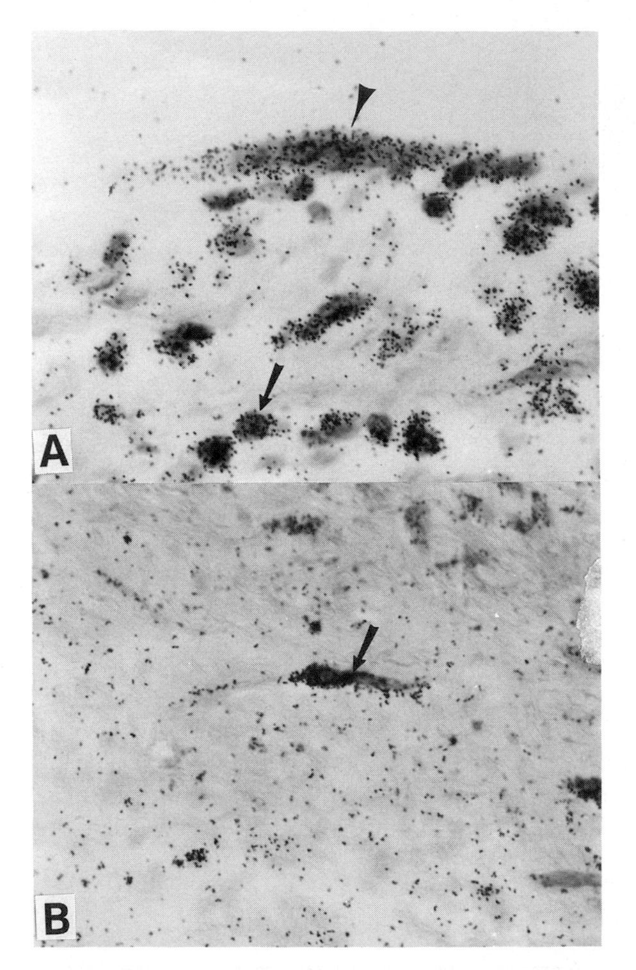

Figure 10 In situ hybridization with the tritium-labeled riboprobe derived from the immediate early gene of CMV. Hybridization to cells morphologically consistent with endothelial (A, arrowhead), mononuclear (A, arrow), and smooth muscle cells (B, arrow) is identified. (From Ref. 22.) (A and B: ×500.)

(b) reduction of the anticoagulant properties of endothelial cells (88), (c) promotion of a chronic allogenic immune response by the upregulation of MHC antigen expression on endothelial and smooth muscle cells (89,90), (d) alteration of lipid metabolism with decreased cholesteryl ester hydrolase production and increased cholesterol and cholesteryl ester accumulation in smooth muscle cells (91), (e) induction of smooth muscle cell proliferation caused by viral DNA insertion into smooth muscle cells (92), and or (f) the process of "molecular mimicry," in which an immune response generated against CMV sequences cross-reacts against self class II antigens (93).

Cytomegalovirus may also interact with the p53 tumor suppressor gene, and this interaction may foster the development of accelerated arteriosclerosis. Speir et al. recently demonstrated a correlation between the accumulation of the p53 gene product and CMV infection in the coronary arteries of nontransplanted patients who developed restenosis following angioplasty (94). The accumulation of p53 gene product is associated with p53 inactivation, and p53 inactivation, in turn, promotes increased cell growth. The mechanism by which CMV inactivates p53 is not clear, but one of the proteins produced by CMV, IE84, has been shown to bind to and inactivate p53. Thus, the production of IE84 in CMV-infected cells in the graft vasculature may lead to the inactivation of the p53 tumor suppressor gene, increased smooth muscle cell growth, and the development of accelerated arteriosclerosis (94).

I. Vascular Tone

Injury to the endothelial cells, whether due to an ischemic insult or one of the immune mechanisms previously outlined, has been shown to have both vasoconstricting and vasodilating potential (95–98). In the early stages of vascular injury, vessels may dilate secondary to the release of vasodilatory agents such as prostacyclin and endothelium-derived relaxing factor (EDRF), allowing for the increased recruitment of inflammatory cells. This vasodilation and the influx of inflammatory cells could, in turn, promote the immunologically mediated proliferative arteriosclerotic lesions commonly seen in heart transplant recipients by the mechanisms previously discussed.

On the other hand, injury to the endothelium may also cause vasoconstriction, via the potent vasoconstrictor endothelin (95). Furthermore, endothelial dysfunction, which often accompanies the development of accelerated arteriosclerosis in the heart transplant recipient, may decrease the production of vasodilatory agents (96). This combination of increased endothelin production and decreased production of vasodilatory agents predisposes the transplant recipient to coronary artery spasm, a common occurrence in vessels with accelerated arteriosclerosis (97,98). This spasm may, in turn, make the lesions functionally much worse than suggested by the vascular anatomy alone.

Remarkably, many of the substances that regulate vascular tone also play a role in cell proliferation. For example, PDGF causes vasoconstriction as well as smooth muscle cell proliferation (99). Thus, it is not surprising that most heart transplant recipients who develop coronary artery spasm also develop accelerated arteriosclerosis (98).

J. Cyclosporine

Although cyclosporine has clearly had an enormous positive impact on the survival of heart-transplant recipients, some researchers have suggested that it is associated with the development of accelerated arteriosclerosis. The introduction of cyclosporine has led to dramatic improvements in 1-year survival rates for heart transplantation, but it has not led to a decrease in the prevalence of accelerated arteriosclerosis. This may not merely be a result of patients surviving long enough to develop the disease but may represent an actual promotion of accelerated arteriosclerosis by cyclosporine.

Cyclosporine is a cyclic polypeptide secreted by the fungus *Tolypocladium inflatum gams*. Cyclosporine inhibits T-helper function and subsequent production of IL-2, thus inhibiting cell-mediated immunity (100). Early studies of cyclosporine's toxicity indicated that the drug has the ability to injure graft vessels directly (101,102). Moreover, when applied to the rat aortic allograft, cyclosporine amplifies transplant-related arteriosclerosis (29). Cyclosporine has also been implicated in causing hyperlipidemia after transplantation (103) by inhibiting corticosteroid clearance through either hepatotoxicity or cytochrome P-450 interaction (104).

Cramer has proposed an additional explanation for the possible association between cyclosporine and accelerated arteriosclerosis. He suggests that since the introduction of cyclosporine, many cases of mild rejection are no longer treated because of the toxicity of cyclosporine. The decreased treatment of mild rejection episodes may increase the cumulative amount of rejection in the graft, thereby promoting the development of the vascular lesions (105). As new immunosuppression agents are introduced, their effects on the development of accelerated arteriosclerosis must be assessed to determine their true effect on graft survival.

K. Endothelial Injury

Clearly, there are a wide variety of mechanisms by which coronary artery endothelium can be injured following transplantation, and there is a large body of evidence suggesting that endothelial injury does in fact occur. Once this injury has occurred, there are a variety of ways it can promote the development of accelerated arteriosclerosis. These include the release of endothelial-derived factors, increased platelet aggregation, the release of vasoactive substances by the endothelium, loss of the endothelial barrier with lipid accumulation, and the upregulation of adhesion molecules.

First, injured endothelial cells can produce and release cytokines and growth factors, thus promoting the development of accelerated arteriosclerosis. In particular, injured endothelial cells have been shown to express PDGF (44), IL-1, and human leukocyte antigens (HLA) (60). PDGF is a potent smooth muscle cell and fibroblast mitogen, and IL-1 promotes the response of T lymphocytes. The increased expression of HLA may result in increased humoral and cellular rejection, thus perpetuating the cycle of vascular injury (58–60).

Second, endothelial injury results in loss of endothelial integrity and in the deposition of platelets and fibrin (33). In addition to directly causing luminal reduction by thrombosis, platelet aggregation may promote arteriosclerosis by the release of a variety of growth factors, again the foremost being PDGF and IL-1 (60,87).

Third, injury to endothelial cells can promote vasoconstriction (95,98). Once arteriosclerosis has developed, transplant recipients are predisposed to develop coronary artery spasm via vasoconstriction (96,98).

Fourth, when the endothelial barrier is broken, the vessels become very susceptible to lipid damage and accumulation. Lipids preferentially accumulate in areas of endothelial injury (106), promote foam cell formation (107), and are chemotactic for monocytes (81). This problem is compounded by the fact that hyperlipidemia is a common occurrence in transplant recipients who receive corticosteroids and cyclosporine (14).

Last, the expression of inflammatory cell adhesion molecules, such as VCAM-1 and ICAM-1, is upregulated on endothelial surfaces following stimulation by cytokines (52,55). As a result of adhesion molecule upregulation, endothelial injury is enhanced secondary to increased leukocyte binding and further cytokine release.

Thus, although it is clear that the development of accelerated arteriosclerosis has many causes, we believe that chronic injury to the endothelium is central to this process.

VII. THERAPEUTIC INTERVENTION

Currently, treatment options for accelerated arteriosclerosis are limited and the only definitive therapeutic alternative available is retransplantation. However, due to limited organ availability, the high rate of recurrence of accelerated arteriosclerosis in second grafts, and the low 1-year survival seen with a second transplant (1,9,108), new treatment strategies must be developed. Recent advances in our understanding of the pathogenesis of accelerated arteriosclerosis suggest a variety of novel methods for intervening at a number of different levels in the development of these vascular lesions. This section discusses new therapeutic options to inhibit the development of accelerated arteriosclerosis, with emphasis on each of the mechanisms previously discussed.

A. Ischemia

Increasing evidence indicates that ischemia-associated organ injury is related to the production of free oxygen radicals either within affected tissues or by phagocytes (109,110). Because this ischemic injury is the first injury the transplanted heart sustains, intervention at this level could dramatically decrease the subsequent development of accelerated arteriosclerosis (37).

More specifically, ischemia-reperfusion injury is associated with conversion of ATP to hypoxanthine and with the proteolytic conversion of xanthine deoxygenase to xanthine oxidase. Upon reperfusion of the ischemic tissue, xanthine oxidase metabolizes hypoxanthine and xanthine to uric acid with the generation of superoxide anion (O_2^-) and hydrogen peroxide. Thus, antioxidants such as superoxide dismutase (SOD, which catabolizes the dismutation of superoxide anions to hydrogen peroxide and oxygen), allopurinol (which inhibits the activity of xanthine oxidase and thereby blocks the generation of both hydrogen peroxide and superoxide anion), and catalase (which catabolizes the divalent reduction of hydrogen peroxide to water) could all conceivably limit peritransplant ischemia and thereby decrease the development of accelerated arteriosclerosis (23).

Indeed, each of these treatments has been evaluated. Human recombinant superoxide dismutase (rh-SOD), given at the time of transplantation, has been shown to significantly reduce first acute rejection episodes and chronic rejection in renal transplant recipients (37). Likewise, other antioxidants such as allopurinol may be effective for the cold storage of the cardiac allograft (111–113). Finally, in several studies, catalase has also been shown to be effective in the prevention of peritransplant cardiac ischemia (114,115).

In addition to the direct inhibition of ischemia-reperfusion injury, antioxidants may play a role in the reduction of previously mentioned macrophage-induced oxidation of lipoproteins, which causes endothelial and smooth muscle cell injury and promotes foam cell formation (80,81). Additionally, the use of the University of Wisconsin preservation solution has been reported to prevent the ischemia-induced upregulation of adhesion and major histocompatibility antigen molecules (116). Last, antioxidants have also been demonstrated to inhibit human and murine T-cell proliferation in vitro (117). Hence, antioxidants may represent a means of inhibiting accelerated arteriosclerosis by decreasing peritransplant ischemic injury, suppressing macrophage oxidative damage, limiting upregulation of cellular adhesion molecules and HLA, and modulating the immune response to the graft.

B. Platelet Activation

Since platelet activation—with subsequent aggregation, degranulation, thrombus formation (33,35,39,40), and growth factor release (42–44)—has been associated with the development of accelerated arteriosclerosis, there have been a number of attempts to prevent accelerated arteriosclerosis by inhibiting platelets with antiplatelet drugs and cyclooxygenase inhibitors. While not all of these studies have demonstrated a beneficial effect of platelet inhibitors (118,119), Lurie et al. reported that in a rat model of heart transplantation, dipyridamole, in association with cyclosporine immunosuppression, resulted in complete prevention of transplant-related arteriosclerosis (120). More recently, Häyry et al. demonstrated the beneficial effect of blockers of the platelet activating factor receptor on smooth muscle cell replication in vitro and allograft arteriosclerosis in vivo (121). Similarly, heparin therapy has been shown to be beneficial in organ transplantation (122), perhaps by its ability to prevent smooth muscle cell proliferation caused by PDGF (123,124). Finally, although yet to be conclusively demonstrated in cardiac transplantation, it is reasonable to assume that with the increased platelet aggregation after transplantation, there may be a beneficial role for daily aspirin therapy (122,125).

C. Complement

As noted previously, activation of complement can promote the formation of vascular lesions seen in accelerated arteriosclerosis (45–48). Several different lines of research indicate a possible application for complement inhibitors, particularly in organ preservation solutions. For example, complement inhibitors such as cobra venom factor (126) and soluble human complement receptor type 1 (SCR1) (46) have been shown to decrease reperfusion injury. SCR1 is a truncated form of the naturally occurring complement regulatory membrane protein. It inhibits classic activity both by binding C3b and C4b of the multisubunit C3 and C5 convertases and by promoting the dissociation of the catalytic subunits C2a and Bb. SCR1 also promotes the degradation of C3b and C4b to inactive forms. SCR1 has already been shown to prolong xenograft survival (127), and substances such as SCR1 have the potential to decrease accelerated arteriosclerosis. Likewise, the beneficial effects of heparin in organ preservation solutions may, in part, also be related to its ability to inhibit complement activity (122,128).

D. Upregulation of Adhesion Molecules and HLA

Local accumulation of inflammatory cells in chronic organ rejection is promoted by the upregulation of inflammatory cell adhesion molecules, such as vascular cell adhesion molecule-1 (VCAM-1) and intercellular adhesion molecule-1 (ICAM-1) (53–56), as well as increased major histocompatibility complex antigen expression (57) on endothelial surfaces. In animal models, antibodies directed at the ICAM-1 molecule have been shown to significantly delay rejection (129,130). Furthermore, as previously discussed, Isobe et al. demonstrated that antibodies directed against ICAM-1 and its ligand, LFA-1, can induce a donor-specific tolerance to heart grafts, resulting in indefinite survival and the complete prevention of accelerated arteriosclerosis in mice (56). Alternatively, Ardehali et al. have demonstrated that the upregulation of adhesion molecules can be prevented with the use of the antioxidant allopurinol (116).

Recent advances in our understanding of the molecular basis for the upregulation of HLA may provide novel strategies for downregulating the expression of these genes (131,132). For example, Song et al. have identified NF-X1, a cysteine-rich transcription factor, which binds to class II MHC genes. When applied to a retroviral construct, over-expression of NF-X1 strongly decreases transcription from the HLA-DRA promoter (132).

E. Antibody and Cell-Mediated Rejection

While the ability of cyclosporine-based immunosuppression to control cell-mediated immune responses has been well documented (133), the drug is associated with several adverse systemic effects, such as nephrotoxicity and increased susceptibility of the recipient to infections and to the development of posttransplant lymphoproliferative disorders. Clearly there is a need for *graft-specific* immunosuppression, which would be relatively free of these systemic effects. The local expression of immunosuppressive cytokines may fill this role and could be accomplished by linking the expression of genes for these substances to constitutive promoters (134).

Genes coding for immunosuppressive molecules such as IL-10, IL-4, and $CTLA_4Ig$ (a soluble fusion protein of $CTLA_4$ and immunoglobulin G1 Fc region), could potentially be transferred to allografted hearts during the period of time between explantation and implantation. As a result, only the allograft would be transfected, resulting in *graft-specific gene expression* and selective protection of the graft.

This approach to immunosuppression is not as far-fetched as it may seem. Zweibel et al. (135), Nabel et al. (136–138), Ohno et al. (139), Dichek et al. (140,141), and Guzman (142) have all demonstrated that genes can be efficiently transferred to endothelial and smooth muscle cells using a variety of gene transfer techniques. Zweibel et al. first described the retroviral transfer and subsequent expression of recombinant genes into cultured endothelial cells (135). In 1989, Nabel et al., using a specially designed double-balloon catheter, established that endothelial cells transferred in vitro could be implanted onto vessels (136). Later, they showed that vessels could be transferred directly by instilling viral vectors into the vessels and that smooth muscle cells can also be transfected (137–139). Dichek et al. were able to genetically alter endothelial cells in vitro to express increased levels of tissue-type plasminogen activator, thereby potentially reducing the atherogenicity of the endothelium (141). Most recently, Ohno and coworkers have shown that smooth muscle cells can be kept from proliferating by a suicide approach using gene transfer of thymidine kinase and ganciclovir treatment (139). These findings demonstrate that gene transfer technology can be used to deliver stable recombinant gene products to the endothelial cells of specific vessels.

In our experience, it is possible to transduce cardiac tissue with viral vectors expressing the marker gene for β-galactosidase (lacZ). The vector of choice for our experiments has been adeno-associated virus (AAV), because of the high infectivity in nondividing cells and stable integration of virus (143). The utility of this technique is shown in Figs. 11 and 12 (see also color plate). These findings illustrate an experiment in which embryonic hearts were grown in culture as tissue explants (144). The hearts were exposed to an AAV lacZ construct using the respiratory syncytial virus promoter. After 48 hr of expression, the

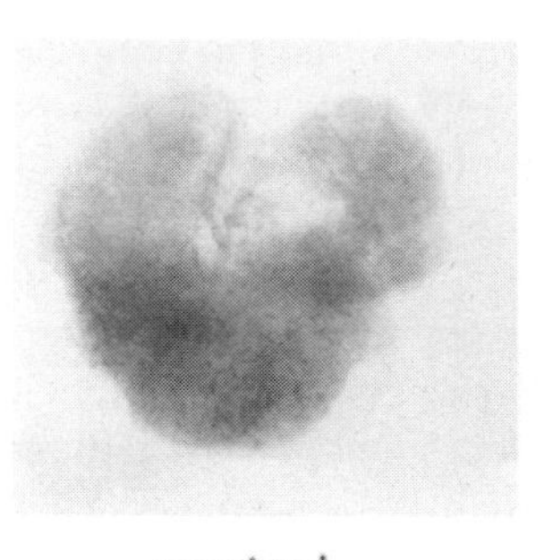

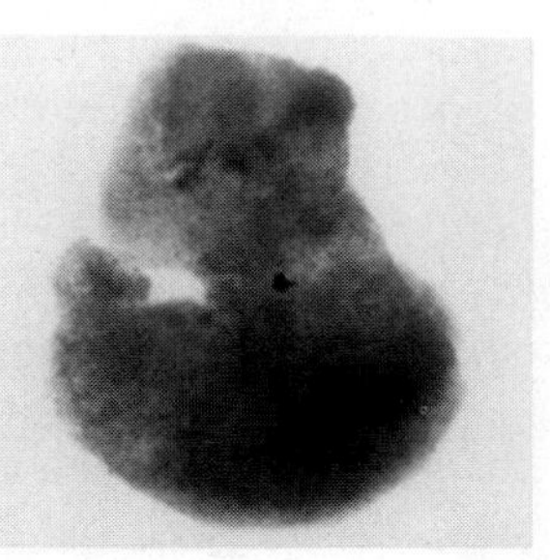

Figure 11 Intact embryonic hearts grown in tissue culture as tissue explants. Successful transduction is demonstrated by the blue staining of the heart transfected with AAV lacZ. (For optimal reproduction, see color plate.)

hearts were stained for β-galactosidase activity. Figure 11 is a photograph of intact hearts, and Fig. 12 is a micrograph of isolated cardiomyocytes transduced with AAV lacZ, demonstrating the successful transfection of cardiac tissue. The proposed targets for gene therapy in cardiac transplantation and accelerated arteriosclerosis include: (a) the endothelial cell, which may be programmed to express recipient antigens or factors that block lymphocyte entry into the intima; (b) the smooth muscle cell, which proliferates and contributes to vascular narrowing; and (c) lymphocytes, which may be influenced by cytokines produced in the graft (145).

Recently, Shaked et al. applied gene therapy to the transplant setting. They were able to use retroviral vectors for gene transfer into rat liver grafts under conditions similar to those of liver transplantation (146). Specifically, liver grafts were perfused with a retrovirus-containing medium that harbored human IL-7 and neomycin phosphotransferase genes during the period of cold ischemia before transplantation. Gene expression was observed up to 21 days after transplantation in the liver grafts (146).

These studies indicate the feasibility of directly targeting the endothelium of the graft

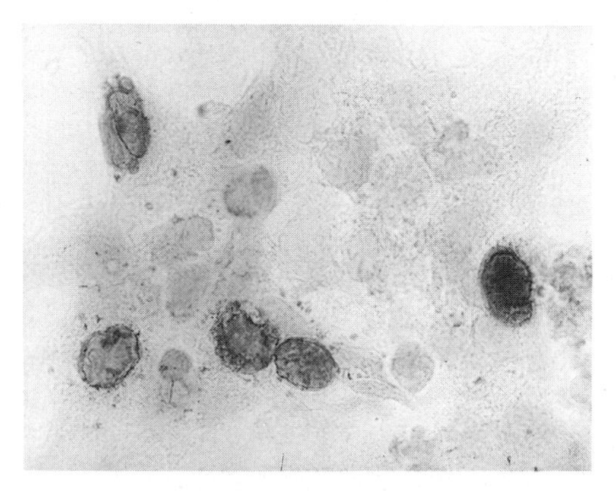

Figure 12 Isolated cardiomyocytes transduced with AAV lacZ. (For optimal reproduction, see color plate.)

with gene therapy to either induce immunotolerance or to suppress the atherogenicity of vascular endothelium. The real promise of these techniques is the possibility of specifically transferring genes to the allograft, thereby resulting in graft-specific immunosuppression.

F. Cytomegalovirus

Cytomegalovirus (CMV) remains a major contributor to the development of accelerated arteriosclerosis. The incidence of CMV disease in the combination of a seronegative heart recipient and a seropositive donor has been reported to be 89%, and 29% with seronegative heart recipients and seronegative donors (147). While proper identification of CMV status prior to transplantation is imperative, avoidance of CMV transmission to CMV seronegative donors is often not possible for a critically ill transplant candidate. Clearly, methods are needed to prevent CMV infection and its accompanying acute and long-term complications.

Ganciclovir (148,149) and anti-CMV immunoglobulin have emerged as effective prophylactic regimens in heart transplant recipients (150,151). In a randomized, placebo-controlled study, Merigan et al. were able to demonstrate that ganciclovir at a dose of 5 mg/kg IV for the first 28 days posttransplantation could reduce the incidence of CMV infection from 46 to 9% at 4 months after heart transplantation (149). Although effective in both the prevention and treatment of CMV infection, ganciclovir carries the potential risk of ganciclovir-resistant strains (152) and the development of myelosuppression. Furthermore, CMV may reactivate at a later time, after treatment has stopped. Also promising for the prevention of CMV-associated accelerated arteriosclerosis is passive immunization with anti-CMV immunoglobulins. In a study by Metselaar et al., prophylactic use of anti-CMV immunoglobulin resulted in a 13% incidence of CMV infection in CMV seronegative heart recipients from a seropositive donor (150), much less than the 89% incidence rate reported by Wreghitt et al. for untreated patients (147). Thus, these findings suggest that prophylaxis against CMV, whether with ganciclovir or IV immunoglobulins, can be a powerful tool in preventing both the acute and long-term complications of CMV particularly that of accelerated arteriosclerosis.

G. Vascular Tone and Cyclosporine

Calcium channel blockers, long known to decrease the contractile force and oxygen requirements of the myocardium, cause vasodilation, and slow conduction through the atrioventricular node, have recently been shown to be effective in the prevention of accelerated arteriosclerosis. In a preliminary report of 57 heart-transplant recipients by Schroeder et al., 17% of the patients treated with diltiazem had coronary artery disease at 2 years, as compared to 50% in the group not treated with diltiazem (153). These findings support earlier observations that calcium channel blockers inhibit the development of atherosclerosis in nontransplant patients (154–156).

The mechanisms by which calcium channel blockers prevent the development of accelerated arteriosclerosis have not been fully elucidated; however, several possibilities exist. First, calcium channel blockers cause direct arteriolar vasodilation by selective inhibition of the slow inward calcium channel current in vascular smooth muscle. This vasodilatory effect could be particularly useful in the later stages of accelerated arteriosclerosis, when endothelial dysfunction results in impaired vasodilatation (96). Second, calcium channel blockers tend to stabilize vascular smooth muscle cells, thereby inhibiting coronary artery vasospasm, a common problem in arteries affected with accelerated arteriosclerosis (98). Third, Dumont et al. have demonstrated that calcium channel blockers act synergistically with cyclosporine, thus potentially reducing the cyclosporine dosage needed to attain adequate immunosuppression and thereby decreasing cyclosporine-induced endothelial injury (157). Calcium channel blockers interfere with the renal excretion of cyclosporine such that the same serum levels of cyclosporine can be achieved with lower doses of the drug. Fourth, in nontransplanted animals, it appears that calcium channel blockers cause increased receptor uptake of low-density lipoproteins (158,159), inhibition of cholesteryl ester deposition in macrophages (160), and increased cholesteryl ester hydrolytic activity in arterial smooth muscle cells (161). Last, calcium channel blockers have been shown to have an immunosuppressive effect, which has been attributed to their ability to inhibit T-cells by regulation of intracellular calcium levels (162). Thus, calcium channel blockers could affect the pathogenesis of accelerated arteriosclerosis by their effect on the vascular tone, cyclosporine synergism, hyperlipidemia, and immunosuppression.

Finally, recently developed, novel antirejection drugs such as rapamycin and leflunomide may be more effective than cyclosporine in preventing accelerated arteriosclerosis because, in addition to their immunosuppressive effects, these drugs may suppress PDGF-induced smooth muscle cell proliferation.

VIII. CONCLUSION

Accelerated arteriosclerosis has emerged as the major long-term complication of heart transplantation. While it is clear that accelerated arteriosclerosis has multiple causes—including ischemia, platelet activation, complement deposition, upregulation of adhesion molecules and HLA antigens, antibody- and cell-mediated rejection, macrophage accumulation, CMV infection, and changes in vascular tone—we believe that ischemia initiates many of these processes and that it is the subtle, chronic injury to the vascular endothelium, particularly by repeated injury from chronic immune-mediated rejection of the graft endothelium, that primarily leads to the development of accelerated arteriosclerosis.

ACKNOWLEDGMENTS

The authors would like to thank Amanda Schlott Lietman, Jane Ann Day, and Rick M. Tracey, R.B.P., for their assistance with this manuscript.

REFERENCES

1. Hosenpud JD, Novick RJ, Breen TJ, Daily OP. The Registry of the International Society for Heart and Lung Transplantation: Eleventh official report—1994. J Heart Lung Transplant 1994; 13:561–570.
2. Thomson JG. Production of severe atheroma in a transplanted human heart. Lancet 1969; 2:1088–1092.
3. Gao S-Z, Alderman EL, Schroeder JS, et al. Progressive coronary luminal narrowing after cardiac transplantation. Circulation 1990; 82:IV269–275.
4. Pascoe EA, Barnhart GR, Carter WH Jr, et al. The prevalence of cardiac allograft arteriosclerosis. Transplantation 1987; 44:838–839.
5. Billingham ME. Graft coronary disease: The lesions and the patients. Transplant Proc 1989; 21:3665–3666.
6. Starnes VA, Stinson EB, Oyer PE, et al. Cardiac transplantation in children and adolescents. Circulation 1987; 76:V43–V47.

7. Taylor SR, Yunis EJ, Fricker FJ. Cardiac transplantation in children. Perspect Pediatr Pathol 1991; 14:60–93.
8. Braunlin EA, Hunter DW, Canter CE, et al. Coronary artery disease in pediatric cardiac transplant recipients receiving triple-drug immunosuppression. Circulation 1991; 84(suppl III): 303–309.
9. Gao S-Z, Schroeder JS, Hunt SA, Stinson EB. Retransplantation for severe accelerated coronary artery disease in heart transplant recipients. Am J Cardiol 1988; 62:876–881.
10. Gao S-Z, Schroeder JS, Alderman EL, et al. Clinical and laboratory correlates of accelerated coronary artery disease in the cardiac transplant patient. Circulation 1987; 76:V56–V61.
11. Uretsky BF, Murali S, Reddy PS, et al. Development of coronary artery disease in cardiac transplant patients receiving immunosuppressive therapy with cyclosporine and prednisone. Circulation 1987; 76:827–834.
12. Billingham ME. Histopathology of graft coronary disease. J Heart Lung Transplant 1992; 11:S38–44.
13. Valantine H, Pinto FJ, St.Goar FG, et al. Intracoronary ultrasound imaging in heart transplant recipients: the Stanford experience. J Heart Lung Transplant 1992; 11:S60–S64.
14. Johnson MR. Transplant coronary disease: nonimmunologic risk factors. J Heart Lung Transplant 1992; 11:S124–132.
15. Olivari MT, Homans DC, Wilson RF, et al. Coronary artery disease in cardiac transplant patients receiving triple-drug immunosuppressive therapy. Circulation 1989; 80(suppl III): 111–115.
16. Sharples LD, Caine N, Mullins P, et al. Risk factor analysis for the major hazards following heart transplantation—Rejection, infection, and coronary occlusive disease. Transplantation 1991; 52:244–252.
17. Pahl E, Fricker FJ, Armitage J, et al. Coronary arteriosclerosis in pediatric heart transplant survivors: Limitation of long-term survival. J Pediatr 1990; 116:177–183.
18. Winters GL, Kendall TJ, Radio SJ, et al. Post-transplant obesity and hyperlipidemia: Major predictors of severity of coronary arteriopathy in failed human heart allografts. J Heart Transplant 1990; 9:364–371.
19. Eich D, Thompson JA, Ko KJ, et al. Hypercholesterolemia in long term survivors of heart transplantation. An early marker of accelerated coronary artery disease. J Heart Lung Transplant 1991; 10:45–49.
20. Grattan MT, Moreno-Cabral CE, Starnes VA, et al. Cytomegalovirus infection is associated with cardiac allograft rejection and atherosclerosis. JAMA 1989; 261:3561–3566.
21. Cameron DE, Greene PS, Alejo D, et al. Postoperative cytomegalovirus infection and older donor age predisposes to coronary atherosclerosis after heart transplantation (abstr). Circulation 1989; 80(suppl II):526.
22. Wu TC, Hruban RH, Ambinder RF, et al. Demonstration of cytomegalovirus nucleic acids in the coronary arteries of transplanted hearts. Am J Pathol 1992; 140:739–747.
23. Gaudin PB, Rayburn BK, Hutchins GM, et al. Peritransplant injury to the myocardium associated with the development of accelerated arteriosclerosis in heart transplant recipients. Am J Surg Pathol 1994; 18:338–346.
24. Costanzo-Nordin MR. Cardiac allograft vasculopathy: Relationship with acute cellular rejection and histocompatibility. J Heart Lung Transplant 1992; 11:S90–S103.
25. Cramer DV, Qian SQ, Harnaha J, et al. Cardiac transplantation in the rat: I. The effect of histocompatibility differences on graft arteriosclerosis. Transplantation 1989; 47:414–419.
26. Cramer DV, Chapman FA, Harnaha JB, et al. Cardiac transplantation in the rat: II. Alteration of the severity of donor graft arteriosclerosis by modulation of the host immune response. Transplantation 1990; 50:554–558.
27. Ono K, Lindsey ES. Improved technique of heart transplantation in rats. J Thorac Cardiovasc Surg 1969; 57:225–229.

28. Bieber CP, Hunt SA, Schwinn DA, et al. Complications in long-term survivors of cardiac transplantation. Transplant Proc 1981; 13:207–211.
29. Mennander A, Tiisala S, Paavonen T, et al. Chronic rejection of rat aortic allograft: II. Administration of cyclosporine induces accelerated allograft arteriosclerosis. Transplant Int 1991; 4:173–179.
30. Billingham ME. The pathologic changes in long-term heart and lung transplant survivors. J Heart Lung Transplant 1992; 11:S252–S257.
31. Porter KA, Thomson WB, Owen K, et al. Obliterative vascular changes in four human kidney homotransplants. Br Med J 1963; 2:639–645.
32. Hruban RH, Beschorner WE, Baumgartner WA, et al. Accelerated arteriosclerosis in heart transplant recipients is associated with a T-lymphocyte-mediated endothelialitis. Am J Pathol 1990; 137:871–882.
33. Young-Ramsaran JO, Hruban RH, Hutchins GM, et al. Ultrastructural evidence of cell-mediated endothelial cell injury in cardiac transplant-related accelerated arteriosclerosis. Ultrastruct Pathol 1993; 17:125–136.
34. Uchino T, Belboul A, El Gatit A, et al. Assessment of myocardial damage by circulating cardiac myosin light chain I after heart transplantation. J Heart Lung Transplant 1994; 13: 418–423.
35. Billingham ME, Baumgartner WA, Watson DC, et al. Distant heart procurement for human transplantation: Ultrastructural studies. Circulation 1980; 62(suppl I):11–19.
36. Yilmaz S, Paavonen T, Häyry P. Chronic rejection of rat renal allografts. Transplantation 1992; 53:823–827.
37. Land W, Schneeberger H, Schleibner S, et al. The beneficial effect of human recombinant superoxide dismutase on acute and chronic rejection events in recipients of cadaveric renal transplants. Transplantation 1994; 57:211–217.
38. Hruban RH, Gaudin PB, Hutchins GM. Ischemia and the development of accelerated arteriosclerosis (letter). Am J Surg Pathol 1995; 19:728–730.
39. Chomette G, Ariol M, Cabrol C. Chronic rejection in human heart transplantation. J Heart Transplant 1988; 7:292–297.
40. Cywes R, Mullen JBM, Stratis MA, et al. Prediction of the outcome of transplantation in man by platelet adherence in donor liver allografts. Evidence of the importance of prepreservation injury. Transplantation 1993; 56:316–323.
41. Alonso DR, Starek PK, Minick CR. Studies on the pathogenesis of atheroarteriosclerosis induced in rabbit cardiac allografts by the synergy of graft rejection and hypercholesterolemia. Am J Pathol 1977; 87:415–442.
42. Ross R, Raines EW, Bowen-Pope DF. The biology of platelet-derived growth factor. Cell 1986; 46:155–169.
43. Ross R, Masuda J, Raines EW, et al. Localization of PDGF-β protein in macrophages in all phases of atherogenesis. Science 1990; 248:1009–1012.
44. Fellstrom B, Dimeny E, Larsson E, et al. Importance of PDGF receptor expression in accelerated atherosclerosis chronic rejection. Transplant Proc 1989; 21:3689–3691.
45. Baldwin WM III, Pruitt SK, Brauer RB, et al. Complement in organ transplantation: Contributions to inflammation, injury and rejection. Transplantation 1995; 59:797–808
46. Weisman HF, Bartow T, Leppo MK, et al. Soluble human complement receptor type 1: In vivo inhibitor of complement suppressing post-ischemic myocardial inflammation and necrosis. Science 1990; 249:146–151.
47. Litt MR, Jeremy RW, Weisman HF, et al. Neutrophil depletion limited to reperfusion reduces myocardial infarct size after 90 minutes of ischemia: Evidence for neutrophil-mediated reperfusion injury. Circulation 1989; 80:1816–1827.
48. Benzaquen LR, Nicholson-Weller A, Halperin JA. Terminal complement proteins C5b-9 release basic fibroblast growth factor and platelet-derived growth factor from endothelial cells. J Exp Med 1994; 179:985–992.

49. Libby P, Warner SJ, Friedman GB. Interleukin-1: A mitogen for human vascular smooth muscle cells that induces the release of growth-inhibitory prostanoids. J Clin Invest 1988; 81: 487–498.
50. Platt JL, Dalmasso AP, Lindman BJ, et al. The role of C5a and antibody in the release of heparan sulfate from endothelial cells. Eur J Immunol 1991; 21:2887–2890.
51. Carson SD, Johnson DR. Consecutive enzyme cascades: Complement activation at the cell surface triggers increased tissue factor activity. Blood 1990; 76:361–367.
52. Lucchesi BR, Mullane KM. Leukocytes and ischemia-induced myocardial injury. Annu Rev Pharmacol Toxicol 1986; 26:201–224.
53. Carlos TM, Harlan JH. Membrane proteins involved in phagocyte adherence to endothelium. Immunol Rev 1990; 114:5–28.
54. Briscoe DM, Schoen FJ, Rice GE, et al. Induced expression of endothelial-leukocyte adhesion molecules in human cardiac allografts. Transplantation 1991; 51:537–539.
55. Youker K, Smith CW, Anderson DC, et al. Neutrophil adherence to isolated adult cardiac myocytes: Induction by cardiac lymph collected during ischemia and reperfusion. J Clin Invest 1992; 89:602–609.
56. Isobe M, Yagita H, Okumura K, Ihara A. Specific acceptance of cardiac allograft after treatment with antibodies to ICAM-1 and LFA-1. Science 1992; 255:1125–1127.
57. Shoskes DA, Parfrey NA, Halloran PF. Increased major histocompatibility complex antigen expression in unilateral ischemic acute tubular necrosis in the mouse. Transplantation 1990; 49:201–207.
58. Cherry R, Nielsen H, Reed E, et al. Vascular (humoral) rejection in human cardiac allograft biopsies: Relation to circulating anti-HLA antibodies. J Heart Lung Transplant 1992; 11:24–29.
59. Rose EA, Pepino P, Barr ML, et al. Relation of HLA antibodies and graft atherosclerosis in human cardiac allograft recipients. J Heart Lung Transplant 1992; 11:S120–123.
60. Libby P, Salomon RN, Payne DD, et al. Functions of vascular wall cells related to development of transplantation-associated coronary arteriosclerosis. Transplant Proc 1989; 21:3677–3684.
61. Paul LC, van Es LA, van Rood JJ, et al. Antibodies directed against antigens on the endothelium of peritubular capillaries in patients with rejecting renal allografts. Transplantation 1979; 27:175–179.
62. Hammond EH, Yowell RL, Nunoda S, et al. Vascular (humoral) rejection in heart transplantation, pathologic observations and clinical implications. J Heart Transplant 1989; 8:430–443.
63. Hammond EH, Yowell RL, Price GD, et al. Vascular rejection and its relationship to allograft coronary artery disease. J Heart Lung Transplant 1992; 11:S111–119.
64. Hess ML, Hastillo A, Mohanakumar T, et al. Accelerated atherosclerosis in cardiac transplantation: Role of cytotoxic B-cell antibodies and hyperlipidemia. Circulation 1983; 68(suppl II): 94–101.
65. Rose EA, Smith CR, Petrossian GA, et al. Humoral immune responses after cardiac transplantation: Correlation with fatal rejection and graft atherosclerosis. Surgery 1989; 106:203–207.
66. Dunn MJ, Crisp SJ, Rose ML, et al. Anti-endothelial antibodies and coronary artery disease after cardiac transplantation. Lancet 1992; 339:1566–1570.
67. Cerilli J, Bassile L, Clark J, et al. Vascular endothelial cell-specific antibody in the pathogenesis of early cardiac allograft rejection. Transplant Proc 1988; 20(suppl I):755–757.
68. Peerschke EI, Reid KB, Ghebrehiwet B. Platelet activation by C1q results in the induction of alpha IIb/beta 3 integrins (GPIIb-IIIa) and the expression of P-selectin and procoagulant activity. J Exp Med 1993; 178:579–587.
69. Hruban RH, Long PP, Perlman EJ, et al. Fluorescence in situ hybridization for the Y-chromosome can be used to detect cells of recipient origin in allografted hearts following cardiac transplantation. Am J Pathol 1993; 142:975–980.
70. Salomon RN, Hughes CCW, Schoen FJ, et al. Human coronary transplantation-associated arteriosclerosis: Evidence for a chronic immune reaction to activated graft endothelial cells. Am J Pathol 1991; 138:791–798.

71. Fox WM III, Hameed A, Hutchins GM, et al. Perforin expression localizing cytotoxic lymphocytes in the intimas of coronary arteries with transplant-related accelerated arteriosclerosis. Hum Pathol 1993; 24:477–482.
72. Young JD, Liu CC, Persechini PM, Cohn ZA. Perforin-dependent and -independent pathways of cytotoxicity mediated by lymphocytes. Immunol Rev 1988; 103:161–202.
73. Peters PJ, Borst J, Oorschot V, et al. Cytotoxic T lymphocyte granules are secretory lysosomes containing both perforin and granzymes. J Exp Med 1991; 173:1099–1109.
74. Ojcius DM, Young JD. Cell-mediated killing: Effector mechanisms and mediators. Cancer Cells 1990; 2:138–145.
75. Berke G, Rosen D. Highly lytic in vivo primed cytolytic T lymphocytes devoid of lytic granules and BLT-esterase activity acquire these constituents in the presence of T cell growth factors upon blast transformation in vitro. J Immunol 1988; 141:1429–1436.
76. Dennert G, Podack ER. Cytolysis by H-2 specific T killer cells: Assembly of tubular complexes on target membranes. J Exp Med 1983; 157:1483–1495.
77. Shinkai Y, Takio K, Okumura K. Homology of perforin to the ninth component of complement (C9). Nature 1988; 334:525–527.
78. Cramer DV, Wu G-D, Chapman FA, et al. Lymphocytic subsets and histopathologic changes associated with the development of heart transplant arteriosclerosis. J Heart Lung Transplant 1992; 11:458–466.
79. Gerrity RG. The role of the monocyte in atherogenesis: I. Transition of blood-borne monocytes into foam cells in fatty lesions. Am J Pathol 1981; 103:181–190.
80. Steinberg D, Witztum JL. Lipoproteins and atherogenesis: Current concepts. JAMA 1990; 264:3047–3052.
81. Quinn MT, Parthasarathy S, Fong LG, Steinberg D. Oxidatively modified low-density lipoproteins: A potential role in recruitment and retention of monocyte/macrophages during atherogenesis. Proc Natl Acad Sci USA 1987; 84:2995–2998.
82. Stemme S, Jonasson L, Holm J, Hansson GK. Immunologic control of vascular cell growth in arterial response to injury and atherosclerosis. Transplant Proc 1989; 21:3697–3699.
83. Dummer JS, White LT, Ho M, et al. Morbidity of cytomegalovirus infection in recipients of heart or heart-lung transplants who received cyclosporine. J Infect Dis 1985; 152:1182–1191.
84. Everett JP, Hershberger RE, Norman DJ, et al. Prolonged cytomegalovirus infection with viremia is associated with development of cardiac allograft vasculopathy. J Heart Lung Transplant 1992; 11:S133–137.
85. Preiksaitis JK, Rosno S, Grumet C, Merigan TC. Infections due to herpesviruses in cardiac transplant recipients: Role of the donor heart and immunosuppressive therapy. J Infect Dis 1983; 147:974–981.
86. Adam E, Melnick JL, Probtsfield JL, et al. High levels of cytomegalovirus antibody in patients requiring vascular surgery for arteriosclerosis. Lancet 1987; 2:291–293.
87. Ross R. Mechanisms of atherosclerosis—A review. Adv Nephrol Necker Hosp 1990; 19: 79–86.
88. Etingin OR, Silverstein RL, Freidman HM, Hajjar DP. Viral activation of the coagulation cascade: Molecular interactions at the surface of infected endothelial cells. Cell 1990; 61: 657–662.
89. Hosenpud JD, Chou SW, Wagner CR. Cytomegalovirus induced regulation of major histocompatibility complex class I antigen expression in human aortic smooth muscle cells. Transplantation 1991; 52:896–903.
90. van Es A, Baldwin WM, Oljans PJ, et al. Expression of HLA-DR on T-lymphocytes following renal transplantation, and association with graft-rejection episodes and cytomegalovirus infection. Transplantation 1984; 37:65–69.
91. Fabricant CG, Hajjar DP, Minick CR, Fabricant J. Herpesvirus infection enhances cholesterol and cholesteryl ester accumulation in cultured arterial smooth muscle cells. Am J Pathol 1981; 105:176–184.

92. Benditt EP. Implications of the monoclonal character of human atherosclerotic plaques. Ann NY Acad Sci 1976; 275:96–100.
93. Fujinami RS, Nelson JA, Walker L, Oldstone MB. Sequence homology and immunologic cross-reactivity of human cytomegalovirus with HLA-DR β chain: A means for graft rejection and immunosuppression. J Virol 1988; 62:100–105.
94. Speir E, Modali R, Huang E-S, et al. Potential role of human cytomegalovirus and p53 interaction in coronary restenosis. Science 1994; 265:391–394.
95. Yanagisawa M, Kurihara H, Kimura S, et al. A novel potent vasoconstrictor peptide produced by vascular endothelial cells. Nature 1988; 332:411–415.
96. Vanhoutte PM, Shimokawa H. Endothelium-derived relaxing factor and coronary artery vasospasm. Circulation 1989; 80:1–9.
97. McFadden EP, Clarke JG, Davies GJ, et al. Effect of intracoronary serotonin on coronary vessels in patients with stable angina and patients with variant angina. N Engl J Med 1991; 324:648–654.
98. Hruban RH, Kasper EK, Gaudin PB, et al. Severe lymphocytic endothelialitis associated with coronary artery spasm in a heart transplant recipient. J Heart Lung Transplant 1992; 11:42–47.
99. Berk BC, Alexander RW. Vasoactive effects of growth factors. Biochem Pharmacol 1989; 38:219–225.
100. Herold KC, Lancki DW, Moldwin RL, Fitch FW. Immunosuppressive effects of cyclosporin A on cloned T cells. J Immunol 1986; 136:1315–1321.
101. Sommer BG, Innes JT, Whitehurst RM, et al. Cyclosporine-associated renal arteriopathy resulting in loss of allograft function. Am J Surg 1985; 149:756–764.
102. Mihatsch MJ, Thiel G, Basler V, et al. Morphological patterns in cyclosporine-treated renal transplant recipients. Transplant Proc 1985; 17:101–116.
103. Becker DM, Chamberlain B, Swank R, et al. Relationship between corticosteroid exposure and plasma lipid levels in heart transplant recipients. Am J Med 1988; 85:632–638.
104. Ost L. Effects of cyclosporine on prednisolone metabolism (letter). Lancet 1984; 1:451.
105. Cramer DV. In: Graft Arteriosclerosis in Heart Transplantation. Austin, TX: R. G. Landes, 1993:48–49.
106. Hardin NJ, Minick CR, Murphy GE. Experimental induction of atheroarteriosclerosis by the synergy of allergic injury to arteries and lipid-rich diet. Am J Pathol 1973; 73:301–326.
107. Gerrity RG. Vesicular transport and intimal accumulation of macromolecules in atherosclerosis-susceptible areas is augmented by hyperlipidemia. Circulation 1987; 76(suppl IV):295.
108. Kaye MP. The Registry of the International Society for Heart and Lung Transplantation: Tenth official report—1993. J Heart Lung Transplant 1993; 12:541–548.
109. Stewart JR, Frist WH, Merrill WH. Oxygen scavengers in myocardial preservation during transplantation. Methods Enzymol 1990; 186:742–748.
110. Green CJ, Healing GM, Lunec J, et al. Evidence of free-radical-induced damage in rabbit kidneys after single hypothermic preservation and autotransplantation. Transplantation 1986; 41:161–165.
111. Stringham JC, Paulsen KL, Southard JH, et al. Prolonging myocardial preservation with a modified University of Wisconsin solution containing 2,3-butanedione monoxine and calcium. J Thorac Cardiovasc Surg 1994; 107:764–775.
112. Yano H, Takenaka H, Onitsuka T, et al. Cardioplegic effect of University of Wisconsin solution on hypothermic ischemia of rat myocardium assessed by mitochondrial oxidative phosphorylation. J Thorac Cardiovasc Surg 1993; 106:502–510.
113. Oz MC, Pinsky DJ, Koga S, et al. Novel preservation solution permits 24-hour preservation in rat and baboon cardiac transplant models. Circulation 1993; 88(suppl II):291–297.
114. Sun SC, Appleyard R, Masetti P, et al. Improved recovery of heart transplants by combined use of oxygen-derived free radical scavengers and energy enhancement. J Thorac Cardiovasc Surg 1992; 104:830–837.

115. Cederna J, Bandlien K, Toledo-Pereyra LH, et al. Effect of allopurinol and/or catalase on hemorrhagic shock and their potential application to multiple organ harvesting. Transplant Proc 1990; 22:444–445.
116. Ardehali A, Laks H, Drinkwater DC Jr, et al. Expression of major histocompatibility antigens and vascular adhesion molecules on human cardiac allografts preserved in University of Wisconsin solution. J Heart Lung Transplant 1993; 12:1044–1051.
117. Hunt NH, Fragonas JC. Effects of anti-oxidants on ornithine decarboxylase in mitogenically-activated T lymphocytes. Biochim Biophys Acta 1992; 1133:261–267.
118. Hoyt G, Gollin G, Billingham ME, Miller DC, Jamieson SW. Effect of anti-platelet regimens in combination with cyclosporin on heart allograft vessel disease. J Heart Transplant 1984; 4:54–55.
119. Muskett A, Burton NA, Eichwald EJ, et al. The effect of antiplatelet drugs on graft atherosclerosis in rat heterotopic cardiac allografts. Transplant Proc 1987; 19:74–76.
120. Lurie KG, Billingham ME, Jamieson SW, et al. Pathogenesis and prevention of graft arteriosclerosis in an experimental heart transplantation model. Transplantation 1981; 31:41–47.
121. Häyry P, Mennander A, Räisänen-Sokolowski A, et al. Pathophysiology of vascular wall changes in chronic allograft rejection. Transplant Rev 1993; 7:1–20.
122. Saunder A, Southard JH, Belzer FO. Beneficial effect of aspirin and heparin in three-day dog kidney preservation. Transplantation 1993; 56:1044–1045.
123. Clowes AW, Karnovsky MJ. Suppression by heparin of smooth muscle cell proliferation in injured arteries. Nature 1977; 265:625–626.
124. Guyton JR, Rosenberg RD, Clowes AW, Kanovsky MJ. Inhibition of rat arterial smooth muscle cell proliferation by heparin: In vivo studies with anticoagulant and nonanticoagulant heparin. Circ Res 1980; 46:625–634.
125. de Lorgeril M, Dureau G, Boissonnat P, et al. Increased platelet aggregation after heart transplantation: Influence of aspirin. J Heart Lung Transplant 1991; 10:600–603.
126. Maroko PR, Carpenter CD, Chiariello M, et al. Reduction by cobra venom factor of myocardial necrosis after coronary artery occlusion. J Clin Invest 1987; 61:661–670.
127. Pruitt SK, Baldwin WM III, Marsh HC Jr, et al. The effect of soluble complement receptor type 1 on hyperacute xenograft rejection. Transplantation 1991; 52:868–873.
128. Weiler JM, Linhardt RJ. Comparison of the activity of polyanions and polycations on the classical and alternative pathways of complement. Immunopharmacology 1989; 17:65–72.
129. Cosimi AB, Conti D, Delmonico FL, et al. In vivo effects of monoclonal antibody to ICAM-1 (CD54) in nonhuman primates with renal allografts. J Immunol 1990; 144:4604–4612.
130. Flavin T, Ivens K, Rothlein R, et al. Monoclonal antibodies against intracellular adhesion molecule 1 prolong cardiac allograft survival in cynomolgus monkeys. Transplant Proc 1991; 23:533–534.
131. Collins T, Korman AJ, Wake CT, et al. Immune interferon activates multiple class II major histocompatibility complex genes and the associated invariant chain gene in human endothelial cells and dermal fibroblasts. Proc Natl Acad Sci USA 1984; 81:4917–4921.
132. Song Z, Krishna S, Thanos D, et al. A novel cysteine-rich sequence-specific DNA-binding protein interacts with the conserved X-box motif of the human MHC class II genes via a repeated cys-his domain and functions as a transcriptional repressor. J Exp Med 1994; 180:1763–1774.
133. Rose EA, Addonizio LJ. Immunosuppression in cardiac transplantation. Bibl Cardiol 1988; 43:1–9.
134. Anderson WF. Prospects for human gene therapy. Science 1984; 226:401–409.
135. Zweibel JA, Freeman SM, Kantoff PW, et al. High-level recombinant gene expression in rabbit endothelial cells transduced by retroviral vectors. Science 1989; 243:220–222.
136. Nabel EG, Plautz G, Boyce FM, et al. Recombinant gene expression in vivo within endothelial cells of the arterial wall. Science 1989; 244:1342–1344.
137. Nabel EG, Plautz G, Nabel GJ. Site-specific gene expression in vivo by direct gene transfer into the arterial wall. Science 1990; 249:1285–1288.

138. Nabel EG, Plautz G, Nabel GJ. Gene transfer into vascular cells. JACC 1991; 17:189B–194B.
139. Ohno T, Gordon D, San H, et al. Gene therapy for vascular smooth muscle cell proliferation after arterial injury. Science 1994; 265:781–784.
140. Dichek DA. Retroviral vector-mediated gene transfer into endothelial cells. Mol Biol Med 1991; 8:257–266.
141. Dichek DA, Neville RF, Zweibel JA, et al. Seeding of intravascular stents with genetically engineered endothelial cells. Circulation 1989; 80:1347–1353.
142. Guzman RJ, Lemarchand P, Crystal RG, et al. Efficient and selective adenovirus-mediated gene transfer into vascular neointima. Circulation 1993; 88:2838–2848.
143. Kotin RM, Siniscalco M, Samulski RJ, et al. Site-specific integration by adeno-associated virus. Proc Natl Acad Sci USA 1990; 87:2211–2215.
144. Kourtis AP, Deyesu EE, Hruban RH, Byrne BJ. Cardiac gene therapy with adeno-associated virus as a means of achieving graft-specific immunosuppression. Mod Pathol 1995; 8:33A.
145. Philip R, Brunette E, Kilinski L, et al. Efficient and sustained gene expression in primary T lymphocytes and primary and cultured tumor cells mediated by adeno-associated virus plasmid DNA complexed to cationic liposomes. Mol Cell Biol 1994; 14:2411–2418.
146. Shaked A, Csete ME, Shiraishi M, et al. Retroviral-mediated gene transfer into rat experimental liver transplant. Transplantation 1994; 57:32–34.
147. Wreghitt TG, Hakim M, Gray JJ, et al. A detailed study of cytomegalovirus infections in the first 160 heart and heart/lung transplant recipients at Papworth Hospital, Cambridge, England. Transplant Proc 1987; 19:2495–2496.
148. Laske A, Gallino A, Carrell T, et al. Cytomegalovirus infection and prophylaxis in heart transplantation. Transplant Proc 1993; 25:1427–1428.
149. Merigan TC, Renlund DG, Keay S, et al. A controlled trial of ganciclovir to prevent cytomegalovirus disease after heart transplantation. N Engl J Med 1992; 326:1182–1186.
150. Metselaar HJ, Balk AH, Mochtar B, et al. Cytomegalovirus seronegative heart transplant recipients: Prophylactic use of anti-CMV immunoglobulin. Chest 1990; 97:396–399.
151. Tinelli M, Percivalle E, Zambelli A, et al. Cytomegalovirus prophylaxis by intravenous immunoglobulins in five heart transplanted patients. Bol Ist Sieroter Milan 1990; 69:459–467.
152. Hirsch MS, Schooley RT. Resistance to antiviral drugs: The end of innocence. N Engl J Med 1989; 320:313–314.
153. Schroeder JS, Gao S-Z, Alderman EL, et al. A preliminary study of diltiazem in the prevention of coronary artery disease in heart-transplant recipients. N Engl J Med 1993; 328:164–170.
154. Lichtlen PR, Hugenholtz PG, Rafflenbeul W, et al. Retardation of angiographic progression of coronary artery disease by nifedipine: Results of the International Nifedipine Trial on Anti-atherosclerotic Therapy (INTACT). Lancet 1990; 335:1109–1113.
155. Loaldi A, Polese A, Montorsi P, et al. Comparison of nifedipine, propranolol and isosorbide dinitrate on angiographic progression and regression of coronary arterial narrowings in angina pectoris. Am J Cardiol 1989; 64:433–439.
156. Waters D, Lesperance J, Francetich M, et al. A controlled clinical trial to assess the effect of a calcium channel blocker on the progression of coronary atherosclerosis. Circulation 1990; 82:1940–1953.
157. Dumont L, Chen H, Daloze P, et al. Immunosuppressive properties of the benzothiazepine calcium antagonists diltiazem and clentiazem, with and without cyclosporine, in heterotopic rat heart transplantation. Transplantation 1993; 56:181–184.
158. Paoletti R, Bernini F, Fumagalli R, et al. Calcium antagonists and low density lipoprotein receptors. Ann NY Acad Sci 1988; 522:390–398.
159. Stein O, Leitersdorf E, Stein Y. Verapamil enhances receptor-mediated endocytosis of low density lipoproteins by aortic cells in culture. Arteriosclerosis 1985; 5:35–44.
160. Daugherty A, Rateri DL, Schonfeld G, Sobel BE. Inhibition of cholesteryl ester deposition in macrophages by calcium channel blockers: An effect dissociable from calcium entry blockade. Br J Pharmacol 1987; 91:113–118.

161. Etingin OR, Hajjar DP. Nifedipine increases cholesteryl ester hydrolytic activity in lipid-laden rabbit arterial smooth muscle cells: A possible mechanism for its antiatherogenic effect. J Clin Invest 1985; 75:1554–1558.
162. McMillen MA, Lewis T, Jaffe BM, Wait RB. Verapamil inhibition of lymphocyte proliferation and function in vitro. J Surg Res 1985; 39:76–80.
163. Hruban RH, Beschorner WE, Baumgartner WA, et al. Accelerated arteriosclerosis in heart transplant recipients: An immunopathology study of 22 transplanted hearts. Transplant Proc 1991; 23:1230–1232.

6

Pathology of Heart Transplantation

Margaret E. Billingham
Stanford University School of Medicine, Stanford, California

I. INTRODUCTION

Heart transplantation has now entered its third decade. The first successful clinical cardiac transplantation was performed in South Africa in 1968 by Christiaan Barnard (1). For approximately the next ten years, heart transplantation was continued throughout the world at a slow rate until 1984, when cyclosporine became widely available to cardiothoracic transplant centers and there was a resurgence of interest in cardiothoracic transplantation. In 1981, the first successful combined heart–lung operation was performed by Reitz et al. at Stanford (2). The 1994 Registry of Heart and Lung Transplantation reported 26,704 heart transplants in 251 centers. In addition, 1567 combined heart–lung transplants were being performed in 93 centers worldwide. Pediatric heart transplantation (0 to 18 years) now number 1918, performed in over 200 centers (see Table 1). More recently, cardiac transplantation has included neonates, infants, and children, although fewer than 7% of heart transplants to date have been in infants and children (3). Results from infant heart transplantation have revealed a 5-year patient survival of 82% in infants receiving hearts within the first month of life (3). The 5-year survival in older children who receive heart transplants is reported to be 72%. Cardiac recipients in the sixth and seventh decades have also been reported with satisfactory survival. The overall 1-year survival for cardiac transplantation is now more than 85% in most major centers worldwide.

Over the years, different immunosuppressive regimens have been used and these, in turn, have affected not only the pathology of the transplanted heart but also the temporal relationship of rejection patterns. At this time, 1994, most centers are using a mixture of azathioprine, steroids, and cyclosporine with or without OKT3 or ATG induction. This has allowed many patients to return to satisfying and productive lives. Despite the wealth of experience over the last 25 years, the major cause of death in cardiac allografts remains acute cardiac rejection or infection in the early years or chronic graft vascular disease in the later years. Acute cardiac rejection may not manifest itself clinically until it is quite severe and difficult to reverse. For this reason, the diagnosis of acute cardiac rejection has been monitored morphologically using the endomyocardial biopsy. Although new noninvasive methods are being developed and many others have been tried, especially immunological ones, to monitor cardiac rejection, it is true at present that the most reliable method for

Table 1 Heart Transplantation Worldwide

Total heart transplants	26,704	251 centers
Pediatric heart transplants	1,918	200 centers
Heterotopic heart transplants	403	
Heart-lung transplants	1,567	93 centers
Xenograft heart transplants	4	

Source: From Ref. 42.

diagnosing acute rejection is still the morphological one. This is true also for children; however, in small infants, the endomyocardial biopsy is much more dangerous and should be used only if no other method is available. In a recent study, echocardiography was found to be 98% accurate for primary rejection surveillance in infants; right ventricular biopsy is required infrequently (4).

The pathology of cardiac transplantation described in this chapter is similar for heterotopic heart transplants as well as for the donor hearts in combined heart–lung transplantation and for children. The pathology of cardiac transplantation can best be summarized in a temporal fashion.

II. DIAGNOSIS OF ACUTE REJECTION

A. Endomyocardial Biopsy

Although noninvasive methods have been tried, at present the endomyocardial biopsy is still the most reliable method for diagnosing acute rejection in cardiac allografts. The biopsy technique has been described and reported in depth in the literature (5,6). The original Konno-Sakakibara bioptome was modified in 1971 so that it could be passed by the right external jugular vein into the apex of the right ventricle to obtain myocardial biopsies from orthotopically transplanted canine hearts. After the encouraging results in dogs, the biopsy technique was modified for use via a percutaneous transvenous (jugular) approach in humans. This technique was first introduced into clinical cardiac transplantation using the new modified Caves-Stanford catheter bioptome in 1972 (7). Since that time, the biopsy method has been used almost continuously to monitor cardiac transplant recipients for acute rejection and infection. The percutaneous transvenous method for obtaining right ventricular biopsies has remained the most popular method, although some centers use the femoral approach. Occasionally, the bioptome will pass into the right atrium and out through the inferior vena cava, so that a small liver biopsy is obtained inadvertently (Fig. 1). New bioptome catheters have been designed ranging in size from 5F to 9F, but the transvenous approach has remained the same. In general, right-sided biopsies are used for monitoring cardiac rejection, although it is possible to do left-sided biopsies if necessary.

B. Indications for Biopsy

The endomyocardial biopsy is also used for pretransplant evaluation and to direct therapy in transplant recipients. Pretransplant endomyocardial biopsy is important because certain diseases may recur (see Table 2), either from the recipient (e.g., amyloid) or from the donor (e.g., using a donor seropositive for cytomegalovirus or, inadvertently, human immunodefi-

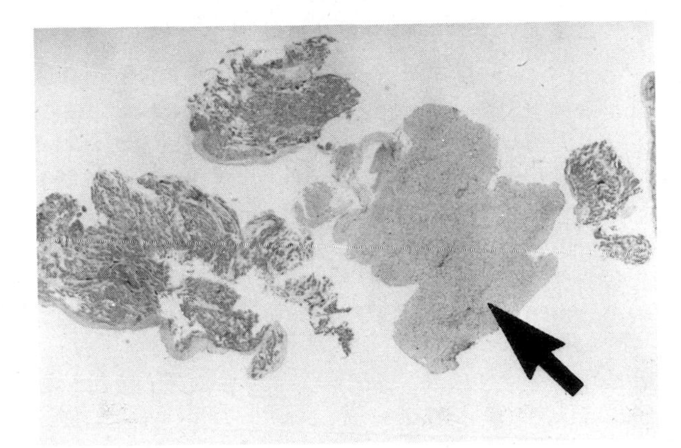

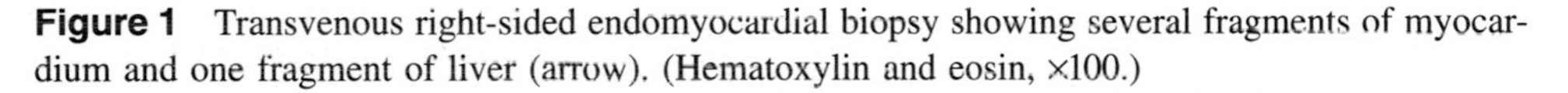

Figure 1 Transvenous right-sided endomyocardial biopsy showing several fragments of myocardium and one fragment of liver (arrow). (Hematoxylin and eosin, ×100.)

ciency virus can result in the disease manifesting itself in the recipient of the donor heart). Amyloid, myocarditis, sarcoidosis, and other diseases cannot always be diagnosed clinically and may be mistaken for idiopathic cardiomyopathy. Hypersensitivity myocarditis (possibly drug-related) has also been found in explanted recipient hearts (8). It is believed, therefore, that a confirmatory diagnostic endomyocardial biopsy should be performed prior to cardiac transplantation to avoid these pitfalls, especially in view of the current donor shortage. Additionally, some transplant centers like to take endomyocardial biopsies of the donor heart either prior to transplantation or during surgery to use as a control for that recipient in the future.

C. Safety

Many patients have had more than forty endomyocardial biopsies spread over the years without adverse sequelae. More than 25,000 endomyocardial biopsies have been performed on more than 740 human cardiac transplant recipients at Stanford since 1972, and there have been no deaths as a result of the biopsy in adults; morbidity has been negligible (less than 0.2%). There was one death as a result of coronary artery rupture in a 3-month-old child who was having a routine biopsy. Since that time, children under 1 year of age are usually biopsied only if symptoms require it and not for routine management.

Table 2 Diseases that Have Recurred in the Donor Heart

From recipient	From donor
Amyloidosis	Melanoma
Sarcoidosis	Cytomegalovirus
Chagas' disease	Toxoplasmosis
Giant-cell myocarditis	Human immunodeficiency virus

D. Tissue Handling and Fixation

Due to the inevitability of sampling error in small biopsy specimens, the International Society for Heart and Lung Transplantation (ISHLT) grading system requires a minimum of four pieces of tissue, of which at least 50% are evaluable (9,10). The tissue should be obtained without dividing by cutting or damaging the small pieces with forceps. The biopsy should be removed carefully from the bioptomes to avoid crush artifact. The biopsy specimen should be fixed immediately in 10% buffered formalin at room temperature (to prevent further contraction artifact). One piece can be frozen in liquid nitrogen or by another standard method for use for immunohistology, in situ hybridization, or frozen section diagnosis.

After fixation, the biopsy should be processed in the usual way by paraffin or plastic embedding and the sections should be cut at 4 μ thickness if possible. Thicker sections make the biopsy more cellular and more difficult to interpret. It is recommended that the biopsies be "step-sectioned" for at least four levels and sometimes right through the paraffin block. This is to prevent further sampling error; also, it is often not feasible to reface the blocks later if more cuts are required because the fragments are so small. For this reason, we usually make one hematoxylin and eosin (H&E) at the first level, the second level being either left blank for future staining or stained with Masson's trichrome. The other levels are also stained with H&E. Different institutions have different methods for doing this, but the reasoning is usually the same. We find that the trichrome stain is particularly useful for highlighting myocyte damage, to show whether or not an inflammatory infiltrate is trapped within a scar, and also to delineate the endocardium in a "Quilty" effect. Although a few centers use electron microscopy, most centers find it not useful for the day-to-day diagnosis of acute rejection, since it takes too long to process. In many cardiac transplant centers today, more than 10 to 20 biopsies are being performed daily, and this is an unwieldly number from the point of view of electron microscopy.

Endomyocardial biopsies can be used for research purposes—for example, new studies involving preservation techniques in which the endomyocardial biopsy will show endothelial damage of capillaries and other vessels. Frozen sections can be used for diagnostic purposes but are prone to artifact such as ice crystal formation, which may make diagnosis more difficult. Rapid fixation and processing (Ultratechnicon method) is quite satisfactory with endomyocardial biopsies, since they are so small that they fix rapidly. Immunohistochemistry can be performed to rule out cytomegalovirus (CMV) infection or to detect lymphocyte markers for target-selective immunosuppression. Immunofluorescence is also used to diagnose acute vascular rejection (11). Because the biopsy cuts across vessels and endothelial integrity is often disturbed in ischemia, false-positive results for immunoglobulins may be present on immunofluorescence (12). The routine use of immunofluorescence as an adjunct to endomyocardial biopsy diagnosis is still a controversial issue, but is dealt with later on in this chapter.

E. Frequency of Endomyocardial Biopsies

Biopsies are usually performed weekly following cardiac transplantation; after discharge, they are performed once every 3 weeks for the first 3 months. Later, they are performed once every 3 months for 1 year, and then annually at the routine yearly checkups or, of course, at any time when there is a suspicion of rejection.

III. IMMEDIATE PATHOLOGY OF ACUTE REJECTION

As mentioned earlier, the pathology of acute rejection is most easily described in a temporal fashion according to the sequence in which the pathology arises (see Table 3), although there may be a good deal of overlap in these changes. In this section, immediate changes, occurring within 24 hours, are described.

A. Right Ventricular Failure

Rarely, following cardiac transplantation, the donor heart will fail to function before the patient leaves the operating room. Ventricular contraction is weak if it exists at all, and the right ventricle dilates and may assume a dark cyanotic hue. This may be due to a number of factors, the most common of which is pulmonary hypertension with a high pulmonary vascular resistance. The normal, nonhypertrophied right ventricle of the donor cannot function against significant pulmonary resistance. Nowadays it is unusual for this to occur, since patients are carefully studied prior to transplantation so that this situation is usually avoided. If there are indications of pulmonary hypertension, then a combined heart-lung block may be the procedure of choice. In the case of known severe pulmonary hypertension, if a heart-lung block is not available, the already hypertrophied heart from another recipient of a heart-lung transplant for pulmonary hypertension can be used (so-called domino transplant).

Occasionally, the donor heart is damaged by direct trauma if the donor is an accident victim, and occasionally myocardial damage results from overloading of the myocardium with the drugs used in resuscitating the donor. In the extreme event where another donor is not available, the patient may be supported with a left ventricular assist device (e.g., Novacor-Baxter) or other extracorporeal means (ECHMO), to keep the circulation going

Table 3 Pathology of Heart Transplantation—Outline of the Temporal Sequence

Immediate (1 to 24 hr posttransplantation)
Right ventricular failure
Hyperacute rejection
Early (1 to 3 weeks posttransplantation)
Ischemia and/or reperfusion injury
Effect of vasopressors
Early acute rejection
Intermediate (1 month to 1 year posttransplantation)
Acute cellular rejection
Infection
Humoral or acute vascular rejection
Lymphoproliferative EBV-related lesions
Late (1 to 22 years posttransplantation)
Hypertrophy and fibrosis
Late acute rejection
Effects of denervation
Graft vascular disease

until another donor heart can be found or the function improves. Histopathologically, the allograft that fails as described above shows only diffuse hemorrhage in the right ventricle; occasionally, fibrin thrombi may be seen in the small vessels, but the pathology is often quite unremarkable and the cause of failure unclear.

B. Hyperacute Rejection

Hyperacute rejection is relatively uncommon, occurring immediately following transplantation (13–15). The heart assumes a dark red color and may dilate and cease to contract. It is usually the result of a major blood group incompatibility between the donor and recipient (ABO mismatch) or may be due to other major histocompatibility differences. One group reported four cases of hyperacute rejection resulting from circulating antiendothelial antibodies (14). The heart rapidly dilates, ventricular arrhythmias develop, and cardiac failure ensures. The pathology of hyperacute rejection shows massive interstitial hemorrhage similar to that seen in an infarct except that it is global in distribution. If the patient is able to survive for a few hours by mechanical means or otherwise, a neutrophilic infiltrate may also be seen. "Sludging" of red cells within small vessels and fibrin thrombi may also be seen in hyperacute rejection. There may be evidence of marked interstitial edema as well. The patient will not survive this condition unless another donor is obtained immediately or mechanical "bridge to retransplant" is instituted until another donor is found. Hyperacute rejection is further described in Chapter 2 of this book.

IV. EARLY PATHOLOGY OF HEART TRANSPLANTATION

This section covers the pathology in the first month following heart transplantation.

A. Reperfusion and/or Ischemic Injury

Often the first biopsy 1 week following cardiac transplantation or any biopsy within the first 3 or 4 weeks will show evidence of focal ischemia, usually subendocardial. These changes may be due to a long ischemic time for the donor heart, though good correlation with ischemic time is often not present, or it may be due to reperfusion injury. Occasionally, small infarcts are seen, some of which are thought to be due to inability to remove air bubbles adequately from the coronary circulation at the time of transplantation. The area of ischemia is often delineated by shrinkage of the myocytes, which appear to have a larger space around them, with pyknotic nuclei and minimal lymphocytic or other inflammatory infiltrates. These changes can be highlighted by the use of Masson's trichrome stain, which colors the affected myocytes a dull gray color rather than the deep red of normal myocardium stained with trichrome (Fig. 2). If the biopsy is later than 1 week, granulation tissue and a few inflammatory cells may be seen (Fig. 3). Very occasionally, frank infarcts can be seen following transplantation, most likely due to a mechanical interruption of the coronary arteries inadvertently at surgery. It is a general rule, however, that in the case of ischemia, there is more myocyte damage than there is inflammatory infiltrate, while the opposite is true of acute rejection; therefore the two should not be confused.

B. Reperfusion Injury

This is similar to ischemic injury but may be seen more focally within the myocardium rather than in the subendocardial areas (16).

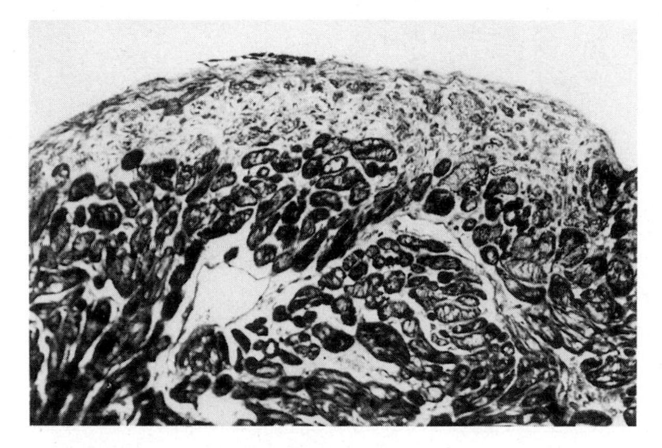

Figure 2 Recent postcardiac transplant biopsy showing a band of subendocardial ischemia (paler area). (Masson's trichrome, ×200.)

C. Pressor Effect Damage

The donor heart may be subjected to high-dose vasopressor agents to sustain it prior to transplantation or as part of resuscitative efforts following the placement of the donor heart, which has been already treated with vasopressors. The donor heart may then be further subjected to high-dose vasopressors to sustain the recipient in the early postoperative course. The effect of these large doses of vasopressors can sometimes be seen in endomyocardial biopsies or at autopsies of hearts that have failed. The pathology is that of a typical "catecholamine effect"—i.e., there is a small focal lesion with a few damaged myocytes surrounded by a mixed inflammatory infiltrate, including neutrophils (Fig. 4). These very small focal insults with minimal inflammatory infiltrates should not be confused with rejection and are usually seen only in the first few weeks following transplantation unless the patient is treated with vasopressors later or resuscitated at a later stage.

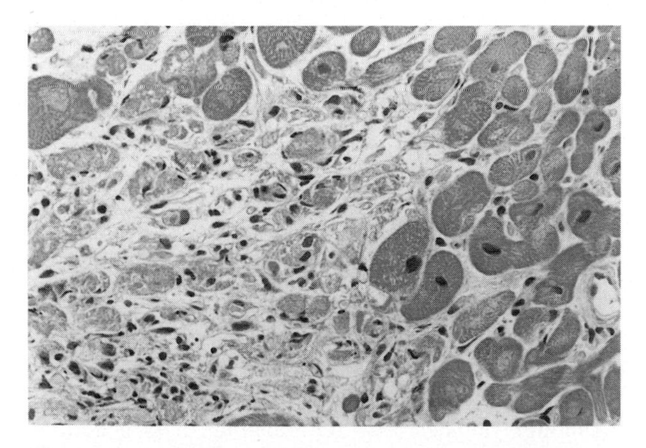

Figure 3 Endomyocardial biopsy showing granulation tissue (paler area) with fewer inflammatory cells and more myocyte damage than is seen in acute rejection. (Hematoxylin and eosin, ×200.)

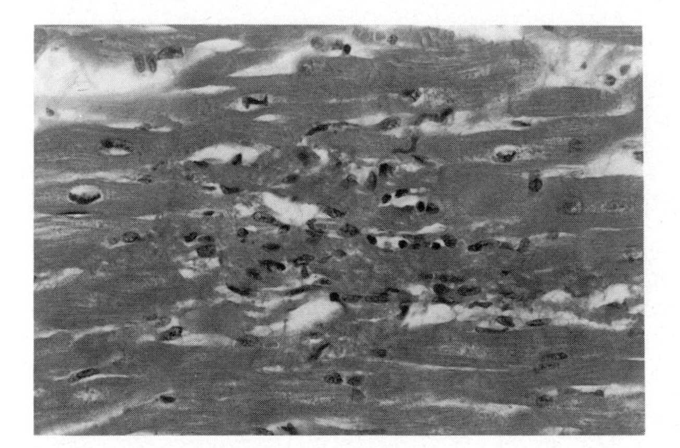

Figure 4 Endomyocardial biopsy showing "catecholamine effect" (central area) with early focal myocyte damage and a sparse inflammatory infiltrate due to high-dose vasopressor agents. (Hematoxylin and eosin, ×200.)

D. Early Acute Rejection

Early acute rejection can occur within the first week or two following cardiac transplantation. In many centers where induction therapy is given, either with or without OKT3 or ATG, the first rejection is "postponed" for 3 or 4 weeks following transplantation. If induction therapy is not given, it is quite possible to see an early acute rejection, particularly if there is a poor match of human leukocyte antigen (HLA) with the donor. The acute rejection seen at this time is exactly similar to that seen later, and is described in the next section.

V. INTERMEDIATE PATHOLOGY

This section covers histopathologic changes seen in endomyocardial biopsies during the first year following transplantation.

A. Acute Rejection

Most acute rejection occurs in the first 3 to 6 months following cardiac transplantation, particularly the first 3 months. Almost all cardiac recipients will have some form of acute rejection, although there are a few who do not.

B. Grading of Acute Rejection

There have been many different grading systems for acute rejection. Because of the dilemma this caused for clinicians and pathologists from center to center (17) and because no two grading systems could be correlated for the purpose of multicenter trials, the International Society for Heart and Lung Transplantation decreed a new standardized grading system (9). The use of this grading system has already allowed many multi-institutional studies to take place. Although not perfectly reproducible, it is generally agreed that the grading system has resulted in much more uniformity among different institutions and pathologists. It is recognized, however, that this grading system may require modification as time goes on. The International Society grading system is shown in Table 4. The main morphological features of acute cardiac rejection are an inflammatory infiltrate, usually mononuclear and either focal or diffuse, with or without myocyte damage. Each of the grades is described briefly below.

1. ISHLT Grade 0

This denotes no evidence of acute rejection and myocardium within normal limits for the donor heart.

2. ISHLT Grade IA and B (Mild Rejection)

This category is subdivided into several grades. Grade 1A represents one or more focal perivascular infiltrates which may be in either one or several of the endomyocardial biopsy pieces seen. There is usually no myocyte damage associated with grade IA (see Fig. 5). Grade IB shows similar focal infiltrates in that they emanate from a small vessel, but spread further into the surrounding myocardium in a "starburst" fashion or "chicken-wire" effect. Although this is described as a diffuse infiltrate, what is meant is a "focally diffuse" infiltrate, not a diffuse infiltrate throughout all the biopsy pieces (see Fig. 6). Again, one or more of these foci may be present, and in many centers these are not treated with augmentation of immunosuppression and the infiltrates disappear spontaneously. A small number of IA or IB grades will progress to a grade II or a higher grade of acute rejection, but

Table 4 Standardized Cardiac Biopsy Grading—International Society for Heart and Lung Transplantation

"Old" Nomenclature	*"New" Nomenclature*	*Grade*
No rejection	No rejection	0
Mild	A = Focal (perivascular or interstitial infiltrate)	I
	B = Diffuse but sparse infiltrate	
"Focal" moderate	One focus only with aggressive infiltration and/or focal myocyte damage	II
Moderate	A = Multifocal aggressive infiltrates	III
	B = Diffuse inflammatory process	
"Severe"	Diffuse, aggressive polymorphous infiltrate ± edema ± hemorrhage ± vasculitis	IV
"Resolving" rejection		Denoted by a lesser grade
"Resolved" rejection		Denoted by grade 0

Additional Required Information

- Biopsy less than four pieces
- Humoral rejection (positive immunofluorescence, vasculitis, or severe edema in absence of cellular infiltrate
- "Quilty" effect A = No myocyte encroachment
  B = With myocyte encroachment
- Ischemia A = Up to 3 weeks posttransplant
  B = Late ischemia
- Infection present
- Lymphoproliferative disorder
- Other

Source: From Ref. 9.

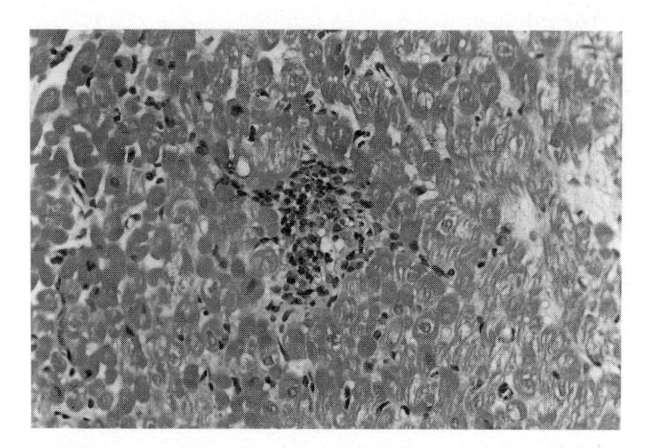

Figure 5 Biopsy showing ISHLT grade 1A rejection: a sparse perivascular infiltrate of activated lymphocytes without myocyte damage. (Hematoxylin and eosin, ×200.)

this is usually in the first year. Following the first year, the incidence of grade I or II proceeding to a higher grade is approximately 4% (18).

3. *ISHLT Grade II*

This represents a single focal inflammatory infiltrate of predominantly activated plump mononuclear cells which is dense enough to cause myocyte damage either by replacement or by direct extension. There should be no more than one focal infiltrate included in all the submitted biopsy pieces (Fig. 7). A recent paper suggests that many of these grade II dense infiltrate are, in fact, intramyocardial portions of a "Quilty" effect (19). This can sometimes be sorted out by a trichrome stain to show fragments of endocardium within the infiltrate or by seeing small vascular spaces that are characteristic of the Quilty effect. In this case, it is recommended that the biopsy paraffin block should be sectioned right through to see if the "grade II focus" meets with a true endocardial infiltrate of Quilty.

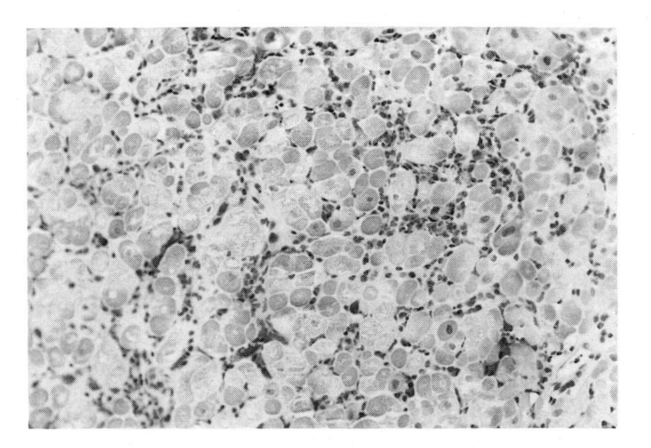

Figure 6 ISHLT grade 1B rejection: a sparse perimyocytic lymphocytic infiltrate ("chicken-wire effect") without myocyte damage. (Hematoxylin and eosin, ×200.)

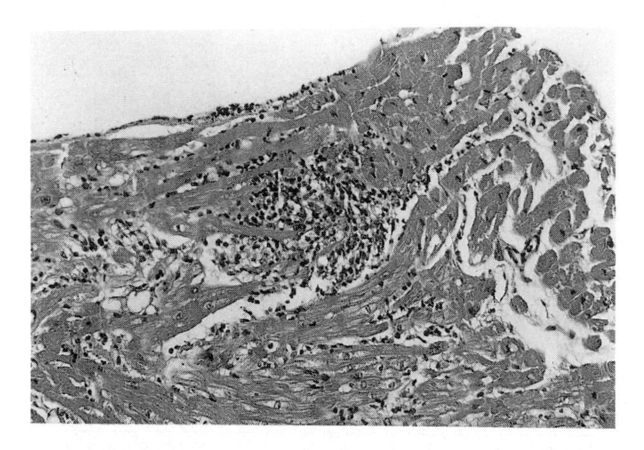

Figure 7 ISHLT grade 2 rejection: an isolated focus of activated lymphocytes with myocyte injury. (Hematoxylin and eosin, ×170.)

4. *ISHLT Grade IIIA and B (Moderate Rejection)*

Grade IIIA represents multifocal lymphocytic infiltrates usually in more than one or two pieces of the total endomyocardial biopsy fragments. At least some of these multifocal infiltrates should include myocyte damage (Fig. 8). In this case, the infiltrates are sometimes accompanied by a sparse but definite endocardial infiltrate that is different from a Quilty effect. The inflammatory infiltrates of a grade IIIA often contain eosinophils and sometimes neutrophils. In ISHLT grade IIIB, the multifocal infiltrates seen in grade IIIA are more confluent, affect a larger number of the biopsy pieces, and contain eosinophils, neutrophils, and sometimes small local hemorrhages in the interstitium due to the usual vasculitis of acute rejection. This grade IIIB is sometimes called "borderline severe." In the case of grade IIIA or B, nearly all transplant centers agree that treatment for acute rejection by increasing the immunosuppression is necessary.

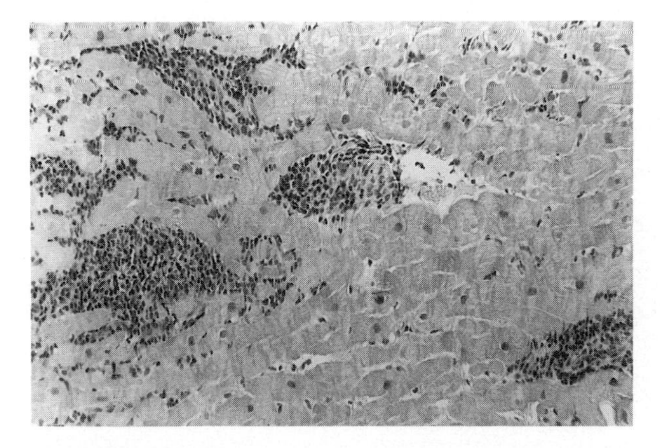

Figure 8 ISHLT grade 3A: many focal areas of lymphocytes with myocyte damage. (Hematoxylin and eosin, ×200.)

5. ISHLT Grade IV

This represents the most severe form of acute rejection, with an obvious vasculitis, interstitial hemorrhage, and, in many cases, edema and a more pronounced neutrophilic or mixed inflammatory infiltrate with myocyte damage (Fig. 9). An endocardial infiltrate that is not a Quilty is also usually seen. These patients should be aggressively treated or the allograft will be lost.

6. Resolving and Resolved Rejection

Because it is based on numerical grades, the ISHLT system does not allow for a diagnosis of "resolving" or a "resolved" acute rejection. Improvement in the rejection pattern should be denoted by assigning a lower numerical grade than that assigned to the previous biopsy. In other words, a grade IIIB, would become a grade I if the biopsy were improved but still contained small lymphocytes with early fibroblasts and pigmented macrophages. This was called a "resolving" rejection in the old system. A "resolved" acute rejection should be designated as numerical grade 0 and should show no evidence of acute rejection, although scar may be present.

C. Phenotyping of Inflammatory Infiltrates

In an attempt to characterize the phenotype of infiltrating mononuclear cells so that target-selective immunosuppression can be given, many centers use immunohistochemistry for quantitating T-cell subsets in serial biopsies. Although trends in the T-cell population have been described by many, the immunophenotyping may not be particularly useful in the actual management or prediction of acute rejection, and it often gives spurious results. It is thought that this is due to sampling error and that if the whole heart were available, immunophenotyping might be more useful and reliable. It is, however, still very useful for basic research. The standardized ISHLT grading system also requires the reporting of the presence of other changes within the endomyocardial biopsy (see Table 4).

As pointed out earlier, it is important to have an adequate biopsy, and the ISHLT grading system requires a minimum of four pieces (at least 50% of each piece should be evaluable and not scar tissue or biopsy site). It has been shown by previous workers that

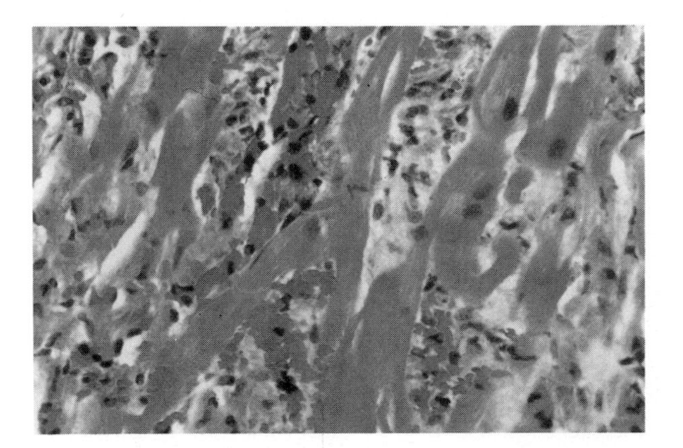

Figure 9 ISHLT grade 4 rejection: diffuse mixed inflammatory infiltrate with hemorrhage and myocyte damage. (Hematoxylin and eosin, ×300.)

there is a 2% false-negative rate in the case of four pieces, whereas there is a 4% rate of false negatives when there are only three pieces (10).

D. Humoral Rejection or Acute Vascular Rejection

In some institutions, immunofluorescence is routinely performed on endomyocardial biopsies to highlight acute vascular rejection (large plump endothelial cells with edema) and the possibility of humoral rejection. Acute vascular rejection has been well documented and described in the literature (11,20). Humoral rejection, on the other hand, is a fairly rare condition. Histopathologically there is edema, prominent endothelial cells, and occasional inflammatory cells, but much less than is seen in cellular rejection. Often the patient shows clinical evidence of heart failure without the usual morphological signs of cellular rejection. Positive immunofluorescence on the biopsy may be present in these situations, reflecting leakage of immunoglobulins (Fig. 10). As pointed out earlier, it is possible to get false-positive as well as false-negative results with this method (12), and this is known to occur particularly when there is ischemia, which may damage the integrity of the endothelial cells, or when the biopsy procedure itself cuts across vessel walls. Prominent endothelial cells are often present as a result of the inevitably contracted state of the myocardium in a biopsy. In most cases, the instance of humoral rejection is very small, although it has been described as high as 40% in some institutions.

E. Quilty Effect

The Quilty effect, described previously, is a focal, dense endocardial infiltrate that may or may not be associated with acute rejection (21,22). Histopathologically, the Quilty effect, so called after the patient in whom it was first described, is an aggregate of mononuclear lymphocytes typically confined to the endocardium (Quilty A) containing small vascular channels (Fig. 11). These aggregates are polyclonal but consist mainly of T cells, and there may be scattered macrophages and nests of B cells as well. Sometimes, the Quilty effect penetrates the underlying endocardium, causing subadjacent myocardial damage. In this case, it is called "Quilty B" for the sake of grading (Fig. 12). Since the ISHLT grading

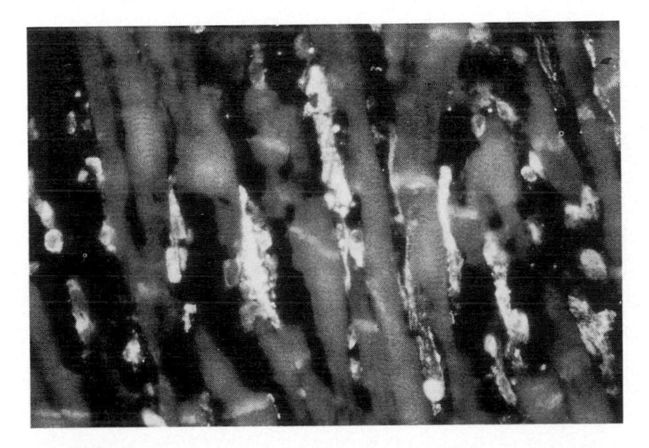

Figure 10 Immunofluorescence for C3 in an endomyocardial biopsy showing small-vessel positivity. (Immunofluorescence, ×300.)

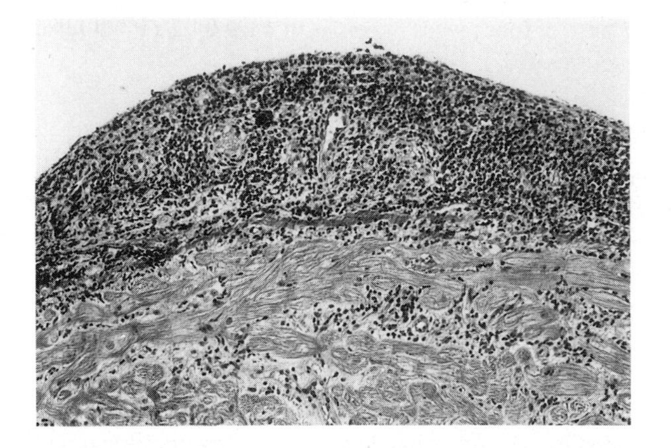

Figure 11 "Quilty A" effect seen on endomyocardial biopsy. Note that most of the infiltrate is within the endocardium (blue line) and contains vascular spaces. (Masson's trichrome, ×180.)

system has been in use, however, it has been shown that there is no clinical difference between Quilty A and Quilty B, and in many institutions neither is treated. Some reports have shown that the Quilty effect is associated with acute cardiac rejection, and others have shown that it is not. It has been seen in animal studies, where the entire endocardium is lined with the Quilty effect but there is no evidence of acute rejection elsewhere. Tangential cuts can be confused with acute rejection on biopsy samples; if this is thought to be the case, it is best to cut right through the block to further delineate the Quilty effect on the endocardium. It can be said, however, that the intensity of the focal infiltrates is much greater than is seen in acute rejection, although it could be confused with lymphoproliferative lesions. The Quilty effect was originally seen when cyclosporine immunosuppression came into use; it was not seen in the previous 10 years, when the immunosuppression used consisted predominantly of corticosteroids, ATG, and azathioprine. It has now been shown that the

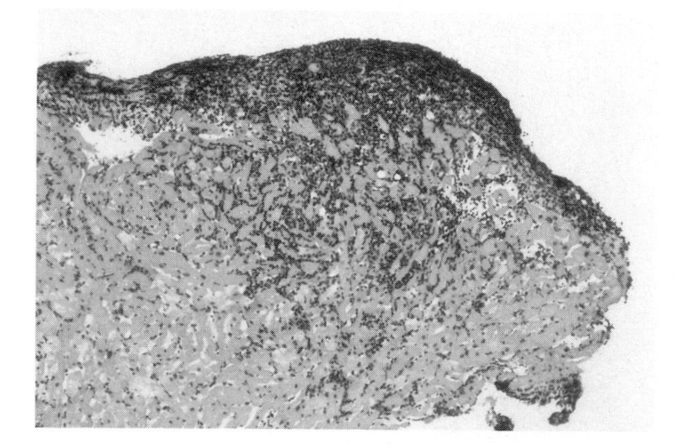

Figure 12 "Quilty B" effect showing lymphocytes spilling over into the subendocardium and surrounding myocytes. (Hematoxylin and eosin, ×170.)

Quilty effect can also be seen with other new immunosuppressant agents becoming available, such as rapamycin and leflunomide (23).

F. Ischemia

Evidence of ischemia in an endomyocardial biopsy should also be listed in the standardized additional required information of the ISHLT cardiac biopsy grading. The histopathologic changes of ischemia have already been described. The ISHLT grading system suggests using ischemia grade A when it is early postcardiac transplantation, denoting a reperfusion or similar etiology. The grading system suggests using ischemia grade B when it is a late manifestation within the graft, and therefore more suggestive of graft coronary disease or other later ischemic insult.

G. Infectious Myocarditis

Because the cardiac recipients are immunosuppressed, infection is a frequent complication of cardiac transplantation. The most common opportunistic infections seen in cardiac allograft recipients are viral, parasitic and fungal. The most common infection seen in endomyocardial biopsies and at autopsy are those involving CMV and *Toxoplasma gondii*. Other bacterial or parasitic infections may also occur, but these are less common. To avoid opportunistic infection, cardiac recipients who are themselves seronegative but who receive donor hearts from seropositive donors for either CMV or toxoplasmosis are often treated prophylactically. It is obviously critical to make the distinction morphologically between acute rejection and infectious myocarditis. In equivocal cases, serology, immunohistochemistry or in situ hybridization may be indicated. In the case of CMV and *Toxoplasma gondii*, the lesions can sometimes be seen without having evoked a surrounding inflammatory infiltrate; this is particularly true in the case of *Toxoplasma gondii* if the cyst is intact (Fig. 13). Cytomegalovirus inclusions will often break into smaller fragments following treatment with DHPG and have a distinctive appearance; they must be looked for carefully (Fig. 14).

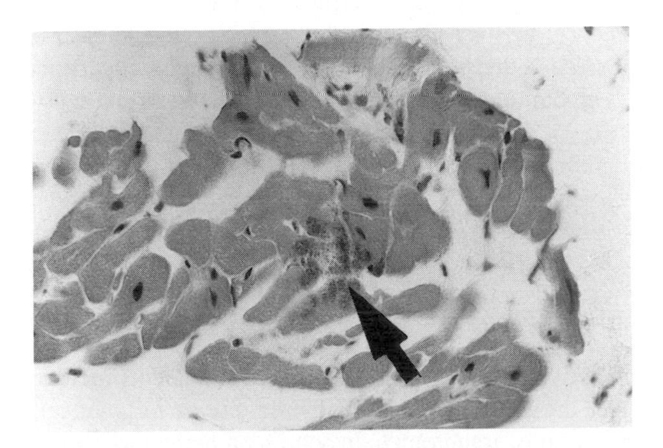

Figure 13 Endomyocardial biopsy showing encysted *Toxoplasma gondii* without an inflammatory reaction. (Hematoxylin and eosin, ×400.)

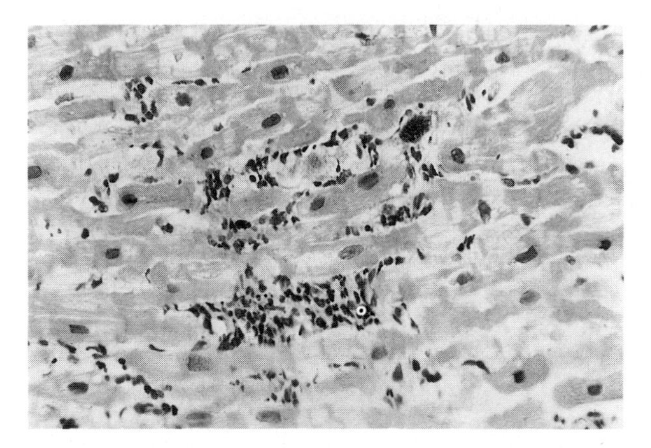

Figure 14 Endomyocardial biopsy showing an inflammatory infiltrate adjacent to CMV inclusions "broken down" by prior treatment with antiviral drugs. (Hematoxylin and eosin, ×300.)

In general, it can be said that infectious myocarditis usually includes a mixed inflammatory infiltrate rather than the monomorphous mononuclear infiltrate of acute rejection. If acute rejection is severe and a mixed infiltrate is then present, one may have to rely on the clinical situation to sort out whether the patient appears to be rejecting or has a severe inflammatory myocarditis, unless the organism can be seen on biopsy. It is possible to have both infection and rejection at the same time; in these cases, it is usual to treat both concomitantly. The hematogenous dissemination of fungus may lead to vascular plaques, causing minute focal infarcts. It goes without saying that infections in immunosuppressed cardiac recipients usually affects other organs in the body as well as the donor heart.

H. Lymphoproliferative Disorder

Lymphoproliferative disease in the immunosuppressed donor-organ recipients is usually EBV-related and may occur in cardiac recipients, particularly in younger patients and children (24,25). These lesions often occur in other organs including the brain and gastrointestinal system and have been described at the site of injections in the thighs in patients who received ATG. Occasionally, lymphoproliferative infiltrates may be seen on endomyocardial biopsies or infiltrating the myocardium at autopsy. Lymphoproliferative lesions are more florid and dense than the infiltrates of acute cardiac rejection (Fig. 15). In situ hybridization for EBV virus is now available to diagnose these lesions, which can then be attenuated by reduction in immunosuppression (particularly cyclosporine) and by instituting antiviral agents such as acyclovir.

I. Other Lesions

Other lesions that may be seen in endomyocardial biopsies in allograft recipients include those due to diseases known to recur in the allograft, such as amyloid disease or giant-cell myocarditis (see Table 2). Also, foreign-body granulomata may be seen in the biopsies of patients who have had many previous biopsies. Other pieces of organ tissue may sometimes be seen: in endomyocardial biopsies performed on the right side, the bioptome, after

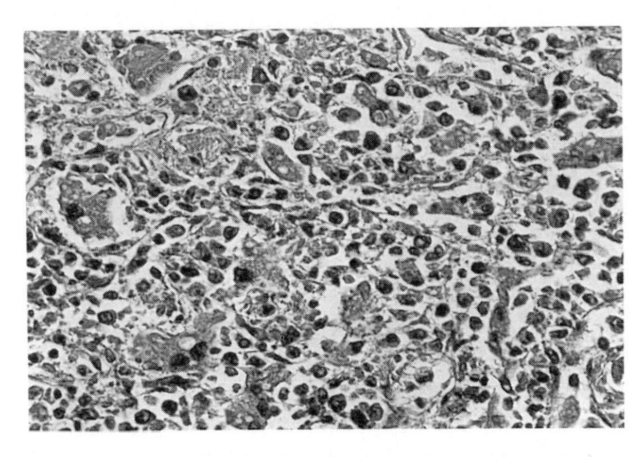

Figure 15 Section showing EBV-related lymphoproliferative infiltrate in a cardiac recipient. (Hematoxylin and eosin, ×200.)

entering the right atrium, may exit through the inferior vena cava into the liver, thus inadvertently obtaining small liver biopsies (Fig. 1).

V. PATHOLOGY OF LONG-TERM CARDIAC TRANSPLANTS

For the purpose of this section, long-term survival is considered to be 1 year or more posttransplantation. Hypertrophy and fibrosis occur in all cardiac recipient hearts, even in very young children. The heart invariably becomes much heavier than normal even without acute rejection. Although occurring mainly in the early postoperative period, acute cardiac rejection may also occur after 1 year, as is also true of episodes of infectious myocarditis. Denervation of the donor heart occurs at surgery and, to date, there has been no good morphological evidence that reinnervation takes place. Finally, the most significant long-term effect of cardiac transplantation is graft vascular disease, which occurs in the donor allograft.

A. Hypertrophy and Fibrosis

It has been observed that transplanted hearts become hypertrophied within 1 week following transplantation. This applies to the hearts of infants and children as well, which become not only bigger but heavier, even in the absence of acute cardiac rejection. Morphometric studies have shown that myocyte width is increased and that there is actual hypertrophy as well as an increase in fibrosis (26). The reason for this is not clear, but it has been postulated that it may be due to reperfusion injury at the time of transplantation, destroying small capillaries, with subsequent replacement by fibrosis; this is similar to the etiology of radiation effect on the heart. The hypertrophy would then be of a compensatory nature. This theory is supported by the fact that, on morphometric examination, there are fewer small vessels per unit area in the myocardium in the allograft than there are in a normal heart (26). The increase in fibrosis may include the pericardium, and this may then cause a restrictive pattern. The pericardium, even if left open at the time of operation, becomes adherent to the epicardium and thickened, and this can cause a restrictive situation. Sometimes fluid may become loculated within the pericardium of cardiac recipients. It should be said, however, than even where fibrosis is increased, as it is in most allografts, this does not appear to restrict increase in growth or size of the heart in infants and children over the ensuing years (27).

B. Acute Cardiac Rejection

Acute cardiac rejection can occur in long-term survivors, but it is much less frequent than during the first year following transplantation. The reasons for the recurrence of acute cardiac rejection in long-term cardiac allograft survivors may be several: (1) The patient may put on undue weight secondary to steroid treatment and thus effectively "dilute" the amount of immunosuppression they receive. (2) Some patients, particularly teenagers, may reduce or not take their immunosuppressants. Some may reduce their medication due to unwanted side effects, such as osteoporosis, acne, and hirsutism. Patients who experiment in this way often do it prior to coming for an annual visit, at which time the biopsies are found to show an unexpected acute rejection. Acute rejection may also follow an episode of CMV myocarditis, as this causes a lowering of the immunological response. Acute cardiac rejection after 1 year is similar morphologically to that occurring at any other time, and the grading should be the same as that occurring soon after transplantation.

C. Denervation

Following cardiac transplantation, the allograft remains denervated and is not under the usual autonomic nervous system control. Heart rate is higher than normal because of the absence of vagal tone. The heart rate in response to dynamic exercise tends to be slower and not to achieve peak levels during maximum exercise as compared with nontransplanted age-matched controls; although the heart rate may increase slowly, it also decreases slowly following rest after activity (28). Morphologically, serial endomyocardial biopsies will show a marked reduction in the number of interstitial nerves, both sensory and sympathetic, within a few weeks or months of cardiac transplantation. This is also shown physiologically by pharmacological challenges and electrophysiological studies on cardiac recipients indicating that the heart remains denervated, at least for some time. Recently, there have been reports that there is some physiological evidence of reinnervation, and there have also been reports that patients have experienced chest pain in response to myocardial infarctions in the allograft. Nevertheless, clear-cut evidence of reinnervation from the morphological standpoint has not been described. Although sparse nerves can be seen in the interstitium on electron microscopy in all allografts, these are thought to be the postganglionic fibers of the intact parasympathetic ganglia that remain in the atrioventricular groove distal to the suture lines at the time of cardiac transplantation. Serial studies up to 11 years following cardiac transplantation have failed to reveal reinnervation, at least to the apex of the heart (29). The sinoatrial and atrial ventricular nodes face a 50% risk of surgical damage during the procurement of the heart in both the recipient and in donor tissue, as described by others (30).

D. Transplant Malignancies

It has been known since the advent of organ transplantation that malignancies develop at a higher rate in immunosuppressed transplant recipients. Unfortunately, this complication also occurs in cardiac allograft recipients (24). The distribution of malignancies is similar to that described in renal and other organ transplants. There is an increase in dermatological cancer. Of particular concern are the lymphoproliferative malignancies due to EBV virus, mentioned earlier. The incidence is higher in cardiac allografts and appears to be slightly higher in children. Some patients with this condition have responded well to radiation, and many have responded well to the reduction of cyclosporine levels and the introduction of acyclovir (31). Extranodal lymphomas have been found in the gastrointestinal tract in cyclosporine-treated patients and at the sites of injection of ATG. Several good publications express the various views on the subject of etiology and also on the phenotype of the malignancies, which are shown to be mainly large cell B-cell lymphomas (Fig. 15) (32,33).

E. Graft Vascular Disease

Graft vascular disease is one of the leading causes of failure of cardiac allografts in the first year following transplantation. Most centers report an incidence of between 30 and 40% in adults at the third year following transplantation as judged by coronary angiography. One study by Gao et al. reported a 91% incidence at 5 years posttransplantation on coronary arteriography; however, actual death from graft coronary disease has been less frequent recently (34). Graft vascular disease may occur as early as 3 months postcardiac transplantation and is seen in cardiac recipients who die of other causes. It can also be quite latent in its appearance, and one cardiac recipient who died after 22 years did so as a result of graft vascular disease. Unfortunately, graft vascular disease does not spare infants or young children or the recipients of combined heart-lung transplants.

The pathology of graft vascular disease has been described previously (35,36) and is that of a concentric intimal proliferation, usually with minimal damage to the elastic lamina and no changes to the smooth muscle media of the vessel wall (Fig. 16). The lesions usually affect all of the coronary vessels in the heart, including the branches (Fig. 17) and even the intramyocardial small vessels (unlike the changes seen in normally occurring atherosclerosis). The intimal thickening may advance quite rapidly between angiographic studies or may occur insidiously. Because small vessels are involved, very small triangular myocardial infarcts may result prior to major infarcts caused by luminal compromise of the larger vessels. In cardiac recipients with older donors, normally occurring atherosclerotic plaques may be observed that are not part of the immune-stimulated intimal proliferation.

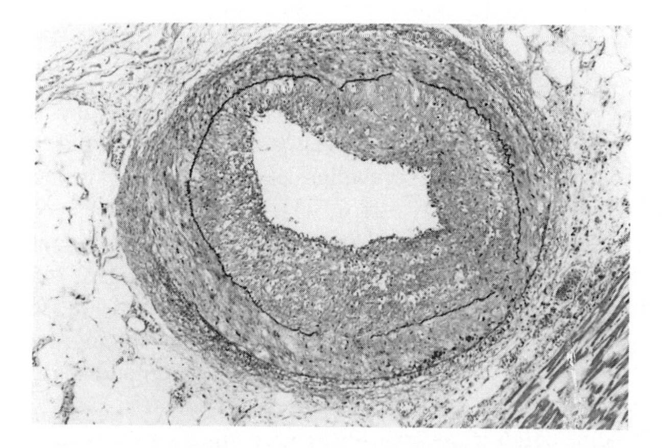

Figure 16 Transverse section of a coronary artery showing a concentric, intimal proliferation characteristic of graft vascular disease. (Elastic van Giesen, ×100.)

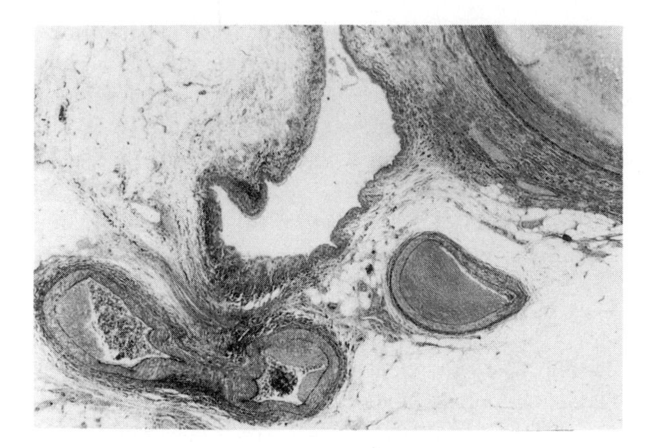

Figure 17 Section of coronary artery branches showing a graft vascular disease. (Elastic van Giesen, ×100.)

In long-term survivors, in whom graft vascular disease has occurred more slowly, it is possible to see superimposed plaques with cholesterol clefts and many foam-filled macrophages (37). In patients who die of acute rejection, there is invariably a vasculitis involving the vessel wall and adventitia. In addition to that, an endothelialitis or aggregation of lymphocytes on the endothelial surface may also be observed in some allografts. Recent work suggests that endothelialitis may be due to CMV infection, which has also been implicated as a cause for graft vascular disease (38). As would be expected, the great vessels that are attached to the donor heart at the time of transplantation, both the aorta and pulmonary artery, may also show intimal proliferation, although it has been observed to be more prevalent in the aorta. The adventitial vessels of both the aorta and the pulmonary artery may be entirely blocked by the typical endocardial proliferation, even in the vessels that are some distance away from the actual suture line and therefore cannot be confused with the endarteritis around the healed incision (39,40). The intimal proliferation appears to consist mainly of modified smooth muscle cells, sparse T lymphocytes, and lipid-filled macrophages. Lymphocytes are not always present within the intimal proliferation and, as mentioned above, small aggregates on the surface (endothelialitis) may or may not be present.

The causes of the intimal proliferation have been extensively reviewed. In brief, it is thought that repetitive immunological injury to the endothelial cells results in activated lymphocytes within the vascular wall and endothelial surface, which cause the release of cytokines and growth factors that ultimately stimulate smooth muscle cell proliferation. The availability of new molecular studies has resulted in a better understanding of the cascade of events that occurs in intimal proliferation (41). These molecular studies have also resulted in the development of new immunosuppressive drugs aimed at reducing the incidence of intimal proliferation. Unfortunately, the development of graft vascular disease does not spare infants or children, and some have been known to die following transplantation from graft coronary disease. In some children, as opposed to adult allograft recipients, vasculitis seems to be more of a feature.

The only treatment for graft coronary disease is retransplantation. Where there are focal lesions, atherectomy and angioplasty have been tried, but the lesions have sometimes recurred.

The pathology and mechanisms of accelerated atherosclerosis in allografts is described at length in Chapter 5.

VI. SUMMARY

Cardiac transplantation is now an accepted form of treatment for end-stage heart disease in all age groups, including neonates with severe congenital heart disease. Long-term cardiac transplant survivors still require immunosuppression, although in some cases this can be modified considerably, particularly in children, to meet growth requirements or mitigate unwanted side effects. In general, acute cardiac rejection can be diagnosed and managed by manipulation of immunosuppression. It is also true that infection in the allograft recipient and in the graft itself can be treated successfully in many cases. Lymphoproliferative disease related to EBV, although an important cause of morbidity, can also be mitigated and to some extent treated. The long-term problem of graft vascular disease is one on which there is great emphasis at the research level at this time, as this seems to be a major cause of loss of the allograft. The only successful treatment is that of retransplantation, which, of course, involves other donors and has proved to be less successful than primary cardiac transplantation. Some patients feel that they do not want to go through a second or third transplantation. Despite the described pathology, cardiac recipients may now live productive and active lives for up to 20 years posttransplantation. Infants who, in the past, could not survive because of hypoplastic left hearts are now growing up to be healthy 5 or 6 years following successful cardiac allograft transplantation.

REFERENCES

1. Barnard CN. A human cardiac transplant: An interim report of successful operation performed at Groote Schuer Hospital, Capetown, S Afr Med J 1967; 41:1271–1274.
2. Reitz BA, Wallwork JL, Hunt SA, et al. Heart-lung transplantation: Successful therapy for patients with pulmonary vascular disease. N Engl J Med 1982; 306:557–564.
3. Kaye MP. Pediatric thoracic transplantation: The world experience. J Heart Lung Transplant 1993; 12:S344–350.
4. Boucek MM, Mathis CM, Boucek RJ Jr, et al. Prospective evaluation of echocardiography for primary rejection surveillance after infant heart transplantation: Comparison with endomyocardial biopsy. J Heart Lung Transplant 1994; 13:66–73.
5. Mason JW. Techniques for right and left endomyocardial biopsy. Am J Cardiol 1978; 41: 887–892.
6. Tilkian AG, Daily EK, eds. Cardiovascular Procedures. St. Louis, MO: Mosby, 1986; 180–203.
7. Caves PK, Stinson EB, Billingham ME, Shumway NE. Percutaneous transvenous endomyocardial biopsy in human heart recipients (experience with a new technique). Ann Thorac Surg 1973; 16:325–336.
8. Gravanis MB, Hertzler GL, Franch RH, et al. Hypersensitivity myocarditis in heart transplant candidates. J Heart Lung Transplant 1991; 10:688–697.
9. Billingham ME, Cary NRB, Hammond ME, et al. A working formulation for the standardization of nomenclature in the diagnosis of heart and lung rejection: Heart rejection study group. J Heart Transplant 1990; 9:587–592.
10. Spiegelhalter DJ, Stovin PGI. An analysis of repeated biopsies following cardiac transplantation. Stat Med 1983; 2:33–40.

11. Hammond EH, Hansen JH, Spencer LS, et al. Vascular rejection in cardiac transplantation: histologic, immunopathologic and ultrastructural features. Cardiovasc Pathol 1993; 2:1–14.
12. Bonnaud EN, Lewis NP, Masek MA, Billingham ME. Reliability and usefulness of immunofluorescence (IF) in cardiac transplantation. J Heart Lung Transplant (accepted for publication).
13. Weil RR, et al. Hyperacute rejection of a transplanted human heart. Transplantation 1981; 32:71–72.
14. Basile L, et al. Identification of the antibody to vascular endothelial cells in patients undergoing cardiac transplantation. Transplantation 1985; 40:672–674.
15. Trento A, Hardesty RL, Griffith BP, et al. Role of the antibody to vascular endothelial cells in hyperacute rejection in patients undergoing cardiac transplantation. J Thorac Cardiovasc Surg 1988; 95:37.
16. Jennings RB, Wartment WB. Reactions of the myocardium to obstruction of the coronary arteries. Med Clin North Am 1962; 46:3–8.
17. Billingham ME. Dilemma of variety of histopathologic grading systems for acute cardiac allograft rejection by endomyocardial biopsy. J Heart Transplant 1990; 9:272–276.
18. Rizeq MN, Masek MA, Billingham ME. Acute rejection: Significance of elapsed time post-transplant. J Heart Lung Transplant. In Press.
19. Bell G, Lones M, Czer LSC, et al. Grade 2 cellular rejection: Does it exist? United States and Canadian Academy of Pathology, Annual Meeting, San Francisco, March 12–18, 1994.
20. Hammond EH, Yowell RL, Nunoda S, et al. Vascular (humoral) rejection in heart transplantation: Pathologic observations and clinical implications. J Heart Transplant 1989; 8:430–443.
21. Joshi A, Masek MA, Brown BW Jr, et al. "Quilty" revisited: A 10-year perspective. Human Pathol. In press.
22. Billingham ME. The post-surgical heart. Am J Cardiovasc Pathol 1988; 1:319–334.
23. Mohacsi P, Joshi A, Wang J, et al. Endocardial mononuclear cell infiltrates (Quilty effect) in heterotopic cardiac allografts in rapamycin-treated rats. Circulation. In press.
24. Penn I. Malignant lymphoma in organ transplantation recipients. Transplant Proc 1981; 13: 736–738.
25. Penn I, ed. University of Cincinnati Roundtable Report on Immunosuppression and Lymphoproliferative Disorders. Raritan, NJ: Ortho Biotech, 1992.
26. Rowan RA, Billingham ME. Pathologic changes in the long-term transplanted heart: A morphometric study of myocardial hypertrophy, vascularity and fibrosis. Hum Pathol 1990; 21:767–772.
27. Boucek MM, Mathis CM, Razzouk A, et al. Indications and contraindications for heart transplantation in infancy. J Heart Lung Transplant 1993; 12:S154–158.
28. Stinson EB, Griepp R, Schroeder JS, et al. Hemodynamic observations one and two years after cardiac transplantation in man. Circulation 1972; 45:1183–1194.
29. Rowan RA, Billingham ME: Myocardial innervation in long-term cardiac transplant survivors: A quantitative ultrastructural survey. J Heart Transplant 1988; 7:448–452.
30. Stovin PGI, Hewitt S. Conduction tissue in the transplanted heart. J Pathol 1986; 149:183–189.
31. Starzl TE, Porter KA, Iwatsukis, et al. Reversibility of lymphomas and lymphoproliferative lesions developing under cyclosporine steroid therapy. Lancet 1994; 1:583–587.
32. Cleary ML, Sklar J. Lymphoproliferative disorders in cardiac transplant recipients are multiclonal lymphomas. Lancet 1982; 2:489–493.
33. Clearly ML, Warnke R, Sklar J. Monoclonality of lymphoproliferative lesions in cardiac transplant recipients: Clonal analysis based on immunoglobulin-gene rearrangements. N Engl J Med 1984; 310:477–482.
34. Gao SZ, Alderman EL, Schroeder JS, et al. Accelerated coronary vascular disease in the heart transplant patient: Coronary arteriographic findings. J Am Coll Cardiol 1988; 12:334–240.
35. Billingham ME. Cardiac transplant atherosclerosis. Transplant Proc 1987; 19:19–25.
36. Billingham ME. Histopathology of graft coronary disease: Presented at the 1991 transplant

Coronary Artery Disease Symposium, St. Louis, Missouri. J Heart Lung Transplant 1992; 11:S38–S44.
37. Pucci AM, Forbes C, Billingham ME. Pathologic features in long-term cardiac allografts. J Heart Transplant 1990; 9:339–345.
38. Speir E, Modali R, Huag E-S, et al. Potential role of human cytomegalovirus and p53 interaction in coronary restenosis. Science 1994; 265:391–394.
39. Russell ME, Fujita M, Masek MA, et al. Cardiac graft vascular disease: Nonselective involvement of large and small vessels. Transplantation 1993; 56:762–764.
40. Fujita M, Russell M, Masek MA, et al. Graft vascular disease in the great vessels and vasa vasorum. Human Pathol 1993; 24:1067–1072.
41. Libby P, Solomon RN, Payne DD, et al. Functions of vascular wall cells related to the development of transplantation-associated coronary arteriosclerosis. Transplant Proc 1989; 21: 3677–3684.
42. 1994 ISHLT Registry Database and UNOS Report at Venice, March 23,1994.

7

Pathology of Lung Transplantation

N. Paul Ohori and Samuel A. Yousem
University of Pittsburgh Medical Center, Pittsburgh, Pennsylvania

I. INTRODUCTION

With the clinical availability of cyclosporine, lung transplantation became a therapeutic option for end-stage pulmonary diseases in the 1980s. Over the past decade, improvements in immunosuppression, donor and recipient matching, organ harvesting and preservation, antimicrobial therapy, and surgical techniques have contributed greatly to increased survival. Currently, survivals of 60 to 70% may be expected over the first 2 posttransplant years (1,2). However, despite improvements in the immunosuppressive regimen, rejection and associated complications are major causes of mortality and morbidity. A thorough understanding of the rejection process along with the ability to distinguish it from other entities and provide appropriate therapies are essential to the long-term survival of the lung allograft recipient. In particular, the awareness of the timing of the graft syndrome is helpful in making the correct diagnosis (Table 1).

II. MECHANISMS OF LUNG TRANSPLANT REJECTION AND OTHER FORMS OF ALLOGRAFT INJURY

A. Allograft Complications Related to the Donor Organ

Although donors are thought to be without severe chronic illnesses, a detailed medical history is often not available due to the acute nature of the transplant procedure. Donor diseases may manifest in the early or late transplant course; fortunately, however, they are not clinically significant in most instances. The most common donor disease noted is related to smoking and the associated pulmonary alterations (i.e., respiratory bronchiolitis, emphysema, chronic bronchitis). Smoker's macrophages from the donor organ may persist in the allograft recipient for up to a year posttransplant and cannot be distinguished from those incurred de novo from the recipient's smoking. Regardless of the donor status prior to implantation, the organ is vulnerable to a number of possible assaults, including trauma, preservation injury, and infection. Preservation (harvest) injury represents organ ischemia and manifests pathologically as diffuse alveolar damage (3,4) with interstitial edema, hyaline membranes, and airspace granulation tissue as organization progresses. In severe cases, extension of damage to involve the airways produces an acute bronchitis/bron-

Table 1 Timetable of Allograft Syndromes

Immediate (0 to 7 days)	Reimplantation response
	Primary graft failure
	?Hyperacute rejection
Early (1 to 4 weeks)	Harvest injury
	Acute cellular rejection
	Infection
Intermediate (1 to 6 months)	Acute cellular rejection
	Infection
	Posttransplant lymphoproliferative disorder
Late (over 6 months)	Bronchiolitis obliterans (chronic airway rejection)
	Infection
	Acute cellular rejection
	Posttransplant lymphoproliferative disorder
	Recurrence of native disease

chiolitis and luminal ingrowth of loose granulation tissue into the airways (5,6). The term "diffuse alveolar damage" implies a diffuse process. In the transplant setting, however, a patchy, temporally homogeneous process has been documented (5) (Fig. 1). For reversible cases, the process resolves over a variable period of time, usually within 1 month post-transplant.

Subclinical donor organ infection may also influence early outcome. While the donor may have a normal chest radiograph and no signs of infection prior to explantation, positive tracheal culture—which may indicate possible aspiration—has been shown to correlate with early infection and lower survival in allograft recipients (7). Although rare, another donor factor that may lead to early graft dysfunction is thromboembolic disease contribut-

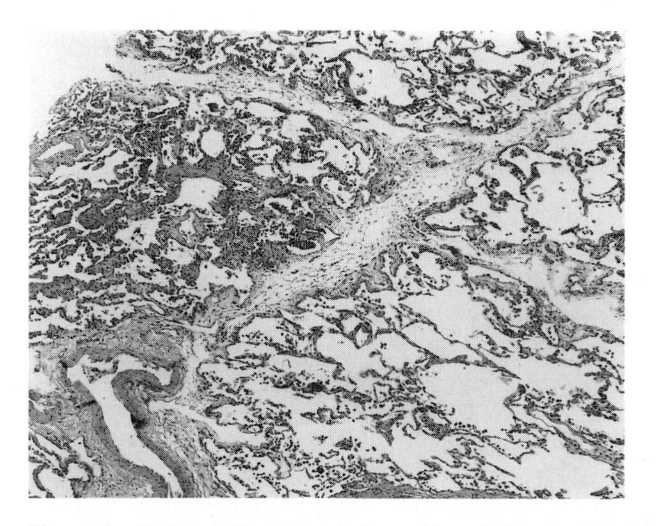

Figure 1 Ischemic damage to the lung allograft from harvest injury may manifest as patchy alveolar damage rather than a diffuse process. Focus of interstitial widening and organization is seen adjacent to relatively normal lung.

ing to significant ischemia. Sources of embolic material include brain (secondary to head trauma) (Fig. 2), bone marrow (presumably due to sternotomy), and cartilage (8). Finally, those cases without a demonstrable etiology are classified as primary graft failure (4). At the University of Pittsburgh Medical Center, primary graft failure was seen in approximately 6% of pulmonary transplants since 1982. In these instances, sepsis or hyperacute rejection was ruled out; an interesting observation was successful transplantation in one instance but not in another when ischemic times, flush solutions, techniques, and donor selection criteria were identical (4).

B. Early Non-Rejection-Related Allograft Complications

Provided that transplantation occurs without significant donor influences, the allograft is then susceptible to a number of host factors. Initially, virtually all grafts are subject to a "reimplantation response" characterized by bilateral opacification on chest radiograph and histological observation of interstitial and alveolar edema and margination of neutrophils (9). The pathogenesis is thought to be related to fluid overload secondary to disruption of the hilar lymphatics. The process resolves within the first week after transplantation, a time period before acute cellular rejection generally takes place.

Early heart/lung transplants were complicated by tracheal dehiscence (10–12). Although, because of improved surgical techniques, this complication is now uncommon, the bronchial artery circulation is sacrificed and bronchomalacia involving the main stem bronchi and their branches is not an uncommon complication (13–16). It has been suggested that this airway ischemic process may contribute to the development of bronchiolitis obliterans (14,16).

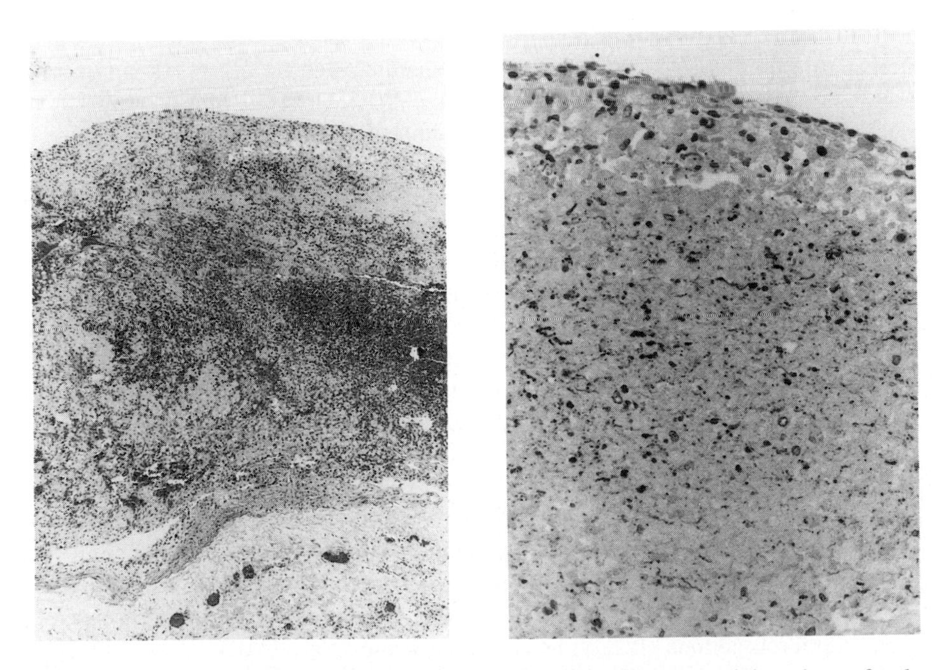

Figure 2 Brain embolism within an artery (left). Neurofilament staining shows focal area of staining supporting the presence of glial elements in embolus (right).

C. Acute Cellular Rejection

Following the first week after transplantation, 30 to 40% of the patients are prone to develop rejection (17). Although hyperacute rejection has been reported in the animal lung transplant model (18) and human kidney and liver transplants, it has not been rigorously documented in human lung transplants. Documentation in the human clinical setting would require demonstration of (1) early graft failure exclusive of alternative clinical or pathological explanation; (2) consistent gross histological, and immunofluorescence findings; (3) demonstration of a presensitized state with a high percentage of panel-reactive antibodies; and (4) the presence of donor-specific antibodies in an eluate from the failed allograft (19).

Acute cellular rejection (ACR) is histopathologically characterized by a perivascular mononuclear cell infiltrate initially surrounding pulmonary veins and later involving arteries and lymphatics (3,20,21). The infiltrate cuffs the vascular structures and often undermines the endothelium. Reactive changes of the endothelium are often noted. The airway mucosa is also a site of mononuclear cell infiltration, and the initial target in the airway is the bronchus-associated lymphoid tissue (BALT). Depletion of the BALT has been documented and has been postulated to play a role in increased susceptibility to graft infection due to the loss of mucosal immunity (22). Later, the infiltrate insinuates itself into the overlying airway mucosa with cytotoxic effects on the individual bronchial cells (apoptosis). Whether the infiltrate involves the perivascular areas, BALT, or peribronchial/bronchiolar areas, the specific target appears to be the major histocompatibility complex (MHC) class II antigens (23–25). The initial phases of the rejection response involve primarily the small vessels, and the pattern of mononuclear cell infiltration varies from rare subtle foci (minimal ACR) to diffuse infiltrates into the interstitium and air spaces with alveolar damage and necrosis, hyaline membranes, and neutrophil and macrophage infiltrates (severe ACR) (26,27) (Fig. 3). In severe cases, the resulting injury may produce a picture of diffuse alveolar damage. Even after resolution of the inflammation, residual interstitial scarring may occur. Although the acute cellular rejection process is typically seen early in the course of transplantation, it may actually occur at any time posttransplant.

Acute cellular rejection is thought to be mediated by an immunological cellular mechanism targeting the donor histocompatibility antigens. Donor lymphoid tissues such as BALT express MHC class II antigens and are predictably the sites of initial immunological response (22,28,29). Infiltration by immunologically active host lymphocytes produces an in situ mixed lymphocyte reaction that initially leads to marked activation and transformation of the lymphocytes, with blastic appearance (Fig. 4), and later results in depletion of the BALT along with markedly diminished IgA and IgG plasma cell populations. Like other solid organs, the transplanted lung also demonstrates an interesting phenomenon of heightened MHC class II antigen expression in the vascular endothelium, bronchial epithelium, and interstitial mesenchymal cells (25,30,31). These sites correspond to foci of mononuclear cell infiltrates that are presumed effector cells of the immunological response. It is now recognized that MHC class II antigen expression is not limited to lymphoid cells and may be seen in the respiratory tract (32). In humans, HLA-DR and DQ expression were found in both the transplanted bronchial epithelium and native tracheal epithelium of the recipient (25,33). However, there was no correlation between the level of expression and episodes of rejection. While the mechanism for this induction is far from being clearly delineated, interferon-gamma (IFN-γ) has been shown to induce MHC class II antigens (34,35). Interferon-gamma is a product of activated $CD4^+$ and $CD8^+$ lymphocytes responding to a variety of rejection and nonrejection stimuli; thus the enhanced MHC class II antigen expression may be both an instigator and a result of the rejection process.

During acute cellular rejection, the major immunophenotypic cell type present is the T lymphocytes, although an occasional B cell may be detected (36,37). This infiltrative cell population has been shown to be of recipient origin by Y chromosomal probe analysis (38). The intensity and numbers of the $CD3^+$ T lymphocytes correlate with the grade of acute cellular rejection. Early in the acute cellular rejection process, the perivascular and peribronchiolar areas are cuffed predominantly by T lymphocytes of CD4 (helper) phenotype, whereas later in the course of acute cellular rejection the population of $CD8^+$ (suppressor/cytotoxic) T cells increases (36,39). At the point of a well-established acute cellular rejection, the CD4/CD8 ratio is less than 1. Furthermore, the infiltrating T cells also express interleukin-2 (IL-2) receptor (CD25), a marker of T-cell activation, which has been shown to correlate with the degree of acute cellular rejection (36,40,41). Other less specific markers expressed during rejection episodes include CD16, CD56, and CD57 (Leu 7), which are expressed in activated lymphocytes, as well as natural killer cells (36,42). Architecturally, peribronchiolar and perivascular lymphocytic cuffs are associated with disruptions of the laminin and type IV collagen basement membrane components, as demonstrated immunohistochemically (43). These alterations probably contribute to irreversible remodeling in the long term allograft.

In addition to immunocompetent lymphocytes, monocyte-macrophages also interact with the allograft. Over the course of graft survival, the BALT sites of secretory immunoglobulin production are depleted and the recipient loses one of the front lines of defense against microbial organisms. The task of defending the graft from infection becomes the onus of other components of the immune system. Most of the alveolar macrophages in the allograft are of recipient origin and must function in removing infectious as well as foreign matter. At the same time, monocyte-macrophages may serve as accessory cells to the recipient lymphocytes in mounting the rejection response. Studies have demonstrated impairment of the chemotactic and phagocytic functions of the alveolar macrophages while the cytotoxic activity remained intact (44). As a consequence, both the hindered antimicrobial activity and augmented rejection responses of the macrophage/monocyte system remain in a precarious balance.

Treatment of ACR also requires balancing between quelling the ACR response and preventing susceptibility to opportunistic infections. Histological response to therapy is characterized initially by the diminution of perivascular infiltrates, while the peribronchiolar and interstitial infiltrates may persist. Clinical improvement may be noted prior to histological resolution, which may take up to 4 weeks (45,46).

D. Chronic Rejection

Repeated episodes of acute cellular rejection, postoperative airway ischemia, and symptomatic cytomegalovirus (CMV) disease predispose the allograft to irreversible changes of bronchiolitis obliterans (OB), manifesting as airway scarring, and graft atherosclerosis not dissimilar to that seen in the heart allograft (47–49). Of the two types of lesions, the airway injury is of greater clinical importance. Specifically, the degree and number of episodes of airway injury during ACR correlates with the risk of OB development (49–51). The airway and vascular lesions are patchy and segmental; they involve both the large and small airways and arteries (3,51). The evolution of OB is marked by inflammatory mucosal

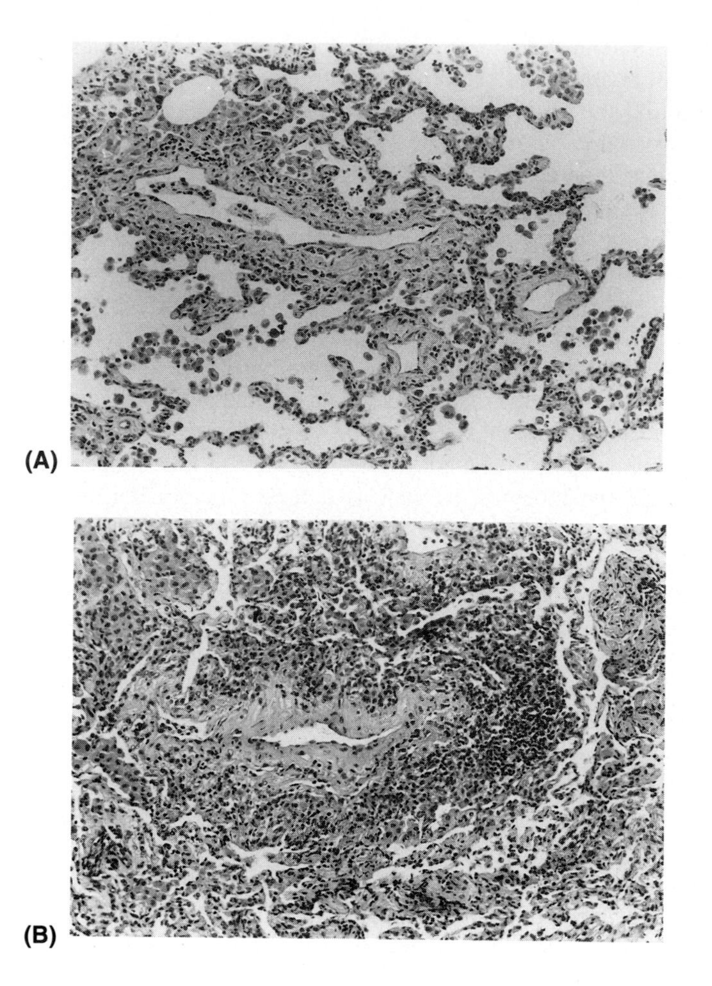

injury, followed by a progressive luminal occlusion by granulation tissue and subsequent scar tissue (Fig. 5). In contrast, chronic inflammatory injury to the larger airways result in cylindrical bronchiectasis (3,51). Early on, the pulmonary functional abnormalities are obstructive; later, restrictive deficits may be superimposed. Although the functional compromise is generally irreversible, the rate of progression of the airway deficit is variable.

In contrast to ACR, where $CD4^{+}$ T-cell infiltrates are associated with MHC class II expression, chronic rejection is characterized by $CD8^{+}$ T-cells located in the peribronchial, perivascular, and interstitial areas with the heightened expression of MHC class I and II antigens in the allograft (52,53). Repeated injury to the airway mucosa leads to disruption of the bronchiolar basement membrane, epithelial cell necrosis, myofibroblastic ingrowth, and finally scarring and terminal obliteration of the airways (43,48–50,54). Initially, active cellular airway infiltrates partially occlude the lumen, whereas older lesions show dense hyalinized, acellular transluminal scars. The process occurs in a temporally heterogeneous manner (3,56), and those airways with dense luminal scar tissue are thought to be irreversibly obstructed; therefore, ventilation depends on the remaining intact airways. While there

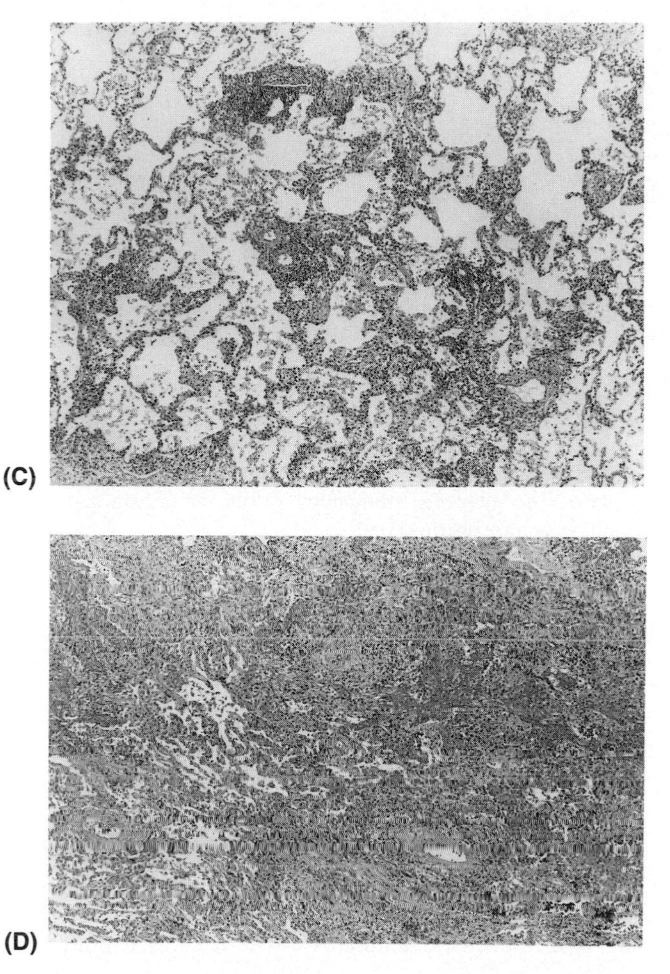

Figure 3 Grades of acute cellular rejection (ACR) are divided by the degrees of mononuclear cell infiltrates. Minimal ACR shows infrequent cuffs of subtle perivascular mononuclear infiltrates (A). In mild ACR, there are dense cuffs of mononuclear cells (5 to 8 cell layers thick) which are readily recognized at low magnification (B). Moderate ACR is characterized by dense infiltrates which are no longer confined to the perivascular areas, but extend into the interstitium and air spaces (C). There is extensive parenchymal damage by the mononuclear cell infiltrates in severe ACR, with hemorrhage and necrosis (D).

is a relationship between ACR and subsequent OB, the mechanism tying the two events is unclear. A "third party" such as CMV may alter the expression of MHC class II to I on the bronchial epithelial cells and subsequently stimulate a new subset of T cells ($CD8^+$) (53).

It should be noted that other processes, such as infection and aspiration, may produce airway injury similar to OB (57). Therefore, the lesions resulting in airway injury and scarring must be taken in the appropriate context—it may be an immunological rejection-related process; rarely, it is a result solely of an infectious, non-rejection-related insult; or it may be due to a spiraling cycle of rejection and infection.

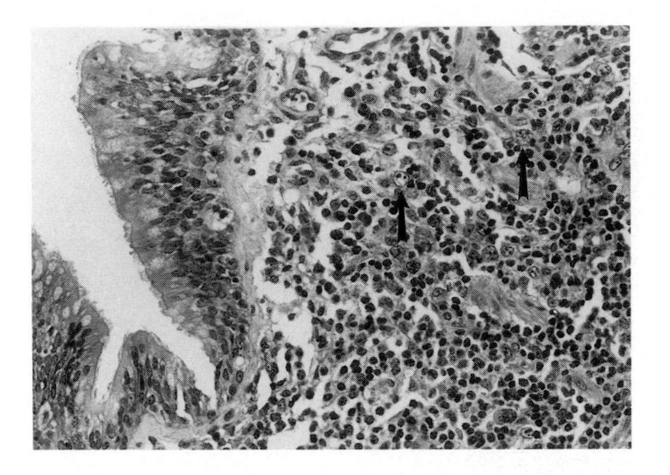

Figure 4 Bronchus-associated lymphoid tissue is one of the initial sites of ACR, where in vivo mixed lymphocyte reaction takes place. The allogenic stimulation results in transformation of lymphocytes, which assume a blastic appearance (arrows).

The other lesion developing in the long-term lung allograft as a manifestation of chronic rejection is graft arteriosclerosis (GAS) (47). The process is patchy and segmental; it involves large elastic arteries and smaller muscular arterioles. The myointimal proliferation and myxoid changes are circumferential, although asymmetry is occasionally noted. The cellular infiltrate is predominantly mononuclear—i.e., lymphocytes (small, round, and activated), plasma cells, and macrophages. The accompanying stromal response in the myxoid plaque consists of fibroblasts, myofibroblasts, endothelial cells, and smooth muscle cells. Although the pathogenesis has not been clearly delineated, the development of GAS probably involves immune mechanisms similar to cardiac transplant vascular rejection. Such extrapolations are based on the correlation between the development of GAS and coronary atherosclerosis in heart-lung transplant recipients (47). In cardiac graft ath-

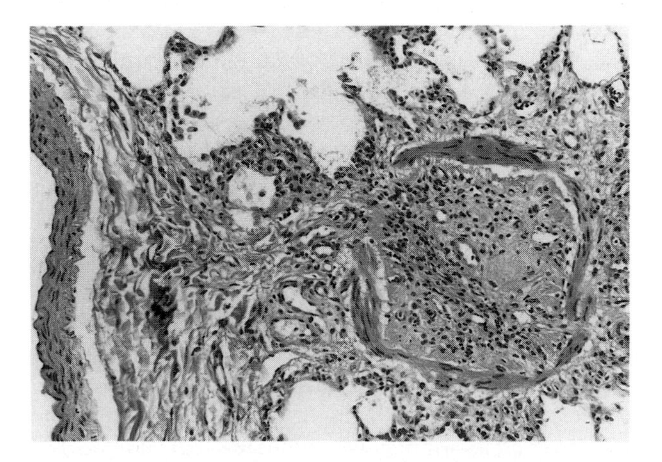

Figure 5 Active bronchiolitis obliterans (OB) with mononuclear infiltrates and intraluminal scarring.

erosclerosis, cellular and humoral responses appear to have roles in its development (58–62). The initiation of the immune response may be related to preceding events such as ischemia or CMV infection (63–65). Ischemic injury with subsequent release of donor antigens could promote cellular and humoral immune responses (66). The tropism of CMV for damaged tissue (67) and its detection in 6 to 50% of the atherosclerotic vessels (64,65) suggest its involvement in the atherogenic process. Cytomegalovirus could contribute to the development of GAS by upregulating MHC antigens (68), activating the coagulation cascade (69), and altering the lipid metabolism of vascular smooth muscle (70).

Although both OB and GAS are thought to represent chronic lung allograft rejection, they may be the result of different pathogenetic mechanisms, as the development of OB does not necessarily correlate with the onset of GAS. Furthermore, there are differences in clinical significance, as pulmonary arterial hypertension is not a major clinical concern in GAS (51).

E. Infections

The major differential diagnosis of rejection is opportunistic infection. This distinction is critical, as the management requires opposing approaches to therapy. While acute cellular rejection is a cellular immunological response with cytotoxicity directed against the donor MHC antigens, infectious processes break down protective epithelial and endothelial barriers and induce inflammatory and fibrogenic reactions in the graft. Since the lung is exposed to the external environment, the route of entry for the infectious organisms is usually through the airways. The types of infectious agents are similar to those of other opportunistic settings, although the clinical manifestations may be different.

Bacterial and fungal infections are complicated by the separation of benign colonizing forms from life-threatening invasive forms. With viral infections such as CMV, the donor and recipient's serological status influences the clinical manifestations of the disease. Reactivation of CMV disease usually does not lead to a serious illness, whereas patients experiencing primary disease have a high mortality and require intense antiviral therapy (71). Morphologically, CMV infections may manifest as diffuse interstitial or miliary pneumonitis with perivascular mononuclear infiltrates (72,73) (Fig. 6). In the absence of identifying the diagnostic intranuclear and cytoplasmic inclusion bodies, distinction from ACR may be difficult. Other viral infections potentially infecting the allograft lung include herpesvirus and adenovirus. Herpes pneumonia also presents with a diffuse or miliary pattern (74) (Fig. 7). However, in contrast to CMV, the inflammatory process is necrotizing, with tracheobronchial involvement or parenchymal disease showing alveolar damage and hyaline membrane formation. The cytopathic changes of Cowdry A and B intranuclear inclusions in cells lacking cytomegaly and cytoplasmic inclusions are helpful in recognizing herpes infection. Adenovirus infections may also affect the allograft, particularly in children (75,76). The morphological background is usually extensive alveolar damage with necrotizing airway involvement. Inclusions, when present, appear as intranuclear Cowdry A–type or smudge cells with absence of clearing between the inclusion and the nuclear membrane.

Prior donor colonization by bacteria and fungi also plays a role in the susceptibility of the allograft to infections. *Pseudomonas* and *Aspergillus* are common colonizers of recipients with cystic fibrosis or chronic obstructive pulmonary disease. Their significance depends on histological evidence of invasion, number of colony forming units in cultures, and clinical manifestations. Invasive aspergillosis protends impending mortality, whereas

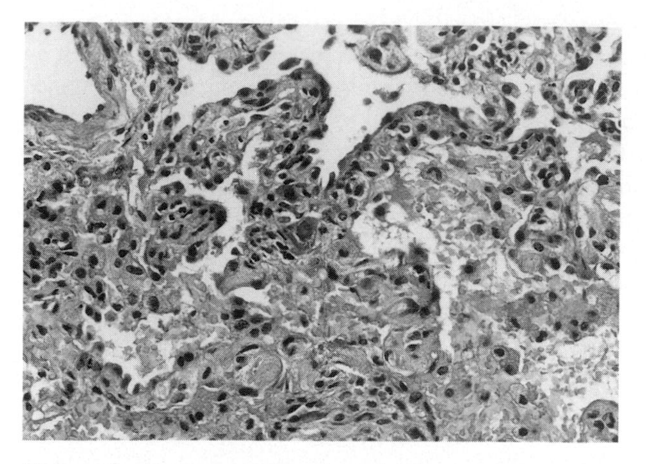

Figure 6 Cytomegalovirus interstitial pneumonia with a diagnostic cytomegalic cell showing intranuclear and cytoplasmic inclusion.

Aspergillus tracheobronchitis follows a relatively benign course when treated early (77). Isolation of organisms such as *Staphylococcus epidermidis* and *Xanthomonas* generally indicates commensal colonization and is thought not to be significant unless found in a clinically suspicious setting. Certain microbes, such as *Mycobacterium tuberculosis*, are recognized to be significant when isolated in any quantity. Once a common pathogen in the lung transplant setting, *Pneumocystis carinii* is now relatively uncommon due to prophylaxis with sulfa medications.

F. Posttransplant Lymphoproliferative Disorders

In addition to rejection and infection, the other major process producing mononuclear cell infiltrates is posttransplant lymphoproliferative disorders (PTLDs). In general, PTLDs are

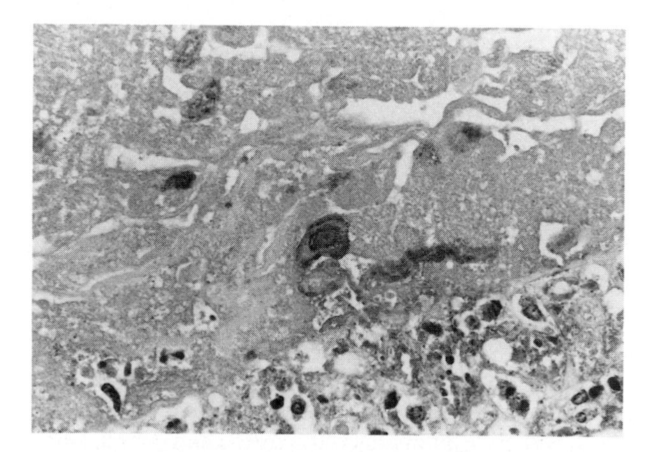

Figure 7 Herpes pneumonia shows a background of necrosis and the characteristic infected cell with Cowdry A intranuclear inclusions.

thought to be a lymphoproliferation of B cells infected with Epstein-Barr virus (EBV) arising in the setting of overimmunosuppression (78). The proliferation may occur anywhere lymphoid tissue resides, although common sites include the gastrointestinal tract, lymph nodes, tonsils, and grafted organ (79–82). As in other solid organ recipients, PTLDs in lung and heart/lung transplant patients may develop either inside or outside of the allograft. An interesting aspect in the lung transplant recipient is the relatively high incidence of PTLDs developing in the allograft itself. At our institution, PTLDs develop in approximately 7% of lung transplant recipients; of these, approximately 60% occur in the allografted lung (83). This latter figure compares with 17% of renal transplant recipients, 8.6% of liver transplant recipients, and rarely in heart transplant recipients (84,85). As PTLD evolves most readily in primary EBV infection (not reactivation), the anatomical and functional aspects of the lung may explain the high incidence of presentation in the allograft. Postulations include the following: (1) the allograft lung being the potential site of direct inoculation; (2) the high doses of immunosuppressives (relative to other grafts), reducing the T-cell population, which under normal conditions would keep the B-cell population in check; and (3) the presence of BALT, which would provide sites to which EBV infected B cells would migrate (83). The occurrence of PTLD in lung allografts tends to be either early or late in the posttransplant course (average 1.7 to 2.2 months). The histological appearance may be broadly subdivided into (1) the polymorphous type, characterized by cells representing the entire spectrum of B-cell differentiation (small lymphocytes, plasma cells, large lymphoid cells, and immunoblasts), and (2) the monomorphous type, characterized by a more uniform population of transformed large cells and immunoblasts (Fig. 8). Most monomorphous types tend to be monoclonal, whereas the polymorphous types are usually polyclonal. The proliferation does not respect anatomical boundaries and infiltrates in a lymphomatous fashion without following the perivascular or peribronchiolar distribution of ACR. Foci of confluent necrosis are not uncommon, reflecting the rapid replication rate of the lymphocytes. In contrast to malignant lymphomas, a subset of PTLDs respond to reduction of immunosuppression (82,84,86).

Patients refractory to the reduction of immunosuppression require additional regimens such as chemotherapy, radiation, or anti–B cell monoclonal antibodies (87). The relationship of chronic airway rejection and PTLD is also of interest, as 83% of patients with PTLD developed OB, whereas only 20 to 30% of non-PTLD long-term survivors developed OB. The reason for this high incidence has not been delineated, although the possibilities would include upregulation of class II antigens secondary to the EBV infection and episodes of high-grade acute cellular rejection following reduction of immunosuppression.

G. Disease Recurrence

While most lung transplants are performed for emphysema, pulmonary hypertension, and interstitial fibrosis, occasionally patients with systemic diseases such as cystic fibrosis, sarcoidosis, lymphangiomyomatosis (LAM), scleroderma, and other connective tissue disorders are transplanted. Of these, recurrence of sarcoidosis and LAM has been documented (88–90). As sarcoidosis is a diagnosis of exclusion, its recurrence is detected by identifying noncaseating granulomas negative for infectious organisms on transbronchial biopsies. The finding of noncaseating granulomas is not diagnostic, and other possibilities must be ruled out clinically. The significance of these findings is as yet uncertain, as the recipients have not shown functional compromise attributed to the recurrent disease and have not had sufficient follow-up to assess the possibility of the development of end-stage

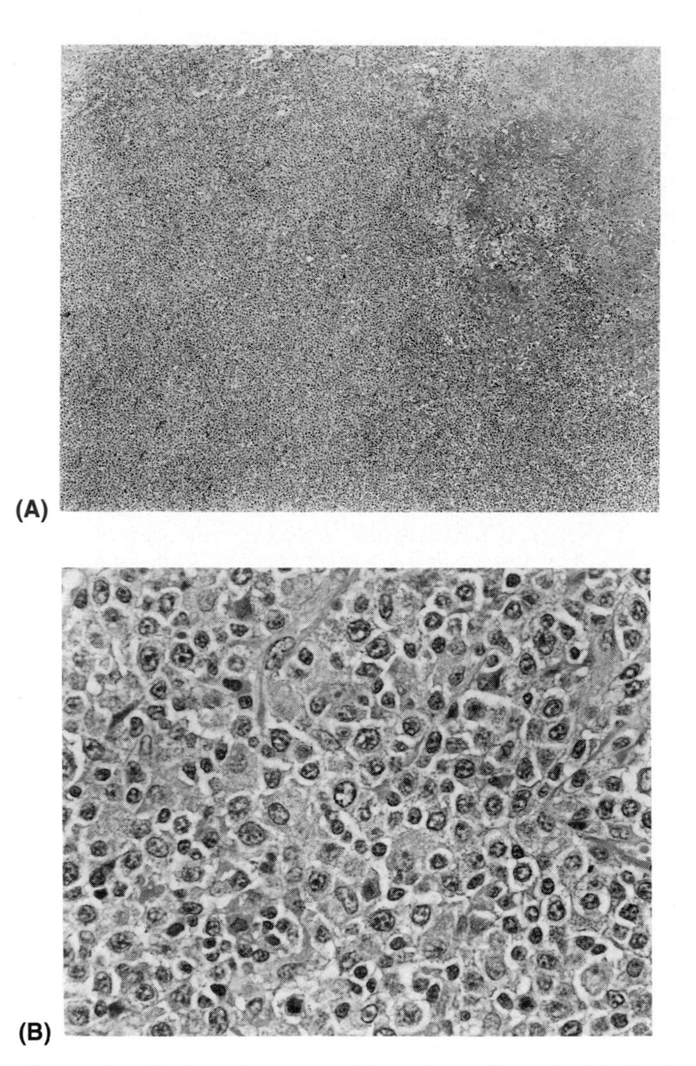

Figure 8 PTLD is characterized by a sheet of lymphoid infiltrate (A), which in this case shows transformed large cells (B).

interstitial disease. A case of recurrent LAM was seen in an autopsy where the donor was male and the recipient female (90) (Fig. 9). In situ hybridization Y-probe analysis showed the recurrent smooth muscle proliferation to be of donor origin, thus suggesting that the pathogenesis of LAM may relate to a circulating factor promoting the growth of myocytes. Rare case reports of giant cell interstitial pneumonia (GIP) have also been documented (91,92). In two reported cases, the procedure performed was a single lung transplant. As GIP is now thought to be a form of pneumoconiosis secondary to occupational exposure to hard metal, recurrence suggests the possibility of residual hard metal in the remaining recipient lung "seeding" the donor lung or the hard metal precipitating a persistent autoimmune reaction in recipient lymphocytes/monocytes.

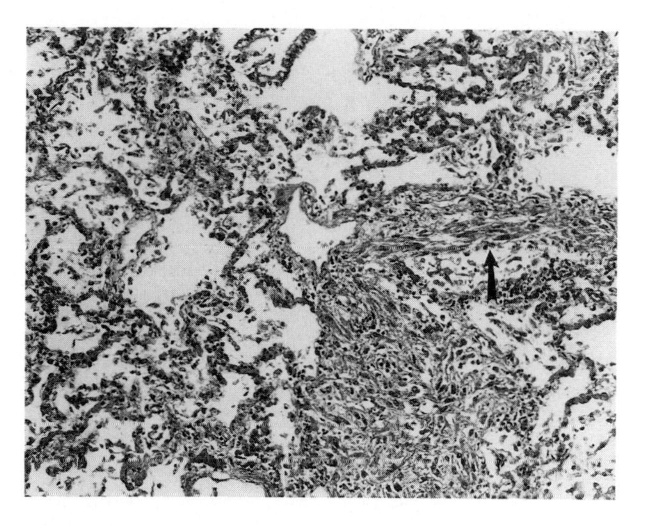

Figure 9 A case of recurrent lymphoangiomyomatosis shows smooth muscle proliferation (arrow) near a vessel.

H. Long-Term Survivors

Finally, long-term survivors approaching 10 years posttransplant have been documented. The clinical course is varied, with some experiencing practically no problems with rejection or infection and others having sustained problems, but the latter have generally adapted to the appropriate immunosuppressive and antimicrobial therapeutic regimen or have developed a symbiotic relationship between the allograft and the host. Routine follow-up biopsies on these patients show little if any pathological alteration. Similarly, autopsy findings in clinically successful transplant patients who died of unrelated causes show relatively unaltered allografts (51). Other long-term survivors may persist despite documentation of OB on multiple occasions. This may reflect the temporally heterogeneous patchy nature of airway damage in the lung allograft.

III. DIAGNOSIS

A. Specimen Requirement

Each procedure for monitoring the lung allograft has its shortcomings, and these must be considered along with the clinical indication for obtaining material for diagnosis. From the diagnostic point of view, the procedure of choice for monitoring lung transplant recipients would be a wedge biopsy obtained by thoracotomy or thoracoscopy (Table 2). However, the morbidity and cost associated with these procedures preclude their routine use. Lung transplant patents are biopsied on multiple occasions, especially early in the transplant course and routinely every 3 to 6 months, depending on the clinical setting. Therefore the procedure used must be reproducible and safe. Fluoroscopic transbronchial biopsies (TBB) along with bronchoalveolar lavage (BAL) provide a good compromise with acceptable sensitivity and specificity for the diagnosis of rejection and other allograft alterations (93). A minimum of five TBBs with three levels of hematoxylin and eosin (H&E) sections, a

Table 2 Procedural Efficiency and Complications

Procedure	Most efficacious	Least efficacious	Complications
TBB	ACR, OB	PTLD, some infections	Occasional pneumothorax
Wedge biopsy	ACR, OB, infections, PTLD	—	Anesthesia, breach of thoracic cavity
BAL (culture, cytology)	Infections	ACR, OB	Relatively minor
BAL (primed lymphocyte test)	?ACR, OB	PTLD, infections	Relatively minor
Fine needle aspiration	PTLD, localized infections	ACR, OB	Occasional pneumothorax

trichrome, and a Grocott stain should provide sufficient sampling for the assessment of the allograft in most cases (93,94). Biopsies may be taken randomly or from areas of clinical suspicion when radiographic infiltrates are present.

B. Diagnosis of Acute Cellular Rejection and Lymphocytic Bronchitis/Bronchiolitis

The TBB is most informative in assessing rejection. As mentioned above, perivascular and peribronchiolar mononuclear cell infiltrates are not specific for rejection and their interpretation must be taken in the appropriate context. Nevertheless, given the absence of other clinical or histological findings suggesting an infectious (e.g., abscess) or lymphoproliferative process, the intensity of infiltrate and extent of alterations may be graded according to the Working Formulation for the Diagnosis of Lung Rejection (94) (Table 3). This formulation was developed to provide a consistent system for promoting patient care, comparison between institutions, and developing alternative therapies. The scheme is divided into five classes: (A) acute cellular rejection, (B) acute airway damage without scarring (lymphocytic bronchitis/bronchiolitis), (C) chronic airway rejection (OB), (D) chronic vascular rejection, and (E) vasculitis. ACR may be graded as minimal to severe, primarily by assessing the perivascular, interstitial, and airspace components. Each grade is further qualified by assessing the presence or absence of airway inflammation. The perivascular and peribronchiolar infiltrates consist of small round lymphocytes, "activated" or "transformed" lymphocytes, plasma cells, and macrophages. In minimal acute cellular rejection, the perivascular infiltrates are subtle (forming a ring of lymphocytes two to three layers thick), rare, and typically do not show accompanying airway inflammation. Mild ACR show a dense, thick perivascular infiltrate of five to seven layers with accompanying features of endothelialitis and frequent airway inflammation. Moderate ACR is characterized by prominent perivascular infiltrates with extension into the adjacent interstitium and air spaces. The inflammatory process affects the majority of tissue sampled and airway inflammation is present in most cases. Although not specific, the presence of eosinophils is a common manifestation of higher grades of ACR and may be helpful in distinguishing it from other inflammatory processes. In severe ACR, there is evidence of extensive alveolar damage with necrosis, hemorrhage, and hyaline membrane formation.

Table 3 Working Formulation for Classification and Grading of Pulmonary Rejection

A. Acute rejection
  0. Grade 0—No significant abnormality
  1. Grade 1—Minimal acute rejection
    a. With evidence of bronchiolar inflammation
    b. Without evidence of bronchiolar inflammation
    c. With large-airway inflammation
    d. No bronchioles present
  2. Grade 2—Mild acute rejection
    a. With evidence of bronchiolar inflammation
    b. Without evidence of bronchiolar inflammation
    c. With large airway inflammation
    d. No bronchioles to evaluate
  3. Grade 3—Moderate acute rejection
    a. With evidence of bronchiolar inflammation
    b. Without evidence of bronchiolar inflammation
    c. With large airway inflammation
    d. No bronchioles to evaluate
  4. Grade 4—Severe acute rejection
    a. With evidence of bronchiolar inflammation
    b. Without evidence of bronchiolar inflammation
    c. With large airway inflammation
    d. No bronchioles to evaluate
B. Active airway damage without scarring
  1. Lymphocytic bronchitis
  2. Lymphocytic bronchiolitis
C. Chronic airway rejection
  1. Bronchiolitis obliterans—subtotal
    a. Active
    b. Inactive
  2. Bronchiolitis obliterans—total
    a. Active
    b. Inactive
D. Chronic vascular rejection
E. Vasculitis

Source: From Ref. 94.

Assessment of the airways is probably one of the more difficult tasks in TBB interpretation. The entire small airway lumen may not be present and the bronchiolar epithelium may be denuded. In addition, the TBB may be oriented at oblique angles, preventing the observation of the airway lumen. Therefore, the detection of an airway may depend on the identification of submucosal smooth muscle bundles. As the routine H&E stain may not be helpful in distinguishing subtle strands of smooth muscle from fibrous tissue on small biopsies, the trichrome stain is helpful in this regard (Fig. 10). Furthermore, the trichrome may be used in assessing the extent of airway scarring.

The term "lymphocytic bronchitis/bronchiolitis" (LBB) (grade B) is used to describe a predominantly lymphocytic infiltrate involving the airways (95) (Fig. 11). In these cases, a

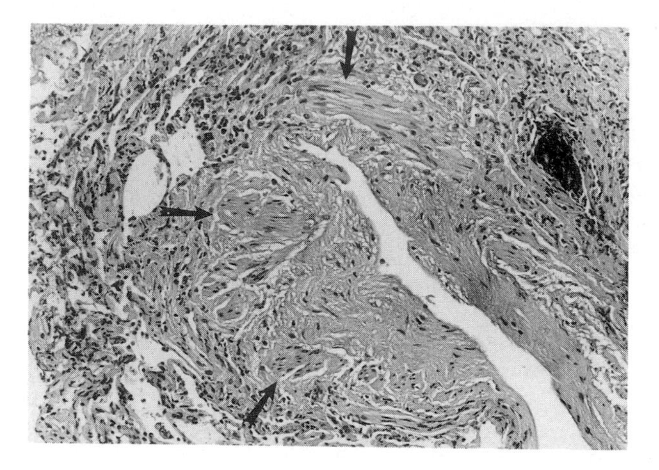

Figure 10 Inactive OB may not show the bronchiolar epithelium; the identification of smooth muscle bundles (arrows) is key to recognizing small airways.

perivascular mononuclear cell infiltrate is not present, and sampling of the uninvolved perivascular areas should be recognized in the biopsies. Therefore, in a given situation, the diagnosis of LBB along with ACR should not be made in the same patient unless the lesions are separated by time or space. As mononuclear infiltrates are not specific, infections should be considered in the differential diagnosis. Biopsies preceding the LBB diagnosis demonstrated ACR in 20 of 26 cases. Follow-up of LBB demonstrated ACR, persistent LBB, OB, or its resolution (95). Thus outside the context of infections, the interpretation of this lesion includes (1) partially treated ACR with resolution of the perivascular but not the airway mononuclear component, (2) ACR where the perivascular infiltrate was not sampled, (3) active airway rejection with predisposition to develop OB, or (4) chronic airway inflammation of unknown significance (95,96). Once the allograft has developed OB and bronchiectasis, airway inflammation by persisting colonizing bacteria (e.g., *Pseudomonas* species) makes the distinction of immunological airway injury from infection difficult.

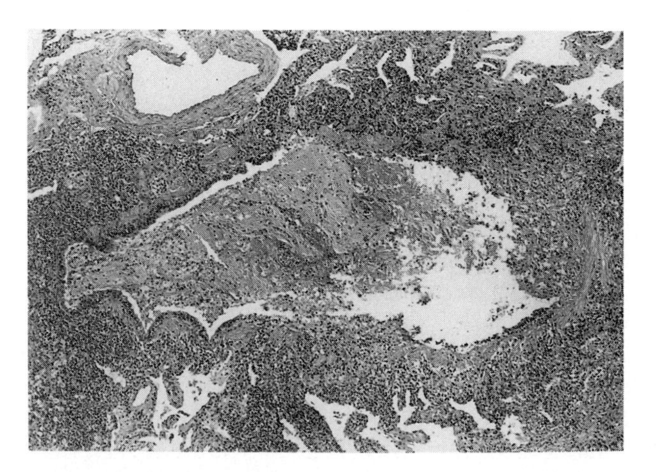

Figure 11 Very active lymphocytic bronchitis, which represented an airway rejection process.

The grading scheme for acute lung rejection by the Working Formulation has been examined in various studies (73,97–99). The issues addressed were the specificity of the diagnosis of acute cellular rejection and the correlation of the degree of perivascular infiltrates with clinical symptoms. Perivascular mononuclear infiltrates by themselves are not specific for acute cellular rejection, as they may be seen in 11 to 42% of CMV cases and 21% of *Pneumocystis* cases (73,99). However, provided that the sampling is adequate, other histological manifestations of that particular infection should be apparent in the biopsies. Cytomegalovirus infections manifest primarily as interstitial neutrophilic infiltrates, and the perivascular involvement is usually secondary and less frequent (99). Diagnostic CMV inclusions are sufficiently characteristic to warrant no further workup. In cases under suspicion, where the inclusion bodies are poorly formed, immunohistochemical stains or in situ hybridization for CMV may provide additional support. *Pneumocystis* penumonia is characterized by the frothy, granular, eosinophilic intraalveolar exudate. The organisms are readily identified on Grocott stains, which should be a routine workup in every lung transplant biopsy. The architectural patterns of mononuclear infiltrates are most specific for ACR when present in the mild to moderate grades. In this setting, the cellular components of the infiltrate are predominantly lymphocytic, plasmacytic, and mononuclear; the location of the infiltrates is primarily confined to perivascular, peribronchial/bronchiolar, and interstitial areas, with some spillage into the air spaces. Neutrophils, if present, would be very few. At the extremes of the spectrum, changes of minimal ACR (A1) overlap with other low-grade infectious, physical, and chemical injuries, which—regardless of cause—are probably not worth treating. Even if it were due to rejection, considering the degree of infiltrate, minimal ACR (A1) is of uncertain significance. Clinically, 61 to 72% of A1 patients were asymptomatic. Of these, 31 to 39% demonstrated persistent mononuclear cell infiltrates on follow-up biopsies, but only a small minority (4%) went on to develop OB. When symptomatic, approximately half responded to enhanced immunosuppression. Possibilities for interpretation would thus include (a) very low grade clinically symptomatic ACR, (2) very early and thus clinically asymptomatic ACR (precursor to a higher-grade lesion), and (3) very low grade clinically asymptomatic ACR which, if allowed to persist, would lead to chronic rejection (significant but indolent lesion) (83). Furthermore, as ACR is a patchy process with lesions developing at different stages, there is a possibility of a sampling problem with undetected higher grades of ACR. In an individual case, any of these possibilities may occur, although most commonly minimal ACR (A1) occurs in an asymptomatic, clinically stable patient and carries no significant risk of further lung injury.

At the other extreme, severe ACR (A4) poses a differential diagnostic problem due to the extensive and diffuse damage produced. The background histological change is similar to diffuse alveolar damage and there is no longer a specific localization of the mononuclear infiltrates to the perivascular and peribronchial/bronchiolar areas. Furthermore, the extensive damage attracts other inflammatory cell types, including large numbers of neutrophils and macrophages; moreover, the etiological possibilities are expanded to include ischemic, infectious, chemical, drug, and physical injuries.

Immunohistochemical analysis of lymphocytic mononuclear cell populations is generally not contributory to the diagnosis and classification of rejection. It may, however, serve in distinguishing rejection infiltrates from PTLD (predominantly a B-cell process). In general, a lymphoid population of greater than 25% B cells with greater than 30% large lymphoid cells favors PTLD over rejection (100). Immunohistochemical stain for EBV–latent membrane protein (LM) is also seen in much greater frequency in PTLD than ACR and may aid in this distinction. In practice, however, alternative procedures to TBB, such as fine needle aspiration (to obtain material from the center of the lesion) or a wedge lung biopsy may be necessary, especially when there is a clinical concern of more than one process. A larger tissue sampling provides an opportunity to study the architectural alterations, which would be helpful in distinguishing rejection from other processes.

C. Diagnosis of Chronic Rejection

From the pathologist's point of view, the diagnosis of bronchiolitis obliterans is probably the most challenging, especially on TBB. Small airway damage of varying degrees and different etiologies may be noted in the allograft. The diagnosis of OB in the lung transplant setting carries the connotation of chronic lung rejection, which is thought to be irreversible. If there is an active component to the OB process, some of the functional compromise may be ameliorated by enhanced immunosuppression, although residual functional deficit is almost inevitable. Therefore, in the transplant setting, the diagnostic term "OB" should be reserved for those instances when additional clinicopathological findings support a rejection process, as it may dictate therapy. When airway fibrosis is found in the context of another process (e.g., infectious organizing pneumonia, aspiration or cicatricial diffuse alveolar damage) qualifications should be made in the pathology report to indicate that the process is not due to rejection-related "OB." The biopsy findings should reflect irreversible small airway damage, and the criteria stated in the Working Formulation mention the identification of submucosal scarring that may be eccentric, concentric, or associated with total obliteration of the bronchiolar lumens (94). Specifically, the bronchioles contain submucosal plaques of dense eosinophilic collagen and are further qualified as to their total or subtotal occlusion and active or inactive cellular infiltrates.

Transbronchial biopsies have been very useful in the diagnosis of OB; their sensitivity for the diagnosis of OB is 87%, while their specificity is 99% (101). The histological lesion of OB may precede the decline in pulmonary function and the detection of an early lesion may provide the opportunity to treat the patient with enhanced immunosuppression to stabilize the rejection process. As mentioned above, the trichrome stain is particularly useful in identifying and assessing airway scarring. This special stain is also helpful in distinguishing the ingrowth of loose myxoid granulation tissue into the alveolar ducts and bronchioles from such processes as diffuse alveolar damage. At times, the biopsies show a partially scarred wall of an airway, which would not be conclusive of a diagnosis of OB. In cases with a high index of suspicion, a repeat TBB or wedge biopsy may demonstrate the diagnostic lesion (5,102). Upon identification, the lesion must be put in the appropriate context. Obstructive processes may be due to nonrejection processes (infection, aspiration, diffuse alveolar damage) or other forms of rejection (ACR, LB), and histological OB may be seen in those without functional deficits, underscoring the importance of clinical correlation (101).

With the progressive scarring and remodeling of the lung parenchyma due to OB, there is increasing difficulty in obtaining adequate TBBs; under such circumstances, it may not be possible to demonstrate OB by TBB alone. To increase the sensitivity of OB detection, a set of criteria using the results of pulmonary function testing was recently established by the International Society for Heart and Lung Transplantation (103). Using forced expiratory volume in 1 sec (FEV_1) as a major criterion, allograft recipients may be placed into mild to severe OB syndrome. The term "bronchiolitis obliterans syndrome" was defined as progressive obstructive functional deficit with or without histological demonstration of OB. As with histological OB, the use of the term "bronchiolitis obliterans syndrome" requires excluding other etiologies leading to small airway disease.

D. Diagnosis of Infection

In contrast to other solid organ transplants, the primary infections in the allograft itself is a relatively common occurrence in the lung transplant. Of the potentially life-threatening infections, 67% occurred in the lung or thoracic cavity (104). The diagnosis may be established by histopathological examination, BAL cytology, culture, or other techniques. As mentioned above, TBB is most sensitive and specific for diagnosing rejection. The detection of bacterial and fungal infections is relatively low by TBB unless florid pneumonic type infiltrates are seen. For this reason, BAL cultures are often performed simultaneously with biopsies to enhance the yield of diagnosing infections. The isolation of microorganisms must be taken in the appropriate context to determine its significance. For bacterial infections, high colony counts (greater than 100,000 colony forming units) are taken as significant and of the opportunistic bacteria; *Pseudomonas* species are particularly problematic in those patients with the primary diagnosis of cystic fibrosis, chronic obstructive pulmonary disease, or OB.

Common viral infections such as CMV and herpes simplex virus (HSV) may be detected on biopsies, cytology, or cultures. As in bacterial and fungal infections, histopathology is less sensitive than culture methods. Here also, positive culture results must be taken in context. While the identification of HSV by any means usually implies significant disease, the significance of finding CMV depends on the methodology used. Identification of CMV by histology or cytologic examination is considered most significant, while culture methods, especially the shell vial assay, although sensitive, are not specific. Additional methodologies such as in situ hybridization and the polymerase chain reaction (PCR) for detecting the viral genome provide alternative means for identifying microorganisms (105–107). The advantage of PCR lies in the rapid and earlier detection of viral infections; however, correlation between the results and clinical manifestations is required to arrive at their significance.

E. Additional Modalities of Allograft Assessment

While biopsies offer an opportunity to assess the architectural alterations, they do not provide the optimal means for studying the cell type and function of the infiltrating cellular population. In this regard, the primed lymphocyte test (PLT) and cell-mediated lympholysis (CML) on lymphocytes obtained by BAL provide a means to investigate cellular mechanisms (108–114). Growth of donor antigen–specific lymphocytes may be seen in impending or ongoing ACR, active OB, and with pneumocystis and CMV infections (115–117). Although the PLT response correlates with disease activity, its use as a distinctive indicator of rejection has been challenged as there is much overlap with episodes of infection (114). However, in the setting of known or suspected rejection, PLT reactivity demonstrating a $CD4^{+}$ population with class II antigen specificity correlates with ACR, while a $CD8^{+}$ population specific for class I antigen correlates with active OB. This and other related techniques will undoubtedly provide further insights into the cellular events of allograft rejection.

Currently, the histopathological assessment of TBB and wedge lung biopsies with BAL material are the mainstay for assessing the posttransplant course of allograft recipients, especially vis-à-vis rejection. Nevertheless, it is important to realize the limitations of histopathological analysis and to continue to test alternative methodologies in order to enhance diagnostic precision.

REFERENCES

1. Fragomeni LS, Kaye MP. The registry of the international society of heart transplantation: Fifth official report—1988. J Heart Transplant 1988; 7:249.
2. Hutter JA, Despins P, Higenbottam T, et al. Heart-lung transplantation: Better use of resources. Am J Med 1988; 85:4–11.
3. Yousem SA, Burke CM, Billingham ME. Pathologic pulmonary alterations in long-term human heart-lung transplantation. Hum Pathol 1985; 16:911–923.
4. Zenati M, Yousem SA, Dowling RD, et al. Primary graft failure following pulmonary transplantation. Transplantation 1990; 50:165–167.
5. Yousem SA, Duncan SR, Griffith BP. Interstitial and airspace granulation tissue reactions in lung transplant recipients. Am J Surg Pathol 1992; 16:877–884.
6. Ohori NP, Iacono AT, Grgurich WF, Yousem SA. Significance of acute bronchitis/bronchiolitis in the lung transplant recipient. Lab Invest 1994; 79:153A.
7. Zenati M, Dowling RD, Dummer JS, et al. Influence of the donor lung on development of early infections in lung transplant recipients. J Heart Transplant 1990; 9:502–509.
8. Rosendale BE, Keenan RJ, Duncan SR, et al. Donor cerebral emboli as a cause of acute graft dysfunction in lung transplantation. J Heart Lung Transplant 1992; 11:72
9. Prop JM, Ehrie MG, Carpo JD, et al. Reimplantation response in isografted rat lungs. J Thorac Cardiovasc Surg 1984; 87:702–711.
10. Hardy JD, Webb WR, Dalton ML Jr, et al. Lung homotransplantation in man. JAMA 1963; 186:1065–1074.
11. Deffebach ME, Charan NB, Lakshminarayan S, Butler J. The bronchial circulation: Small, but a vital attribute of the lung. Am Rev Respir Dis 1987; 135:463–468.
12. Griffith BP, Hardesty RL, Trento A, et al. Heart-lung transplantation: Lessons learned and future hopes. Ann Thorac Surg 1987; 43:6–16.
13. Morgan E, Lima O, Goldberg M, et al. Successful revascularization of totally ischemic bronchial autografts with omental pedicle flaps in dogs. J Thorac Cardiovasc Surg 2982; 84:204–210.
14. Novick RJ, Ahmad D, Menkis AH, et al. The importance of acquired diffuse bronchomalacia in heart-lung transplant recipients with obliterative bronchiolitis. J Thorac Cardiovasc Surg 1991; 101:643–648.
15. Yousem SA, Dauber JH, Griffith BP. Bronchial cartilage alterations in lung transplantation. Chest 1990; 98:1121–1124.
16. Frost AE, Keller CA, Cagle PT. The Multi-Organ Transplant Group. Severe ischemic injury to the proximal airway following lung transplantation. Chest 1993; 103:1899–1901.
17. Griffith BP, Paradis IL, Zeevi A, et al. Immunologically mediated disease of the airways after pulmonary transplantation. Ann Surg 1988; 208:371–378.
18. Tavakoli R, Devaux TY, Nonmenmacher L, et al. Xenogeneic hyperacute rejection in the lung in rats. Chirurgie 1990; 116:684–689.
19. Demetris AJ, Jaffe R, Tzakis A, et al. Antibody-mediated rejection of human orthotopic liver allografts. Am J Pathol 1988; 132:489–502.
20. Veith FJ, Sinha SBP, Daughtery JC, et al. Nature and evolution of lung allograft rejection with and without immunosuppression. J Thorac Cardiovasc Surg 1972; 63:509.
21. Veith FJ, Koerner SK, Siegelman SS, et al. Diagnosis and reversal of rejection in experimental and clinical lung allografts. Ann Thorac Surg 1973; 16:172.

22. Hruban RH, Beschorner WE, Baumgartner WA, et al. Depletion of bronchus-associated lymphoid tissue associated with lung allograft rejection. Am J Pathol 1988; 132:6–11.
23. Spits H, Yassel H, Thompson A, de Vries JE. Human T4+ and T8+ cytotoxic T lymphocyte clones directed at products of different class II major histocompatibility complex loci. J Immunol 1983; 131:678.
24. Meuer SC, Schlossman SF, Reinherz EL. Clonal analysis of human cytotoxic T lymphocytes: T4 and T8+ effector T cells recognize products of different major histocompatibility complex regions. Proc Natl Acad Sci USA 1982; 79:4395.
25. Yousem SA, Curley JM, Dauber J, et al. HLA-class II antigen expression in human heart-lung allografts. Transplantation 1990; 49:991–995.
26. Veith F, Sinha S, Blumcke S, et al. Nature and evolution of lung allograft rejection with and without immunosuppression. J Thorac Cardiovasc Surg 1972; 63:509.
27. Halasz NA, Catanzaro A, Trummer MJ, et al. Transplantation of the lung: Correlation of physiologic, immunologic, and histologic findings. J Thorac Cardiovasc Surg 1973; 66: 581–587.
28. Prop J, Wildevuur CRH, Nieuwenhuis P. Lung allograft rejection in the rat: Specific immunologic properties of lung grafts. Transplantation 1985; 40:126–131.
29. Prop J, Wildevuur CRH, Nieuwenhuis P. Lung allograft rejection in the rat: Corresponding morphologic rejection phases in various rat strain combinations. Transplantation 1985; 40:132–136.
30. Romaniuk A, Prop J, Petersen AH, et al. Expression of class II major histocompatibility complex antigens by bronchial epithelium in rat lung allografts. Transplantation 1987; 44: 209–214.
31. Pober JS, Collins T, Gimbrone MA Jr, et al. Inducible expression of class II major histocompatibility complex antigens and the immunogenicity of vascular endothelium. Transplantation 1986; 41:141–146.
32. Glanville AR, Tazelaar HD, Theodore J, et al. The distribution of MHC class I and II antigens on bronchial epithelium. Am Rev Respir Dis 1989; 139:330–334.
33. Hruban RH, Beschorner WE, Baumgartner WA, et al. Evidence that the expression of class II MHC antigens is not diagnostic of lung allograft rejection. Transplantation 1989; 48:529–530.
34. Steeg PS, Sztein MB, Mann DL, et al. Interferon regulation of DR antigen expression and alloantigen-presenting capabilities of the promyelocytic cell line HL60. Scand J Immunol 1985; 21:425.
35. Wong GHW, Clark-Lewis I, McKimm-Breschkin JL, et al. Interferon-gamma induces enhanced expression of Ia and H-2 antigens on B lymphoid, macrophage, and myeloid cell lines. J Immunol 1983; 131:788.
36. De Blic J, Peuchmaur M, Carnot F, et al. Rejection in lung transplantation—An immunohistochemical study of transbronchial biopsies. Transplantation 1992; 54:639–644.
37. Martin T, Yousem SA. Can immunohistochemical studies of graft infiltrating cells predict steroid responsiveness in moderate acute cellular rejection in lung allograft recipients? Lab Invest 1994; 70:152A.
38. Yousem SA, Sonmez-Alpan E. Use of a biotinylated DNA probe specific for the human Y chromosome in the evaluation of the allograft lung. Chest 1991; 99:275–279.
39. Yamamoto R, Kinoshita H, Kinoshita Y, et al. Immunohistochemical aspects of acute rejection of the allografted rat lung. Transplantation 1990; 49:631–632.
40. Kamholz S, Roslin M, Mondragon M, et al. IL-2 activated killer cell activity is associated with the early phase of allograft rejection. Transplant Proc 1991; 23:597–598.
41. Lawrence EC, Holland VA, Young JB, et al. Dynamic changes in soluble interleukin-2 receptor levels after lung or heart-lung transplantation. Am Rev Respir Dis 1989; 140:789–796.
42. Hruban RH, Beschorner WE, Baumgartner WA, et al. Diagnosis of lung allograft rejection by bronchial intraepithelial Leu-7 positive T lymphocytes. J Thorac Cardiovasc Surg 1988; 96:939–946.

43. Yousem SA, Duncan SR, Ohori NP, Sonmez-Alpan E. Architectural remodeling of lung allografts in acute and chronic rejection. Arch Pathol Lab Med 1992; 116:1175–1180.
44. Paradis I, Rabinowich H, Zeevi A, et al. Life in the allogeneic environment after lung transplantation. Lung 1990; (suppl):1172–1181.
45. Starnes VA, Theodore J, Oyer PE, et al. Evaluation of heart-lung transplant recipients with prospective serial transbronchial biopsies and pulmonary function studies. J Thorac Cardiovascular Surg 1989; 98:683–695.
46. Starnes VA, Theodore J, Oyer PE, et al. Pulmonary infiltrates after heart-lung transplantation: Evaluation by serial transbronchial biopsies. J Thorac Cardiovasc Surg 1989; 98:945–950.
47. Yousem SA, Paradis IL, Dauber JH, et al. Pulmonary arteriosclerosis in long-term human heart-lung transplant recipients. Transplantation 1989; 47:564–569.
48. Clelland C, Higenbottam T, Otulana B, et al. Histologic prognostic indicators for the lung allografts of heart-lung transplants. J Heart Transplant 1990; 9:177–186.
49. Bando K, Paradis IL, Konishi H, et al. Obliterative bronchiolitis after lung and heart-lung transplantation: An analysis of risk factors and management. In press.
50. Yousem SA, Dauber JA, Keenan R, et al. Does histologic acute rejection in lung allografts predict the development of bronchiolitis obliterans? Transplantation 1991; 52:306–309.
51. Tazelaar HD, Yousem SA. The pathology of combined heart-lung transplantation: An autopsy study. Hum Pathol 1988; 19:1403–1416.
52. Holland V, Cagle PT, Windsor NT, et al. Lymphocyte subset populations in bronchiolitis obliterans after heart-lung transplantation. Transplantation 1990; 50:955–959.
53. Taylor PM, Rose ML, Yacoub MH. Expression of MHC antigen in normal human lung and transplanted lungs with obliterative bronchiolitis. Transplantation 1989; 48:506–510.
54. Scott JP, Higenbottam TW, Sharples L, et al. Risk factors for obliterative bronchiolitis in heart-lung transplant recipients. Transplantation 1991; 51:813–817.
55. Yousem SA. Small airway injury in heart-lung transplant recipients. Semin Respir Med 1992; 13:85–93.
56. Burke C, Theodore J, Dawkins KD, et al. Post-transplant obliterative bronchiolitis and other late lung sequelae in human heart-lung transplantation. Chest 1986; 6:824–829.
57. Abernathy EC, Hruban RH, Baumgartner WA, et al. The two forms of bronchiolitis obliterans in heart-lung transplant recipients. Hum Pathol 1991; 22:1102–1110.
58. Rose EA, Smith CR, Petrossian GA, et al. Humoral immune response after cardiac transplantation: Correlation with fatal rejection and graft atherosclerosis. 1989; 106:203–208.
59. Rose EA, Pepino P, Barr ML, et al. Relation of HLA antibodies and graft atherosclerosis in human cardiac allograft recipients. J Heart Lung Transplant 1992; 11:S120–S123.
60. Hammond EH, Yowell RL, Nunoda S, et al. Vascular (humoral) rejection in heart transplantation: Pathologic observations and clinical implications. J Heart Transplant 1989; 8:430–443.
61. Hruban RH, Beschorner WE, Baumgartner WA, et al. Accelerated arteriosclerosis in heart transplant recipients: An immunopathology study of 22 transplanted hearts. Transplant Proc 1991; 23:1230–1232.
62. Hruban RH, Beschorner WE, Baumgartner WA, et al. Accelerated arteriosclerosis in heart transplant recipients is associated with a T-lymphocyte-mediated endothelialitis. Am J Pathol 1990; 137:871–882.
63. Gaudin PB, Rayburn BK, Hutchins GM, et al. Peritransplant injury to the myocardium associated with the development of accelerated arteriosclerosis in heart transplant recipients. Am J Surg Pathol 1994; 18:338–346.
64. Dresdale AR, Kraft PL, Paone G, et al. Reduced incidence and severity of accelerated graft atherosclerosis in cardiac transplant recipients treated with prophylactic antilymphocyte globulin. J Cardiovasc Surg (Torino) 1992: 33:746–753.
65. Wu T-C, Hruban RH, Ambinder RF, et al. Demonstration of cytomegalovirus nucleic acids in the coronary arteries of transplanted heart. Am J Pathol 1992; 140:739–747.

66. Foerster A, Abdelnoor M, Geiran O, et al. Morbidity risk factors in human cardiac transplantation: Histocompatibility and protracted graft ischemia entail high risk of rejection and infection. Scand J Thorac Cardiovasc Surg 1992; 26:169–176.
67. Goodman ZD, Boitnott JK, Yardley JH. Perforation of the colon associated with cytomegalovirus infection. Dig Dis Sci 1979; 24:376–380.
68. von Willebrand E, Pettersson E, Ahonen J, Hayry P. CMV infection, class II antigen expression and human kidney allograft rejection. Transplantation 1986; 42:364–367.
69. Etingin OR, Silverstein RL, Friedman HM, Hajjar DP. Viral activation of the coagulation cascade: Molecular interactions at the surface of infected endothelial cells. Cell 1990; 61: 657–662.
70. Hajjar DP, Fabricant CG, Minick CR, Fabricant J. Virus-induced atherosclerosis: Herpesvirus infection alters aortic cholesterol metabolism and accumulation. Am J Pathol 1986; 122: 62–70.
71. Duncan AJ, Dummer JS, Paradis IL, et al. Cytomegalovirus infection and survival in lung transplant recipients. J Heart Transplant. In press.
72. Smyth RL, Sinclair J, Scott JP, et al. Infection and reactivation with cytomegalovirus strains in lung transplant recipients. Transplantation 1991; 52:480–482.
73. Tazelaar HD. Perivascular inflammation in pulmonary infections: Implications for the diagnosis of lung rejection. J Heart Lung Transplant 1991; 10:437–441.
74. Smyth RL, Higenbottam TW, Scott JP, et al. Herpes simplex virus infection in heart-lung transplant recipients. Transplantation 1990; 49:735–739.
75. Becroft DMO. Histopathology of fatal adenovirus infection of the respiratory tract in young children. J Clin Pathol 1967; 20:561–569.
76. Thurlbeck WM, ed. Pathology of the lung. Am J Med 1980; 68:725–732.
77. Solans E, Yeldandi V, Garrity E, et al. Patterns of aspergillus infection in lung transplant. Lab Invest 1994; 70:155A.
78. Randhawa PS, Yousem SA, Paradis IL, et al. The clinical spectrum, pathology, and clonal analysis of Epstein-Barr virus-associated lymphoproliferative disorders in heart-lung transplant recipients. Am J Clin Pathol 1989; 92:177–185.
79. Cleary ML, Warnke R, Sklar J. Monoclonality of lymphoproliferative lesions in cardiac transplant recipients: Clinical analysis based on immunoglobulin gene rearrangements. N Engl J Med 1984; 30:477–482.
80. Hanto DW, Sakamoto K, Purtilo DT, et al. The Epstein-Barr virus in the pathogenesis of post-transplant lymphoproliferative disorders. Surgery 1981; 90:204–213.
81. Shapiro RS, McClain K, Blazar B, et al. EBV related B-cell lymphoproliferative disease after T depleted mismatched bone marrow transplantation. In: Levine PH, Ablashi DV, Nanoyama M, et al., eds. Epstein-Barr Virus and Human Disease. Clifton, NJ: Humana Press, 1987; 91–95.
82. Starzl TE, Nalesnik MA, Porter KA, et al. Reversibility of lymphomas and lymphoproliferative lesions developing under cyclosporine steroid therapy. Lancet 1984; 1:584–587.
83. Yousem, SA, Randhawa P, Locker J, et al. Post-transplant lymphoproliferative disorders in heart-lung transplant recipients: Primary presentation in the allograft. Hum Pathol 1989; 20:361–369.
84. Nalesnik MA, Jaffe R, Starzl TE, et al. The pathology of post-transplant lymphoproliferative disorders occurring in the setting of cyclosporine A-prednisone immunosuppression. Am J Pathol 1988; 133:173–192.
85. Abu-Farsakh H, Cagle PT, Buffone GJ, et al. Heart allograft involvement with Epstein-Barr virus-associated post-transplant lymphoproliferative disorder. Arch Pathol Lab Med 1992; 116:93–95.
86. Cohen JI. Epstein-Barr virus lymphoproliferative disease associated with acquired immunodeficiency. Medicine 1991; 70:137–160.

87. Fischer A, Blanche S, Le Bidois J, et al. Anti-B-cell monoclonal antibodies in the treatment of severe B-cell lymphoproliferative syndrome following bone marrow and organ transplantation. N Engl J Med 1991; 324:1451–1456.
88. Stewart S. Pathology of lung transplantation. Semin Diag Pathol 1992; 9:210–213.
89. Johnson BA, Duncan DR, Ohori NP, et al. Recurrence of sarcoidosis in pulmonary allograft recipients. Am Rev Respir Dis 1993; 148:1373–1377.
90. Nine JS, Ohori NP, Yousem SA. Recurrence of original disease in lung allografts. Lab Invest 1994; 70:153A.
91. Frost AE, Kellar CA, Brown RW, et al. Single lung transplantation for giant cell interstitial pneumonitis: Recurrence of original disease in the transplanted lung. In press.
92. Barberis M, Harari S, Tironi A, Lampertico P. Recurrence of primary disease in a single lung transplant recipient. Transplant Proc 1992; 24:2660–2662.
93. Higenbottam T, Stewart S, Penketh A, Wallwork J. Transbronchial lung biopsy for the diagnosis of rejection in heart-lung transplant patients. Transplantation 1988; 46:532–539.
94. Yousem SA, Berry GJ, Brunt EM, et al. A working formulation of the standardization of nomenclature in the diagnosis of heart and lung rejection: Lung rejection study group. J Heart Lung Transplant 1990; 9:593–601.
95. Yousem SA. Lymphocytic bronchitis/bronchiolitis in lung allograft recipients. Am J Surg Pathol 1993; 17:491–496.
96. Yousem SA, Paradis IL, Dauber JA, et al. Large airway inflammation in heart-lung transplant recipients—Its significance and prognostic implications. Transplantation 1990; 49:654–656.
97. Sibley RK, Berry GJ, Tazelaar HD, et al. The role of transbronchial biopsies in the management of lung transplant recipients. J Heart Lung Transplant 1993; 12:308–324.
98. DeHoyos A, Chamberlain D, Schvartzman R, et al. Prospective assessment of a standardized pathologic grading system for acute rejection in lung transplantation. Chest 1993; 103:1813–1818.
99. Nakhleh RE, Bolman RM, Henke CA, Hertz MI. Lung transplant pathology: A comparative study of pulmonary acute rejection and cytomegalovirus infection. Am J Surg Pathol 1991; 15:1197–1201.
100. Rosendale B, Yousem SA. Discrimination of EBV related post-transplant lymphoproliferations (PTLD) from acute rejection in lung allograft recipients. Lab Invest 1994; 70:154A.
101. Yousem SA. Can transbronchial biopsy aid in the diagnosis of bronchiolitis obliterans in lung transplant recipients? Transplantation 1994; 57:151–153.
102. Cagle PT, Brown RW, Yousem SA. Diagnosis of chronic lung transplant rejection by transbronchial biopsy. Lab Invest 1993; 68:129A.
103. Cooper JD, Billingham M, Egan T, et al. A working formulation for the standardization of nomenclature and for clinical staging of chronic dysfunction in lung allografts. J Heart Lung Transplant 1993; 12:713–716.
104. Dummer JS, Montero CG, Griffith BP, et al. Infections in heart-lung transplant recipients. Transplantation 1986; 41:725–729.
105. Weiss LM, Movahed LA, Berry GJ, et al. In situ hybridization studies for viral nuclei acids in heart and lung allograft biopsies. Am J Clin Pathol 1990; 93:675–679.
106. Niedobitek G, Finn T, Herbst H, et al. Detection of cytomegalovirus by in-situ hybridization and histochemistry using a monoclonal antibody CCH2: A comparison of methods. J Clin Pathol 198; 41:1005–1009.
107. Buffone GJ, Frost A, Samo T, et al. The diagnosis of CMV pneumonitis in lung and heart/lung transplant patients by PCR compared with traditional laboratory criteria. Transplantation 1993; 6:342–347.
108. Rabinowich H, Zeevi A, Yousem SA, et al. Alloreactivity of lung biopsy and bronchoalveolar lavage-derived lymphocytes from pulmonary transplant patients: Correlation with acute rejection and bronchiolitis obliterans. Clin Transplant 1990; 4:376.

109. Paradis IL, Marrari M, Zeevi A, et al. HLA phenotype of lung lavage cells following heart-lung transplantation. Heart Transplant 1985; 4:422.
110. Zeevi A, Fung JJ, Paradis IL, et al. Lymphocytes of bronchoalveolar lavages from heart-lung transplant recipients. Heart Transplant 1985; 4:417.
111. Fung JJ, Zeevi A, Kaufman C, et al. Interactions between bronchoalveolar lymphocytes and macrophages in heart-lung transplant recipients. Hum Immunol 1985; 14:287.
112. Rabinowich H, Zeevi A, Paradis IL, et al. Proliferative response of bronchoalveolar lavage lymphocytes from heart-lung transplant patients. Transplantation 1990; 49:115.
113. Zeevi A, Keenan R, Duquesnoy RJ. Lung transplantation bronchoalveolar lavage diagnosis of lung rejection. Crit Care Rev 1991; 2:228.
114. Reinsmoen NL, Boman RM, Savik K, et al. Differentiation of class I- and class II-directed donor-specific alloreactivity in bronchoalveolar lavage lymphocytes from lung transplant recipients. Transplantation 1992; 53:181–189.
115. Zeevi A, Fung JJ, Paradis IL. Bronchoalveolar macrophage lymphocyte reactivity in heart-lung transplant recipients. Transplant Proc 1987; 19:2537.
116. Zeevi A, Rabinowich H, Paradis IL, et al. Lymphocyte activation in bronchoalveolar lavages from heart-lung transplant recipients. Transplant Proc 1988; 20:189.
117. Zeevi A, Uknis ME, Spichty KJ, et al. Proliferation of cytomegalovirus-primed lymphocytes in bronchoalveolar lavages from lung transplant patients. Transplantation 1992; 54:635–639.

8

Pathology of Liver Transplantation

Dale Craig Snover
University of Minnesota Medical School, Minneapolis, Minnesota

As with all solid organ allografts, rejection of the liver may be manifest as hyperacute, acute, or chronic rejection. Hyperacute rejection is a rare and uncommonly encountered practical issue. It is diagnosed by a combination of clinical, immunological, and histological parameters. Histological features are integral to the diagnosis. Acute and chronic rejection are much more common and practical problems. Acute rejection occurs in from 50 to 80% of liver allografts. The diagnosis of acute rejection relies heavily on the biopsy, and the role of clinical assessment in diagnosis has been somewhat controversial. Chronic rejection continues to be a considerable problem, occurring in approximately 6 to 16% of grafts. Significant issues exist in the definition of this entity (if it is a single entity) and in meaningful diagnosis. Biopsy is rarely diagnostic of chronic rejection, although histology is an important adjunct to diagnosis in conjunction with clinical features.

Interpretation of the biopsies from liver allografts requires consideration of the full range of possible problems that can arise in this setting. These include technical, infectious, and drug-induced diseases and recurrence of the original disease as well as rejection. These processes tend to occur at characteristic times following transplantation, as illustrated in Table 1. Although this chapter deals mainly with the pathology of rejection, these other possible diagnoses are discussed, as they are relevant to the differential diagnosis of rejection.

I. HYPERACUTE (HUMORALLY MEDIATED) REJECTION

Hyperacute rejection is defined as rejection resulting from preformed antidonor antibodies—antibodies that are usually directed at vascular elements of the graft and hence cause arteritis ad extensive ischemic damage to the affected organ. There has been some debate about the terminology of "hyperacute rejection" and its distinction from "accelerated acute rejection." The term "hyperacute" implies a very rapid onset of dysfunction and organ failure, as seen in the hyperacutely rejected kidney. Such extremely rapid failure is not typical of this process in the liver, perhaps due to its size and reserve capacity. Therefore another term may be preferable. However, the term "accelerated acute" rejection would imply to this author rejection with a mechanism similar to that of typical acute rejection and

Table 1 Differential Diagnosis of Liver Dysfunction following Liver Transplantation

Time period	Common diagnoses	Less likely diagnoses
First week	Technical problems (especially vascular anastomoses) Acute rejection Primary graft failure	Hyperacute rejection Drug reactions Opportunistic infections
1 week to 2 months	Acute rejection Opportunistic infections Drug reactions Technical problems (especially biliary anastomosis)	Chronic vascular rejection Vanishing bile duct syndrome
2 months and beyond	Chronic vascular rejection Vanishing bile duct syndrome Recurrence of original disease Transfusion-related viral infections (hepatitis B or C)	Acute rejection Drug reaction Opportunistic infection Technical problems

Source: From Ref. 56.

hence may be misleading as well. Certainly the term "humorally mediated" rejection defines the process. However, there may well be a component of humorally mediated rejection in severe acute rejection and even in chronic rejection. Therefore, although the term "hyperacute rejection" is flawed, it seems a reasonable and generally understood one that acts as a reasonable shorthand for this process.

Absolute identification of hyperacute rejection requires the identification of antibodies in the blood of the recipient which are directed at antigens known to be expressed on cells of the donor organ, or observation of these antibodies in the damaged donated organ, with evidence of arteritis and ischemic damage to the organ as a result of this immunoglobulin and complement deposition. The fact that in some experimental models of hyperacute rejection the defining feature (i.e. deposition of immunoglobulin and complement in the graft) is lost after a few hours indicates that a problem may exist in diagnosis even if frozen tissue is available for analysis (1). The pathology of hyperacute rejection has not been the subject of extensive study in the human liver, in large part because of the rarity of the phenomenon and because of difficulty in its clinical distinction from other causes of liver failure in the immediate posttransplant period, in particular so-called primary graft failure. Although it was originally reported that transplantation of the liver in the face of preformed antibodies or across the ABO barrier did not result in hyperacute rejection or excessive loss of grafts, more recent data indicate that there is decreased survival for such patients (2,3). In addition, there are now several reports of hyperacute rejection associated with preformed anti-HLA antibodies (4–6). It has been suggested that at least some of the cases reported in the literature as primary graft failure are likely manifestations of hyperacute rejection in which the immunological nature of the lesion has not been recognized. Since the liver is a vital organ and cannot be removed as soon as it starts failing, as the transplanted kidney can, livers with hyperacute rejection are more likely to reach an uninterpretable stage of necrosis prior to death of the patient or retransplantation, masking the usual histopathological correlates of arteritis and a neutrophilic infiltrate.

In the first human case of hyperacute rejection reported in a patient with preformed anti-HLA antibodies, biopsy taken 30 min after anastomosis of the organ showed focal neutrophilic infiltration around the central veins associated with fibrin deposition (4). These changes were initially interpreted as preservation effect but, in retrospect, probably represented the earliest manifestation of the hyperacute rejection that was to follow. Biopsy at 5 days, during which time the organ never functioned well, showed arteritis and an intense portal tract neutrophilic infiltrate, along with extensive ischemic lobular necrosis (Fig. 1). At the time of autopsy there was extensive necrosis with superimposed acute rejection, since prophylactic immunosuppression was discontinued. Several similar cases have subsequently been reported (5,6). In some primate model systems of hyperacute rejection, there has been more apparent hemorrhage with little inflammation and no mention of arteritis (7,8). Interestingly, some series of primary graft failure with similar hemorrhagic features have been reported in humans, although it has been claimed that these cases are unlikely to represent hyperacute rejection (9).

As a practical matter, hyperacute rejection should be considered in any graft with early severe dysfunction, and a portion of any biopsy in this setting ideally should be snap-frozen for immunofluorescence studies, although the latter is not a necessity and, as implied above, may not be sufficient to rule out hyperacute rejection. If a biopsy shows a heavy neutrophilic portal infiltrate, the differential diagnosis will include obstructive biliary tract disease and sepsis. The presence of arteritis and/or ischemic necrosis would militate against either of these diagnoses. The clinical features, laboratory findings, and radiologic findings would also not support biliary obstruction. Necrosis and hemorrhage may also be caused by ischemia related to thrombosis or stricture of the arterial anastomosis. This problem may have to be assessed radiologically, although on biopsy purely technical ischemia will not in general result in the type of portal infiltrate typically seen in hyperacute rejection. However, if hyperacute rejection manifests without this portal infiltrate (as suggested by some of the animal models), the distinction from other causes of ischemia will require radiological examination.

II. ACUTE (CELLULAR) REJECTION

Acute rejection is usually defined as a predominantly cell-mediated form of rejection that is often reversible with increased immunosuppression. Time considerations do not enter into the definition of this process, since on occasion reversible cellular rejection can occur years after transplantation, especially in noncompliant patients who discontinue their immunosuppression. In general, however, acute rejection occurs in the first few months following transplantation. Obviously the above definition is a clinically and histologically imprecise one, since the inclusion of reversibility implies that the diagnosis can be made only after immunosuppression halts the process (i.e., technically speaking, one cannot lose the graft or die of acute rejection if it is truly reversible). Such semantic issues aside, there is general consensus on the occurrence and diagnosis of this process.

Acute rejection is the most common consideration in biopsy diagnosis of the liver transplant patient, especially in the period from about 2 weeks until several months following transplantation. Interpretation of the liver biopsy with possible acute rejection will depend on the clinical context of the case and in particular the reason the biopsy was taken. Biopsies in which acute rejection may be seen may be obtained because of clinical manifestations of rejection or may be detected using a protocol biopsy—i.e., biopsy taken at a prespecified interval regardless of the clinical status of the patient. A biopsy taken to ascertain the cause of liver dysfunction can be viewed to a certain degree as a biopsy taken

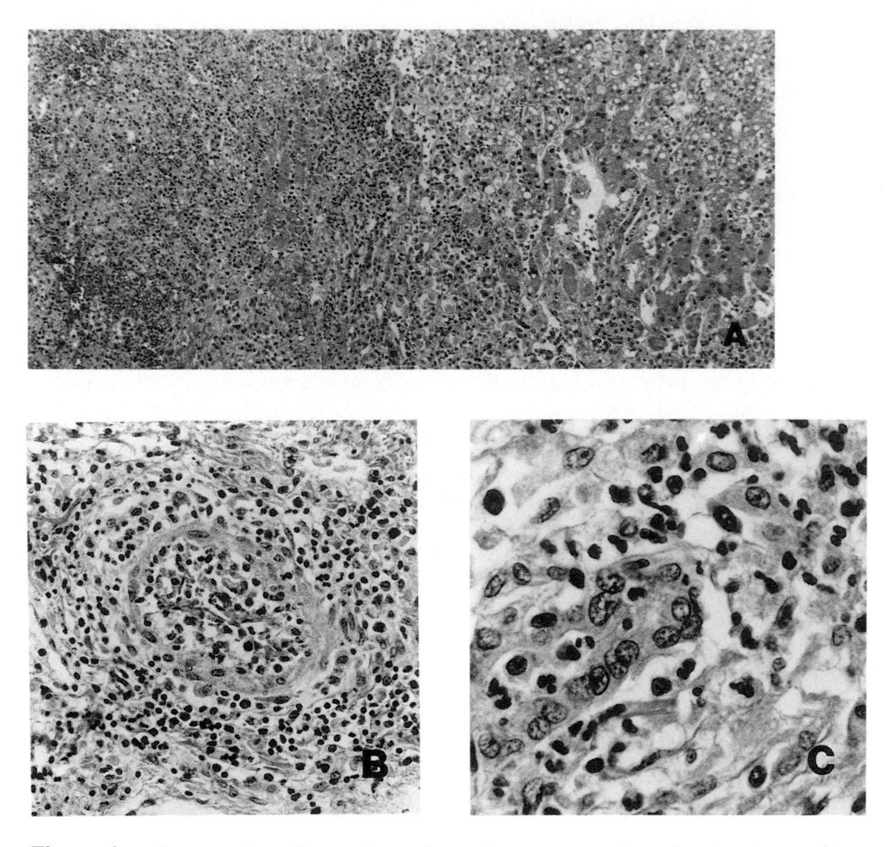

Figure 1 Biopsy at day 5 in a patient who underwent transplantation despite a positive crossmatch. A. Confluent ischemic necrosis is evident in the left part of the field. (Hematoxylin and eosin, ×100.) B. Portal tract showing occlusive arteritis and a dense predominately polymorphonuclear infiltrate. (Hematoxylin and eosin, ×190.) C. Bile duct showing intraepithelial lymphocytes and intraluminal PMNs. Note the surrounding polymorphonuclear infiltrate. (Hematoxylin and eosin, ×480.) (From Ref. 60.)

to rule out causes of liver disease other than rejection, for which rejection therapy would be contraindicated. As such, it may be appropriate to treat a patient as if he or she had rejection even if the biopsy is not considered diagnostic but only consistent with rejection. On the other hand, the protocol biopsy is used to predict that the patient will develop liver dysfunction if not treated and as such should be called rejection only if there is a high degree of certainty of the diagnosis. Therefore, in order to avoid unnecessary administration of immunosuppressive agents to patients with no need for them, rejection in this setting should be diagnosed only by using the most stringent of criteria. As a rule of thumb, if you are at an institution that utilizes the protocol biopsy and cases where biopsies diagnosed as rejection frequently resolve spontaneously without augmented immunosuppression, the diagnostic criteria being used are probably too liberal and should be reconsidered.

The histological diagnostic features of acute rejection are generally considered well defined and relatively reproducible (10–14). The diagnostic triad used by most centers includes a portal infiltrate, usually composed of lymphocytes and eosinophils with some neutrophils but no or few plasma cells; evidence of damage to interlobular bile ducts; and inflammation and damage to the endothelium of venous structures (endothelialitis or endotheliitis). Although in principle the application of these diagnostic criteria seems simple, in practice there are considerable problems in some cases. A prototypical case in which all three elements are present in abundance (Fig. 2) should cause no diagnostic problems, will usually be accompanied by some evidence of liver dysfunction, and should in general be treated. Problems in diagnosis arise in four areas: (1) the definition of bile duct damage, (2) the extent of bile duct damage considered necessary to allow a diagnosis of rejection, (3) the recognition and definition of endothelialitis, and (4) the diagnostic significance of a biopsy without all three elements of the triad.

The definition of bile duct damage is not straightforward and the fine details have not been well studied. A "normal" interlobular bile duct generally accompanies an arteriole of

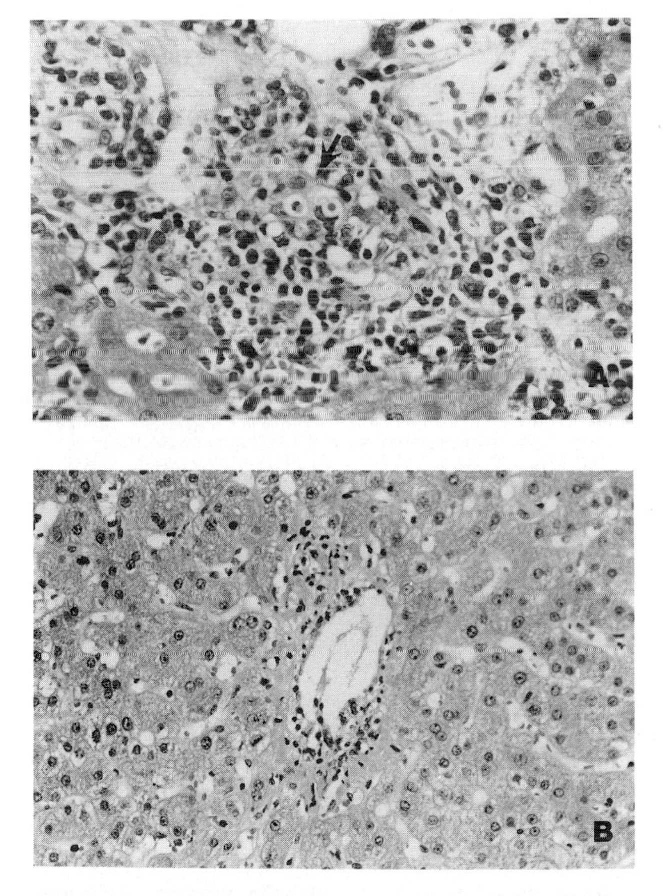

Figure 2 Acute (cellular) rejection. A. Portal tract showing an inflammatory infiltrate composed mainly of lymphocytes with lesser numbers of eosinophils and neutrophils. Near the center of the tract there is a bile duct (arrow) with cytoplasmic vacuolation, nuclear variability, an irregular margin, and infiltration by lymphocytes, features of rejection damage. (Hematoxylin and eosin, ×240.) B. The central vein shows damage to the endothelium with elevation and an infiltrate of lymphocytes (endothelialitis). (Hematoxylin and eosin, ×240.)

similar size (15). When cut in cross section, it is round, with a uniform distribution of nonoverlapping nuclei, and has a clear-cut lumen. The nuclei are round to slightly oval with evenly distributed chromatin without apparent nucleoli. In occasional otherwise normal ducts there will be an apparent missing nucleus, which should cause no alarm. The cytoplasm of normal bile duct cells is usually moderate in amount and mildly eosinophilic. When damaged in rejection, the bile ducts usually have some vacuolation of their cytoplasm, with overlapping and/or missing nuclei. There may be pseudostratification, although this is not common. Often the nuclei are enlarged, with a vesicular appearance. Nucleoli may be prominent and occasional mitoses may be seen. Since there is an infiltrate associated with this damage, there are usually lymphocytes and even neutrophils in the walls of the ducts as well as occasionally in the lumen. It is important to note that the presence of neutrophils in the lumen does not constitute sufficient grounds for a diagnosis of ascending cholangitis in this setting.

Using this definition of damage, one will encounter damaged ducts in a large number of inflammatory diseases of the liver. Such damage is well recognized in viral infections (particularly hepatitis C), primary biliary cirrhosis, primary sclerosing cholangitis, autoimmune hepatitis, and some drug reactions; occasional lesions indistinguishable from damaged ducts may be seen in many conditions and hence certainly are of no diagnostic value. How, then, does one determine whether duct damage is "significant" or not? In large part, the significance of damage is determined by the proportion of ducts that are in such a state as well as by the company that the duct keeps in terms of the type of inflammation and/or the presence of endothelialitis. In my opinion, a few damaged ducts accompanied by a mixed inflammatory infiltrate and endothelialitis are important diagnostically, whereas a larger number of damaged ducts without endothelialitis and with a purely lymphocytic infiltrate may be less significant. We have used the figure of 50% as a significant percentage of damaged ducts (this percentage can usually be estimated) since most reactive conditions—including primary bile duct–damaging processes such as primary biliary cirrhosis—will usually have only a minority of ducts damaged. In our experience, biopsies with less that 50% damaged ducts without accompanying endothelialitis will often resolve spontaneously (16). This may represent a "self-healing" form of rejection, but since treatment is not required, we prefer not to apply a designation of rejection for cases such as this. Such a biopsy in the presence of clinical dysfunction with no other likely cause may represent grounds for rejection therapy, however. Biopsies with more than 50% damaged ducts are usually associated with clinical liver dysfunction and require therapy. Hence, we will diagnose a liver with an infiltrate and greater than 50% bile duct damage as rejection even in the absence of endothelialitis.

The definition of endothelialitis has been refined over the years, with the realization that the original oversimplified definition (of attachment of lymphocytes to the endothelium of veins) led to an overdiagnosis of this lesion. In order to interpret a lesion as endothelialitis, there should be evidence of damage to the endothelium in addition to the presence of lymphocytes (Fig. 2). This damage usually takes the form of enlargement of the endothelial cells (which often look plump and somewhat rounded), which are lifted off from their basement membrane. In many cases, strands of cytoplasm connect the lymphocytes and endothelium. A common artifact that may simulate endothelialitis is a tearing of the specimen, with the formation of a hole the size of a central vein (Fig. 3). Cellular debris at the periphery of the hole may simulate lymphocytes and damaged endothelium if not viewed critically. To the question of how many veins need to be involved to diagnose endothelialitis, the answer depends on the severity of the process. One vein with unequivo-

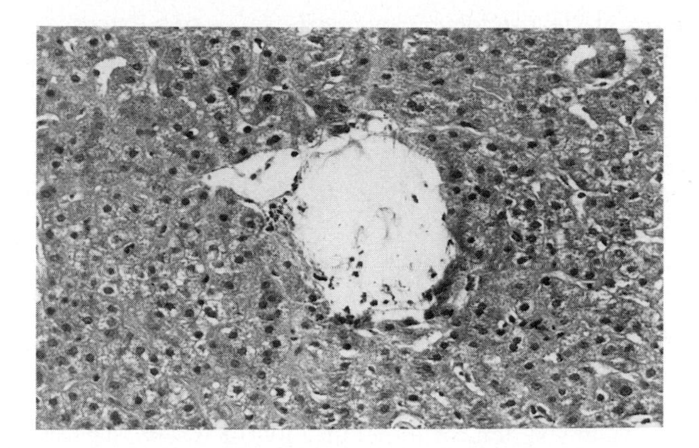

Figure 3 Pseudoendothelialitis of a central vein caused by tearing of the tissue. Note that the true central vein is adjacent to the hole with the apparent endothelialitis and that there is no endothelium in the hole. (Hematoxylin and eosin, ×192). (From Ref. 11.)

cal endothelialitis is adequate. However, in cases where the endoethelialitis is more equivocal, I like to see it in several veins before interpreting it as "significant."

To summarize, minimal criteria for the diagnosis of rejection are as follows. First, the presence of an infiltrate is a sine qua non for the diagnosis of rejection, although in itself it is obviously not diagnostic. Given an appropriate infiltrate, rejection may be diagnosed if there is clear-cut endothelialitis with any degree of bile duct damage or if there is greater than 50% bile duct damage in the absence of endothelialitis. Lesser degrees of duct damage indicate a process that in our experience will often resolve spontaneously and thus is not a strict indication for immunosuppressive therapy. On the other hand, in the face of clinical indications of liver dysfunction, such nondiagnostic findings may be sufficient to initiate rejection therapy if there are no other clinical contraindications to increasing immunosuppression, such as infection.

The question of acute rejection in the absence of clinical or laboratory signs of disease has been raised previously. In general, if strict diagnostic criteria for rejection are used, most cases of biopsy-diagnosed rejection will occur in patients with signs or symptoms of rejection. As a corollary to this statement, if you find yourself diagnosing rejection in a significant proportion of patients without such signs, you should reevaluate your diagnostic criteria for specificity. There is a body of literature indicating that some cases of biopsy-proven rejection resolve spontaneously (17). This may be true in a limited number of cases. It is also possible that the diagnostic criteria will have to be modified because of idiosyncrasies of immune modulation in individual treatment centers. Therefore, rather than adopt the published diagnostic criteria absolutely, one should make whatever modifications are necessary to provide accurate diagnoses in one's own institution.

A. Grading of Acute Rejection

The issue of grading of acute rejection is one of considerable debate and interest. However, in general the accurate diagnosis of rejection is much more important than the grade. Although we and others have used grading to modulate therapy with good results, no trial has been done to illustrate the efficacy of the histological approach over a more empirical approach of graduated doses of immunosuppression following an accurate diagnosis of rejection. Until such trials are performed, there will be continued calls for pathologists to provide a grade of rejection.

There are several grading systems in the literature (12,16,18–20). None of them has fulfilled all of the basic criteria for a good grading system in that none has been demonstrated to be reproducible by its creator or others and to predict behavior of rejection or response to therapy in a prospective fashion. The system we devised and use was designed based on retrospective analysis of histological features that were found in patients with poor outcomes of their rejection either in the form of acute failure or by the development of chronic rejection. The system is simple in design and is generally reproducible between individuals in my own institution, although formal reproducibility testing has not been performed. Others have reported using this system or a modification of it with success (Phillips MJ, personal communication). This system as well as others in the literature are described and critiqued in Table 2. The one singular and somewhat unifying theme of most of these systems is the recognition that the presence of centrilobular necrosis is usually a sign of poor outcome (21). Perhaps lesser degrees of rejection, for which there is less consensus, are also less important to recognize.

It is important to remember that although severe rejection is characterized by centrilobular necrosis, this necrosis is a manifestation of ischemia and will be mimicked by other processes, including nonrejection causes of ischemia and occasionally by drug toxicity and viral infection. Therefore, the diagnosis of severe acute rejection should be made only if there is concomitant evidence of rejection; if there is any doubt that the ischemia is caused by rejection, evaluation of blood flow through the arterial and venous anastomoses should be performed. Drug reactions that may simulate ischemia include reactions to hyperalimentation and azathioprine (22,23). Of the viruses involving the liver, recurrent hepatitis C would appear to be the one that most often causes centrilobular ballooning simulating ischemia (24). With both drugs and viruses, however, there is usually little of the hepatocellular dropout that is seen with ischemia.

B. Acute Rejection Following Therapy for Rejection

Following treatment for rejection, there are several histological changes that may occur and may lead to problems in diagnosis. Effective treatment will usually lead to a decrease in or elimination of inflammation from the liver. Biopsies following treatment may be categorized as showing no rejection (resolution), improved rejection, no change, or worsening rejection. Even with improvement, there may be some residual bile duct damage depending on the time after treatment that the biopsy is taken and the severity of damage that was present prior to treatment. If treatment is less than totally effective, however, histological resolution may be even less complete. In general, endothelialitis is the first feature to disappear, followed by the portal infiltrate and bile duct damage (16). Attempting to diagnosis rejection following treatment is more difficult than making the diagnosis in the untreated liver; hence it is generally considered imperative that biopsy be taken prior to therapy, regardless of how certain the clinician is that the patient is suffering rejection, unless there is a strong clinical contraindication to biopsy.

In some treated patients, a pattern suggestive of obstructive liver disease develops. This lesion, which we previously called prolonged rejection, is characterized by expansion of the portal tracts with bile ductular proliferation, a mixed infiltrate often containing a

Table 2 Published Grading Systems for Acute Rejection

Grade	Williams et al. (12)	Snover et al. (16)	Kemnitz et al. (18)	Demetris et al. (19)	Hubscher et al. (20)[a]
No rejection					score 0–2
Consistent with, nondiagnostic		Infiltrate with damage to <50% of bile ducts	Slight infiltrate and bile duct damage, no endothelialitis	Mononuclear infiltrate with "blastic" lymphocytes, little evidence of tissue damage	score 3
Mild rejection	Minimal portal infiltrate with minimal subendothelial infiltration	Infiltrate with damage to <50% of bile ducts with endothelialitis	Slight infiltrate with endothelialitis, bile duct damage, <10% hepatocyte necrosis	Mild infiltrate with bile duct damage, with or without endothelialitis	score 4–5
Moderate rejection	"More extensive" infiltration of portal tracts and parenchyma with focal nonbridging necrosis of parenchyma	Infiltrate with damage to >50% of bile ducts	Mild rejection but hepatocyte necrosis 10–30%	Portal expansion secondary to infiltrate with bile duct damage and "spill-over" into the lobule	score 6–7
Severe rejection	Marked mononuclear infiltration of portal tracts and parenchyma with bridging necrosis	Mild or moderate rejection with paucity of bile ducts, arteritis and/or centrilobular ballooning and necrosis	Mild rejection but with hepatocyte necrosis >30% with bridging	Mild or moderate rejection with evidence of interstitial hemorrhage or ischemic hepatocyte necrosis or inflammatory arteritis	score 8–9

[a]This grading system relies on grading of the portal infiltrate, bile duct damage, and endothelialitis on a scale of 0 to 3, then summing the results of each for a total score from 0 to 9.

prominent component of neutrophils, and sometimes cholangiolar cholestasis (10). If this histological pattern is seen, it is prudent to recommend radiological evaluation of the biliary tree, although—if the patient has been recently treated for a known episode of rejection—it will almost invariably be secondary to the rejection.

C. Variation of the Histology of Acute Rejection (Theoretical Mechanistic Possibilities)

Although we generally think of acute rejections as a single process, it is possible if not probable that the histological features that we think of as acute rejection reflect a variety of immunological mechanisms that are influenced by various factors in the donor organ and the host. These might include the degree of histocompatibility between donor and host, the specific types of incompatibilies (e.g., differences in class I antigens may lead to rejection affecting bile ducts, whereas differences in antigens specific to vascular structures may lead to more vascular damage), the presence of antidonor antibodies in the recipient (perhaps determining if arteritis and severe rejection are to occur), the occurrence of simultaneous or prior infections (such as the possible link between cytomegalovirus (CMV) infection and chronic vascular rejection), and the specific immunosuppressive regimens used (e.g., we already know that increased immunosuppression will result in decreased incidence of endothelialitis). The reported association between vanishing bile duct syndrome and mismatches at class I loci and matching at class II may represent such a mechanistic variation (25,26). The various histological patterns of acute rejection that we have identified include cases with abundant endothelialitis and minimal bile duct damage, cases with marked bile duct damage with little or no endothelialitis, and cases with arteritis. Although we have chosen to use these variation as grades of rejection, it is possible that they relate to different mechanisms that are more or less susceptible to the immunosuppressive agents in use, leading to a correlation with outcome (23). It is possible that there are additional histological subtypes not yet identified as rejection, including involvement of large bile ducts (too large to be seen in a needle biopsy, giving a sclerosing cholangitis-like pattern) or a purely large-vessel type resulting in ischemic damage to the liver without concomitant histological changes of rejection in the biopsy. While these possibilities remain to be explored, correlation of histological factors with immunological parameters may provide insight into these mechanisms.

III. CHRONIC REJECTION

The diagnosis of chronic rejection of the liver is not as well defined as that of acute rejection, in part because a totally satisfactory definition of chronic rejection does not exist. To most clinicians, chronic rejection represents an irreversible form of rejection which is not responsive to increased immunosuppressive therapy. However, defining irreversibility is not an easy task, since the only treatment for chronic rejection of the liver is retransplantation, a procedure that by definition renders the process in the graft irreversible. There is no time parameter implied by the use of the term "chronic" in this context, and chronic rejection has been diagnosed in the first few months posttransplant, although most cases will occur more than 6 months out. In addition to problems with definition of the process, several of the terms used in the literature for this process are often confusing. Terms used as synonyms for "chronic rejection" include "vanishing bile duct syndrome" and "ductopenic rejection." Both of these terms emphasize the loss of bile ducts seen with chronic rejection. Although loss of bile ducts is a feature of chronic rejection, it also occurs in acute reversible rejection as well as in a late-occurring form that is not necessarily irreversible, a process that is described below. Since there is no absolute level of bile duct loss below which the loss is irreversible, we consider these terms somewhat misleading. Also, as described below, in some cases these terms are used to describe two quite different processes.

A number of papers have addressed the pathological features of chronic rejection, and—as a general statement—there is agreement that the diagnosis of chronic rejection is not an isolated pathological diagnosis on biopsy (11,13,19,20,24,28,29). One type of chronic rejection, chronic vascular rejection characterized by obliterative endarteritis resulting in irreversible ischemic damage to the liver, is generally recognized by all groups who have studied this process. The characteristic lesion of this process, subintimal accumulation of foamy histiocytes in medium to large arteries leading to narrowing of the lumen, is usually not present on biopsy because of the size of the vessels involved. In resection specimens, this lesion is relatively easy to identify, although it may be focal (Fig. 4). Although the diagnostic lesion is not seen, biopsy of the liver in chronic vascular rejection will show progressive central ischemic changes over time. These consist of centrilobular hepatocellular ballooning, often accompanied by dropout of clusters of hepatocytes (Fig. 5). With time, lipofuscin tends to accumulate in the damaged cells and centrilobular pericentral fibrosis develops. These changes generally develop in livers that have shown previous evidence of acute rejection and have failed to respond to therapy. Since ischemic change is also a feature of severe acute rejection (as well as technical causes of ischemia, as noted above), it is never diagnostic of chronic rejection in and of itself. Rather, it is consistent with that diagnosis. We have suggested that a diagnosis of chronic vascular rejection should be made by a combination of clinical and pathological factors, including a series of biopsies consistent with progressive ischemic disease, failure of this process to show improvement with "maximal" immunosuppressive therapy, and evidence of synthetic liver failure (28). The last of these criteria is critical, since it is our opinion that retransplantation should not be performed if the liver is not in synthetic failure.

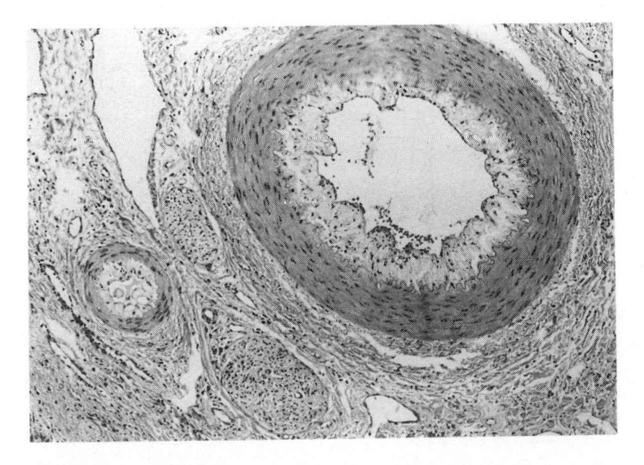

Figure 4 Hepatectomy specimen of chronic vascular rejection. The arteries demonstrate variable degrees of luminal occlusion caused by subintimal accumulation of foamy histiocytes. (Hematoxylin and eosin, ×120.)

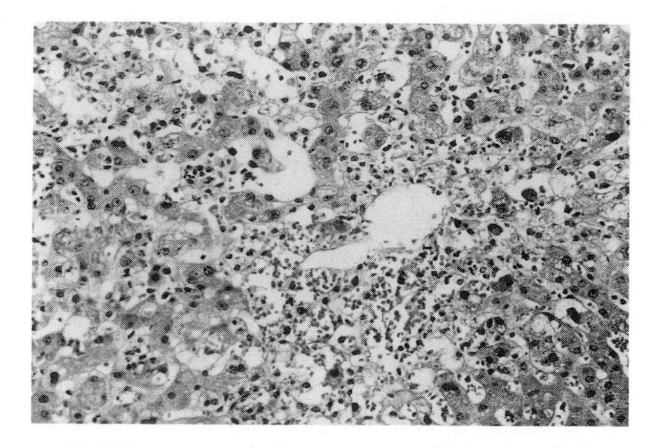

Figure 5 Biopsy of a liver that was eventually resected for chronic vascular rejection. The central region demonstrates dropout of hepatocytes with associated ballooning degeneration and a scant lymphoplasmacellular infiltrate. (Hematoxylin and eosin, ×240.)

In addition to the ischemic hepatocellular changes, the portal tracts in chronic vascular rejection are usually mildly inflamed and the bile ducts are damaged or destroyed, leading to a paucity of ducts (hence the synonyms "vanishing bile duct syndrome" and "ductopenic rejection"). The character of the damaged ducts is somewhat different from the damaged ducts of acute rejection (29) in that the ducts are often not vacuolated but rather have "hard"-appearing eosinophilic cytoplasm with loss of nuclei (Fig. 6). It is likely that at least part of this bile duct damage is due to ischemia (30). Other features of chronic vascular rejection include severe cholestasis and often a centrilobular lymphoplasmacellular infiltrate associated with the hepatocellular ballooning and fibrosis. The significance of this infiltrate is unknown, although it raises the interesting possibility that there is cell-mediated as well as ischemic damage to hepatocytes in chronic vascular rejection. In

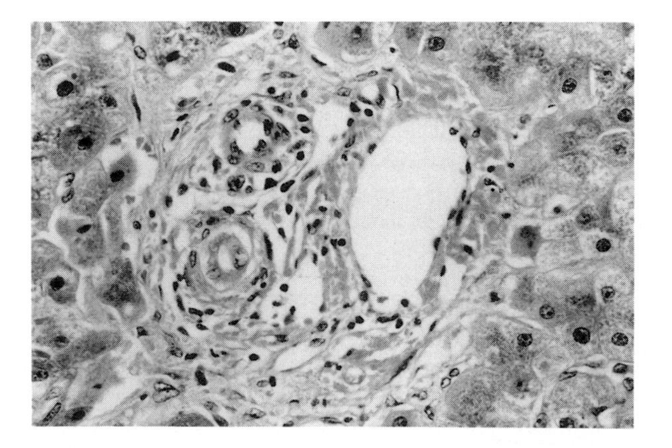

Figure 6 Hepatectomy specimen with chronic vascular rejection. The bile duct in this tract is generally intact, with loss of all except two of its nuclei, which are vesicular with prominent small nucleoli. The cytoplasm of the bile duct cells is eosinophilic. (Hematoxylin and eosin, ×480.)

general, hepatocytes are not targets of the rejection process, a feature usually explained by the failure of hepatocytes to express MHC antigens in the resting state (31–34). However, in a variety of inflammatory conditions including rejection, there is evidence of induced hepatocellular expression of class I MHC antigens, and possibly class II as well (33–37). It is possible that this increased expression leads to inflammatory destruction of hepatocytes which, if not reversed, may play a role in the cascade leading to chronic rejection. This hypothesis is supported by evidence of more class I expression in chronic than in acute rejection (38).

A more controversial type of chronic rejection is that characterized by loss of interlobular bile ducts without ischemic change (28). This process has been implied by terms such as "vanishing bile duct syndrome" and "ductopenic rejection," although, as mentioned above, these terms have been used in a somewhat ambiguous fashion to include livers with chronic vascular rejection. We therefore recommend that these terms (particularly the term "vanishing bile duct syndrome") not be used. This form of "chronic" rejection, defined by persistent liver dysfunction (usually in the form of elevated bilirubin, with retained synthetic function) that fails to respond to immunosuppressive therapy, is characterized histologically by progressive loss of interlobular bile ducts without ischemic changes (Fig. 7). Interestingly, as the ducts disappear, the inflammatory infiltrate of the acute rejection disappears and the portal tracts take on a very characteristic empty appearance, a feature first reported by Portmann et al. (39). Fibrosis usually does not develop.

Although it would appear from the literature that patients have undergone retransplantation because of this lesion, our experience has been that many of these patients will regrow their bile ducts, with eventual return to normal liver function and structure. Interestingly, during the regrowth phase, there is a reappearance of proliferating bile ductules, first at the periphery of the portal tracts in the general location of the embryological ductal plate, with subsequent reappearance of interlobular ducts, loss of the proliferative ductules, and loss of the cholestasis that is usually present at the peak of disease (Fig. 8) (28). This regrowth has taken as long as 6 months to begin and a year to complete; therefore patience is of the essence in handling these patients. Since synthetic failure does not occur,

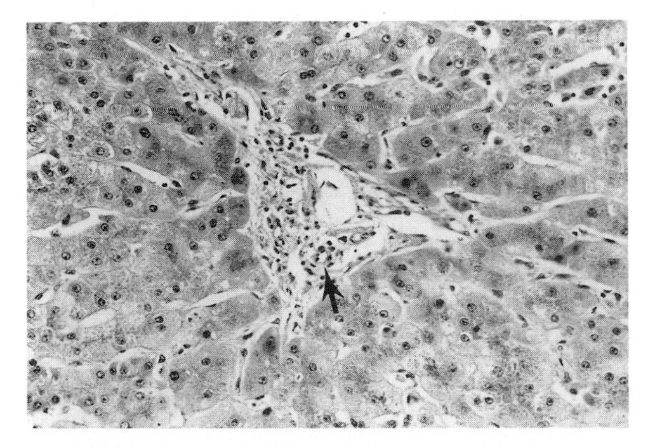

Figure 7 Chronic rejection with paucity of bile ducts ("pure vanishing bile duct syndrome"). This portal tract has no identifiable interlobular bile duct despite the presence of an identifiable arteriole (arrow). (Hematoxylin and eosin, ×240.)

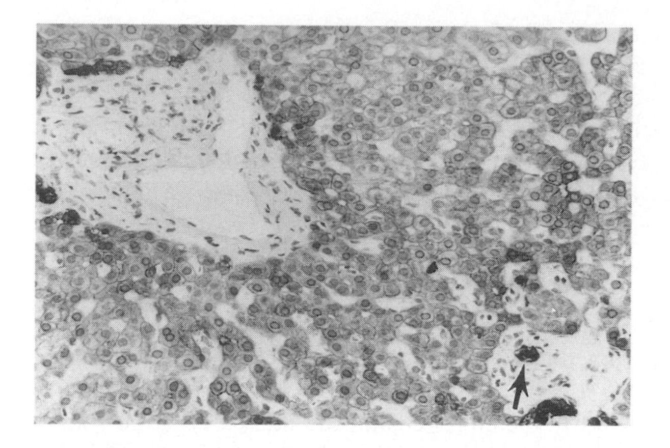

Figure 8 Regrowth of bile ducts in a patient with chronic rejection with paucity of bile ducts ("pure vanishing bile duct syndrome"). Note the presence of cytokeratin-positive proliferating ducts at the periphery of the portal tracts (in the location of the embryological ductal plate) with the presence of only one interlobular bile duct (arrow). (Cytokeratin AE1/AE3 by PAP technique, ×240.)

these patients are clinically stable although often quite jaundiced. Although our observations have not been formally confirmed by others, there are several reports in the literature of resolution of "vanishing bile duct syndrome" and "ductopenic rejection" that are similar to our cases (20,40). At least some of the patients published from the Mayo Clinic as having resolution of their ductopenic rejection have followed a histological course very similar to that of our cases (R. Weisner, personal communication). This phenomenon has not been seen in some centers with a large experience in transplantation; therefore there may be some geographic variable at play in determining the presence and incidence of this form of rejection versus chronic vascular rejection (B. Portmann, personal communication).

Several factors have been reported to be associated with the development of chronic rejection. These include various types of HLA mismatches, the presence of anti–class I antibodies, and the presence of prior CMV infection (25,26,41). The latter factor is particularly intriguing, because a similar association has been noted in heart allografts (42). There is not consensus on this point, however (43). Given the variation in definition of chronic rejection in the liver, this is perhaps not surprising. It is of some interest, however, that the group reporting the strongest association between CMV and chronic rejection ("vanishing bile duct syndrome," in their parlance) states that all of their cases are associated with vascular obliterative lesions (i.e., are chronic vascular rejection) (25,26). On the other hand, a large group reporting a lack of association combined cases of chronic vascular rejection and "chronic" rejection with paucity of ducts alone under one heading as "ductopenic rejection" (44). Data from our experience with the separation of these two groups suggest (without statistical significance) that there is an association between CMV infection and chronic vascular rejection and that there is no association with the nonvascular form of "chronic" rejection (28). By mixing the two groups, the significance of the infection may be masked. The association of CMV with the vascular form of chronic rejection would be in keeping with the findings in cardiac allografts.

IV. OTHER DISEASES OCCURRING IN THE LIVER GRAFT AND THEIR DISTINCTION FROM REJECTION

A. Primary Graft Failure

The term "primary graft failure" (PGF) refers to a poorly defined condition in which the newly grafted liver fails to function properly, starting in the immediate posttransplant period. By definition, there is no obvious cause for this failure, such as arterial thrombosis or rejection. In general, there is no problem distinguishing PGF from acute rejection. However, as mentioned above, it is not always possible to distinguish PGF from hyperacute rejection.

Given the reported incidence of PGF of about 6%, attempts have been made to find histological factors that will predict its occurrence (45–49). Several reports have suggested that the presence of marked macrovesicular steatosis (defined as greater than 60% of the parenchyma affected with the fatty change) at the time of transplantation is predictive, and it has become the policy at many centers to reject such livers for transplantation. Review of the data fails to support the degree of support that this criterion enjoys. There have been few true comparative data of the effect of fatty change on graft failure, since it appears that, based on a report of two cases, most centers have stopped using such grafts (49). Although there is a statistical connection between PGF and fatty change, the degree of PGF in fatty livers in one study was only 6% (14% for massive steatosis) and would therefore at best represent only a relative contraindication to transplantation, not the absolute contraindication that many centers employ (47). This fact has recently been reemphasized (48). Other factors reported to be predictive have included massive hydropic degeneration and centrilobular necrosis, although again neither of these factors would appear to represent an absolute contraindication to use of the organ.

B. Technical Complications (Biliary and Vascular)

Technical problems consists mainly of stricture of the biliary tree, breakdown of the biliary anastomosis, and stricture or thrombosis of the vascular anastomoses (50,51). In general, none of these problems will cause differential diagnostic problems with rejection, assuming that the diagnosis of rejection is always made on a biopsy taken prior to initiation of any antirejection therapy.

There are several patterns of treated rejection that will simulate technical problems. Partially treated rejection will sometimes show a pattern of bile ductular proliferation with cholestasis histologically nearly identical to cholestasis of sepsis but also compatible with large-duct obstruction (10). It may be appropriate to perform radiological studies for obstruction when such a pattern is seen; however, if this pattern occurs in the weeks following treatment for rejection and sepsis can be excluded clinically, it is reasonable to ascribe it to the rejection process.

The development of severe acute rejection or chronic vascular rejection is associated with ischemic changes that mimic technical anastomotic problems. As with the issue of treated rejection and biliary obstruction, if the sequence of events and associated histological findings are taken into account, the correct diagnosis can usually be made. Ischemic change in isolation, not associated with other more typical changes of rejection, should be considered highly indicative of technical problems and evaluated radiologically. On the other hand, if there have been a series of biopsies showing rejection which are now beginning to demonstrate central ischemic changes, almost invariably the ischemic changes will be due to rejection. Although radiological assessment of the anastomoses may still be done, they are not as mandatory as in the more typical ischemic case.

C. Viral Hepatitis (Cytomegalovirus, Hepatitis B and C, Including Recurrence)

The opportunistic viral infections that involve the liver posttransplant—such as CMV, HSV, and adenovirus—do not typically produce changes that are likely to be confused with rejection. There is nothing inherent in these infections that prevents the occurrence of rejection, however; therefore the presence of one of these viruses should not exclude the diagnosis of simultaneous rejection.

On occasion Epstein-Barr virus (EBV) infection has caused confusion with rejection. Epstein-Barr virus may result in a predominantly portal infiltrate of mononuclear cells with entrapment and occasionally even damage to interlobular bile ducts (52). Endothelialitis is not typically considered a part of the histology of EBV infection. In addition, the portal infiltrate, while being predominantly mononuclear, usually contains plasma cells and immunoblasts and does not contain many eosinophils, features in contrast to rejection. In addition, typical EBV-related lymphoid proliferations occur later in the course of transplant than most rejection episodes. Therefore, if one encounters a late biopsy showing a portal infiltrate containing plasma cells with mild bile duct damage but no endothelialitis, the diagnosis of EBV-related disease should be considered more likely than the diagnosis of rejection.

Hepatitis B and C can occur either as de novo infections or as recurrence in those patients transplanted for chronic hepatitis with cirrhosis. Typical infections with these viruses do not cause problems with the histological diagnosis of rejection, although—clinically—rejection is usually in the differential. In most cases there is more lobular inflammation and hepatocellular damage than in rejection. Occasionally one will encounter recurrent hepatitis C presenting with a histological picture characterized by centrilobular hepatocellular ballooning with a mild portal infiltrate that may demonstrate a mild degree of bile duct damage (24). In such cases the possibility of chronic vascular rejection may be suggested if the central ballooning is interpreted as an ischemic change. In general, there is no significant necrosis in these areas, and other features of chronic vascular rejection—including loss of bile ducts as well as a previous diagnosis of rejection—are often missing.

D. Recurrent Disease Other Than Infection

Of all the diseases that may recur following transplantation, the one causing the most controversy regarding recurrence versus chronic rejection is primary biliary cirrhosis (PBC) (53–55). This controversy has been caused in large part because of difficulty in defining recurrence of PBC in the allografted liver as well as by crossover in histological features. Although there is not absolute concurrence, the bulk of data would support the contention that PBC does recur in the allografted liver. The absolute frequency of this recurrence is quite variable in the literature, but a recent well-documented publication places the risk at about 16%, which is in keeping with an unpublished rate of about 10% at the University of Minnesota (55).

Histological features common to both chronic rejection and PBC include the type of portal infiltrate, bile duct damage, and bile duct loss. The major feature found in chronic vascular rejection but not PBC is central ischemic change. Granulomas would appear to be a feature of PBC not yet documented in chronic rejection (although I should hasten to add that in our experience, most granulomas in the transplanted liver are not associated with PBC either). Utilizing the concept that the diagnosis of chronic rejection requires not only a consistent biopsy but also a series of biopsies, starting with acute rejection and showing progression to chronic vascular rejection, the differential from PBC should not be difficult in most cases. Primary biliary cirrhosis should occur without progression from rejection, may have granulomas, and should not have ischemic change.

E. Drug Reactions

Although a plethora of drugs are commonly taken by transplant patients, none have led to the development of histological features likely to be confused with rejection, either acute or chronic. Drugs with demonstrated toxicity to the liver include cyclosporine, azathioprine, steroids, numerous antibiotics, and hyperalimentation (Table 3) (56).

It is often difficult to specifically assign a drug as a cause of disease in the transplanted organ. Hyperalimentation may cause cholestasis associated with centrilobular ballooning degeneration (23). Portal tract changes are rare, although in occasional cases in which the hyperalimentation has not been discontinued we have suspected that portal fibrosis with bile ductular proliferation and cholangiolar cholestasis have resulted from this agent. The only way to prove the association in an individual patient is to discontinue the parenteral

Table 3 Drugs Commonly Administered to Transplant Patients and Their Reported Hepatotoxicity

Drug	Reported toxicity
Cyclosporine	Cholestasis
Azathioprine	Cholestatic hepatitis
	Venoocclusive disease
	Peliosis hepatis
Corticosteroids	Fatty change
	Sinusoidal dilatation
	Nodular regenerative hyperplasia
Trimethoprim-sulfamethoxazole	Hepatitis
	Cholestatic hepatitis
Penicillin and derivatives	Hepatitis
	Cholestatic hepatitis
Cephalosporins	Rare hepatitis
	Rare cholestatic hepatitis
Amphotericin	Rare hepatitis
	Sinusoidal dilatation
	Nodular regenerative hyperplasia
Ketoconazole	Hepatitis
	Cholestatic hepatitis
Fluconazole	Rare hepatitis (one case)
Hyperalimentation preparations	Cholestatic hepatitis
	Portal fibrosis with obstructive features
	Central ballooning degeneration

Source: From Ref. 56.

feedings and rebiopsy. Although hyperalimentation effect does not simulate rejection, distinction from ischemia may be more difficult.

Azathioprine also causes cholestatic hepatitis with histological features not too different from hyperalimentation, although the degree of ballooning is often less (22).

Cyclosporine (CSA) hepatotoxicity is still difficult to define absolutely. While there is no doubt that clinically apparent cholestasis is associated with CSA, the histological features have not been well defined (57). Canalicular cholestasis has been seen in some patients with high CSA levels as well as in some animal model systems (58). However, minor histological cholestasis is so common in the transplanted liver that it is of no significance as a diagnostic feature. Wisecarver et al. have described accumulation of cellular debris in the sinusoids as a feature associated with CSA toxicity (59). This finding has yet to be confirmed, however.

REFERENCES

1. Forbes RDC, Guttman RD. Pathogenetic studies of cardiac allograft rejection using inbred rat models. Immunol Rev 1984; 77:5–29.
2. Gordon RD, Fung JJ, Markus B, et al. The antibody crossmatch in liver transplantation. Surgery 1986; 100:705–715.
3. Demetris AJ, Jaffe R, Tzakis A, et al. Antibody mediated rejection of human orthotopic liver allografts: A study of liver transplantation across ABO blood group barriers. Am J Pathol 1988; 132:489–502.
3b. Demetris AJ, Nakamura K, Yagihashi A, et al. A clinicopathological study of human liver allograft recipients harboring preformed IgG lymphocytic antibodies. Hepatology 1992; 16: 671–681.
4. Hanto DW, Snover DC, Noreen HJ, et al. Hyperacute rejection of a human orthotopic liver allograft in a presensitized recipient. Clin Transplant 1987; 1:304–310.
5. Bird G, Friend P, Donaldson P, et al. Hyperacute rejection in liver transplantation: A case report. Transplant Proc 1989; 21:3742–3744.
6. Gubernatis G, Kemnitz J, Bornscheuer A, et al. Potential various appearances of hyperacute rejection in human liver transplantation. Langenbechs Arch Chir 1989; 374:240–244.
7. Knechtle SJ, Kolbeck PC, Tsuchimoto S, et al. Hepatic transplantation into sensitized recipients: Demonstration of hyperacute rejection. Transplantation 1987; 43:8–12.
8. Gubernatis G, Lauchart W, Jonker M, et al. Signs of hyperacute rejection of liver grafts in Rhesus monkeys after donor-specific presensitization. Transplant Proc 1987; 19:1082–1083.
9. Hubscher SG, Adams DH, Buckels JAC, et al. Massive hemorrhagic necrosis of the liver after liver transplantation. J Clin Pathol 1989; 42:360–370.
10. Snover DC, Sibley RK, Freese DK, et al. Orthotopic liver transplantation: A pathological study of 63 serial liver biopsies from 17 patients with specific reference to the diagnostic features and natural history of rejection. Hepatology 1984; 4:1212–1222.
11. Snover DC. The pathology of liver transplantation. In: Sale GE, ed. The Pathology of Organ Transplantation. Boston: Butterworths, 1990.
12. Williams JW, Peters TG, Vera SP, et al. Biopsy directed immunosuppression following hepatic transplantation in man. Transplantation 1985; 39:589–596.
13. Demetris AJ, Lasky S, Van Thiel DH, et al. Pathology of hepatic transplantation: A review of 62 adult allograft recipients immunosuppressed with a cyclosporine/steroid regimen. Am J Pathol 1985; 118:151–161.
14. Demetris AJ, Belle SH, Hart J, et al. Intraobserver and interobserver variation in the histopathological assessment of liver allograft rejection. Hepatology 1991; 14:751–755.
15. Nakanuma Y, Ohta G. Histometric and serial section observations of the intrahepatic bile ducts in primary biliary cirrhosis. Gastroenterology 1979; 76:1326–1332.

16. Snover DC, Freese DK, Sharp HL, et al. Liver allograft rejection: An analysis of the use of biopsy in determining outcome of rejection. Am J Surg Pathol 1987; 11:1–10.
17. Dousset B, Hubscher SG, Padbury RT, et al. Acute liver allograft rejection—Is treatment always necessary? Transplantation 1993; 55:529–534.
18. Kemnitz J, Ringe B, Cohnert TR, et al. Bile duct injury as part of diagnostic criteria for liver allograft rejection. Hum Pathol 1989; 20:132–143.
19. Demetris AJ, Qian S, Sun H, Fung JJ. Liver allograft rejection: An overview of morphologic findings. Am J Surg Pathol 1990; 14(suppl 1):49–63.
20. Hubscher SG, Buckels JAC, Elias E, et al. Vanishing bile duct syndrome following liver transplantation—Is it reversible? Transplantation 1991; 51:1004–1010.
21. Ludwig J, Gross JB Jr, Perkins JD, Moore SB. Persistent centrilobular necroses in hepatic allografts. Hum Pathol 1990; 21:656–661.
22. De Pinho R, Goldberg CS, Lefkowitch JH. Azathioprine and the liver: Evidence favoring idiosyncratic mixed cholestasis-hepatocellular injury in humans. Gastroenterology 1984; 86:162–165.
23. Dahms BB, Halpin TC Jr. Serial liver biopsies in parenteral nutrition-associated cholestasis of early infancy. Gastroenterology 1981; 81:136–144.
24. Ferrell LD, Wright TL, Roberts J, et al. Hepatitis C viral infection in liver transplant recipients. Hepatology 1992; 16:865–876.
25. Donaldson PT, Alexander GJ, O'Grady, et al. Evidence for an immune response to HLA class I antigens in the vanishing-bile duct syndrome after liver transplantation. Lancet 1987; 1:945–951.
26. O'Grady JG, Alexander GJ, Sutherland S, et al. Cytomegalovirus infection and donor/recipient HLA antigens: Interdependent co-factors in pathogenesis of vanishing bile-duct syndrome after liver transplantation. Lancet 1988; 2:302–305.
27. Gubernatis G, Kemnitz J, Tusch G, et al. Different features of acute liver allograft rejection, their outcome and possible relationship to HLA-compatibility. Transplant Proc 1989; 21:2213–2214.
28. Freese DK, Snover DC, Sharp H, et al. Chronic rejection after liver transplant: A study of clinical, histopathologic, and immunologic features. Hepatology 1991; 13:882–891.
29. Ludwig J, Weisner RH, Batts KP, et al. The acute vanishing bile duct syndrome (acute irreversible rejection) after orthotopic liver transplantation. Hepatology 1987; 7:476–483.
30. Oguma S, Belle S, Starzl TE, Demetris AJ. A histometric analysis of chronically rejected human liver allografts. Insights into the mechanisms of bile duct loss: Direct immunologic and ischemic factors. Hepatology 1989; 9:204–209.
31. Daar SA, Fuggle SV, Fabre JW, et al. The detailed distribution of HLA-A, B, C, antigens in normal human organs. Transplantation 1984; 38:289–292.
32. Daar AS, Fuggle SV, Fabre JW, et al. The detailed distribution of MHC class II antigens in normal human organs. Transplantation 1984; 38:293–298.
33. Steinhoff G. Major histocompatibility complex antigens in human liver transplants. J Hepatol 1990; 11:9–15.
34. Vierling JM. Immunologic mechanisms of hepatic allograft rejection. Semin Liver Dis 1992; 12:16–27.
35. So SKS, Platt JL, Ascher NL, Snover DC. Increased expression of class I antigens on hepatocytes in rejecting liver allografts. Transplantation 1987; 43:79–85.
36. Steinhoff G, Wonigeit K, Pichlmayr R. Analysis of sequential changes in major histocompatibility complex expression in human liver grafts after transplantation. Transplantation 1988; 45:394–401.
37. Hubscher SG, Adams DH, Elias E. Changes in the expression of major histocompatibility complex class II antigens in liver allograft rejection. J Pathol 1990; 162:165–171.
38. Rouger P, Gugenheim J, Gane P, et al. Distribution of the MHC antigens after liver transplantation: relationship with biochemical and histological parameters. Clin Exp Immunol 1990; 80:404–408.
39. Portmann B, Neuberger JM, Williams R. Intrahepatic bile duct lesions. In: Calne RV, ed. Liver transplantation. London: Grune & Stratton, 1983: 279–287.

40. van Hoek B, Weisner RH, Krom RAF, et al. Severe ductopenic rejection following liver transplantation: Incidence, time of onset, risk factors, treatment, and outcome. Semin Liver Dis 1992; 12:41–50.
41. Batts KP, Moore SB, Perkins JD, et al. Influence of positive lymphocyte crossmatch and HLA mismatching on vanishing bile duct syndrome in human liver allografts. Transplantation 1988; 45:376–379.
42. McDonald K, Rector TS, Braulin EA, et al. Association of coronary artery disease in cardiac transplant recipients with cytomegalovirus. Am J Cardiol 1989; 64:359.
43. Stovin PG, Sharples L, Hutter JA, et al. Some prognostic factors for the development of transplant-related coronary artery disease in human cardiac allografts. J Heart Lung Transplant 1991; 10:38–44.
44. Paya CV, Wiesner RH, Hermans PE, et al. Lack of association between cytomegalovirus infection, HLA matching and the vanishing bile duct syndrome after liver transplantation. Hepatology 1992; 16:66–70.
45. Quiroga J, Colina I, Demetris AJ, et al. Cause and timing of first allograft failure in orthotopic liver transplantation: a study of 177 consecutive patients. Hepatology 1991; 14:1054–1062.
46. d'Alessandro AM, Kalayoglu M, Sollinger HW, et al. The predictive value of donor liver biopsies for the development of primary nonfunction after orthotopic liver transplantation. Transplantation 1991; 51:157–163.
47. Adams R, Reynes M, Johan M, et al. The outcome of steatotic grafts in liver transplantation. Transplant Proc 1991; 23:1538–1540.
48. Karayalcin K, Mirza DF, Harrison RF, et al. The role of dynamic and morphological studies in the assessment of potential liver donors. Transplantation 1994; 57:1323–1327.
49. Todo S, Demetris AJ, Makowka L, et al. Primary nonfunction of hepatic allografts with preexisting fatty infiltration. Transplantation 1990; 47:903–905.
50. Lerut J, Gordon RD, Iwatsuki S, et al. Biliary tract complications in human orthotopic liver transplantation. Transplantation 1987; 43:47–51.
51. Wozney P, Zajko AB, Bron KM, et al. Vascular complications after liver transplantation: A 5-year experience. AJR 1986; 147:657–663.
52. Randhawa PS, Markin RS, Starzl TE, Demetris AJ. Epstein-Barr virus–associated syndromes in immunosuppressed liver transplant recipients: Clinical profile and recognition on routine allograft biopsy. Am J Surg Pathol 1990; 14:538–547.
53. Demetris AJ, Markus BH, Esquivel C, et al. Pathologic analysis of liver transplantation for primary biliary cirrhosis. Hepatology 1988; 8:939–947.
54. Polson RJ, Portmann B, Neuberger J, et al. Evidence for disease recurrence after liver transplantation for primary biliary cirrhosis: Clinical and histologic follow-up studies. Gastroenterology 1989; 97:715–725.
55. Hubscher SG, Elias E, Buckels JA, et al. Primary biliary cirrhosis: Histological evidence of disease recurrence after liver transplantation. J Hepatol 1993; 18:173–184.
56. Snover DC. Biopsy Diagnosis of Liver Disease. Chapt. 10. Baltimore: Williams & Wilkins, 1992.
57. Lorber MI, Van Buren CT, Flechner SM, et al. Hepatobiliary and pancreatic complications of cyclosporine therapy in 466 renal transplant recipients. Transplantation 1987; 43:35–40.
58. Ryffel B, Donatsch P, Madorin M, et al. Toxicological evaluation of cyclosporin A. Arch Toxicol 1983; 53:107–141.
59. Wisecarver JL, Earl RA, Haven MC, et al. Histologic changes in liver allograft biopsies associated with elevated whole blood and tissue cyclosporin concentrations. Mod Pathol 1992; 5:611–616.
60. Snover DC. The pathology of acute rejection. Transplant Proc 1986; 18(suppl 4):123–127.

9

Pathology of Kidney Transplantation

Lorraine C. Racusen
Johns Hopkins University School of Medicine, Baltimore, Maryland

Kim Solez
University of Alberta, Edmonton, Alberta, Canada

Steen Olsen
University Institute of Pathology, Municipal Hospital, Århus, Denmark

I. INTRODUCTION

Evaluation of renal allograft status posttransplantation is often difficult, and the allograft biopsy may play a critical role in the posttransplant management of the renal allograft patient. Until very recently, however, there had been no standardized approach to histopathological evaluation of renal allograft biopsies or to grading of severity of rejection-related changes in those biopsies. Standardized schema for grading of heart and lung allografts were developed and published in 1990. Following these models, an international meeting was held in Banff, Canada, in 1991 to draft a formulation for a schema for histological evaluation and grading of rejection-related changes in renal allograft biopsies. This Banff schema was revised by contributing authors and published in August 1993 (1) and is currently in use for central slide review of allograft biopsies in a number of large international trials of immunosuppressive agents as well as in many medical centers worldwide. In this chapter, we review the classification system, discuss ongoing studies on reproducibility and clinical validation of the schema, point out areas of the grading system that will require further refinement, and discuss future directions in pathological evaluation of the renal allograft.

II. SPECIMEN ADEQUACY AND PROCESSING

Before any definitive evaluation of the renal allograft biopsy can be performed, issues related to specimen adequacy and recommendations for processing of specimens must be addressed. While changes in the renal medulla may reflect changes in the renal cortex and may be adequate to establish the presence of rejection, a reasonable sample of cortex should be obtained to grade and/or rule out rejection with a significant degree of certainty. Therefore, an adequate sample is defined as one containing seven or more glomeruli and at least one artery. Specimens with one to six glomeruli and at least one artery would be marginally adequate. If there are no glomeruli and/or no arteries in the biopsy, the specimen is inadequate to rule out rejection or to adequately grade an ongoing rejection process, though it may be possible to establish a diagnosis of rejection.

It is recommended that each specimen be mounted with multiple sections on each of a total of seven slides, three stained with hemotoxylin and eosin (H&E), three with periodic acid-Schiff reagent (PAS), and one with a trichrome stain. The PAS and/or silver stains are particularly useful for defining tubular basement membranes (TBM) to accurately assess severity of tubulitis, in which intraepithelial inflammatory infiltrates must by definition breach the TBM, and for evaluating glomerulitis. The PAS stain is also very useful for rapid identification of atrophic tubules and for identifying hyalinosis lesions in renal arterioles—lesions which are graded in the Banff schema. Trichrome stains aid in assessing chronic fibrosing changes in the interstitium and in vessel walls.

III. SEMIQUANTITATIVE ASSESSMENT OF HISTOLOGIC CHANGES—ACUTE

The criteria for rejection diagnosis in the Banff schema focus on inflammatory infiltration of tubules and/or vessel walls to establish the diagnosis and grade the severity of rejection. While interstitial inflammatory infiltrates are a constant feature in renal allograft rejection, such infiltrates, even if diffuse in a given biopsy, must be regarded as not specific for rejection, since they have not infrequently been demonstrated in protocol biopsies in well-functioning grafts (2–6). Moreover, there is no correlation between degree of interstitial inflammation and response to antirejection therapy (7–9). Failure of the extent of inflammatory infiltrate on biopsy to correlate with either renal dysfunction or response to therapy is almost surely due to sampling error. The relatively small needle biopsies that are typically obtained from these allografts may lead to over- or underestimation of extent of inflammation in the entire graft. Indeed, sampling error has been recognized as a problem since the very early days of allograft biopsy (10).

On histological evaluation, each of the major parenchymal components of the kidney—glomeruli, interstitum, tubules, and vessels—are assessed for both acute and chronic changes. Acute and chronic histological findings are graded on a semiquantitative scale (see Table 1). A numerical code is then developed, which, for acute changes, combines "g" (glomerulus), "i" (interstitium), "t" (tubules), and "v" (vessels) with a numerical score for each. Thus, a completely normal biopsy would be graded g0, i0, t0, v0. Chronic changes are coded similarly, with a "c" prefix for each category and a numerical score for each. A biopsy lacking any chronic change, therefore, would be graded cg0, ci0, ct0, cv0.

Semiquantitative assessment of histological changes, whether formal or informal, deliberate or subconscious, serves as the basis for a diagnosis of rejection made by any pathologist interpreting a renal allograft biopsy. The numerical scoring system of the Banff schema provides a relatively objective way of recording a short-hand summary of these semiquantitative findings. Regardless of subsequent changes in summary classification of rejection, the criteria for which may evolve over time, or the narrative wording utilized at individual centers to describe biopsy findings, the numerical scores would remain unaltered. While coding is not a mandatory feature of the system for general use, it is mandatory for allograft assessment in international and multicenter trials.

Table 1 Numerical Codes for Semiquantitative Assessment of Acute and Chronic Changes in the Allograft Biopsy[a]

Acute changes (see text)		
g	0, 1, 2, 3	No, mild, moderate, severe glomerulitis (g3 = mononuclear cells in capillaries of all or nearly all glomeruli with endothelial enlargement and luminal occlusion)
i	0, 1, 2, 3	No, mild, moderate, severe interstitial mononuclear cell infiltration (in rejection edema and lymphocyte activation usually accompany mononuclear cell infiltration; i3 = >50% of parenchyma inflamed)
t	0, 1, 2, 3	No, mild, moderate, severe tubulitis (t3 = >10 mononuclear cells per tubule or per 10 tubular cells in several tubules)
v	0, 1, 2, 3	No, mild, moderate, severe intimal arteritis (assessed in most involved vessel) (v3 = severe intimal arteritis and/or transmural arteritis and/or hemorrhage and recent infarction)
ah	0, 1, 2, 3	No, mild, moderate, severe nodular hyaline afferent arteriolar thickening suggestive of cyclosporine toxicity (ah3 = severe PAS-positive thickening in many arterioles)
Chronic changes (see text)		
cg	0, 1, 2, 3	No, mild, moderate, severe chronic transplant glomerulopathy (% glomeruli)
ci	0, 1, 2, 3	No, mild, moderate, severe interstitial fibrosis, often with mononuclear cell inflammation (% total interstitial area)
ct	0, 1, 2, 3	No, mild, moderate, severe tubular atrophy and loss (% tubular area)
cv	0, 1, 2, 3	No, mild, moderate, severe fibrous intimal thickening often with elastica fragmentation (cv3 indicates complete occlusion); (cg and cv lesions suggest the presence of chronic rejection) (assessed in most damaged vessel)

[a]Both acute and chronic codes can be used together if the situation warrants.
Modified from Ref. 1.

In the following section, we briefly consider the criteria for the numerical codes employed for acute lesions occurring in each of the major histological components in the kidney.

A. Glomeruli

Acute inflammatory changes may occur in the glomerulus posttransplant, so-called glomerulitis. Endocapillary glomerulitis is defined as an increase in number of mononuclear cells in the glomerular capillary lumina. The first report of this lesion (11) in the renal allograft proposed that it might be due to active cytomegalovirus (CMV) infection, an association that could not be confirmed by later authors. Moderate or severe glomerulitis occurs in about 13% of graft biopsies from the early posttransplant period (12). The light microscopic picture resembles that of acute immune complex glomerulonephritis, but neutrophils are usually not present in the glomeruli; on electron microscopy and immunofluorescence microscopy, no immunodeposits are seen (Marcussen and Olsen, unpublished data). There is some correlation between glomerulitis and acute rejection, but many biopsies with glomerulitis have no rejection and most biopsies with rejection have no glomerulitis (12). Graft function seems not be influenced by its presence and even severe glomerulitis is compatible with a functioning graft. An adverse effect on graft survival has been presumed (13), but in our material graft survival did not seem to be influenced by the presence of glomerulitis per se (12) if acute rejection in the early posttransplant course was taken into consideration. Transition from endocapillary glomerulitis to chronic glomerular transplant disease has also been suggested (14,15). We did not find such an association (12), but a larger number of patients and a longer observation period is necessary to determine whether glomerulitis has any prognostic impact on graft survival. Early posttransplant endocapillary glomerulitis may be a particular pattern of rejection due to pathogenic mechanisms other than conventional rejection, but the available data do not justify its inclusion in the lesions used for grading of acute rejection. Therefore, it is evaluated but not included as a diagnostic criterion for rejection. A summary of criteria for semiquantitative grading of glomerulitis is shown in Table 2. A glomerulus with glomerulitis graded g3 is shown in Fig. 1.

B. Interstitium

Interstitial inflammation is graded by the extent of parenchyma infiltrated by mononuclear cells (see Table 3). While severity of interstitial inflammation is not part of the semiquantitative assessment, in general its severity is reflected in the degree of inflammatory infiltration of tubules, which is assessed separately and should be viewed as one of the cardinal features for the diagnosis of acute rejection. As noted above, mild-to-moderate interstitial inflammation must be regarded as not specific for rejection, since such infiltrates may be seen in autografts (16) as well as well-functioning transplants (2–6). If severe or diffuse, however, it is certainly suggestive if not diagnostic of rejection. Relatively large perivenous aggregates may be seen in renal allograft biopsies (see Fig. 2). In general, these aggregates do not appear to be as significant as extension of the infiltrate into the renal parenchyma. These large aggregates, as well as inflammatory infiltrates in the subcapsular cortex related to handling and "healing in" of the allograft, (see below, Sec. IV.B) should not be weighted as heavily in the scoring as infiltrates into renal parenchyma and away from the immediate subcapsular zone.

The mononuclear cellular infiltrate in renal allograft rejection has been evaluated by light and electron microscopy (17) and immunohistochemistry. It typically consists of approximately 50% lymphocytes, 25% macrophages, and 12% plasma cells. Large, blast-like lymphocytes as well as plasma cells may be particularly numerous in early rejection. The majority of cells infiltrating the graft express T-cell markers, generally a mixture of $CD4^+$ and $CD8^+$ cells. There is some evidence for a predominance of CD8 and CD45R0 cells in acute rejection of the renal allograft (18), but the ratio of CD4 to CD8 cells may vary in early versus later acute rejection (19,20). Leu-7–positive natural killer cells and macrophages have also been identified in rejecting renal allografts (21,22); the presence of Leu-7–positive cells infiltrating the tubular epithelium is a reliable marker of rejection (21) (see Fig. 3). The presence of B cells in substantial numbers may indicate inflammation related to infection rather than rejection; when associated with clusters of atypical plasma cells, post-

Table 2 Quantitative Criteria for the Early Type of Allograft Glomerulitis ("g") (0 to 3+)[a]

0 = No glomerulitis
1 = Glomerulitis in a minority of glomeruli
2 = Segmental or global glomerulitis in 25 to 75% of glomeruli
3 = Glomerulitis (mostly global) in all or almost all glomeruli

[a]Accumulation of monocytes and lymphocytes in glomerular capillaries with endothelial swelling

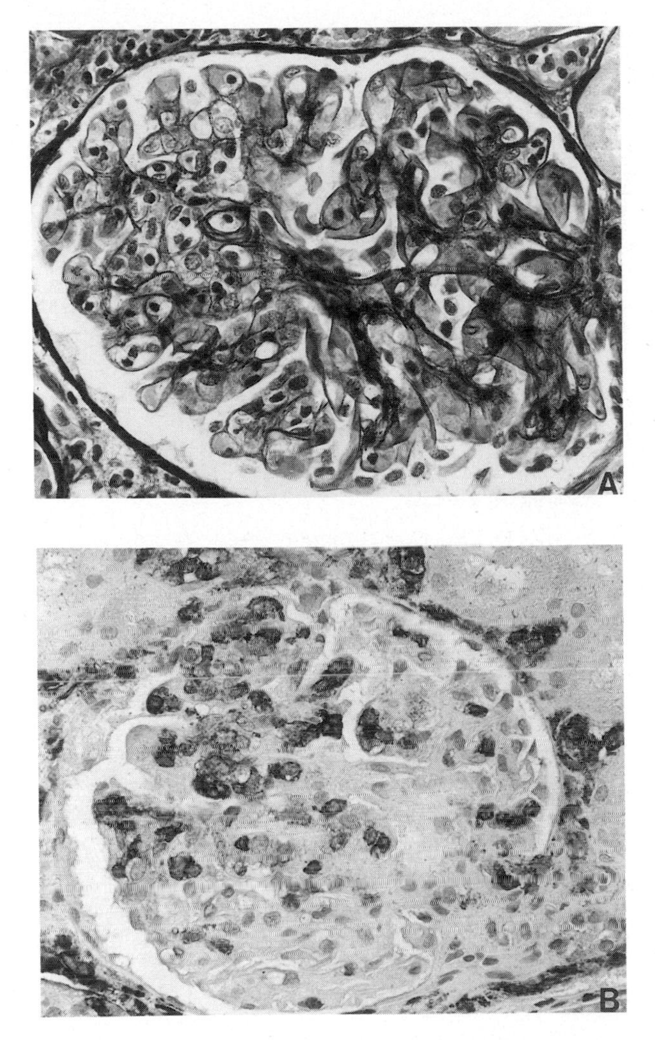

Figure 1 A. Glomerulus with severe glomerulitis (g3). Most capillary loops contain lymphocytes, macrophages, and/or swollen endothelial cells. (PAS, ×400.) B. Immunoperoxidase stain for common leukocyte antigen in the same case, demonstrating numerous leukocytes in the glomerulus and surrounding interstitium. (×400).

Table 3 Quantitative Criteria for Mononuclear Cell Interstitial Inflammation ("i") (0 to 3+)

0 = No or trivial interstitial inflammation
1 = up to 25% of parenchyma inflamed
2 = 26 to 50% of parenchyma inflamed
3 = >50% of parenchyma inflamed

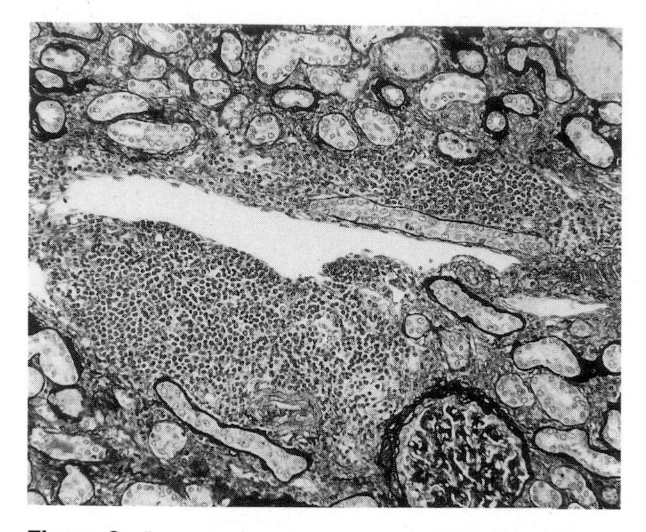

Figure 2 Large perivenous aggregate of bland lymphocytes. (PAS/MS, ×160.)

transplant lymphoproliferative disorder must be ruled out. Immuno-phenotyping of mononuclear infiltrates may eventually prove to be a reliable and widely applicable technique enabling more precise diagnosis and grading of rejection and may ultimately be formally incorporated into a rejection schema. For the moment, however, immunophenotyping remains an ancillary technique that may be useful in equivocal cases (see Chap. 3).

Polymorphonuclear leukocytes and/or eosinophils may be present in the inflammatory infiltrate of acute rejection. When these cells are numerous, the rejection may be aggressive, responding poorly to therapy (23). Polymorphonuclear leukocytes may be seen in cases of antibody-mediated rejection (24,25) and are commonly seen in ABO-incompatible grafts. Infiltrates of polymorphs also occur around recent infarcts and may therefore be

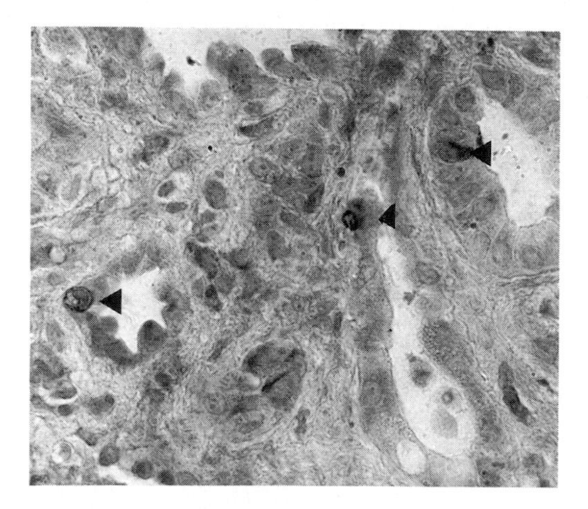

Figure 3 Several Leu-7+ intraepithelial lymphocytes in renal tubules (arrowheads). (Immunoperoxidase stain, ×500.)

numerous in cases of hyperacute or acute rejection with arteritis and infarction. We now designate an interstitial infiltrate with more than occasional polymorphs and/or eosinophils or those with large numbers of typical or atypical plasma cells with an asterisk in the coding system—e.g., i2*.

Interstitial edema almost invariably accompanies the inflammatory infiltrate and is not graded separately, though it may be noted in the narrative description.

C. Tubules

The tubules in the renal allograft are a major target of the rejection process. Inflammatory infiltration of the tubular epithelium, or tubulitis, is a typical feature of acute rejection (26–28). While mild tubulitis (1 to 4 lymphocytes per most affected tubules) may occur in allografts with stable function or acute tubular necrosis (3), more severe tubulitis appears to be quite specific for rejection (1). Criteria for semiquantitative grading of tubulitis based on severity of infiltrate in the most involved tubules, are shown in Table 4. Tubulitis is defined as invasion of mononuclear cells across the tubular basement membrane; these cells generally lie below or between the tubular epithelial cells (see Fig. 4). Localization of inflammatory cells may be difficult in sections stained with H&E. However, definition of true tubulitis may be markedly enhanced by PAS or silver stain, which highlight tubular basement membranes preferentially and also allow morphological identification of infiltrating mononuclear cells. The infiltrating cells typically have a small clear area around them and can be differentiated from the surrounding tubular cells morphologically. In general, significant tubulitis tends to occur in areas of interstitial inflammation and should be sought in those areas, though in occasional cases tubulitis is more extensive than interstitial inflammation. With very aggressive inflammation, tubular basement membranes may be disrupted; this change can be defined with PAS or silver stains, which highlight tubular basement membrane. Recent studies on segmental localization of tubulitis in allograft biopsies have demonstrated that tubulitis is most severe in the distal convoluted tubule and the cortical collecting system, followed by proximal tubules and distal straight tubules (29).

Immunohistochemistry, if available, may enhance identification and quantitation of tubulitis. Staining for common leukocyte antigen serves to mark infiltrating leukocytes. Immunophenotyping of the lymphocytes invading the tubule may provide greater specificity in diagnosing a rejection process. As noted above, the presence of Leu-7–positive cells infiltrating the tubular epithelium is a fairly reliable marker of rejection (21) (see Fig. 3). Identification of cytotoxic cells using antibodies to granzyme B and/or perforin (30–32) or identification of cytotoxic T lymphocyte–specific gene transcripts (33) may ultimately also be useful adjuncts in identifying effector cells of the rejection response in the allograft biopsy. Other potentially useful tubular markers include enhanced tubular cell expression of HLA antigens (34,35) and/or adhesion molecules (36,37), which may contribute to targeting of the tubular epithelium for immunological attack.

Table 4 Quantitative Criteria for Tubulitis ("t") (0 to 3+)

0 = No mononuclear cells in tubules
1 = Foci with 1 to 4 cells/tubular cross section or 10 tubular cells
2 = Foci with 5 to 10 cells/tubular cross section
3 = Foci with >10 cells/tubular cross section

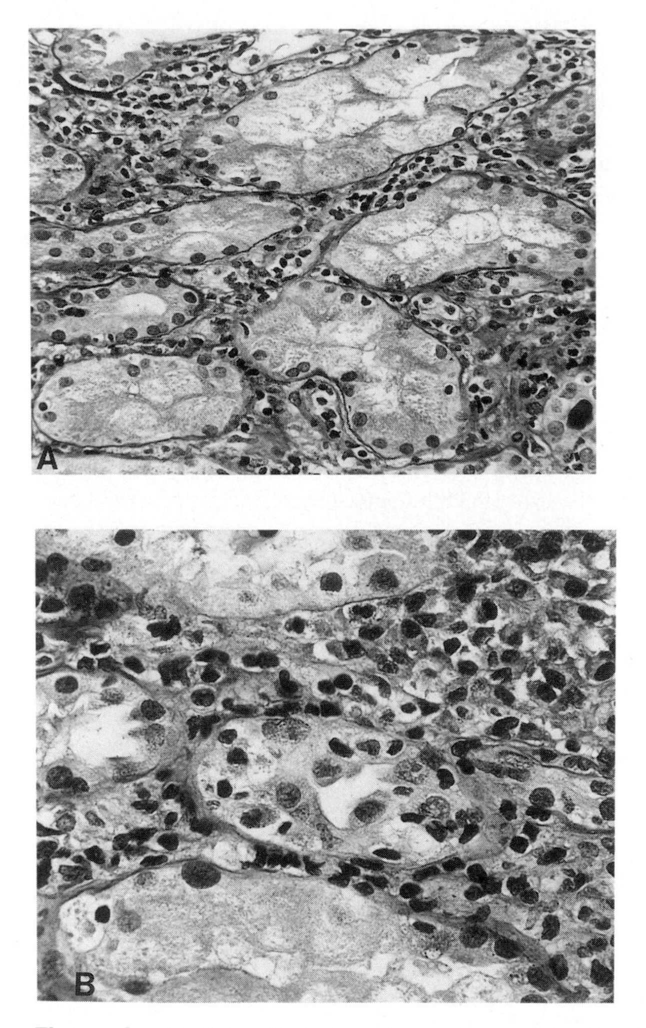

Figure 4 Tubulitis with intraepithelial lymphocytes that have crossed the tubular basement membrane. A. Mild, t1. (PAS, ×300.) B. Severe, t3. (PAS, ×600.)

D. Vessels

1. Arteries

Intimal arteritis is the pathognomic lesion of acute rejection and is highly specific for that process in the allograft. This finding was recognized in several early studies of human renal allograft pathology (38–42) and continues to be an important finding in renal allograft biopsies, though the most severe lesions are rarely seen except in nephrectomies performed for irreversible rejection in the era of modern immunosuppressive regimens. The lesion is characterized by intimal thickening due to edema and an inflammatory infiltrate, with mononuclear cells beneath the endothelium (see Figs. 5 and 6). Criteria for quantitation of intimal arteritis are shown in Table 5 and are based on severity of the inflammatory

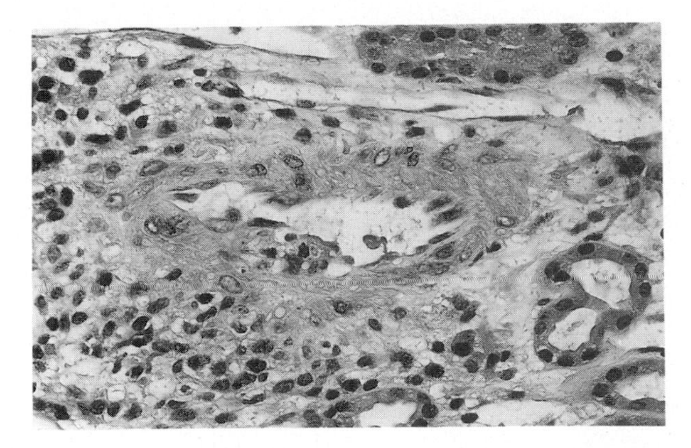

Figure 5 Mild intimal arteritis (v1). Note the focal accumulation of inflammatory cells beneath the intima of this small artery. (H&E, ×400.)

changes in the most involved vessel. Despite its importance as a marker of rejection, however, arteritis is the lesion probably most vulnerable to being missed due to sampling error. Multiple sections must be carefully examined to rule out this process confidently.

With intimal arteritis, endothelial cells are generally enlarged and vacuolated and may be partially or completely detached from the intima. The intima contains edema fluid, matrix material, fibrin, and cells, including infiltrating inflammatory cells and myofibroblasts. Infiltrating cells include lymphocytes, plasma cells, and macrophages. With more severe involvement, cells of the media may become necrotic as the inflammatory process extends to become transmural. Vascular necrosis and thrombosis are features of severe acute rejection graded v3 (see Fig. 6). Infarction, when present as an acute process not dating from the immediate posttransplant period and therefore likely not related to mechanical vascular injury to the graft, can be taken as a reliable marker of severe rejection-related vascular injury.

While many of these vascular changes are quite specific, thrombosis and fibrinoid necrosis in arterioles and small arteries has also been reported as a manifestation of cyclosporine toxicity (43,44) and has occasionally been reported without clinical evidence of rejection in renal allograft patients not receiving cyclosporine (45). Plasma levels of cyclosporine and presence or absence of other features of allograft rejection are helpful in assessing these differential considerations.

Focal hyaline change is occasionally observed in arteries. It appears to have an entirely different significance from similar changes in arterioles (see below). It is sometime seen in continuity with healing intimal arteritis lesions. At least in some instances focal arterial hyaline lesions appear to be a sequel of prior rejection episodes. It may lead eventually to some of the chronic lesions discussed in Sec. IV, below.

Studies of immunohistochemical localization of the vascular cell adhesion molecule VCAM-1 have shown that endothelial cell expression of this molecule may define sites of acute vascular inflammation in renal allograft rejection. However, it is not clear that this finding enhances the diagnosis of rejection above detection of intimal arteritis by light microscopy also, since VCAM expression was increased essentially only in areas with a venulitis or arteritis (46).

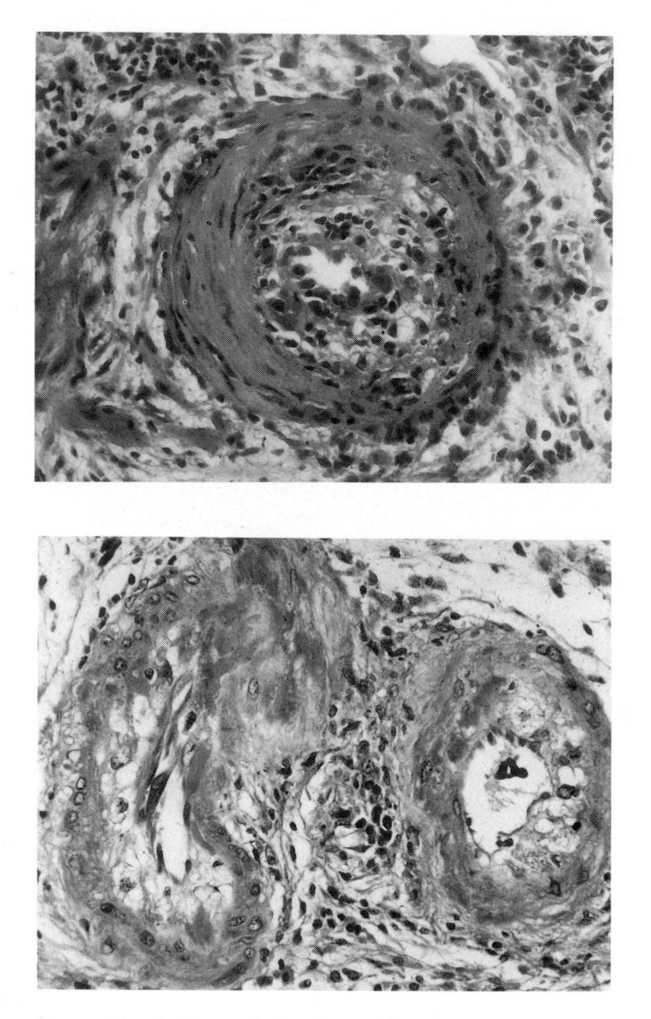

Figure 6 A. Severe intimal arteritis (v3). (H&E, ×400.) B. Fibrinoid necrosis in adjacent vessel. (H&E, ×400.)

Table 5 Quantitative Criteria for Intimal Arteritis ("v") (0 to 3+)

0 = No arteritis
1 = Mild-to-moderate intimal arteritis in at least one arterial cross section
2 = Moderate-to-severe intimal arteritis in at least one arterial cross section
3 = Severe intimal arteritis in at least one arterial cross section and/or "transmural" arteritis, fibrinoid change and medial smooth muscle necrosis, often with patchy infarction and interstitial hemorrhage

Modified from Ref. 1.

2. Arterioles

Occasionally, inflammatory changes in arteries in acute rejection may also be seen in arterioles (and can be graded like the arterial lesions). It is unknown whether this arteriolitis has the same significance as intimal arteritis. An additional feature that may be detected in renal allograft biopsies is the presence of hyaline arteriolar thickening. These lesions are typically PAS-positive and are graded according to severity and extent (see Table 6). If of new onset and especially if occurring in a nodular pattern at the periphery of arterioles, (see Fig. 7) arteriolar hyalinosis lesions are highly suggestive of cyclosporine toxicity (43). These changes may also develop in allografted kidneys, however, with hypertension or diabetes in the recipient. In native kidneys, hyaline change in arterioles is a relatively nonspecific finding which commonly develops as a result of hypertension, diabetes, or aging. Donor kidneys should be biopsied prior to or at the time of implantation to provide a baseline assessment of this and other chronic changes (see below) as well as to rule out hyperacute rejection or other pre-existing disease or injury that may, at least initially, compromise graft function.

IV. SEMIQUANTITATIVE ASSESSMENT OF HISTOLOGICAL CHANGES—CHRONIC

Acute rejection-related changes in the allograft, while interfering with function, are usually treatable with the array of immunosuppressive agents available. Renal allograft loss at the present time is largely due to chronic changes developing in the grafted organ. These chronic changes are also assessed semiquantitatively and are regarded as manifestations of "chronic allograft nephropathy," which may result from a number of processes, including "chronic rejection." Chronic histopathological changes have been detected in systematic biopsies of well-functioning long-term renal allografts as well as in biopsies of grafts with functional impairment; renal functional reserve would presumably be compromised in these kidneys, and these changes are predictive of later graft dysfunction (47). The grading of chronic allograft nephropathy, regardless of underlying causes for the nephropathic changes, is most important for the prediction of long-term graft function and is often important in deciding whether or how to treat any accompanying acute changes in the older allograft.

A. Glomeruli

Chronic glomerular changes that develop in renal allografts have been designated as "chronic transplant glomerulopathy." Changes in the glomerulus include subendothelial widening, mesangial expansion, enlarged endothelial cells, peripheral mesangial interposition, and occasional cellular crescents (14,47–49) (see Fig. 8). Adhesions may form

Table 6 Quantitative Criteria for Arteriolar Hyaline Thickening ("ah") (0 to 3+)

0 = No PAS-positive hyaline thickening
1 = Mild-to-moderate PAS-positive hyaline thickening in at least one arteriole
2 = Moderate-to-severe PAS-positive hyaline thickening in more than one arteriole
3 = Severe PAS-positive hyaline thickening in many artioles

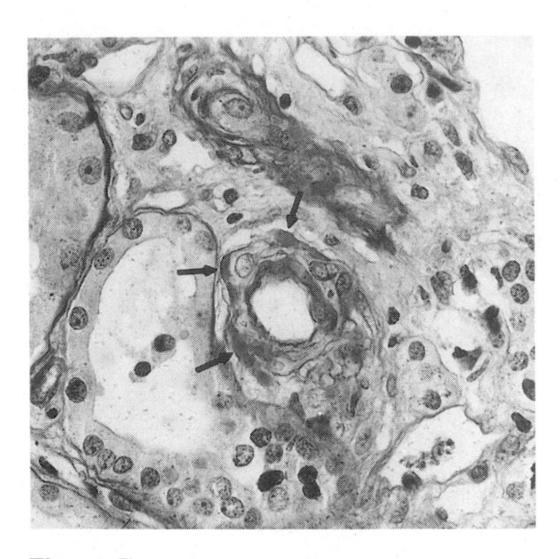

Figure 7 Arteriole with peripheral hyaline nodules (arrows). (PAS, ×300.)

between the glomerular tuft and Bowman's capsule. Periodic acid-Schiff and silver stains may be useful in quantitating mesangial matrix increase and peripheral interposition. Immunofluorescence microscopy may reveal IgM, C_3, and IgG in peripheral capillary loops and mesangial regions, and weak reactions for IgA have also been reported. On electron microscopy, flocculent electron-lucent material may be seen in the widened subendothelial space. This subendothelial widening is also seen in acute rejection. In chronic glomerulopathy in transplants, however, there is a more complex picture, with several types of basement membrane abnormalities. There may also be fine granular electron-dense deposits that may be subendothelial, intramembranous, subepithelial, or mesangial; these are similar in

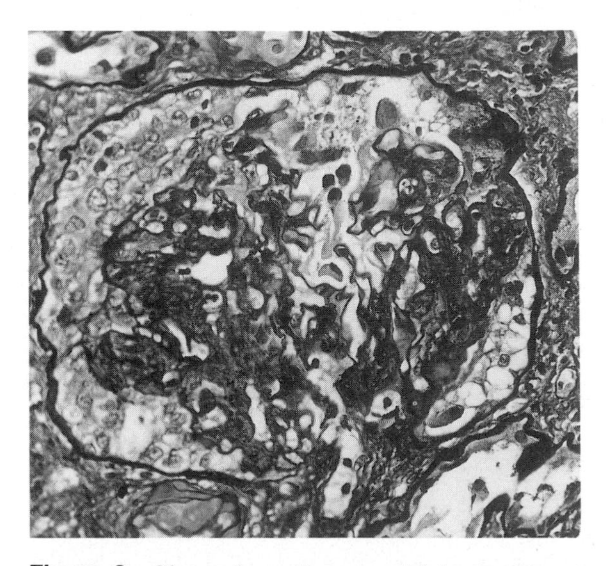

Figure 8 Glomerulus with mesangial interposition, increased mesangial matrix, and crescent formation. (×400.)

appearance to dense deposits of immune complexes (50). If they are numerous, the possibility of a de novo or recurrent glomerulonephritis must be considered. (See below, Sec. V.B.5).

These light microscopic changes are graded as mild, moderate, or severe chronic transplant glomerulopathy based on % of glomeruli showing progressive changes (up to 25% mild, 26–50% moderate >50% severe). While they are assumed to result from chronic immunological injury, the pathogenic mechanisms of these changes are not clear.

Other chronic glomerular changes may be present in the renal allograft. These are most often due to hypertension and/or ischemic changes in allograft vessels. With the use of increasingly older donors, preexisting glomerular sclerosis—usually a bland increase in matrix, collapse of loops, and eventual global scarring—and chronic vascular disease may be present in the donor kidney at the time of grafting (see Fig. 9), and will, of course, persist in the allograft. Many centers do pretransplant biopsies in older donors and/or those with vascular disease to assess the degree of irreversible chronic change. In general, kidneys are considered suitable for transplantation if less than 25% of glomeruli are sclerotic on pretransplant biopsy. In addition to these preexisting changes, late ischemic glomerulopathy with thickening, wrinkling, and collapse of glomerular capillary walls associated with extracapillary fibrotic material may develop in the allografts as occlusive changes develop in allograft vessels due to hypertension, drugs, or "chronic rejection." These glomerular changes are not, directly at least, immune-mediated. While not chronic transplant glomerulopathy in the strictest sense, they are real changes that have implications for allograft function and should be indicated as a % of glomeruli involved.

As discussed below, while glomerular changes tend to correlate with tubulo-interstitial scarring and chronic vascular lesions, they may not. There are grafts that have chronic glomerular changes with no demonstrable vascular lesions, or vice versa; this disassociation may be due in part to sampling error. Moreover, tubular atrophy and interstitial scarring

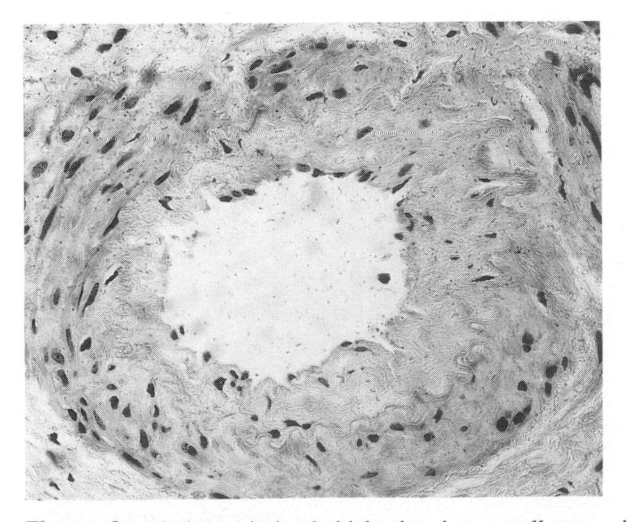

Figure 9 Moderate intimal thickening in a small artery in a biopsy taken immediately after implantation. (H&E, ×400.)

may also be out of proportion to chronic glomerular changes, probably due in part again to sampling error and to the existence of anephric glomeruli. As will be discussed below, it is the tubulointerstitial changes which are used to grade chronic transplant nephropathy, since these latter changes are least susceptible to sampling error and appear to be the best predictor of long-term outcome.

B. Tubulointerstitum

As discussed below, the degree of interstitial fibrosis and tubular atrophy, which almost always correlate very closely, is the critical factor in grading chronic transplant nephropathy. Fibrosis and atrophy are coded semiquantitatively by the extent of chronic changes, varying from mild (ci1 or ct1) to severe (ci3, ct3). A mild grade is assigned when interstitial fibrosis or tubular atrophy involves less than 25% of the parenchyma, moderate with 25 to 50% involvement, and severe when more than 50% of the parenchyma shows these chronic changes. Special stains may be very useful in the quantitation of these changes. In particular, trichrome stains that highlight collagen may help in assessing of interstitial fibrosis, and PAS or silver stains, which preferentially stain tubular basement membranes, may be used to define the thickened and sometimes reduplicated basement membranes surrounding atrophying tubules (Fig. 10). With chronic tubular changes (ct3), actual loss of tubules may occur as atrophy progresses. As with more acute changes, superficial cortical changes reflecting scarring related to perioperative subcapsular injury should be identified as such, if possible, and not graded; such changes do not bode ill for graft survival.

As with glomerular lesions, these chronic tubulointerstitial changes may evolve in the graft secondary to chronic immunologically mediated vascular injury ("chronic rejection"). However, they may also evolve secondary to hypertension- or drug-induced vascular changes or secondary to primary tubulointerstitial processes, including infection, reflux, and drug reactions. More rarely, they may be due to primary glomerular disease in the allograft. In addition, they may be present in the donor kidney, once again emphasizing the

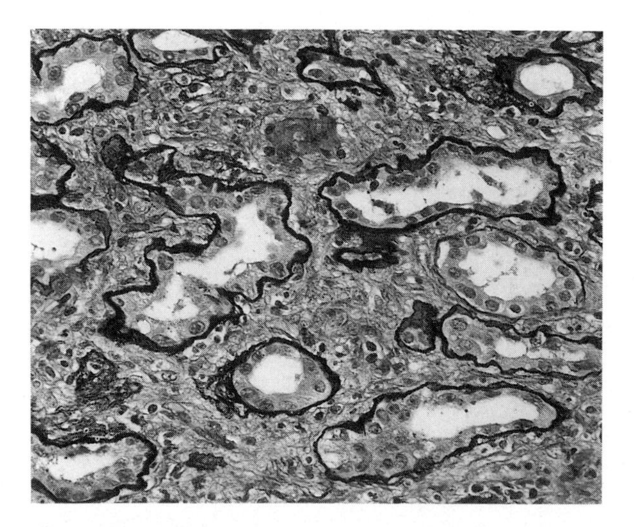

Figure 10 Thickened basement membranes around atrophic tubules. (PAS/MS, ×250.)

importance of a peri-implantation biopsy of the allograft. However, regardless of the cause, these chronic changes have significant implications for graft survival.

C. Vessels

Chronic vascular changes in the renal allograft may be caused by a variety of mechanisms. Repeated episodes of acute rejection, especially with a prominent vascular component, are presumed to lead to chronic vascular changes on an immunological basis, so-called chronic vascular rejection (51–53). In particular, new-onset fibrous intimal thickening is suggestive of chronic rejection (54). However, recipient hypertension must be ruled out, since this process may also produce morphologically identical changes in the arteries. Disruption of the internal elastica may reflect previous inflammatory injury to the vessel. Reduplication of the elastica may also be seen. Grading is based on extent of fibrous intimal thickening in the most involved vessel.

Accelerated arteriosclerosis may be seen in renal allografts, though this lesion is more common in cardiac grafts. In these cases, the intima becomes rapidly thickened with numerous foam cells; occasionally, chronic inflammatory cells may be seen (see Fig. 11). These changes may evolve quickly, within a few months, and lead to relatively rapid graft loss. The etiology of this lesion is unclear but is likely different from the usual mechanisms of arteriosclerosis, since the lesion in kidney as well as in other organs is typically concentric and diffuse (55). This lesion is discussed at length in Chap. 5.

V. THE BANFF WORKING CLASSIFICATION

A. Rejection Diagnosis

Diagnostic categories for renal allograft rejection in the Banff schema are shown in Table 7. As already discussed, the cardinal features used for the diagnosis of acute allograft rejection

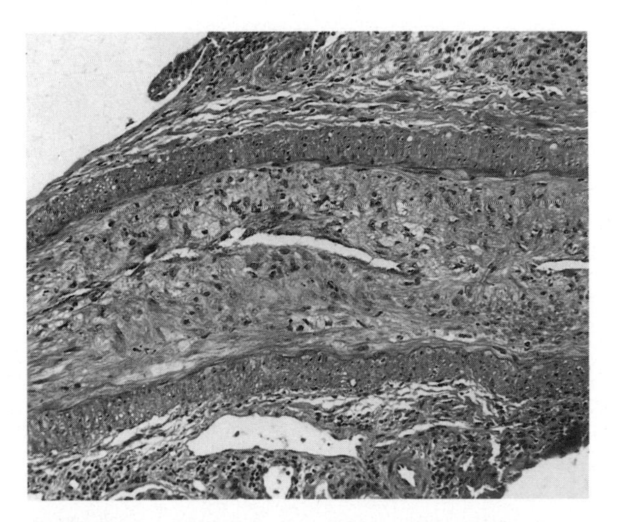

Figure 11 Accelerated atherosclerosis in a biopsy taken less than 4 months post-transplant. There are numerous foam cells and occasional inflammatory cells in the markedly thickened intima. (A. H&E, ×40; B. H&E, ×100.)

Table 7 Diagnostic Categories for Renal Allograft Biopsies

1. Normal
2. Hyperacute rejection (see definitions)
3. Borderline changes ("very mild acute rejection")

   This category is used when no intimal arteritis is present but only mild or moderate focal mononuclear cell infiltration with foci of mild tubulitis (1 to 4 mononucelar cells/tubular cross section).
4. Acute rejection

   Grade I, mild acute rejection

   Cases with significant interstitial infiltration (>25% of parenchyma affected) and foci of moderate tubulitis (>4 mononuclear cells/tubular cross section or group of 10 tubular cells).

   Grade II, moderate acute rejection

   Cases with (A) significant interstitial infiltration and foci of severe tubulitis (>10 mononuclear cells/tubular cross section) and/or (B) mild or moderate intimal arteritis.

   Grade III, severe acute rejection

   Cases with severe intimal arteritis and/or "transmural" arteritis with fibrinoid change and necrosis of medial smooth muscle cells. Recent focal infarction and interstitial hemorrhage without other obvious cause are also regarded as evidence for grade III rejection.
5. Chronic allograft nephropathy

   (Glomerular and vascular lesions help define type of chronic nephropathy; new-onset arterial fibrous intimal thickening suggests the presence of chronic rejection.)

   Grade I — Mild chronic transplant nephropathy
Mild interstitial fibrosis and tubular atrophy

   Grade II — Moderate chronic transplant nephropathy
Moderate interstitial fibrosis and tubular atrophy

   Grade III — Severe chronic transplant nephropathy
Severe interstitial fibrosis and tubular atrophy and tubular loss
6. Other (changes not considered to be due to rejection)

are tubulitis and vasculitis. For chronic transplant nephropathy, severity is graded using tubulointerstitial changes, though glomerular and vascular lesions help define the type and, potentially, etiology of the chronic changes. Each of these categories is discussed briefly.

1. Normal

A normal biopsy is one showing no change or very trivial inflammation or scarring. This category would most often be applied to postimplantation biopsies or protocol biopsies performed in the absence of specific clinical indications.

2. Hyperacute Rejection

Hyperacute rejection occurs very rapidly in the allograft, and morphological changes related to this process are typically seen in the postimplantation biopsy. This form of rejection is due to preformed antibody in a previously sensitized patient and is characterized by polymorphonuclear leukocyte accumulation in glomerular and peritubular capillaries (see Fig. 12). These vessels may be congested, and small thrombi form rapidly as endothelial cell injury ensues. Infarcts of the renal parenchyma then develop, and most of these grafts are lost.

Immunofluorescence stains can demonstrate antibody and complement components in vessels (43,56,57). IgM isohemagglutinins are deposited with ABO incompatibility, while antibodies from presensitization to HLA-A or B antigens are largely IgG (43). Rarely,

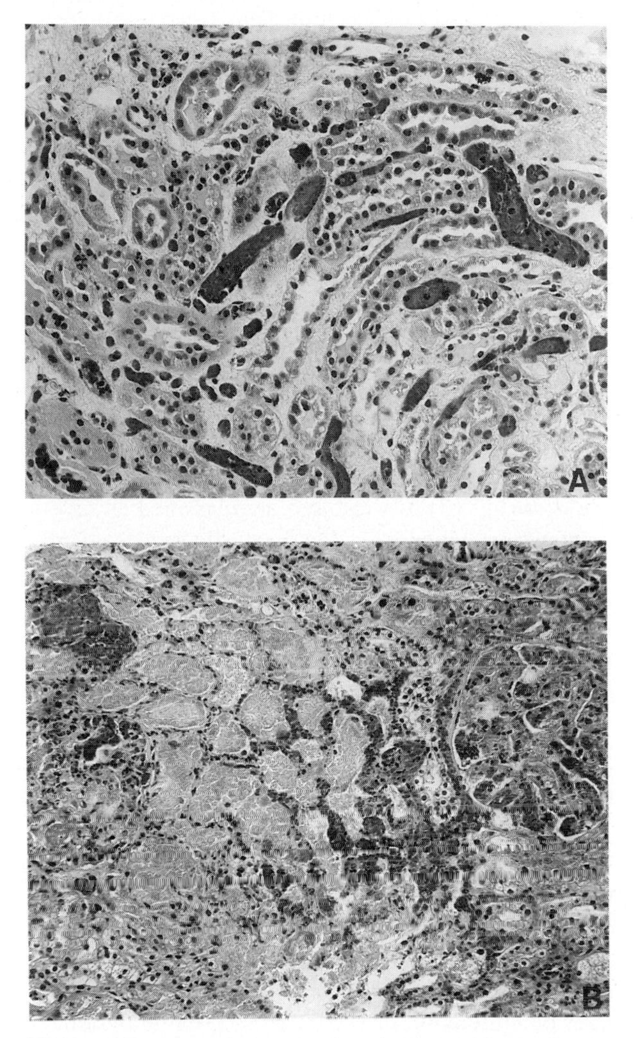

Figure 12 Hyperacute rejection. A. Congestion and numerous polymorphonuclear leukocytes in peritubular capillaries in implantation biopsy. (H&E, ×250.) B. Biopsy taken several days later, showing parenchymal infarction. (H&E, ×160.)

preexisting antibodies to class II MHC antigens (HLA-DR, DQ) have been reported to cause hyperacute or accelerated acute rejection (see Chap. 2), with deposition in arterioles in some of these cases. Activation of complement can occur even with low levels of antibody and may be more reliably identified in allograft vessels than is antibody itself (25,58,59). Fibrinogen may be detected in capillaries as well.

3. Borderline Changes

Synonyms for this category include "very mild acute rejection" and "consistent with early acute rejection." By definition, no intimal arteritis is present. Accompanying a mild or moderate focal interstitial inflammatory infiltrate there is a mild tubulitis (t1). Since well-functioning grafts may show mild tubulitis (t1), this biopsy finding is not in itself an indication for antirejection therapy. However, in the presence of suggestive clinical features of rejection, therapy may be warranted in individual cases.

4. *Acute Rejection*

The changes of acute rejection are assigned to grades I, II, or III (mild, moderate, and severe rejection).

In grade I acute rejection, there is a moderate tubulitis (t2) accompanied by a significant interstitial infiltrate (i2 or i3). The likely clinical response to this finding would be to treat for rejection unless there are no clinical signs.

Moderate acute rejection, grade II, is divided into IIA and IIB, depending on the absence or presence of arteritis. In grade IIA, there is severe tubulitis (t3) with a significant interstitial infiltrate; in grade IIB, there is mild to moderate intimal arteritis (v1 or v2). With these findings on biopsy, the patient should be treated for rejection. If the patient does not respond to steroids, OKT3/ALG should be considered.

When the biopsy reveals severe intimal arteritis and/or transmural arteritis, fibrinoid change, and/or medial smooth muscle necrosis (v3), the changes are classified as severe acute rejection. There may be patchy infarction and/or interstitial hemorrhage as well, and occasionally these latter changes are found without identifying a vascular lesion. If the infarction is new and correlates with clinical signs of rejection, this may be adequate for diagnosis. The patient should be treated aggressively unless the clinical course suggests that the rejection may be irreversible. It has been shown that if infarcts and/or glomerular thrombosis and/or arterial or arteriolar thrombosis were present in a graft biopsy as new findings not dating from the time of transplantation, 100% of affected grafts were lost within 1 year (60).

5. *Chronic Allograft Nephropathy*

As noted above, 90% or more of renal allografts survive for 1 year, despite occasional episodes of acute rejection. It is now the chronic changes, which appear to occur inevitably in many allografts if followed over time, that produce graft loss (61–63). Sometimes chronic changes evolving in the graft are superimposed on preexisting chronic changes present in the donor kidney at the time of transplantation. Implantation biopsy helps define these baseline changes, enabling better determination of progression in the allograft recipient.

In native kidney diseases of various etiologies, including primary glomerular diseases, it is the degree of interstitial scarring and tubular atrophy on biopsy that determines long-term prognosis. This strong correlation is probably due to the fact that biopsies generally capture a great deal of tubulointerstitium, with relatively few glomeruli and even fewer vessels. These same considerations are important in the renal allograft. Therefore, chronic transplant nephropathy is graded on the basis of extent of interstitial fibrosis and tubular atrophy—changes that almost invariably correlate strongly with each other.

In grade I, mild chronic allograft nephropathy, there are mild tubulointerstital changes (ct1, ci1). Moderate chronic change, grade II, shows intermediate changes (ct2, ci2), with 25 to 50% of the parenchyma showing interstitial fibrosis and tubular atrophy. With extension to greater than 50% of the biopsied parenchyma (ct3, ci3), this process is graded as severe, grade III.

As discussed above, a number of processes may converge to produce scarring in the renal allograft. These include vascular disease (immunological or nonimmunological), hypertension, drug toxicity, and reflux/obstruction.

B. Pathological Findings Not Related to Rejection

1. *Posttransplant Lymphoproliferative Disorder*

While uncommon posttransplant, this disorder is an important entity to be distinguished from rejection, and is placed first among differential diagnoses. Early identification of posttransplant lymphoproliferative disorder (PTLD) is critical for patient management. Previously, this disorder was believed not to occur until months to years after transplantation (64). Recently, however, it has been reported considerably earlier, sometimes within weeks of allografting (64–66).

Histologically, PTLD is characterized by a monomorphous or polymorphous infiltrate containing plasma cells, which are usually atypical. There is typically a diffuse interstitial infiltrate (i3) in the absence of concomitant rejection and significant tubulitis or vasculitis. However, the two processes, PTLD and rejection, may coincide. In PTLD, cells in the interstitial infiltrate express B-cell markers, and in situ hybridization or other molecular probes for EBV antigen are almost invariably positive.

The pathology of this disorder is described at length in Chap. 12.

2. *Nonspecific Changes*

There are a variety of changes in renal allograft biopsies that may accompany rejection but in themselves are not diagnostic or even strongly suggestive of rejection. These include nonspecific inflammatory changes and nonspecific vascular changes.

As noted above, focal nodular inflammatory infiltrates and perivascular aggregates of inflammatory cells, especially near the corticomedullary junction, are common findings in allograft kidneys. In the absence of an associated tubulitis (i.e., t0), these changes must be regarded as nonspecific, since they may be seen in well-functioning grafts. If associated with mild tubulitis (t1), these infiltrates would be considered borderline for rejection.

Several vascular changes may also be seen in well-functioning grafts and must be considered nonspecific. These include endothelial reactive changes without true endotheliolitis—i.e., without invasion of inflammatory cells beneath the endothelial cells into the intima. These reactive changes simply reflect endothelial injury or activation; possible causes include ischemia and drug reaction as well as rejection. Vacuolization of smooth muscle cells in the vessel wall may be seen—a change that is nonspecific, reflecting prolonged vasoconstriction and/or drug effect. Venulitis is seen whenever there is trafficking of inflammatory cells into the allograft; as noted, inflammatory infiltrates are commonly seen in allografts whether or not rejection is present.

3. *Acute Tubular Necrosis*

Acute tubular cell injury is very common in the allografted kidney and is a major cause of primary nonfunction of the allograft. Tubular injury may result from in situ injury in the donor; ischemia during harvesting, storage, and transport of the organ; and/or ischemic injury incurred perioperatively in the recipient. The morphology is similar to that of acute tubular cell injury in the native kidney. Histological changes include loss and nonreplacement of tubular cells, cell necrosis, and regenerative changes (see Fig. 13). There may be accompanying interstitial edema and a mild inflammatory infiltrate (i1), but there should be no or only trivial tubulitis. As in native kidneys, there may be accumulation of nucleated cells in the vasa recta of the outer medulla as well. Other changes may include tubular cell vacuolization and blebbing, and tubular dilation reflecting distal tubular obstruction.

While the morphology of acute tubular injury in native and allograft kidneys is similar, there are some differences as well. We have found more extensive tubular cell necrosis, less

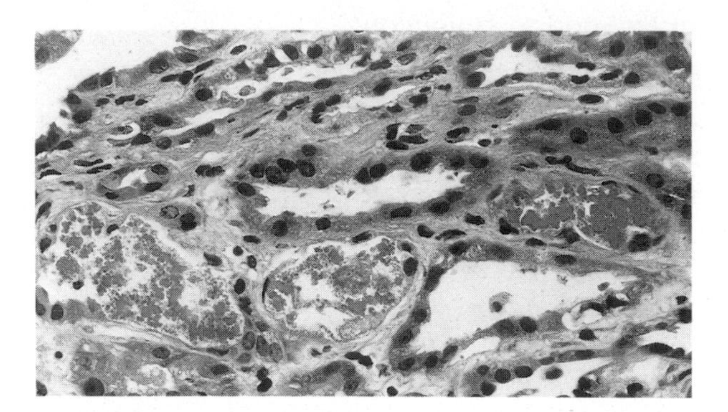

Figure 13 Early posttransplant biopsy showing frank necrosis of tubular cells. (H&E, ×400.)

loss of apical microvilli and basolateral infoldings, and more numerous deposits of calcium oxalate in allograft tubular cell injury compared to native kidney (3). Differences are likely due to important differences in flow, temperature during ischemia time, and other factors.

4. *Acute Interstitial Nephritis*

Non-rejection-related interstitial nephritis may occur in allografts and may be very difficult to differentiate from the rejection response. Neutrophils in an interstitial inflammatory infiltrate and/or leukocyte casts suggest the possibility of infection, and eosinophils could signal a hypersensitivity reaction, perhaps due to drugs. Unfortunately, however, neutrophils and/or eosinophils may be quite numerous in the infiltrates of acute rejection, as noted above. The presence of significant tubulitis and/or vasculitis would strongly suggest rejection but does not necessarily rule out infection or drug reactions, which may occur concomitant with rejection. It is probably best to raise this differential if the interstitial inflammatory infiltrate is not largely mononuclear.

5. *Cyclosporine-Associated Changes*

Cyclosporine-associated changes in the renal allograft may be acute or chronic. They may mimic, to some extent, rejection-related changes, especially in the older allograft, and may, of course, be coincident with rejection.

Tubular cell changes associated with cyclosporine administration are not necessarily a manifestation of cyclosporine *toxicity*, since they may be seen with administration of the parenteral vehicle for cyclosporine in experimental animals (67). Tubular cell changes include vacuolization and especially isometric vacuolization, eosinophilic inclusions in tubular cells, and microfilaments aggregated in the cytoplasm.

There are a range of vascular changes described with cyclosporine (43,67), changes that are important in the pathogenesis of cyclosporine toxicity. These include marked vasoconstriction, which may result in occlusion of arterioles and smooth muscle vacuolization. Progressive injury to the vessel wall leads to necrosis and hyalinosis of individual muscle cells and nodular hyaline afferent arteriolar deposits, which have recently been shown to be renin-rich. These hyaline changes in their most typical form are nodular and peripheral in the arteriole (see Fig. 7), but the entire arteriolar wall may be replaced by hyaline material; hyaline arteriolar change related to cyclosporine can usually be confidently diagnosed only if an early peri-implantation biopsy is available from which to judge preexisting arteriolar hyaline change. In older transplants, similar changes may arise with hypertension or diabetes in the donor. A mucoid intimal thickening in arterioles may occasionally be seen. Finally, cyclosporine may rarely produce a thrombotic microangiopathy, which may be devastating to the allograft.

Interstitial fibrosis has been described as a late sequel of cyclosporine therapy (43,68–70) and is likely the result of ischemia due to chronic vasoconstriction. This chronic change and chronic vascular changes produced by the drug may contribute to the picture of chronic transplant nephropathy. Glomerular sclerosis or ischemic collapse and juxtaglomerular apparatus hyperplasia may also be seen with chronic cyclosporine therapy. Pathological changes produced by cyclosporine and other immunosuppressive agents are discussed in detail and illustrated other chapters.

6. *Subcapsular Injury*

Subcapsular injury may occur at the time of transplantation of the allograft, related to ischemia with loss of capsular blood supply. This process results in acute inflammatory changes and later chronic scarring. Localization to the superficial cortex and absence of other evidence of rejection should enable differentiation from rejection-related changes.

7. *Pretransplant Acute Endothelial Injury*

Pretransplant endothelial injury was historically seen in kidneys perfused prior to transplantation. The histological changes seen included capillary thrombosis, ischemic change, and ultimate infarction in severe cases. This form of injury often led to reduced graft function and, in some cases, graft loss (71). With current preservation methods, this lesion is rarely seen in severe form. Focal glomerular thrombi, presumably due to endothelial injury during harvesting/preservation, no longer portend significant graft dysfunction (72).

8. *Papillary Necrosis*

Rarely, papillary necrosis may be seen in allografted kidneys. If such necrosis is extensive, graft loss invariably ensues.

9. *De Novo Glomerular Disease*

Various types of de novo glomerular diseases occur in allografted kidneys. In many cases, these occur with no greater frequency than in native kidneys; however, a few occur with significantly increased frequency in allografts.

The most common de novo glomerular disease is membranous nephropathy, reported in approximately 1 to 2% of grafts (73,74). Histological evaluation may reveal both the thickened capillary loops and increased mesangial matrix seen in membranous nephropathy and associated rejection and/or vascular changes. There is IgG and C_3 in capillary loops by immunofluroscence and subepithelial dense deposits on electron microscopy (see Fig. 14). It has been postulated that this immune glomerulopathy is produced by a humoral immune response to allograft antigen(s) (75).

Other de novo glomerular diseases that may occur in special circumstances in allografts are anti-GBM disease and acute immune complex glomerulonephritis secondary to administration of antilymphocyte serum. Anti-GBM disease may occur when patients with Alport's disease, who develop glomerular disease due to absence of a normal collagen constituent in the glomerular basement membrane (76,77), receive allografted normal kidneys that contain this antigen. In some of these individuals, a humoral response to this antigen may develop. Anti-GBM antibodies may be detected in the serum of these patients;

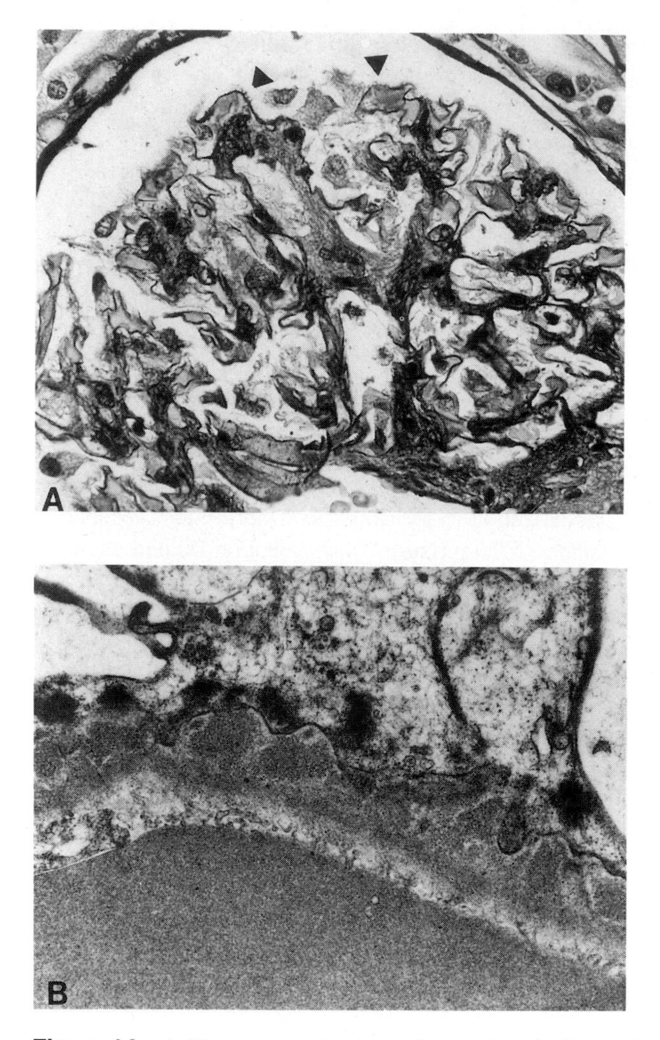

Figure 14 A. De novo membranous glomerulopathy in a patient 3 years after renal transplant. The patient's original disease was IgA nephropathy. Note silver-positive "spikes" (arrowheads). (PAS/MS, ×500.) B. Subepithelial deposits on electron micrograph. (×26,470.)

the renal allograft in these cases may continue to function normally, but a typical crescentic glomerulonephritis with graft loss may occur (78,79), and recurrent anti-GBM disease has been reported in a subsequent allograft (80).

The glomerulonephritis produced by antilymphocyte serum protein/antibody produces a picture analogous to that of acute serum sickness. There is glomerular hypercellularity, and subepithelial immune deposits are seen by immunofluorescence and electron microscopy.

10. Recurrent Disease

Recurrent disease is a significant cause of late allograft dysfunction and should be separated from rejection-related changes. Recurrent disease can, of course, be diagnosed with confidence only when the patient's original disease has been well documented.

Immune complex glomerulonephritis may recur in allografted kidneys. Of these, type II membranoproliferative glomerulonephritis and IgA nephropathy have the highest recurrence rate (81). Membranoproliferative glomerulonephritis (MPGN) and chronic transplant glomerulopathy, described above, may be very difficult to differentiate by light microscopy. Immunofluorescence microscopy, however, should reveal peripheral glomerular staining for C_3 and characteristic deposits by electron microscopy in type I MPGN. With type II MPGN, the distinctive ribbonlike intramembranous deposits are easily identified. In type I MPGN, however, the subepithelial deposits may be sparse, and since rare densities may be seen in transplant glomerulopathy, the differential diagnosis may be difficult; it has been suggested that peripheral staining for C_3 on immunofluorescence should be used to diagnose MPGN in this setting (15). Membranous nephropathy recurs in renal allografts in 3 to 7% of cases but is less common than the de novo membranous nephropathy described above (82,83).

Focal segmental glomerulosclerosis with hyalinosis recurs commonly in renal allografts, with a frequency of from 20 to 100% (81). Recurrence is most likely in younger patients who had rapid progression to end stage (less than 3 years) in their native kidney (84,85). If there is recurrence in an initial allograft, there is a substantially increased risk of recurrence in subsequent allografts (86,87). Light microscopy of recurrent FSGSH has demonstrated an early focal segmental proliferation, which may have a predominance of epithelial cells, followed by typical segmental sclerosis with hyalinosis (88,89) (see Fig. 15).

Anti-GBM disease recurs with clinical symptoms in approximately 25% of patients, but graft loss is rare. Pauci-immune crescentic glomerulonephritis may also recur and may lead to graft loss (90).

There are a variety of systemic diseases that produce pathological changes in the kidney and may produce recurrent disease in the renal allograft. These include Henoch-Schönlein purpura, hemolytic uremic syndrome, amyloidosis, Wegener's granulomatosis, cryoglobulinemia, monoclonal gammopathies, lupus nephritis, and diabetes. Most of these

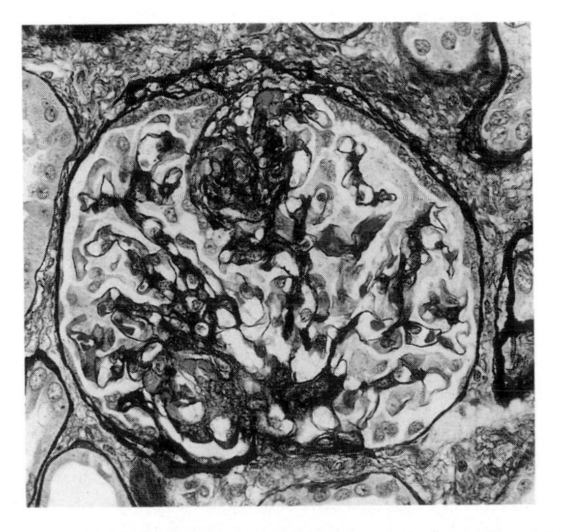

Figure 15 Focal segmental glomerulosclerosis with hyalinosis (FSGSH) 6 months posttransplant in a patient with a rapidly progressive FSGSH in his native kidney. At transplant nephrectomy 18 months posttransplant, many glomeruli showed characteristic lesions of FSGSH. (PAS/MS, ×400.)

recur at rates of 5 to 30% and lead to graft loss relatively rarely; hemolytic uremic syndrome has the highest incidence of graft loss, 40 to 50%. Lupus nephritis recurs rarely (<1% of cases). While diabetic nephropathy occurs in essentially all patients with time, the disease rarely leads to graft loss. In general, the histology of these diseases in the allograft is similar to that in native kidneys. However, diabetic changes progress slowly, so that while thickened glomerular basement membranes, increased mesangial matrix, and arteriolar hyaline change may be seen, full-blown Kimmelsteil-Wilson nodules are rare in renal allografts. The microangiopathic changes of hemolytic uremic syndrome may be mimicked or exacerbated by both cyclosporine and antilymphocytic globulin (ALG), as well as by malignant hypertension and severe acute allograft rejection; these factors should be considered in interpreting microangiopathic changes in the allograft.

Nonglomerular diseases may also recur in the allograft. Most of these—including Alport's syndrome, progressive systemic sclerosis, sickle cell nephropathy, and Fabry's disease—recur with low incidence. Oxalosis, however, historically has recurred in 90 to 100% of grafts and led to graft loss in many; current strategies to deplete oxalate stores and/or provide the absent enzyme or cofactors to prevent oxalate overproduction and deposition in the allograft (91) have improved this bleak prognosis.

11. Preexisting Disease

Disease in the donor kidney may have important effects on allograft function following grafting and must be defined in order to interpret pathological changes in the allografted kidney accurately. In particular, chronic changes may preexist in kidneys from older donors (92), which are being utilized more and more frequently for transplantation. These changes of "nephrosclerosis"—which include glomerulosclerosis, intimal fibrous thickening in arteries and hyaline arteriolar change, and associated interstitial fibrosis and tubular atrophy and are related to age-related vascular disease and/or hypertension—must be assessed in a peri-implantation biopsy, so that pathological changes in subsequent biopsies can be interpreted adequately. Kidneys from diabetic patients are also being harvested and transplanted at some centers, and these, too, should be evaluated histologically for baseline assessment at the time of engraftment.

Other preexisting diseases, especially glomerular diseases, may also be detected in the allograft. This is a particular problem in areas where certain disease are endemic, such as IgA nephropathy and hepatitis B–associated glomerulonephritis in the Orient.

12. Other

Included in this category are a variety of processes that may have important effects on the allograft and may be diagnosed, or at least suggested, by pathological findings on biopsy of the graft.

Bland infarction on biopsy early posttransplant in the absence of evidence of rejection, which may also lead to thrombosis and infarction (see above), may be the result of arterial or venous thrombosis in the graft due to mechanical injury and/or postoperative hypotension. Small segmental infarcts have little impact on allograft function; large infarcts may lead to graft loss. Severe congestion and/or hemorrhagic infarction suggest venous occlusion. It has been reported that fresh infarcts or thrombosis of vessels on biopsy predicts early graft loss (91). Infarcts or thrombosis in very early biopsies, however, which are unlikely to be rejection-related, do not preclude a good graft outcome (93). Absence of collateral circulation in the allograft may modify the typical appearance of infarcts in this setting (94).

Viral infections, to which these immunosuppressed patients are vulnerable, may involve the allografted kidney. Of these, CMV is the most prevalent. Most commonly, CMV is associated with focal mononuclear infiltrates, with some evidence for a preponderance of $CD8^+$ T lymphocytes (95). Cytomegalovirus inclusions may occasionally be seen within tubular cells. Rarely, there is associated tubular damage and atrophy (96). Occasionally, CMV inclusions have been reported in glomerular endothelial and epithelial cells and vascular endothelium as well (97). We have also seen CMV in the wall of the allograft ureter. Epstein-Barr virus–associated B-cell lymphoproliferative disorder may be detected as a graft infiltrate; this entity is described at length above. Finally, stricture of the graft ureter may result from infection with polyomavirus (98). Detection of virus in the allografted kidney or ureter is enhanced by immunostaining and in situ hybridization techniques.

Finally, ureteric complications in the transplanted kidney may produce pathological changes. With obstruction and reflux, tubular dilation, extravasated Tamm-Horsfall protein, interstitial edema, and a bland inflammatory infiltrate may be seen. It is likely that in occasional patients, slowly developing strictures may contribute to the chronic tubulointerstitial changes denoted as chronic transplant nephropathy in the Banff classification scheme.

VI. REPRODUCIBILITY OF THE BANFF CLASSIFICATION

As with any classification system, the value of this schema hinges on reproducibility among pathologists and ultimately on biological significance and clinical relevance.

Even before the Banff classification was finalized, preliminary studies were under way to assess the reproducibility of the schema. This early study was expanded to an international group of five pathologists who had helped to develop the schema. These individuals scored early renal allograft biopsies for acute histopathological findings according to the Banff classification, assessing interobserver and intraobserver variability over a range of specimens. The results of this study have been published (99) and are discussed here. Several other, similar studies are currently under way, assessing reproducibility and comparing use of the schema to assessment methods in place at each institution.

A. Methods

Seventy-seven early graft biopsies, including a range of histopathological findings, were selected for inclusion in the studies. All biopsies were performed and processed at the Aarhus Kommunehospital from 1989 to 1991; all biopsies were obtained less than 90 days posttransplant. All specimens were adequate by the Banff criteria (see above). The biopsies were scored by the Banff schema by five pathologists who had no knowledge of results of scoring by the other pathologists or of clinical information or graft outcome. In addition to semiquantitative scoring and rejection grading, morphometric analysis was performed on the interstitial inflammatory infiltrate using a projecting microscope and a point-counting system.

Kappa analysis was used for statistical evaluation of reproducibility (100). This analytical method corrects for observer agreement by chance, and is, therefore, a rigorous assessment of true agreement. In addition to standard kappa analysis, weighted kappa analysis was also applied. This analysis weights disagreements according to how serious a deviation from exact agreement they are considered to be (101,102). For example, the difference in grading between observers of "normal" versus "grade 2 rejection" is more severe than a difference in grading of "normal" versus "borderline." Discrepancies in assessing the presence or absence of vasculitis were also given greater weight because this feature is so critical for rejection diagnosis. Table 8 shows the weighting scheme devised for these studies.

Interobserver associations were calculated as the probability that a randomly selected case assigned to a specific category by one pathologist would be assigned to the same category by a second randomly selected pathologist. Intraobserver statistics were calculated for all five lesions for the two pathologists who scored all the cases twice.

B. Results

The interobserver statistics for the five observers for the scoring of vasculitis and tubulitis and the grading of rejection are shown in Table 9; the interobserver associations and kappa values for vasculitis scoring and rejection grading are shown in Table 10. For vasculitis scoring, the best reproducibility is seen for v0 and v3, with probabilities of 0.86 and 0.51 and corresponding kappa values of 0.64 and 0.46. Probabilities of agreement of rejection grading varied from 0.29 (kappa 0.24) for grade I to 0.68 (kappa 0.51) for grade II. Weighted kappa values, calculated for vasculitis scoring and rejection grade, were 0.58 and 0.55 respectively. As might be expected, intraobserver agreement was generally higher than interobserver agreement. For both inter- and intraobserver agreement, the best reproducibility was obtained for v and i scores, with less good values for g and t scores. There was good correlation between semiquantitative scoring of interstitial inflammation and morphometric assessment of the volume fraction of inflammatory infiltrate in the cortex.

C. Discussion

While there are no objective criteria for the interpretation of the kappa (κ) value, in general a κ value above 0.60 is considered excellent and below 0.20 poor (103). The reproducibility of various histopathological parameters in the Banff classification varied from 0.18 to 0.47.

Table 8 Weighting of Disagreement Between Two Observers for Intimal Arteritis and Rejection Grading (Values Used for Estimation of Weighted Kappa)

Intimal arteritis:	Score by first observer			
Score by second observer	0	1	2	3
0	0	4	5	6
1	4	0	1	2
2	5	1	0	1
3	6	2	1	0

Rejection grading:	Score by first observer				
Score by second observer	Normal	Borderline	Grade 1	Grade 2	Grade 3
Normal	0	1	3	4	5
Borderline	1	0	2	3	4
Grade 1	3	2	0	1	2
Grade 2	4	3	1	0	1
Grade 3	5	4	2	1	0

Table 9 Interobserver Agreement, Reproducibility (Kappa Values), and Spearman's Correlation Coefficient (Rho) for the 77 Biopsies Scored by Five Observers

	Overall agreement	Kappa	Kappa (95% confidence limits)	Rho[a]
g	0.48	0.26	0.22–0.31	0.64
i	0.54	0.33	0.29–0.38	0.79
t	0.53	0.35	0.31–0.40	0.69
v	0.70	0.47	0.42–0.52	0.75
ah	0.57	0.18	0.13–0.24	0.58
Rejection grade	0.55	0.40	0.36–0.44	0.62

[a]Rho values are calculated as the mean of all pairwise correlations.

For tubulitis and vasculitis, the critical features upon which the diagnosis of rejection is based, values were 0.35 and 0.47 respectively and the κ value for final rejection grading was 0.40. These values are adequate but leave room for improvement. The lowest agreement was found with grading of glomerulitis and arteriolar hyalinosis, parameters not used for diagnosing or grading rejection in the Banff classification.

As noted, the kappa method is a very stringent test of reproducibility. The weighted kappa statistic, which allows distinction between categorical and subcategorical disagreement, was also applied to these data, using a reasonable though arbitrary weighting scheme

Table 10 Interobserver Associations and Chance Corrected Associations (Kappa, in parentheses) Between the Five Pathologists[a]

Vasculitis (v):

Assignment of first observer	Assignment of second observer: 0	1	2	3
0	0.86 (0.64)	0.10 (−0.12)	0.01 (−0.08)	0.03 (−0.09)
1	0.31 (0.79)	0.46 (0.32)	0.15 (0.08)	0.08 (−0.02)
2	0.09 (−1.34)	0.37 (0.21)	0.33 (0.27)	0.21 (0.12)
3	0.16 (−1.18)	0.16 (−0.05)	0.17 (0.09)	0.51 (0.46)

Rejection grade:

Assignment of first observer	Assignment of second observer: Normal	Borderline	Grade I	Grade 2	Grade 3
Normal	0.54 (0.40)	0.31 (0.05)	0.01 (−0.06)	0.12 (−0.33)	0.02 (−0.08)
Borderline	0.25 (0.04)	0.50 (0.31)	0.11 (0.05)	0.10 (−0.36)	0.04 (−0.07)
Grade 1	0.02 (−0.26)	0.47 (0.27)	0.29 (0.24)	0.22 (−0.19)	0 (−0.10)
Grade 2	0.08 (−0.18)	0.09 (−0.26)	0.04 (−0.02)	0.68 (0.51)	0.11 (0.02)
Grade 3	0.05 (−0.23)	0.10 (−0.24)	0 (−0.07)	0.40 (0.09)	0.44 (0.39)

[a]The table shows the probability that after the first observer has scored or graded a given case, a second person who observes randomly will give the same case the same score or grade. The corresponding kappa values are shown in brackets. The sum of each row equals 1.

(see Table 8). As summarized, κ values for vasculitis and rejection grading were substantially improved by this analysis. Reduction of grading categories to "no acute rejection" versus "acute rejection" improved interobserver agreement to 0.78, κ value 0.56; "no or mild rejection" versus "moderate-to-severe rejection" resulted in agreement of 0.81 and a κ value of 0.62.

It is clear that while reproducibility of the Banff classification is adequate, improvements can be made. Formulation of more precise definitions and description of criteria should improve agreement. Based on a small study in which tubulitis was assessed on each of four sections on the same slide by a single observer, it is important to assess all sections on every slide to ensure complete agreement. There will always be a potential problem with observer interpretation, as analysis of reproducibility of the cardiac allograft rejection schema revealed. For example, in the Banff classification, an infarct that one observer ascribes to a non-rejection-related vascular accident and graded v0 may be interpreted by another as a sign of severe rejection, and graded v3. Once again, precise definitions and descriptions may ultimately prevent such discrepancies.

Overall, the Banff classification is fairly reproducible, comparing well with other pathology schema that have been evaluated in this way (104–108). Continued refinement of the classification, other reproducibility studies that are currently under way, and clinical validation studies will all contribute to improvement and eventual finalization of these diagnostic criteria.

VII. CLINICAL VALIDATION OF THE BANFF CLASSIFICATION

The Banff classification is new, and a number of clinical validation studies are just getting under way using the schema. Hansen et al. have published in abstract form a study assessing rejection grading using the schema and corresponding 1/2-year and 1-year renal allograft survivals (109).

A. Models

The study was retrospective, and involved 105 renal transplants biopsied at the Aarhus Kommunehospital during 1989 to July 1991. A total of 320 graft biopsies were performed on these kidneys. Biopsies were done routinely (a) at 3 weeks after transplant, (b) at weekly intervals with graft dysfunction, and (c) weekly in grafts with primary nonfunction. For analysis, patients were divided into two groups, those with no rejection therapy (A), and those treated for rejection (B). The two groups were comparable with regard to age, sex, incidence of retransplant and living related donor transplants, and presence of circulating anti-class I and anti-class II antibodies.

Biopsies were blinded and retrospectively analyzed by the Banff criteria. When more than one biopsy was taken, the most severe changes were used to calculate survival.

B. Results

In group A (no rejection treatment), three grafts with grade 0 changes were lost by 1 year due to patient death from complications of immunosuppression; these patients died with functioning grafts. Three grafts with grade 0 changes were lost in group B as well, again with no histological evidence of rejection at the time of graft nephrectomy or patient death of complications. In contrast, with grade II or grade III changes in the graft, one third of grafts lost function by one year. Results are summarized in Table 11.

Table 11 Severity of Rejection Grade Related to One-Half and 1 Year Graft Survival

Banff class	N	Graft function ½ Year	1 Year
Grade 0	52	47	46
Grade I	8	8	8
Grade II	37	26	25
Grade III	4	2	2
Not classified	4	4	4

C. Discussion

These early results suggest a trend toward clinical relevance of the Banff grading schema. The numbers are small in this preliminary study of validation of the Banff classification. Patients are continuing to accrue, however, in this and other studies designed to assess the clinical validation of the classification. Results from more definitive studies of the schema, in its current form and in modified form, are forthcoming from a number of centers.

VIII. FUTURE DIRECTIONS

Assessment of renal allograft biopsies to detect rejection, define the nature of the process, and/or predict outcome remains an evolving process. There are a number of areas that must be more carefully defined and some new observations that may have to be integrated into the diagnostic schema.

The Banff working classification for diagnosing and grading rejection is currently undergoing testing and reassessment. Based on initial reproducibility studies of acute allograft changes, assessment of glomerulitis and arteriolar hyalinosis have proven to have high interobserver variation. Since these changes are not used to diagnose or grade rejection, they could potentially be dropped from the semiquantitative coding system, or, alternatively, be defined more carefully to reduce discrepancies in grading between observers. Tubulitis, a finding that is essential to the diagnosis and grading of rejection, must also achieve better reproducibility; staining of multiple sections with PAS and/or silver stains and/or immunohistochemical staining to better enumerate intraepithelial inflammatory cells should enhance agreement among observers.

Immunohistology and/or molecular biology may ultimately prove pivotal in defining a rejection process in the renal allograft. As noted above, identification of cytotoxic effector cells—by cell surface markers and/or expression of characteristic enzymes and/or other gene products (21,31–37)—has already been shown to correlate with acute rejection in the graft. Detection of expression of growth factors, cytokines, and their receptors will likely also ultimately prove to be important tools in diagnosing rejection (110). Enhanced expression of adhesion molecules in tubules and vascular endothelium has been detected in acute rejection (36,37,46). However, it remains unclear whether expression of ICAM or VCAM, which correlate with inflammatory changes in the biopsy, adds significantly to histological observations made on routinely prepared sections. Moreover, expression of these adhesion molecules may be seen not only in rejection but also with ischemic injury, for example, and may not be as specifically useful for ruling in rejection in the early posttransplant setting.

Defining the mechanisms underlying a specific rejection process is an area not addressed by the Banff classification in its current form. It is hoped that further studies of the molecular biology of humoral, cell-, and antibody-mediated cell cytotoxicity-mediated rejection processes will enable us to identify morphological and molecular correlates of these processes confidently. In the current formulation, emphasis is on a "typical" cell-mediated process. However, the presence of intracapillary and/or intratubular polymorphonuclear leukocytes and potentially vascular deposition of C_3 with or without immunoglobulin suggests a possible antibody-mediated component of rejection, though other processes, and especially infection, should be ruled out.

While acute rejection grading is being rigorously tested for reproducibility and clinical validity, assessment of chronic changes awaits testing. As noted, it is clearly chronic changes that will determine ultimate outcome of most allografts. It is hoped that the relatively straightforward semiquantitative assessment used in the schema to grade "chronic transplant nephropathy" will provide clinically useful prognostic information. Using a more complex "chronic allograft damage index," Isoniemi et al. have found that chronic changes at 2 years in normally functioning grafts were predictive of functional impairment at 4 years posttransplant (47).

Newly recognized lesions that may have prognostic significance in the renal allograft involve the peritubular capillaries. Peritubular capillary basement membrane splitting and lamination, detectable by light and electron microscopy, have been described an average of 2 years posttransplant (111,112). These changes correlated with the presence of transplant glomerulopathy, and it is assumed that both are the result of immune-mediated endothelial injury. Changes in the peritubular capillaries precede and may be predictive of glomerular changes (112). Potentially related observations have been made in biopsies taken 1 to 12 weeks following transplantation, in which significant increases in endothelial thickness and cross-sectional area and increased adherence and passage of lymphocytes and monocytes through the peritubular capillary endothelium were seen by electron microscopy (113). Whether these alterations will have more prognostic significance than do other routinely evaluated chronic changes remains to be seen.

As newer immunosuppressive agents are introduced, pathological changes and their significance must be reassessed. Some changes, such as the presence in the graft of large numbers of eosinophils as a feature auguring poor prognosis (23), were studied prior to cyclosporine immunosuppression and require reassessment. While many changes will likely be the same, important differences may emerge as clinical experience with these new agents grows. Clearly the field of pathological assessment of renal allograft biopsies will remain a fertile area for investigation for a long time to come.

ACKNOWLEDGMENTS

The authors thank Ms. Kimberly Gill for typing the manuscript. Dr. Racusen is supported in part by grant R01 DK4381103 from the NIH.

REFERENCES

1. Solez K, et al. The Banff classification of kidney transplant pathology. Kidney Int 1993; 44:411–422.

2. D'Ardenne AJ, Dunnill MS, Thompson JF, et al. Cyclosporine and renal graft histology. J Clin Pathol 1986; 39:145–151.
3. Solez K, Racusen LC, Marcussen N, et al. Morphology of ischemic acute renal failure, normal function, and cyclosporine toxicity in cyclosporine-treated renal allograft recipients. Kidney Int. 1993; 43:1058–1067.
4. Burdick JF, Beschorner WE, Smith WJ, et al. Characteristics of early routine renal allograft biopsies. Transplantation 1984; 38:679–684.
5. Neild GH, Taube DH, Hartley RB, et al. Morphological differentiation between rejection and cyclosporine nephrotoxicity in renal allografts. J Clin Pathol 1986; 39:152–159.
6. Matas AJ, Sibley R, Mauer SM, et al. Pre-discharge, post-transplant kidney biopsy does not predict rejection. J Surg Res 1982; 32:269–274.
7. Kiaer H, Hansen HE, Olsen S. The predictive value of percutaneous biopsies from human renal allografts with early impaired function. Clin Nephrol 1980; 13:58–63.
8. Banfi G, Imbasciati E, Tarantino A, Ponticelli C. Prognostic value of renal biopsy in acute rejection of kidney transplantation. Nephron 1981; 28:222–226.
9. Hsu AC, Arbus GS, Noriega E, Huber J. Renal allograft biopsy: A satisfactory adjunct for predicting renal function after graft rejection. Clin Nephrol 1976; 5:260–265.
10. Rapaport FT, Converse JM, Billingham RE. Recent advances in clinical and experimental transplantation. JAMA 1977; 237:2835–2840.
11. Richardson W, Colvin RB, Cheeseman SH. Glomerulopathy associated with cytomegalovirus viremia in renal allografts. N Engl J Med 1981; 305:57–63.
12. Olsen S, Spencer E, Cockburn S, et al. Endocapillary glomerulitis in the renal allograft. Transplantation, 1995; 59:1421–1425.
13. Axelsen RA, Syemour AE, Mathew TH, et al. Glomerular transplant rejection: A distinctive pattern of early graft damage. Clin Nephrol 1985; 23:1–11.
14. Maryniak RK, First MR, Weiss MA. Transplant glomerulopathy: Evolution of morphologically distinct changes. Kidney Int 1985; 27:799–806.
15. Habib R, Zurowska A, Hinglais N, et al. A specific glomerular lesion of the graft: Allograft nephropathy. Kidney Int. 1993; 44(suppl 42):S104–S111.
16. Lund B, Myhre-Jensen O. Renal transplantation in rabbits. II. Morphological alterations in autografts. Acta Pathol Microbiol Scand 1970; 78:701–712.
17. Olsen TS. Pathology of allograft rejection. In: Burdick JF, Racusen LC, Solez K, Williams GM, eds. Kidney Transplant Rejection, 2d ed. New York: Marcel Dekker, 1992: 333–358.
18. Ibrahim S, Dawson DV, Sanfilippo F. Predominant infiltration of rejecting human renal allografts with T cells expressing CD8 and CD45R0. Transplantation 1995; 59:724–728.
19. Ibrahim S, Dawson DV, Van Trigt, P, Sanfilippo F. Differential infiltration by CD45R0 and CD45RA subsets of T cells associated with human heart allograft rejection. Am J Pathol 1993; 142:1794–1803.
20. Hoshinaga K, Mohanakumar T, Goldman MH, et al. Clinical significance of in situ detection of T lymphocyte subsets and monocyte/macrophage lineages in heart allografts. Transplantation 1984; 38:634–637.
21. Beschorner WE, Burdick JF, Williams GM, Solez K. The presence of Leu 7 reactive lymphocytes in renal allografts undergoing acute rejection. Transplant Proc 1985; 17:618–622.
22. Malinowski K, Waltzer WC, Jao S, et al. Homing of CD8CD57 T lymphocytes into acutely rejected renal allografts. Transplantation 1992; 54:1013–1017.
23. Weir MR, Hall-Craggs M, Shen SY, et al. The prognostic value of the eosinophil in acute renal allograft rejection. Transplantation 1986; 41:709–712.
24. Halloran PF, Wadgymar A, Ritchie S, et al. The significance of the anti-class I antibody response: I. Clinical and pathologic features of anti-class I-mediated rejection. Transplantation 1990; 49:85–91.
25. Halloran PF, Schlaut J, Solez K, Srinivasa NS. The significance of the anti-class I response: II.

Clinical and pathologic features of renal transplants with anti-class I-like antibody. Transplantation 1992; 53:550–555.

26. Croker BP, Salomon DR. Pathology of the renal allograft. In: Tisher CC, Brenner BM, eds. Renal Pathology. Philadelphia: Lippincott, 1993:1591–1640.
27. Nadasdy T, Ormas J, Stiller D, et al. Tubular ultrastructure in rejected human renal allografts. Ultrastruct Pathol 1988; 12:195–207.
28. Sibley RK, Rynasiewicz J, Ferguson RM, et al. Morphology of cyclosporine nephrotoxicity and acute rejection in patients immunosuppressed with cyclosporine and prednisone. Surgery 1983; 94:225–234.
29. Ivanyi B, Hansen HE, Olsen S. Segmental localization and quantitative characteristics of tubulitis in kidney biopsies from patients undergoing acute rejection. Transplantation 1993; 56:581–585.
30. Matsuno T, Sakagami K, Saito S, et al. Does perforin mediate the indirect injury of renal allografts in acute rejection? Transplant Proc 1993; 25:879–880.
31. Hameed A, Truong LD, Price V, et al. Immunohistochemical localization of granzyme B antigen in cytotoxic cells in human tissues. Am J Pathol 1991; 138:1069–1075.
32. Kataoka K, Naomoto Y, Shiozaki S, et al. Infiltration of perforin-positive mononuclear cells into the rejected kidney allograft. Transplantation 1992; 53:240–242.
33. Lipman ML, Stevens AC, Bleackley RC, et al. The strong correlation of cytotoxic T lymphocyte-specific serine protease gene transcripts with renal allograft rejection. Transplantation 1992; 53:73–79.
34. Fuggle SV, McWhinnie DL, Chapman JR, et al. Sequential analysis of HLA class II antigen expression in human renal allografts: Induction of tubular class II antigens and correlation with clinical parameters. Transplantation 1986; 42:144–150.
35. Hall BM, Bishop GA, Duggin GG, et al. Increased expression of HLA-DR antigens on renal tubular cells in renal transplants: Relevance to the rejection response. Lancet 1984; 2:247–251.
36. Brockmeyer C, Ulbrecht M, Schendel DJ, et al. Distribution of cell adhesion molecules (ICAM-1, VCAM-1, ELAM-1) in renal tissue during allograft rejection. Transplantation 1993; 55:605–609.
37. Briscoe DM, Pober JS, Harmon WE, Cotran RS. Expression of vascular cell adhesion molecule-1 in human renal allografts. J Am Soc Nephrol 1992; 3:1180–1185.
38. Porter KA, Thomson WB, Owen K, et al. Obliterative vascular changes in four human kidney homotransplants. Br Med J 1963; 2:639–645.
39. Porter KA, Marchioro TL, Starzl TE. Pathological changes in 37 human renal homotransplants treated with immunosuppressive drugs. Br J Urol 1965; 37:250–273.
40. Hamburger J, Crosnier J, Dormont J. Experience with 45 renal homotransplantations in man. Lancet 1965; 1:985–992.
41. Kincaid-Smith P. Histological diagnosis of rejection of renal homografts in man. Lancet 1967; 2:849–852.
42. Busch GJ, Reynolds FS, Galvanek EG, et al. Human renal allografts: The role of vascular injury in early graft failure. Medicine 1971; 50:29–83.
43. Mihatsch MJ, Gudat F, Ryffel B, Thiel G. Cyclosporine nephropathy. In: Tisher CC, Brenner BM, eds. Renal Pathology, 2d ed. Philadelphia: Lippincott, 1994:1641–1681.
44. Van Buren D, Van Buren CT, Flechner SM, et al. De novo hemolytic uremic syndrome in renal transplant recipients immunosuppressed with cyclosporine. Surgery 1985; 98:54–62.
45. Abramowicz D, Pradier O, Marchant A, et al. Induction of thromboses within renal grafts by high-dose prophylactic OKT3. Lancet 1992; 1:777–778.
46. Alpers CE, Hudkins KL, Davis CL, et al. Expression of vascular cell adhesion molecule-1 in kidney allograft rejection. Kidney Int 1993; 44:805–816.
47. Isoniemi HM, Krogerus L, von Willebrand E, et al. Histopathological findings in well-functioning long-term renal allografts. Kidney Int 1992; 41:155–160.

48. Petersen VP, Olsen TS, Kissmeyer-Nielson F, et al. Late failure of human renal transplants: An analysis of transplant disease and graft failure among 125 recipients surviving for one to eight years. Medicine 1975; 54:45–71.
49. Matthew TH, Mathews DC, Hobbes JB, Kincaid-Smith P. Glomerular lesions after renal transplantation. Am J Med 1975; 59:177–190.
50. Olsen S, Bohman S-Q, Petersen V. Ultrastructure of glomerular basement membrane in long term renal allografts with transplant glomerular disease. Lab Invest 1974; 30:176–189.
51. Dennis MJS, Foster MC, Ryan JJ, et al. The increasing importance of chronic rejection as a cause of renal allograft failure. Transplant Int 1989; 2:214–217.
52. Kasiske BL, Kalil RSN, Lee HS, Rao KV. Histopathologic findings associated with a chronic progressive decline in renal allograft function. Kidney Int 1991; 40:514–524.
53. Mihatsch MJ, Ryffel B, Gudat F. Morphological criteria of chronic rejection: Differential diagnosis, including cyclosporine nephropathy. Transplant Proc 1993; 25:2031–2037.
54. Paul LC, Hayry P, Foegh M, Dennis MJ, et al. Diagnostic criteria for chronic rejection/accelerated graft atherosclerosis in heart and kidney transplants. Fourth Alexis Carrel Conference on Chronic Rejection and Accelerated Arteriosclerosis in Transplanted Organs. Transplant Proc 1993; 25:2022–2023.
55. Gao S, Alderman EI, Schroeder JS, et al. Progressive coronary luminal narrowing after cardiac transplantation. Circulation 1990; 82:269–275.
56. Kissmeyer-Nielsen F, Olsen S, Peterson VP, Fjeldborg O. Hyperacute rejection of kidney allografts associated with pre-existing humoral antibodies against donor cells. Lancet 1966; 2:662–665.
57. Williams GM, Hume DM, Hudson RP, et al. "Hyperacute" renal homograft rejection in man. N Engl J Med 1968; 279:611–618.
58. Scornik JC, LeFor WM, Cicciarelli JC, et al. Hyperacute and acute kidney graft rejection due to antibodies against B cells. Transplantation 1992; 54:61–64.
59. Svalander C, Nyberg G, Blohme I, et al. Acute early allograft failure and the C3/macrophage phenomenon. Transplant Proc 1993; 25:903–904.
60. Kiaer H, Hansen NE, Olsen S. The predictive value of percutaneous biopsies from human renal allografts with early impaired function. Clin Nephrol 1980; 13:58–63.
61. Paul LC. Chronic rejection of organ allografts. Magnitude of the problem. Transplant Proc 1993; 25:2024–2025.
62. Foster MC, Rowe PA, Wenham PW, et al. Late results of renal transplantation and the importance of chronic rejection as a cause of late graft loss. Annu Rev Cell Surg Eng 1989; 71:41–44.
63. Knight RJ, Kerman RH, Welsh M, et al. Chronic rejection in primary renal allograft recipients under cyclosporine-prednisone immunosuppressive therapy. Transplantation 1991; 51: 355–359.
64. Penn I. The changing pattern of post-transplant malignancies. Transplant Proc 1991; 23:1101–1103.
65. Cockfield SM, Preiksaitis J, Harvey E, et al. Is sequential use of ALG and OKT3 in renal transplants associated with an increased incidence of fulminant post-transplant lymphoproliferative disorder? Transplant Proc 1991; 23:1106.
66. Alfrey EJ, Friedman AL, Grossman RA, et al. A recent decrease in time to development of monomorphous and polymorphous post-transplant lymphoproliferative disorder. Transplantation 1992; 54:250–253.
67. Racusen LC, Solez K. Nephrotoxicity of cyclosporine and other immunosuppressive and immunotherapeutic agents. In: Hook JB, Goldstein R, eds. Toxicology of the Kidney, 2d ed. New York: Raven Press, 1992:319–360.
68. Myers BD, Ross J, Newton L, et al. Cyclosporine-associated chronic nephropathy. N Engl J Med 1984; 311:699–705.

69. Greenberg A, Egel JW, Thompson ME, et al. Early and late forms of cyclosporine nephrotoxicity: Studies in cardiac allograft recipients. Am J Kidney Dis 1987; 9:12–22.
70. McCauley J, Van Thiel GH, Starzl TE, Puschett JB. Acute and chronic renal failure in liver transplantation. Nephron 1990; 55:121–128.
71. Spector D, Limas C, Frost JL, et al. Perfusion nephropathy in human transplants. N Engl J Med 1976; 295:1217–1221.
72. Gaber LW, Gaber AO, Tolley EA, Hathaway DK. Prediction by post revascularization biopsies of cadaveric kidney allografts of rejection, graft loss, and preservation nephropathy. Transplantation 1992; 53:1219–1225.
73. Montagnino G, Colturi C, Banfi G. Membranous nephropathy in cyclosporine-treated renal transplant recipients. Transplantation 1985; 40:100–102.
74. Truong L, Gelfand J, D'Agati V, et al. De novo membranous glomerulopathy in renal allografts: A report of ten cases and review of the literature. Am J Kidney Dis 1989; 14:131–144.
75. Thoenes GH, Pielsticker K, Schubert G. Transplantation-induced immune complex kidney disease in rats with unilateral manifestation in the allografted kidney. Lab Invest 1979; 41: 321–333.
76. Kashtan C, Fish AJ, Kleppel M, et al. Nephritogenic antigen determinance in epidermal and renal basement membranes of kindreds with Alport-type familial nephritis. J Clin Invest 1986; 78:1035–1044.
77. Kalluri R, Gunwar S, Reeders ST, et al. Goodpasture's syndrome: Localization of the epitope for the autoantibodies to the carboxy terminal region of the L3 (1V) chain of basement membrane collagen. J Biol Chem 1991; 266:24,018–24,024.
78. Shah B, First MR, Mendoza NC, et al. Alport's syndrome: Risk of glomerulonephritis induced by anti-glomerular basement membrane antibody after renal transplantation. Nephron 1990; 50:34–38.
79. Fleming SJ, Savage COS, McWilliams LJ, et al. Anti-glomerular basement membrane antibody-mediated nephritis complicating transplantation in a patient with Alport's syndrome. Transplantation 1988; 46:857–859.
80. Rassoul Z, Al-Khader AA, Al-Sulaiman M, et al. Recurrent allograft antiglomerular basement membrane glomerulonephritis in a patient with Alport's syndrome. Am J Nephrol 1990; 10:73–76.
81. Ramos E, Recurrent diseases in the renal allograft. J Am Soc Nephrol 1991; 2:109–121.
82. Berger BE, Vincenti F, Biava C, et al. De novo and recurrent membranous glomerulopathy following kidney transplantation. Transplantation 1983; 35:315–319.
83. Montagnino C, Colturi C, Banfi G. Membranous nephropathy in cyclosporine-treated renal transplant recipients. Transplantation 1989; 47:725–727.
84. Pinto J, Lacerda G, Cameron JS, et al. Recurrence of focal and segmental glomerulosclerosis in renal allografts. Transplantation 1981; 32:83–89.
85. Habib R, Antignac C, Hinglais N, et al. Glomerular lesions in the transplanted kidney in children. Am J Kidney Dis 1987; 10:198–207.
86. Lewis EJ. Recurrent focal sclerosis after renal transplantation. Kidney Int 1982; 22:315–323.
87. Strigel JE, Sibley RK, Fryd DS, Mauer M. Recurrence of focal segmental sclerosis in children following renal transplantation. Kidney Int 1986; 30:S44–S50.
88. Morales JM, Andres A, Prieto C, et al. Clinical and histological sequence of recurrent focal segmental glomerulosclerosis. Nephron 1988; 48:241–242.
89. Korbet SM, Schwartz MM, Lewis EJ. Recurrent nephrotic syndrome in renal allografts. Am J Kidney Dis 1988; 11:270–276.
90. Matthew TM. Recurrence of disease after renal transplantation. Am J Kidney Dis 1988; 12: 85–96.
91. DePauw W, Gelin M, Danpure CJ, et al. Combined liver-kidney transplantation in primary hyperoxaluria type I. Transplantation 1990; 50:886–887.
92. Niaudet P, Nussenzveig P, Habib R, et al. Systematic one year renal graft biopsy in children

with normal renal function. In: Towaine JL, ed. Transplantation and Clinical Immunology; Evaluation and Monitoring in Transplantation. Vol 24. Amsterdam: Elsevier, 1992:111–115.
93. Solez K, McGraw DI, Beschorner WE, et al. Reflections on use of the renal biopsy as the "gold standard" in distinguishing transplant rejection from cyclosporine nephrotoxicity. Transplant Proc 1985; 17(suppl 1):123–133.
94. Racusen LC, Solez K. Renal infarction, cortical necrosis and athero-embolic disease. In Tisher C, Brenner B, eds. Renal Pathology, 2d ed. Philadelphia: Lippincott, 1994:810–831.
95. Platt JL, Sibley RK, Michael AF. Interstitial nephritis associated with cytomegalovirus infection. Kidney Int 1985; 28:550–552.
96. Cameron J, Rigby RJ, van Deth AG, Petric JJB. Severe tubulointerstitial disease in a renal allograft due to cytomegalovirus infection. Clin Nephrol 1982; 18:321–325.
97. Cameron JS. Glomerulonephritis in renal transplants. Transplantation 1982; 32:237–245.
98. Coleman DV, Mackenzie SD, Gardner SD, et al. Human polyomavirus (BK) infections and ureteric stenosis in renal allograft recipients. J Clin Pathol 1978; 31:338–347.
99. Marcussen N, Olsen TS, Benediktsson H, et al. Reproducibility of the Banff classification of renal allograft pathology: Inter and intraobserver variation. Transplantation 1995. In press.
100. Silcocks PBS. Measuring repeatability and validity of histological diagnosis—A brief review with some practical examples. J Clin Pathol 1983; 36:1269–1275
101. Cohen J. Weighted kappa: Nominal scale agreement with provision for scaled disagreement or partial credit. Psychol Bull 1968; 70:213–230.
102. Ker M. Issues in the use of kappa. Invest Radiol 1991; 26:78–83.
103. Land JR, Koch GG. The measurement of observer agreement for categorical data. Biometrics 1977; 33:159–174.
104. Schwartz MM, Lan SP, Bernstein J, et al. Irreproducibility of the activity and chronicity indices limits their utility in the management of lupus nephritis: Lupus nephritis collaborative study group. Am J Kidney Dis 1993; 21:374–377.
105. Hastrup N, Hamilton-Dutoit S, Ralfkider E, Pallesen G. Peripheral T-cell lymphomas: An evaluation of reproducibility of the updated Kiel classification. Histopathology 1991; 18:99–105.
106. van Lijnschoten G, Arends JW, de la Fuente AA, et al. Intra- and interobserver variation in the interpretation of histological features suggesting chromosomal abnormality in early abortion specimens. Histopathology 1993; 22:25–29.
107. Tezuka F, Namiki T, Higashiwai H. Observer variability in endometrial cytology using K statistics. J Clin Pathol 1992; 45:292–294.
108. Theodossi A, Skene AM, Portmann B, et al. Observer variation in assessment of liver biopsies including analysis by kappa statistics. Gastroenterology 1980; 79:232–241.
109. Solez K, Hansen HE, Kornerup HJ, et al. Clinical validation and reproducibility of the Banff schema for renal allograft pathology. Transplant Proc 1995; 27:1009–1011.
110. Noronha IL, Weis H, Hartley B, et al. Expression of cytokines, growth factors, and their receptors in renal allograft biopsies. Transplant Proc 1993; 25:917–918.
111. Monga G, Mazzucco G, Novara R, Reale L. Intertubular capillary changes in kidney allografts: An ultrastructural study in patients with transplant glomerulopathy. Ultrastruct Pathol 1990; 14:201–209.
112. Monga G, Mazzucco G, Messina M, et al. Intertubular capillary changes in kidney allografts: A morphological investigation on 61 recent specimens. Mod Pathol 1992; 5:125–130.
113. Ivanyi B, Hansen H, Olsen TS. Post-capillary venule-like transformation of peritubular capillaries in acute renal allograft rejection. Arch Pathol Lab Med 1992; 116:1062–1067.

COLOR PLATES

CHAPTER 3

Figure 1 Kidney biopsy 9 days after transplantation. Routine hematoxylin and eosin staining (top left) of formalin-fixed tissue demonstrates marked endothelialitis of an artery, with lymphocytes, monocytes, and neutrophils disrupting the endothelium. Immunofluorescence stains on frozen sections from the same biopsy revealed little IgG but strong linear staining for C4d and C3b on the endothelium of an artery.

Figure 3 Acute heart allograft rejection. Acute rejection is characterized by an intense mononuclear cell infiltrate associated with myocyte necrosis (A). In this case, immunohistochemical staining demonstrated that the infiltrate was composed of a mixture of CD4 (B) and CD8-positive cells, most of which expressed CD45RO (C). The infiltrate was accompanied by the upregulation of class II antigen expression on endothelial cells (D). [A, hematoxylin and eosin; B–D, immunostaining for CD4 (B), CD45RO (C), and HLA-DR(D); all ×400.]

CHAPTER 5

Figure 1 Schematic representation of transplant-related accelerated arteriosclerosis illustrating the diffuse and concentric luminal narrowing characteristic of this lesion. (From Ref. 33.)

Figure 2 Gross photograph of a section of a coronary artery of the heart from a patient with accelerated arteriosclerosis. Note the concentric nature of the luminal narrowing and the diffuse involvement of both the larger epicardial and smaller perforating coronary arteries. (From Ref. 163.)

Figure 6 Fluorescence in situ hybridization for the Y chromosome. Hybridization was not detected in cardiac myocytes (A). In contrast, note the intense focal punctate yellow hybridization present in infiltrating lymphocytes (B) and in subendothelial lymphocytes and macrophages (C and D). C and D: The lumina of the vessels occupies the top third of the photograph, endothelial cells are identified as the single layer of flattened cells immediately lining these lumina, and the subendothelial lymphocytes and macrophages occupy the lower portion of the photograph. (From Ref. 69.)

Figure 7 Immunohistochemical staining demonstrating that the endothelialitis in the coronary arteries of this explanted heart with accelerated arteriosclerosis is composed of macrophages (A) and T lymphocytes (B). The endothelialitis is associated with induced class II major histocompatibility antigen expression on endothelial cells (C), and the T lymphocytes stain as cytotoxic T lymphocytes (D). (From Ref. 32.) (A: Immunohistochemical staining, MAC-387, ×400; B: CD45RO, ×685; C: HLA DR, ×575; D: CD8, ×575.)

Figure 9 $CD8^+$ lymphocytes were identified in the subendothelial spaces of coronary arteries with transplant-related arteriosclerosis (A). In contrast to the diffuse staining seen with the anti-CD8 antibody, a granular cytoplasmic staining was seen when the same cells were stained for perforin (B). (From Ref. 71.) (A: immunohistochemical stain for CD8, ×960; B: immunohistochemical stain for perforin, ×900.)

Figure 11 Intact embryonic hearts grown in tissue culture as tissue explants. Successful transduction is demonstrated by the blue staining of the heart transfected with AAV lacZ.

Figure 12 Isolated cardiomyocytes transduced with AAV lacZ.

Continued

CHAPTER 11

Figure 2 Acute pancreas rejection. This tissue is double-stained with antibodies to chromogranin A (red stain) and leukocyte common antigen (LCA) (brown stain). Chromogranin A demonstrates the islets while LCA shows the inflammatory infiltrates in rejection. Note that the islets are not involved by inflammation. The inflammation is primarily concentrated in fibrous septae but also infiltrates the pancreatic acinar tissue. [Double immunostains; chromogranin A (red) and leukocyte common antigen (brown), no counterstain.]

Figure 13 A pancreas with recurrent diabetes. The lymphocytes (brown) surround and involve islets (red) with destruction of beta cells. [Double immunostain chromogranin A (red) and leukocyte common antigen (brown), no counterstain.]

CHAPTER 13

Figure 1 Inflammatory cells in MGG-stained cytocentrifuge preparations (A–C): A lymphoid blast cell with immature nucleus and cytoplasmic basophilia, a small lymphocyte and a neutrophil (A), a monocyte and two small lymphocytes (B), a macrophage and a lymphocyte (C). Kidney parenchymal cells in MGG-stained cytopreparations (D–F): A group of normal tubular cells (D), swelling, degeneration and vacuolation in tubular cells in ATN (E), isometric vacuolation and swelling in a tubular cell during CyA toxicity (F). Liver parenchymal cells in MGG-stained cytocentrifuge preparations (G–I): A group of normal hepatocytes (G), degenerative changes in hepatocytes (H), accumulation of bile in the hepatocytes indicating cholestasis (I).

CHAPTER 15

Figure 35 Allograft rejection. (A) Photomicrograph of a histological section in an animal with graft ejection shows areas of inflammatory cell infiltration with associated myocyte necrosis, particularly affecting the interventricular septum (S) and right ventricular (RV) free wall. (B) and (C) Corresponding T_1-weighted images, respectively, before (PRE) and after (POST) Gd-DTPA administration, show zones of intense myocardial enhancement corresponding to the sites of histological rejection. S = interventricular septum; RV = right ventricular free wall. (From Ref. 75.)

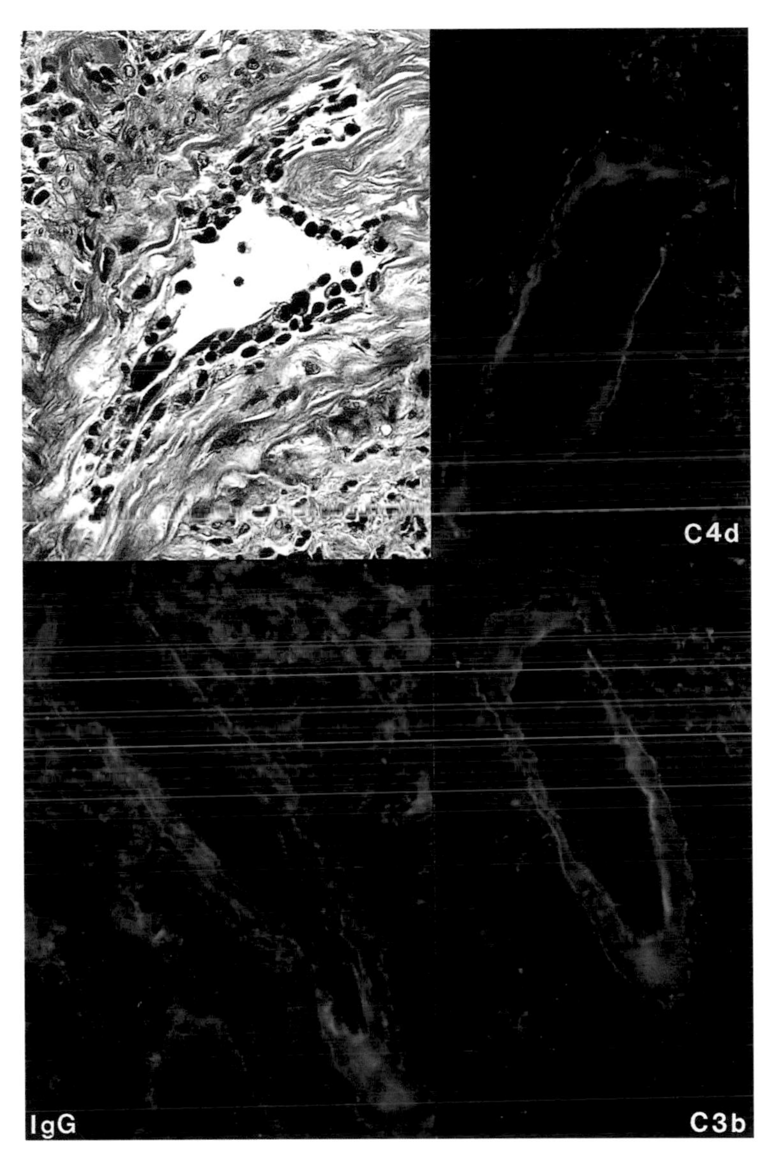

Figure 3.1

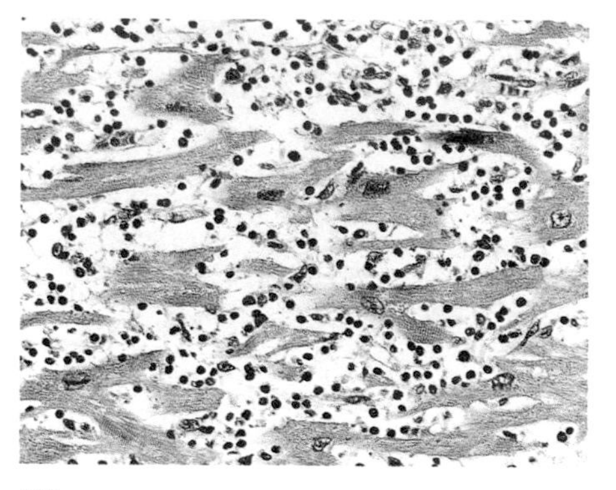

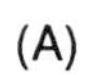

(A)

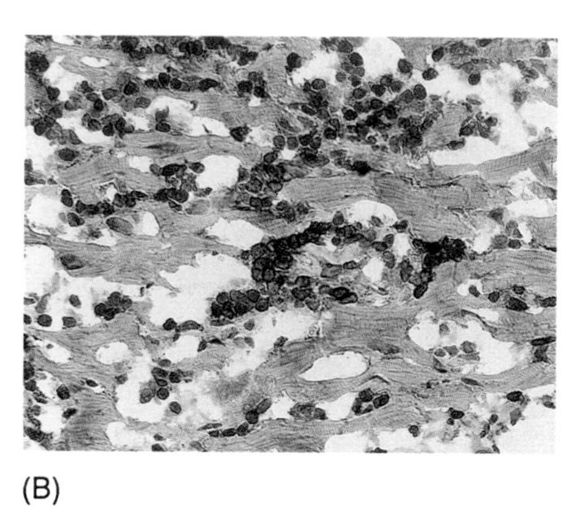

(B)

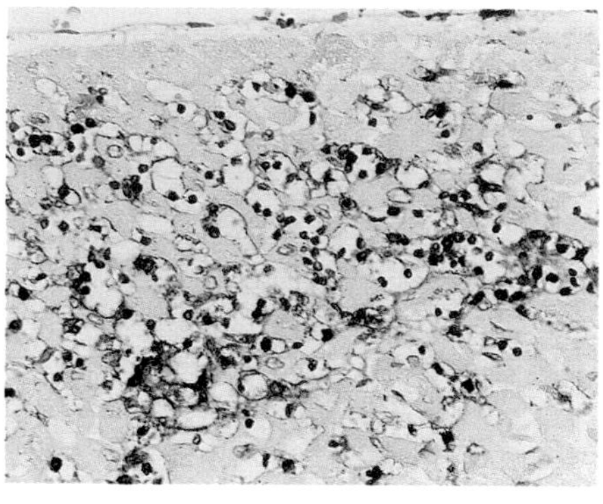

(C)

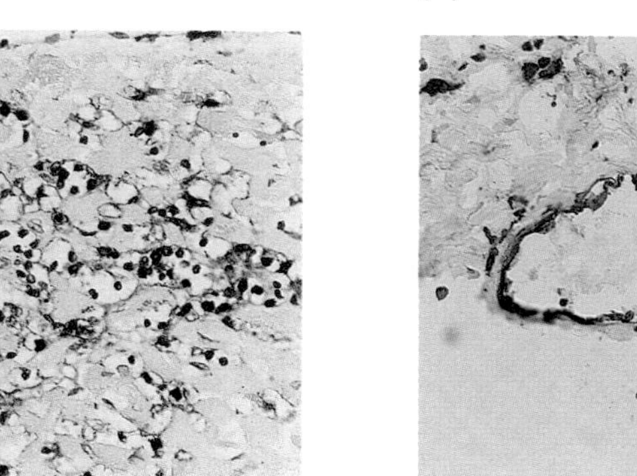

(D)

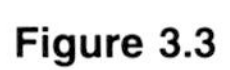

Figure 3.3

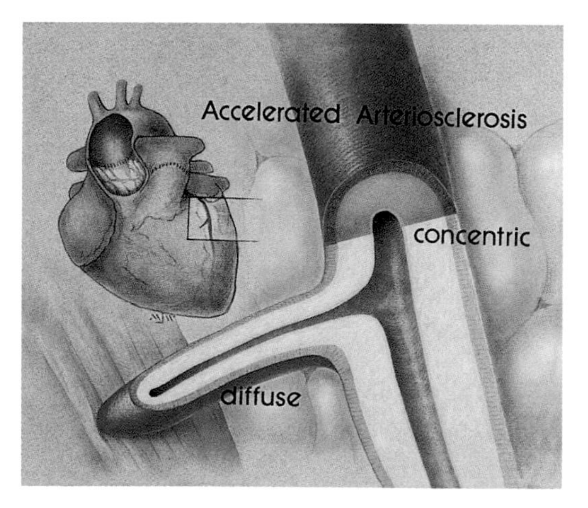

Figure 5.1

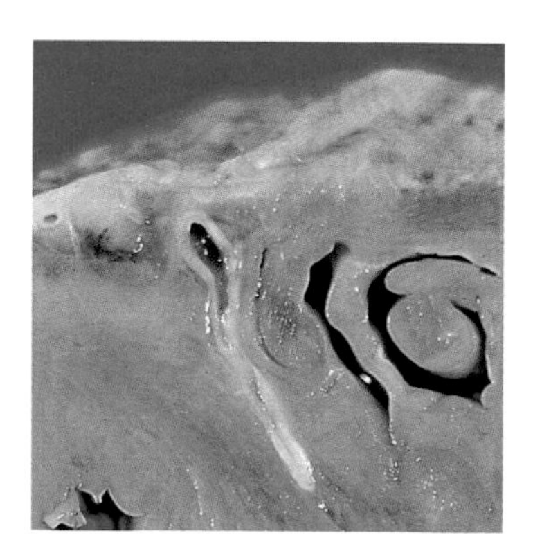

Figure 5.2

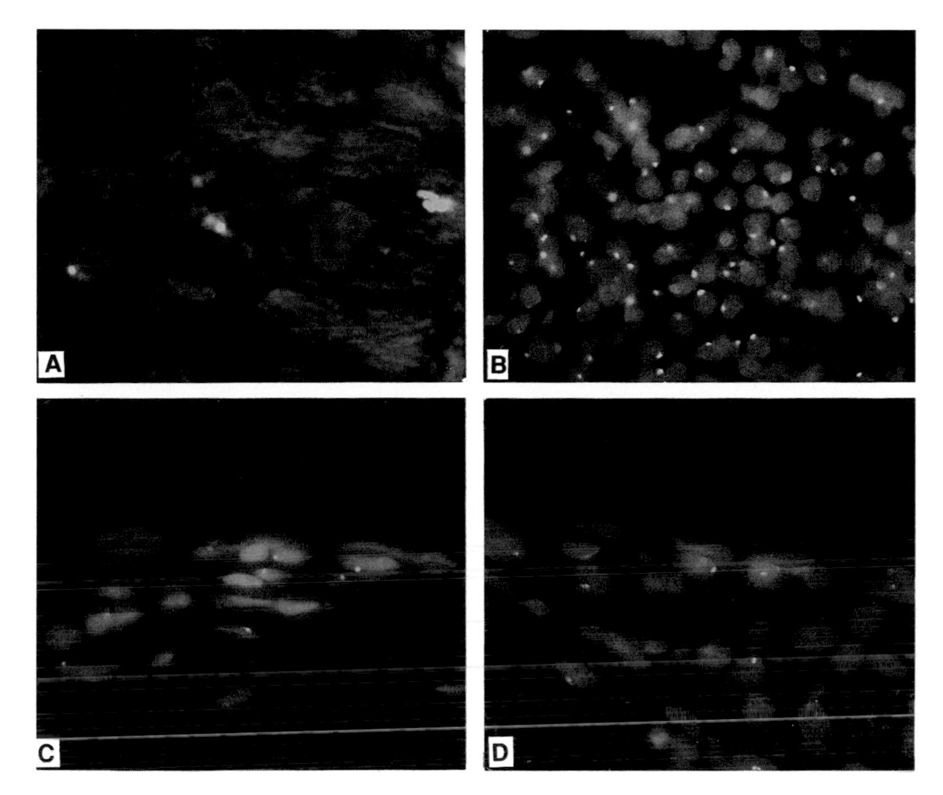

Figure 5.6

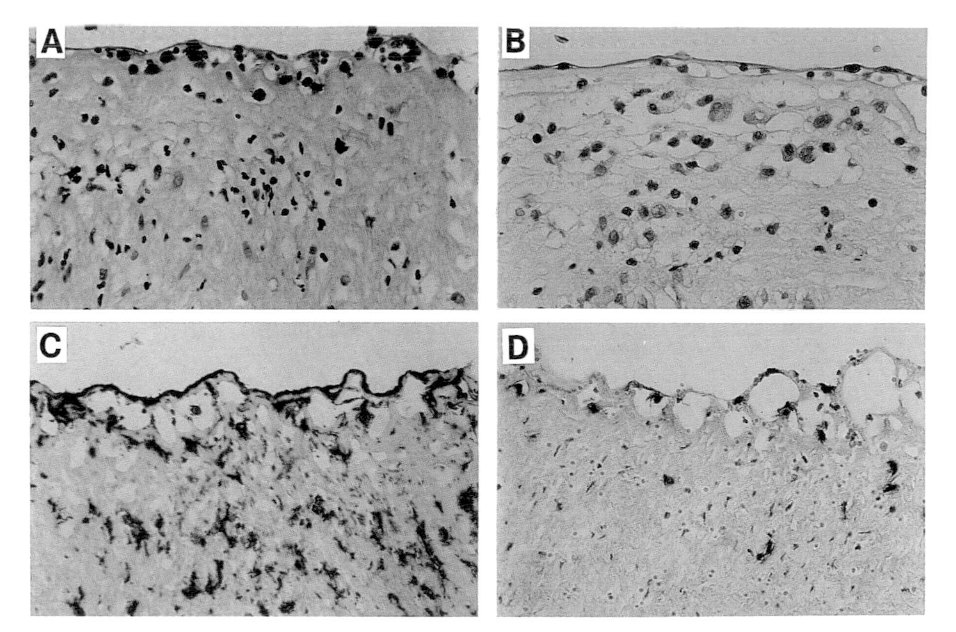

Figure 5.7

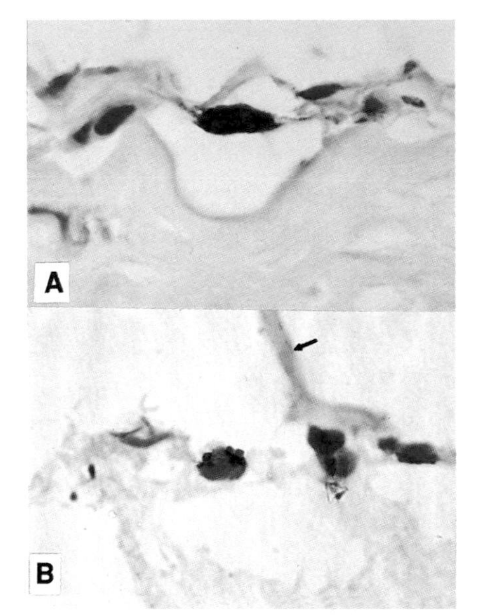

Figure 5.9

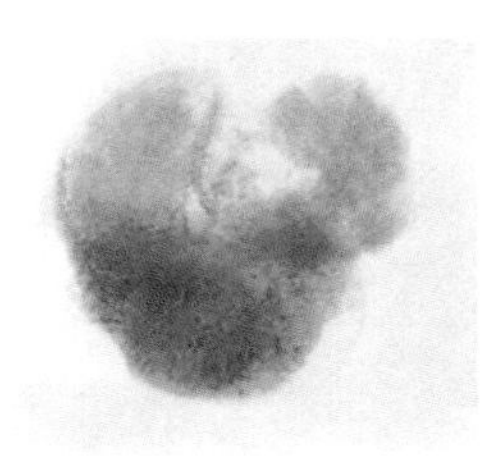

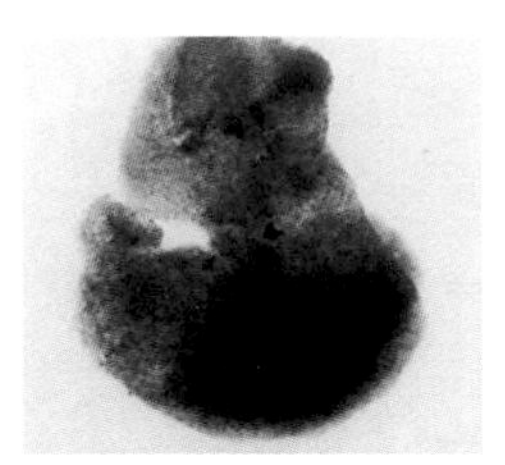

Figure 5.11

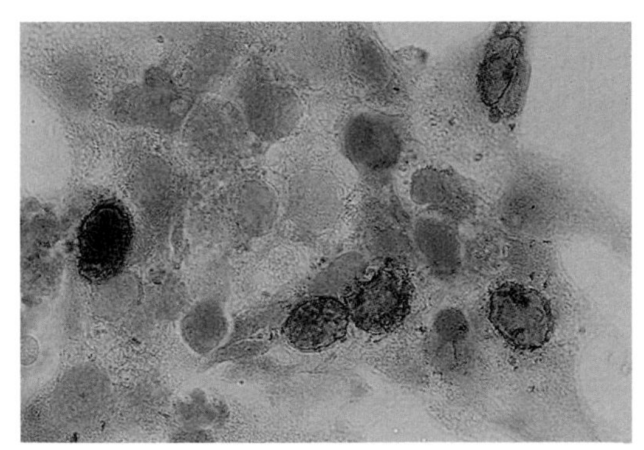

Figure 5.12

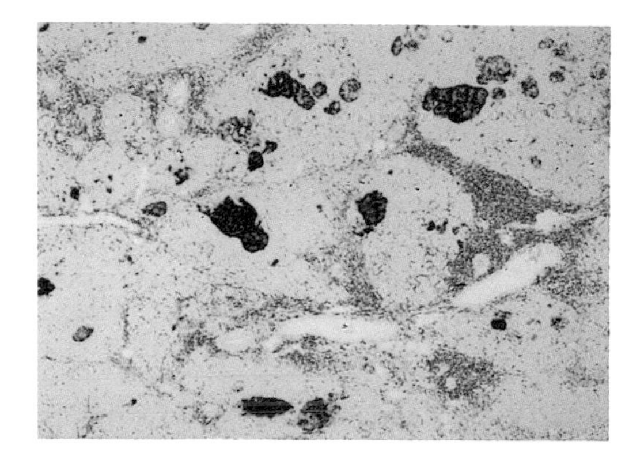

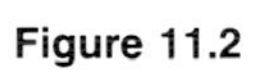

Figure 11.2

Figure 11.13

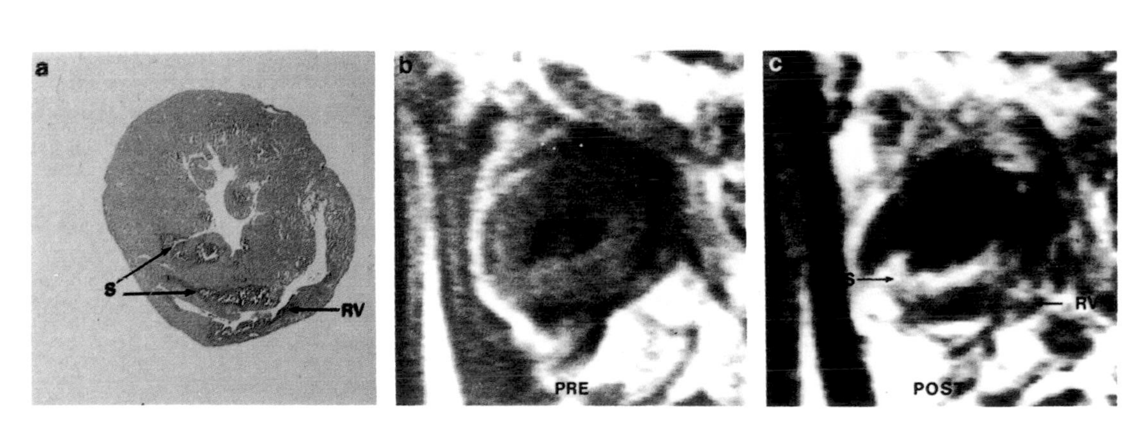

Figure 15.35

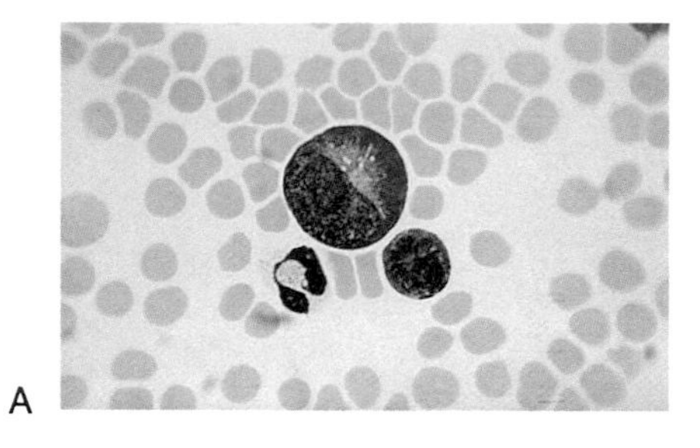

A

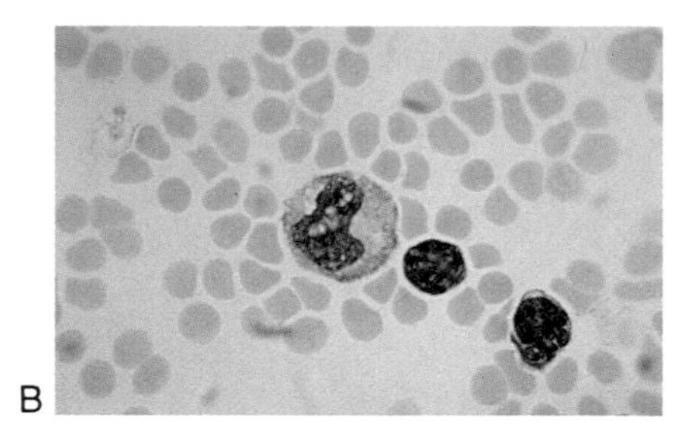

B

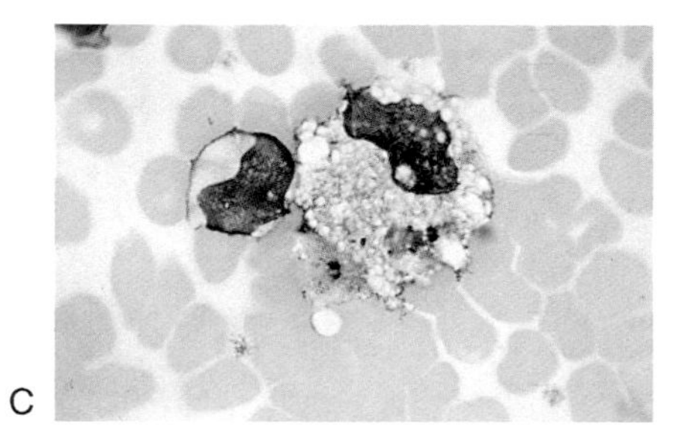

C

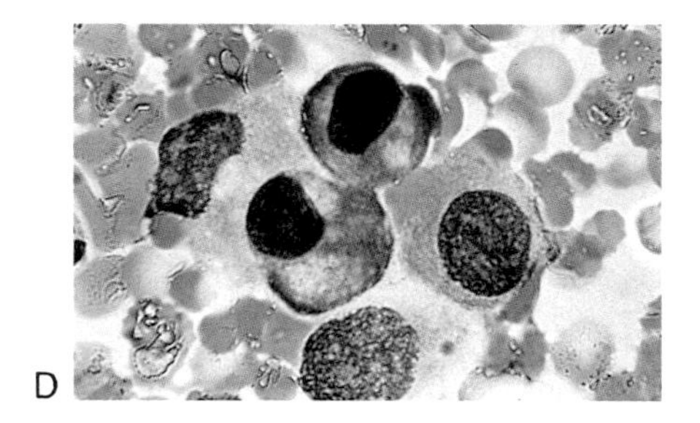

D

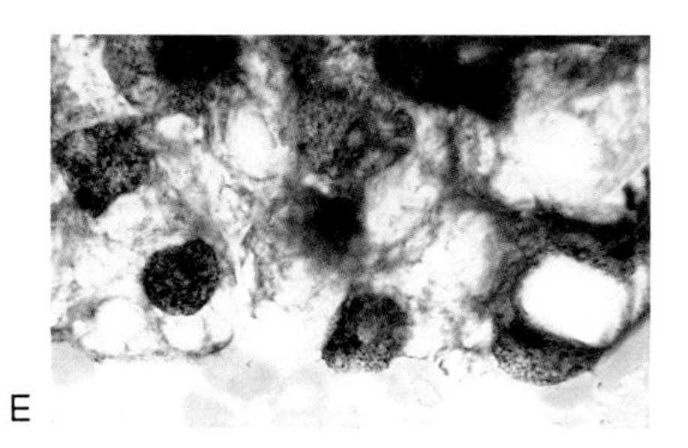

E

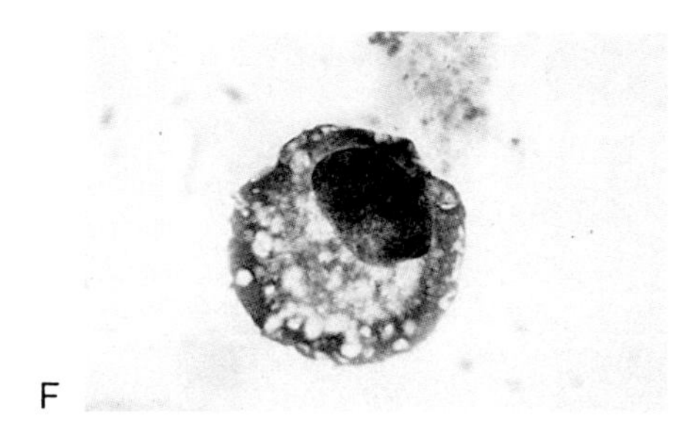

F

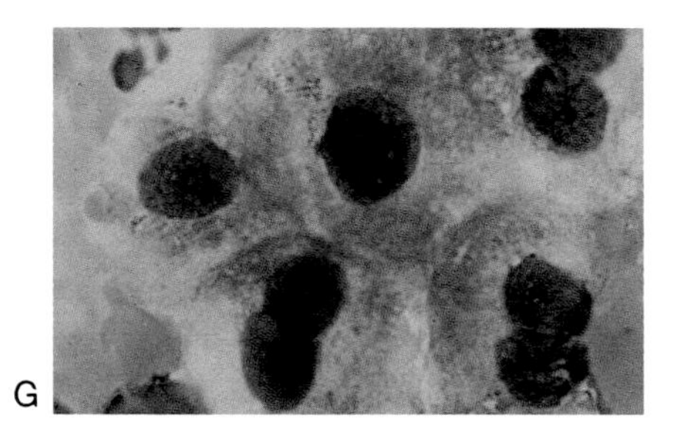

G

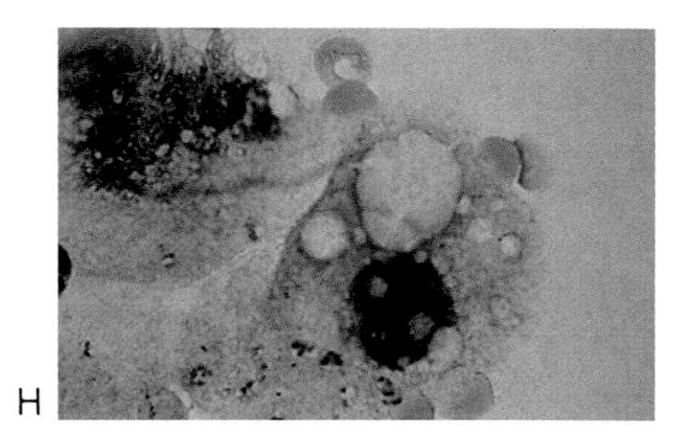

H

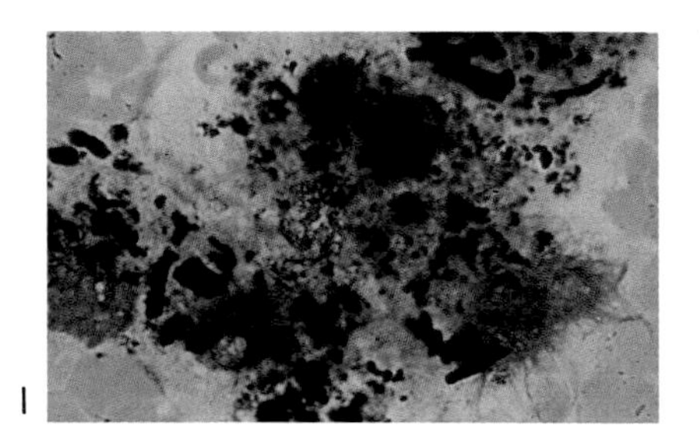

I

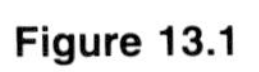

Figure 13.1

10

Pathology of Intestinal Transplantation

Barbara F. Banner
University of Massachusetts Medical Center, Worcester, Massachusetts

I. INTRODUCTION: HISTORICAL PERSPECTIVE

A. Animal Models

The techniques for small bowel transplantation have been developed in animal models for nearly 40 years. The first successful small bowel autografts and allografts were performed by Lillehei et al. in the 1950s (1,2). These studies provided baseline data about bowel preservation, surgical techniques, and rate of recovery of bowel function. It was noted that animals with a full intestinal allograft died with a systemic syndrome of wasting and enlarged lymph nodes, while the allograft remained free of inflammation. It was suggested that the homograft rejected the host or in some manner caused a metabolic upset that led to the host's demise (2). When the allograft segments were shortened (2), or radiated (3), the wasting graft-versus-host disease (GVHD) decreased and the bowel segments were rejected. During the 1960s and 70s, surgical techniques were refined and various immunosuppression regimens using azathioprine, steroids, antilymphocyte globulin, cyclosporin A (CyA), and radiation were investigated (3–8). A landmark study from this period was that of Monchik and Russell (9), who showed that rejection and GVHD could be separated by using inbred strains of rats and their F1 hybrid offspring as donor-recipient pairs. This made it possible to construct unidirectional models in which either rejection or GVHD would occur or bidirectional models in which both reactions could occur. Recently, emphasis has been on using immunophenotypic markers to define the cellular constituents and mechanisms of the rejection and GVH reaction (10–19).

B. Human Trials

The first small bowel transplants in humans were performed in the 1960s (20). The initial experience with small bowel transplantation in humans was not encouraging. Most of the patients died in the early posttransplant period due to technical problems, rejection, or sepsis. The longest survival was 176 days in a woman who received a bowel from her HLA-identical sister. In 1986, Cohen et al. (21) reported a 26-year-old woman who lived for 11 days after small bowel transplant under CyA immunosuppression. Of note was the fact that she was followed by daily stomal mucosal biopsies. In 1988 Goulet et al. reported long-term survival (205 days) in a child using CyA immunosuppression (22). This was the first reported attempt to study immunophenotypic markers and class II antigen expression in biopsies posttransplant. In 1989 there were two reports of successful multivisceral transplants with long-term (4 to 6 months) survival and death due to posttransplant lymphoproliferative disorder (23,24). Since 1988 there have been continuing reports of clinical trials of total small bowel, small bowel/liver, and multivisceral transplants from Pittsburgh (25,26), the University of Western Ontario in Canada (27,28), the University of Kiel in Germany (29), and the Hopital Necker-Enfants Malades in Paris (30).

In the animal and human studies, the major problems involved in small bowel transplantation are rejection, GVHD, and preservation injury. In long-term survivors, ischemia, infection, posttransplant lymphoproliferative disorder (PTLD), and possibly toxic effects of drugs on the allograft become important. These problems are described in a number of reviews (20,31–34).

II. ANATOMICAL CONSIDERATIONS IN SMALL BOWEL TRANSPLANTATION

A. Vascular and Nerve Supply

The small bowel measures about 20 ft from the gastric pylorus to the ileocecal valve (35). The arterial supply to the duodenum includes the celiac and superior mesenteric arteries (SMA). The remainder of small bowel, cecum, appendix, and right colon are supplied by the SMA or its branches. The branches of the SMA form several tiers of arcades in the mesentery before the vasa recta, which penetrate the bowel wall. The venous blood supply parallels the arteries. From the submucosal venous plexi, veins emerge that drain into the superior mesenteric vein (SMV) and ultimately the portal vein. Thus, the most physiological anastomoses for the transplanted bowel are the SMA to aorta and the SMV to portal vein. Studies comparing portal to inferior vena cava anastomosis for small bowel allografts note no difference in the timing or histological appearance of rejection but do note that recipients appear to be in better metabolic status if the graft is drained into the portal rather than the systemic circulation (36,37).

The lymphatic drainage consists of the central lacteals of the villi coalescing into a submucosal plexus and thence into larger channels, which drain into lymph nodes distributed along the arteries. Eventually, drainage reaches the root of the mesentery. Lillehei's group (2,38) demonstrated by methylene blue injection studies that the lymphatic drainage became reestablished between 2 and 6 weeks after small bowel autotransplants in dogs. Schmid et al. (39), using similar techniques in rats, found that some lymphatic collaterals were established by day 3, and that full drainage of methylene blue and chylomicrons to host retroperitoneum was resumed by day 14.

The nerve supply of the small bowel is distributed with the arteries. Along with branches of the SMA are sympathetic nerve fibers, parasympathetic fibers from the vagus, and afferent pain fibers from receptors in the serosa, peritoneum, and adventitia. There are extrinsic branches of the nerves around the myenteric and submucosal plexi. After transplantation, these nerves may not regenerate. Abnormal motility, intraluminal pressures, and intramural electrical activity after bowel transplantation have been described (40,41). These factors may all contribute to the poor tone, decreased peristalsis, and hypertrophy of muscle that have been observed in long-term survivors of small bowel transplantation (42,43).

B. Microscopic Anatomy

Microscopically, villous structure varies slightly in different regions of the small intestine. In the duodenum, the villi may be branched or fused, whereas in the jejunum and ileum they are tall and straight. Villous/crypt ratio, as estimated in routine hematoxylin and eosin (H&E) sections is about 3 to 5/1 in the duodenum and 6/1 in the ileum. In all regions, the villi are covered by a single layer of columnar epithelium, which includes absorptive cells and goblet cells, seen in routine H&E sections, and "cup" cells, "tuft" cells, and neuroendocrine cells identified with special techniques. Also normally present within the epithelial layer are scattered lymphocytes, amounting to one or two per villus. The epithelium is supported by a basement membrane that is in intimate association with the capillary plexus. In addition to capillaries, the stroma of the villus contains a central lacteal, a few nerve and smooth muscle fibers, and rare lymphocytes and plasma cells. For practical purposes, villi away from dome areas appear devoid of inflammatory cells. Most of the digestive enzymes are situated in the brush border of the villi. In well-fixed and processed pathological specimens, dissolution of the villous brush border, cytoplasmic vacuoles, large intercellular spaces, and large numbers of intraepithelial lymphocytes may be taken as signs of mucosal injury.

The mitotically active proliferation zone is in the lower third of the crypts of Lieberkuhn. From here newly formed cells literally migrate up the sides of the crypts and villi toward the villous tips, from which they slough. The cells differentiate by producing different enzymes, mucins, and surface binding proteins at different levels of their migration up the sides of the villi. This renewal traffic normally takes 3 to 5 days. Cell migration and differentiation resume after small bowel transplantation. In fact, villous architecture may be normal for a considerable time after small bowel transplant (42,43). Long-term survivors of small bowel transplantation recover and maintain good nutritional status (43,44).

In addition to proliferating cells, the crypts contain goblet cells, Paneth cells, endocrine cells, and I cells. Goblet cells secrete mucin, water, and ions. IgA is secreted in the crypts. Paneth cells store and secrete lysozyme, which has bactericidal action. Neuroendocrine cells are detected by silver stains or immunhistochemical techniques. Normally there are one to three neuroendocrine cells per crypt and per villus in microscopic sections. A large number of hormones has been detected in these cells (35), the most frequent of which are serotonin and somatostatin. These cells function as growth promotors and regulators of bowel function and motility. They are known to be increased in actively inflamed mucosas in inflammatory bowel disease, but they have not been studied in bowels posttransplant.

The crypts are supported by the lamina propria stroma and particularly by the fibrolamellar sheath that encompasses each crypt. The pericryptal fibroblasts are known to synthesize collagen. They have been found to express class II antigen (45). Normally there are lymphocytes, plasma cells, mononuclear cells, and rare eosinophils in the lamina propria. They are loosely distributed and do not fill the space between the crypts. After small bowel transplantation, crypt structure and the lamina propria relationships are restored. The status of specific crypt components, such as the neuroendocrine cells and Paneth cells, has not been studied. Changes in the relative number of these cells and their function after transplantation are not documented. Nor is it known what volume, mass, or number of crypt cells may be destroyed by rejection before the mucosa loses the capacity to regenerate.

III. MUCOSAL IMMUNE SYSTEM AND ITS ROLE IN REJECTION REACTIONS

A. GALT System Structure and Function

The structure and function of the gut-associated lymphoid tissue (GALT) have been extensively studied, and there are recent, excellent reviews of the subject (35,46). Lymphoid follicles are present in the mucosa along the entire length of the gastrointestinal (GI) tract. These follicles are most prominent as the Peyer's patches in the ileum. The follicles straddle the muscularis mucosa and are supported at their base by a plexus of vessels and lymphatics. The follicles are covered by epithelium to form a dome area, which is adapted for absorption and presentation of antigens by the "M cells," or microfold cells, located in the dome areas. Their apical surface is less regular than that of the absorptive cells, and the microvilli are smaller, broader, and less regular; they appear as ridges or "microfolds." This structure permits the M cells to transport large molecules and antigens, bacteria, and viruses into the underlying lymphoid tissue. Normally both T and B lymphocytes are present in the lamina propria, although B cells are rare away from the GALT areas. The lymphocytes are present in both the epithelium and the lamina propria. The IELs are primarily T suppressor cells ($CD8^+$, T8 phenotype), while the LPLs are predominantly T-helper cells ($CD4^+$, T4 phenotype). Normally there is a population of $CD68^+$ (KP1) cells of monocyte/macrophage lineage in the lamina propria. Class II antigen (HLA-DR) is expressed on endothelium, some inflammatory cells, and variably on epithelium (Fig. 1).

B. Cells Involved in Rejection Reactions

The techniques for tracking donor and recipient cells in the bowel after transplant are still in the experimental stage, so the role of the various lymphocyte and macrophage subpopulations in the rejection process has not been entirely worked out. In 1988 Goulet et al. (22) noted a pericryptal infiltrate of $CD3^+$ $CD4^+$ (T-helper cells) in mucosal biopsies as early as day 3 after small bowel transplant in a child. Activated ($CD25^+$) T cells increased proportionately by day 7, and expression of HLA-DR was noted on crypt enterocytes. All of these changes were noted prior to any change in the clinical status or light microscopic features of the biopsies. In a subsequent study from this group, Brousse et al. (10) noted similar findings in mucosal biopsies from three additional children after small bowel transplant. Lamina propria lymphocytes and expression of HLA-DR on crypt cells decreased with response to antirejection therapy. Others have also noted infiltration of stimulated macrophages and lymphocytes and increased class II antigen expression on crypt cells prior to histological evidence of rejection (12–16). Oberhuber et al. (15) found increased $CD4^-$ and $CD8^-$ intraepithelial lymphocytes (IELs) in rejected grafts and speculated that these cells may be precursors of the $CD8^+$ cells. Similar cells seem to be involved in both acute and chronic rejection reactions. Tilney et al. (33) noted that the cells mediating rejection were T lymphocytes and macrophages regardless of the stage of the rejection process, although their proportions varied.

C. Distribution of Donor and Recipient Cells in the Allograft

In 1990 Clark et al. (17) used donor-specific antibodies to show that graft lymphoid tissues became infiltrated with host lymphocytes within 1 day posttransplant. Lamina propria lymphocytes (LPLs) were replaced by day 5 with no evidence of damage. During the rejection process, 50% of the total cells in the lamina propria were macrophages, indicat-

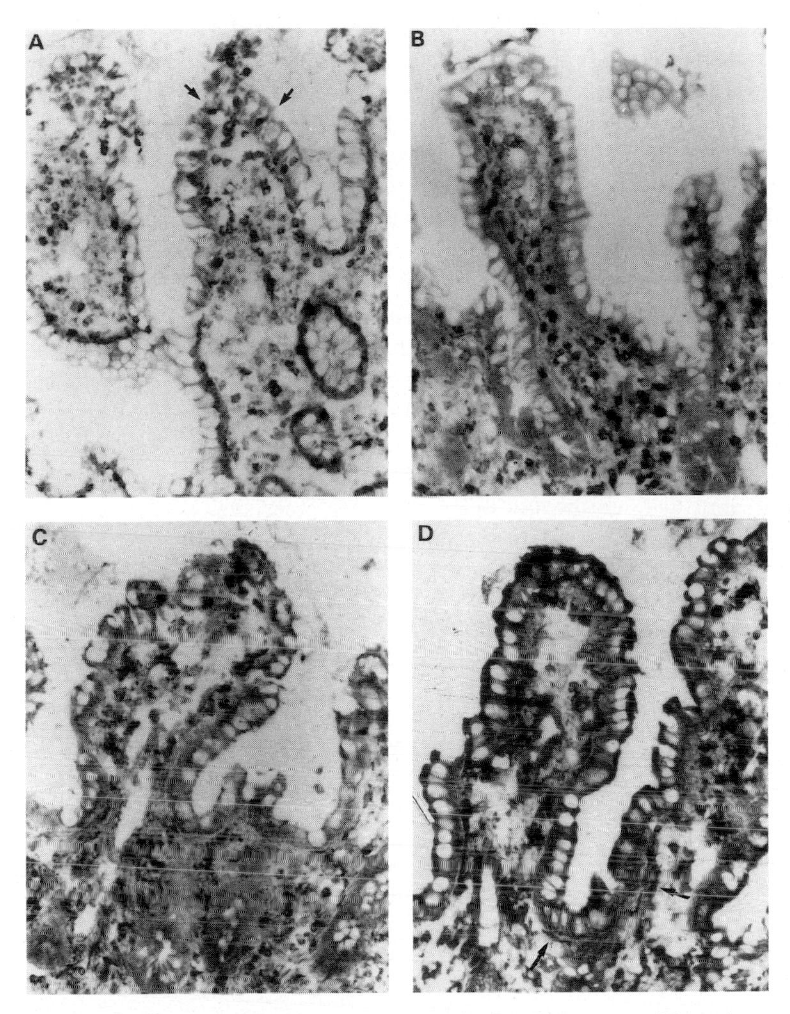

Figure 1 Immunostained frozen sections of normal human small bowel mucosa. (×200.) A. $CD8^+$ cells in the lamina propria and epithelium (arrows). B. $CD4^+$ cells in the lamina propria. C. $CD68^+$ (KP1) cells in the lamina propria. D. HLA-DR expression on epithelium, lymphocytes, vessel and rare stromal cells (arrows).

ing a primary role for them in rejection. Therapy with CyA delayed but did not abolish the process. Iwaki et al. (19) studied three patients with small bowel transplant or small bowel-liver transplant under FK506. They found that donor lymphocytes appeared transiently in the peripheral blood of the recipients in the immediate posttransplant period. Lymphocytes of recipient phenotype replaced the donor lymphocytes in the lamina propria of the small bowel allograft, and replacement was complete by 10 to 12 weeks.

In 1990 Murase et al. (47) made a new and significant observation that lymphocytic infiltrates and epithelial injury occurred in Peyer's patches before they were detected elsewhere in the mucosa. They described expansion of the T-cell zone of Peyer's patches by infiltration of lymphoblasts as early as day 4 posttransplant. The dome epithelium was disrupted. Also noted was expansion and replacement of T-cell zones in the mesenteric lymph nodes. Over the next 2 days, the Peyer's patches were replaced by histiocytes, and lymphocytic cryptitis was first noted remote from the Peyer's patches. Peyer's patches were progressively destroyed by necrosis and abscess formation. These studies are important because they suggest that the sequence of events in rejection of small bowel grafts may follow the expected routes of lymphocyte traffic in the small bowel. This has implications for understanding the mechanism of rejection and possibly the mechanisms of other inflammatory disorders of the small bowel. There are implications also for biopsy sampling during clinical follow-up (Demetris AJ, personal communication). Subsequently, these authors, using recipient-specific monoclonal antibody against class II MHC antigens, showed that the Peyer's patches, lamina propria, and mesenteric nodes of the graft were populated by recipient cells starting within day 12 of multivisceral transplants, and the recipient cells did not appear to be involved in rejection reactions, as the epithelial compartment was normal (48). In a follow-up study, Nakamura et al. (49) studied two cases with male/female discrepancy between donor and recipient using a fluorescence-labeled DNA probe for the Y chromosome. They found that although the inflammatory cells in the lamina propria of the graft were genetically those of the recipient, their relationships to each other were normal and the structure of the mucosa was normal.

IV. COMPLICATIONS OF SMALL BOWEL TRANSPLANT

A. Ischemia

Unlike other organs such as kidney, the acceptable period of cold ischemia for bowel is 5 to 7 hr (1,50). Pathological changes in the graft due to ischemia during the transplant procedure are seen within the first 3 days. They consist of sloughing of villous epithelium and congestion and hemorrhages in the lamina propria (50,51). These changes are reversible. In long-term survivors, ischemia due to pathological changes in the graft vessels is a major component of chronic rejection.

B. Rejection

1. Acute Cellular Rejection

a. Incidence. In humans the incidence of rejection is not well established, since the number of cases reported in human trials is still small. Prior to 1990, the experience was limited to single case reports. Rejection was documented by biopsy upon clinical suspicion in some patients, but the frequency of occurrence of either rejection or GVHD is not known for any of the initial cases. Rejection occurred acutely (<12 days), or was delayed (2 to 5 months) in all five children receiving small bowel transplants in the series by Goulet et al. (30). Interestingly, the two long-term survivors with multivisceral transplants reported in 1989 (23,24) did not show evidence of rejection. From the data available, it appears that rejection occurred to some degree in most of the cases of total small bowel transplant reported after 1990. The largest series to date from Pittsburgh cites at least one episode of rejection in 21 of 24 grafts (87.5%) (26). Several studies suggest that rejection may be less frequent or less severe with combined small bowel-liver allografts than with a small bowel allograft alone (25,47,52).

b. Pathological Features of Acute Cellular Rejection (Table 1). The first systematic pathological study and classic description of the changes in allografts of small bowels was that of Holmes et al. (51). In a detailed histological analysis of mucosal biopsies obtained

Table 1 Microscopic Features of Acute Cellular Rejection

Phase	Interval posttransplant	Histology	Comment	Ref. #
	1 hr	Edema, congestion, denuded villous tips	Reversible changes due to ischemia	51
	1.8 days	Increased lymphs/plasma cells in lamina propria		57
	3 days	Endothelial and epithelial cell injury	Changes seen by EM	55
Phase I	4–5 days	Increased lymphs/plasma cells in lamina propria, increased Ia+ cells in lamina propia, increased OX8+ and ED1+ cells in muscle	"Suspicious" for rejection	16,51,53,54
Phase II	6–7 days	Increased lymphs/plasma cells/ polys, villous blunting, crypt hyperplasia, apoptosis in crypts	Diagnostic	51,53,55
Phase III	8–10 days	Villous/mucosal slough, diffuse lymphs/polys, increased WBCs in deeper layers, vasculitis	Diagnostic	51, 53, 54

daily or twice weekly from segmental jejunal allografts in dogs receiving azathioprine and prednisone, these authors noted that grafts in the untreated animals became grossly congested and edematous after day 4 and progressed to necrosis by day 8. Grafts in the immunosuppressed animals slowly became pale and lost their normal mucosal architecture. Survival times of these grafts varied from 5 to 125 days. Microscopically, immediate changes noted (within 1 hr of transplant) were edema and congestion, loss of epithelium at the villus tips, and increased number of crypt mitoses. These changes were reversible and were probably due to injury sustained during the transplant procedure. The earliest changes the authors could attribute to rejection were first noted on day 4. These included increased lymphocytes and plasma cells in the lamina propria around the crypts. Necrosis of crypt cells and increased mitoses were noted. Over the next few days, crypts became longer and villi shorter. As the process progressed to completion over the next 3 to 4 days, deeper layers of the bowel wall became involved by inflammation, and the mucosa became necrotic and eventually sloughed. Holmes et al. noted that the changes were patchy in nature and that they occurred in all of the transplanted animals, with immunosuppression merely delaying the process.

Subsequently, three phases of histopathological changes in acute cellular rejection were described (53,54). These phases are illustrated in Fig. 2. "Phase I" (days 4 to 5) consists of increased numbers of lymphocytes and plasma cells in the lamina propria without distortion of villous architecture. "Phase II" (days 6 to 7) consists of increased inflammation in lamina propria with extension into muscularis propria, increased mitoses, crypt apoptoses, and villous blunting. Perivascular lymphocyte cuffing and outright vasculitis have been noted. "Phase III" (day 10) consists of mucosal destruction and sloughing and transmural inflammation (Fig. 2). Thus, the rejection process unmodified by immuno-

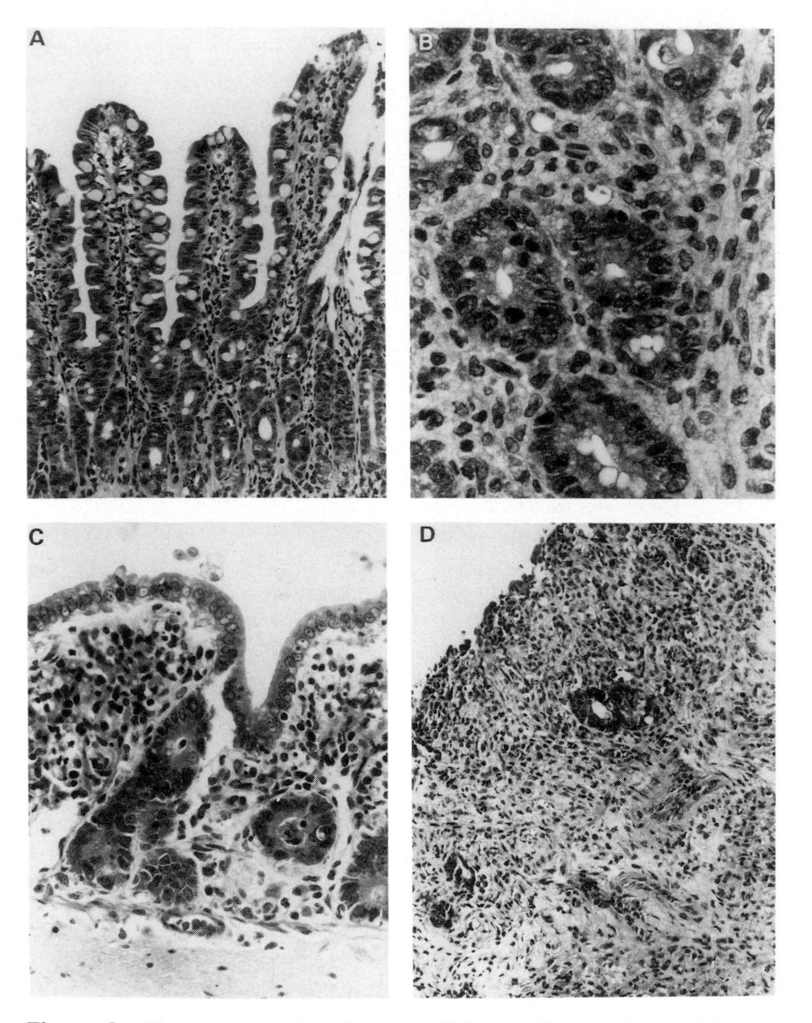

Figure 2 Photomicrographs of a rat small bowel allograft showing three phases of acute cellular rejection. A. Phase I, day 4, with increased lymphocytes in the lamina propria, particularly around the crypts. (H&E, ×200.) B. Phase I at high power showing lymphocytic cryptitis. (H&E, ×400.) C. Phase II, day 6, with villous blunting, lymphocytic cryptitis and sloughed cells in a crypt lumen. (H&E, ×200.) D. Phase III, day 10, with inflammatory destruction of the mucosa, and only rare glands remaining. (H&E, ×200.)

suppression produces histological changes in the graft from day 4 to 5 which progress to mucosal destruction by day 9 to 10. More sophisticated studies have documented changes as early as day 3, including endothelial cell injury (55) and infiltration by immunocompetent cells (14,16,18,22).

Studies that include the pathological changes in the early posttransplant period all describe the same morphological changes regardless of the animal studied or the type of immunosuppression. Evidence suggests that the small bowel is involved diffusely in rejection. Yamataka et al. (56) serially sectioned allograft segments and noted that, in the early stages (day 4 biopsies), rejection was present throughout the graft, but in patchy distribution. Cohen et al. (57) showed no difference between proximal and distal biopsy samples in their small bowel allografts. Stengl et al. (58) compared ileal and jejunal segment allografts and found no difference between them in terms of survival or histological changes.

2. Chronic Rejection

a. Incidence. The definition of chronic rejection is not established. Should the definition be based on arbitrary time period or on specific histological or clinical features? Should chronic rejection be defined solely as the end-stage, fibrotic graft, or is there a preceding, subacute process that could be potentially reversible? Since most studies have not focused on chronic rejection, the incidence and frequency of rejection episodes in long-term survivors after transplantation is not known. In most studies, chronic rejection has been suspected on the basis of a combination of clinical features of graft failure (inanition, diarrhea, malabsorption, failure to thrive) and progressive inflammation and fibrosis in graft biopsies. Subclinical rejection reactions identified pathologically may persist in allografts and eventually lead to graft failure (42,59).

In humans, rejection episodes were diagnosed clinically in four of five patients reported by Goulet et al. (30). These episodes occurred between 2 and 5 months post-transplant. One graft was removed at 17 months due to chronic rejection. A rejection reaction was documented by stomal biopsy at 166 days in 1 of the 23 patients reported by Todo et al. (25,26). Rejection was less severe in patients receiving bowel-liver allografts in that series.

b. Pathogenetic Mechanisms. An excellent overview of mechanisms involved in chronic rejection in many organs is by Tilney et al. (33). Unlike acute rejection reactions where specific cell-mediated epithelial cell injury occurs, many factors contribute to the end-stage fibrotic graft in small bowel, as in liver and kidney. Continuing cellular rejection, ischemia, and poor motility are the most important contributing factors. Cell-mediated damage to epithelium and endothelium continues in the allograft (8,42,43,51,53). Rosemurgy and Schraut noted that chronically rejecting grafts in immunosuppressed animals exhibited the three histological phases of rejection, but they occurred over a longer period of time compared to the changes in acutely rejecting, nonimmunosuppressed grafts (53). In the study of Williams et al. (8), inflammation was found in biopsies of 17 of 27 dogs with long-term survival (mean 112 days) after small bowel transplant. This inflammation was attributed to rejection and was felt to be a major contributing factor in the demise of 6 dogs. The immunophenotypic profile of the inflammatory cells in chronic rejection was studied by Brousse et al. (10), who noted increased T-suppressor cells in the lamina propria and strong expression of HLA-DR antigen on crypt cells.

In addition to cell-mediated injury to the epithelial compartment, long-surviving grafts are also vulnerable to damage from ischemia. Ischemia may result from vascular thrombosis, arteriosclerosis of graft arteries, or rejection-related endothelialitis and vasculitis with eventual endarteritis obliterans (42,43,60,61). Langrehr et al. (43) studied the clinical and pathological features of chronic rejection and the ameliorating effects of CyA and FK506 in an animal model. Chronic rejection was defined as diarrhea and 50-g weight loss after 4 weeks of maintenance CyA therapy. In this model, villous architecture was maintained. Mucosal infiltrates of mononuclear cells and lymphocytic cryptitis were noted. Most striking were endothelialitis and vasculitis involving submucosal and mesenteric vessels. Peyer's patches and mesenteric lymph nodes showed lymphocytic depletion and fibrosis.

Decreased motility due to denervation leads to bacterial overgrowth, muscle hypertrophy, and obstruction (40,43,59). Less directly, inanition due to poor bowel function contributes to the eventual decline in clinical status and possibly promotes bacterial translocation and sepsis.

c. Pathological Features of Chronic Rejection (Table 2). Criteria have not been established for the diagnosis of chronic rejection in small bowel. The following changes have been described in long-surviving (>100 days) animals and humans under immunosuppression with CyA or FK506 (42,43,60,61). Grossly, the bowel is thick due to muscle hypertrophy and fibrosis. Peyer's patches can be seen as scars. Mesenteric fibrosis, vascular thrombi, and adhesions have also been noted. Cobblestone appearance of the mucosa has been described.

Microscopic changes in chronic rejection are shown in Table 2 and illustrated in Fig. 3. They include the following:

Mucosa: Villi are normal initially, then blunted or flat. There is crypt dropout. Remaining crypts show regenerative changes with increased mitoses and gastric or Paneth cell metaplasia. Lymphocytic cryptitis, crypt abscesses, or apoptosis may be present. Chronic inflammation, acute inflammation, and fibrosis are present in the lamina propria. There may be evidence of edema and dilated lacteals.

Submucosa: Acute and/or chronic inflammation, fibrosis, and lymphocytic infiltrates are present around vessels and nerves. Endothelialitis, active vasculitis and endarteritis obliterans have been described.

Table 2 Microscopic Features of Chronic Rejection

Mucosa
Villi blunt or flat
Crypts show lymphocytic cryptitis
Apoptosis/satellitosis
Lymphocytic crypt abscesses
Crypt dropout
Regenerative changes
Lamina propria contains lymphocytes, plasma cells, and monocytes
Fibrosis
Telangiectasia/lymphangiectasia
Submucosa/muscle
Chronic inflammation around vessels and nerves
Fibrosis
Endothelialitis
Endarteritis obliterans
Lymphoid tissue
Lymphocytic atrophy
Fibrosis/obliteration
Mesentery
Chronic inflammation
Lymphocytic vasculitis
Fibrosis
Atrophy of fat

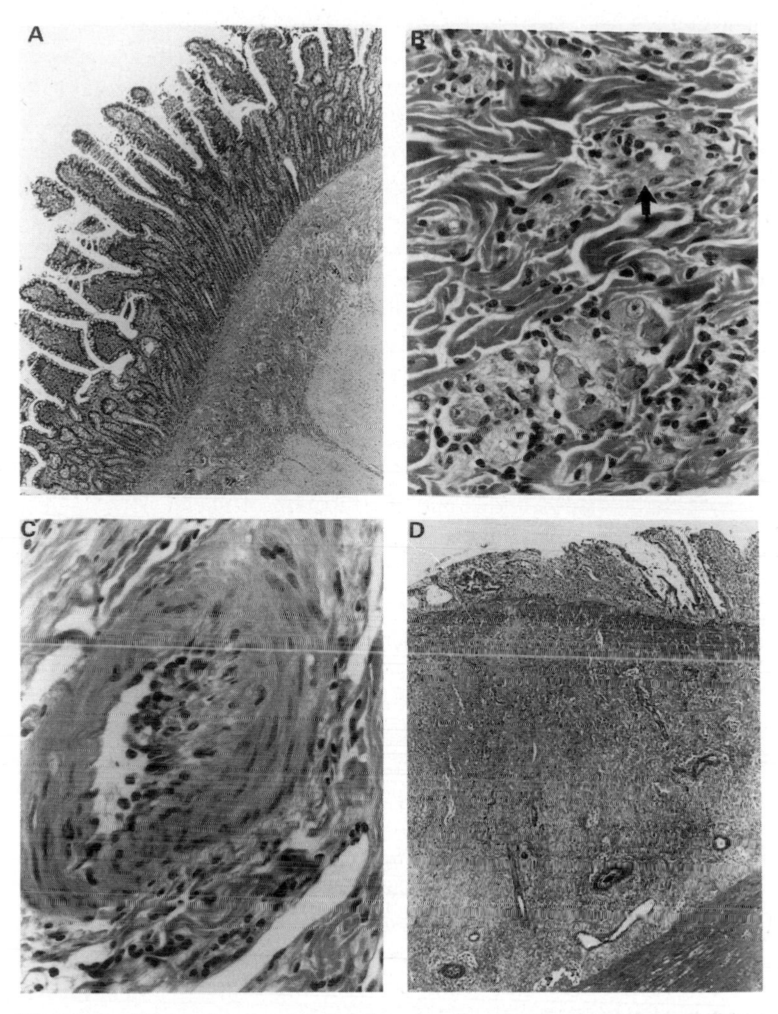

Figure 3 Photomicrographs showing chronic rejection in canine small bowel allografts. A. Allograft wall at 3 months with normal villous architecture and fibrosis in the submucosa. Chronic inflammation, not easily seen here, is present also. (H&E, ×40.) B. Higher power of submucosa showing a ganglion of Meissner's plexus infiltrated by lymphocytes and plasma cells. Note endothelialitis in a nearby arteriole (arrow). (H&E, ×400.) C. Higher power of submucosa showing intimal inflammation in an artery. (H&E, ×400.) D. Allograft at 6 months showing crypt loss and fibrous thickening of the wall. (H&E, ×40.)

Lymphoid tissue: Peyer's patches and lymph nodes may be infiltrated by blasts and activated lymphocytes with corresponding loss of native lymphoid tissue. Eventually lymph nodes become atrophic and fibrotic.

Mesentery: Atrophy of fat, inflammation, fibrosis and lymphocytic vasculitis have been described.

3. Role of Mucosal Biopsy in the Diagnosis of Rejection

Since acute cellular rejection in part, if not entirely, involves mucosal structures, it is becoming increasingly clear that mucosal biopsy is an adequate means to diagnose acute cellular rejection. Cohen et al. (57) created exteriorized blind pouches at the proximal and distal ends of small bowel allografts. They noted that mucosal biopsies from the deeper part of the pouches exhibited changes identical to those in the in-continuity bowel and suggested that pouches could be used to monitor the graft with biopsies. Although there are numerous studies using biopsies to monitor the course of rejection after transplantation, currently there are no studies to determine the diagnostic accuracy or predictive value of mucosal biopsies compared to other techniques for diagnosing rejection.

At the University of Pittsburgh, endoscopic mucosal biopsies were part of the follow-up of the 23 patients with small bowel transplant and immunosuppression by FK506 (50,62). The biopsies were obtained weekly for the first 3 months and then as needed. Fever, abdominal pain, vomiting, watery diarrhea, and increased stomal output constituted the clinical signs of rejection. During these episodes, the endoscopic appearance of the mucosa was dusky and ischemic, with ulcerations and poor peristalsis. Biopsies showed increasing lymphocytic infiltration of the lamina propria and walls of venules and crypts. Necrosis of crypt epithelial cells, mucus depletion, and loss of Paneth cells was followed by reparative changes of irregularly shaped crypts and stratification of nuclei. Histological changes interpreted as showing more severe rejection included ulcers, polymorphonuclear leukocytes plugging capillaries, villous blunting, pseudomembranes, and bacterial superinfection. These histological features interpreted as due to rejection resolved with additional immunosuppression. The authors noted that rejection was more accurately diagnosed in the early (<1 month) transplant period, when biopsy changes were often accompanied by clinical signs of rejection and response to increased immunosuppression was more reliable.

Doubts about the usefulness of mucosal biopsies in the diagnosis of rejection have been raised. Schmid et al. (54) note that inflammatory infiltrates and changes in the villi may be seen in a number of disease processes and may not be specific for rejection. They also note that consecutive biopsies, rather than a single biopsy, may be necessary to establish a diagnosis of rejection. Another pitfall in using biopsies to detect rejection is that the mucosa near the exteriorized end of the bowel at a stoma exhibits acute and chronic inflammation and fibrosis, and may mimic rejection (50). Several studies of long-term survivors on both CyA and FK605 describe destructive inflammation in the submucosa and muscularis propria (42,60,61) and even the mesentery (43) when the mucosa appears structurally normal, and the reliability of mucosal biopsies in diagnosing chronic rejection has been questioned.

C. Graft-Versus-Host Disease

1. *Incidence*

Graft-versus-host disease is a systemic syndrome characterized by destruction of host tissues by donor lymphocytes. Prerequisite for this are immunocompromise of the host, immunocompetent donor lymphocytes, and some degree of alloantigen mismatch between the donor and host tissues. The bowel has the greatest potential of any engrafted organ except the bone marrow for mounting a GVH reaction due to its large amount of lymphoid tissue.

A GVH reaction may occur concurrently with rejection and may be evident in host tissue without being clinically apparent (8,60,62–64). Studies of GVHD reactions in fully allogeneic donor/recipient combinations in bidirectional animal models of small bowel transplant show that whether GVHD or rejection predominates depends on the type of immunosuppression used (3,62,65–67). Langrehr et al. (65) tested the factors influencing

GVHD in a bidirectional animal model and noted that GVHD occurred only when the donor had been presensitized to host antigens and the recipient was immunosuppressed. Reports of GVHD in humans are rare. In the Pittsburgh series (62), one patient of 24 had GVHD. Theoretically, a controlled GVH reaction could work to the recipient's advantage, since the effect of a GVH reaction on host lymph nodes would be to diminish the host's ability to mount a rejection reaction (60,68).

2. *Pathology*

GVHD is noticeable experimentally at day 10 (16,69) when T helper cells, macrophages and lymphoblasts of donor origin infiltrate host lymphoid tissue and organs. Clinically, GVHD may be suspected when the patient has skin rash, diarrhea, or wasting. Biopsies of skin or liver reveal the diagnostic lesion of lymphocyte killing of epithelial cells and eventual destruction of the epithelium. The criteria for the diagnosis of GVHD in the skin, liver and GI tract are well established (70,71). Lymphocytes around and within the crypts without much inflammation elsewhere in the lamina propria and scattered apoptotic crypt cells are presumptive evidence of a GVH reaction. These findings alone are nonspecific (42). Like other sites such as the skin and liver, the finding characteristic of GVHD in the bowel is satellitosis, i.e., a lymphocyte associated with a necrotic epithelial cell (70–72). More advanced lesions may exhibit crypt abscesses, with necrotic epithelial and inflammatory cells in the crypt lumens. The most severe GVHD reactions cause necrosis and sloughing of the mucosa. The findings of early or mild GVHD in the bowel are subtle and may not be identified easily at low power, since the lymphocytic infiltrate is sparse and concentrated around the crypts. Histologic changes of GVH reaction in skin and host bowel are shown in Fig. 4.

D. Infection

The most common infectious complication in animals after small bowel transplant is bacterial translocation and sepsis (73). Infection by other agents has been surprisingly infrequent. Williams et al. (8) reported histoplasmosis in long-surviving dogs. In the Pittsburgh series, nine patients with infectious complications were reported (74). The complications included positive blood cultures for enterococci, *S. aureus*, *Enterobacter cloacae*, *Candida albicans*, and *Clostridium difficile*; pseudomembranous colitis; and enterococcal wound infection. Three patients were found to have CMV, adenovirus, herpes stomatitis, and Epstein-Barr virus meningoencephalitis. All infections responded to therapy.

E. Drug Effects

Toxic effects of CyA and FK506 on small bowel have been investigated but not proven. Crane et al. (75) demonstrated a reduction in intestinal wall vasculature of CyA-treated rats by high-resolution radiographic techniques. In studies using FK506 immunosuppression, no toxicity of FK506 has been described (43,63).

F. Causes of Death—Autopsy Studies

Deaths in the immediate posttransplant period are usually due to infarction of the graft due to vascular thrombosis (8,59), or mechanical problems such as volvulus (8,59). Without immunosuppression, the bowel allograft survives 6 to 12 days and the animals quickly die

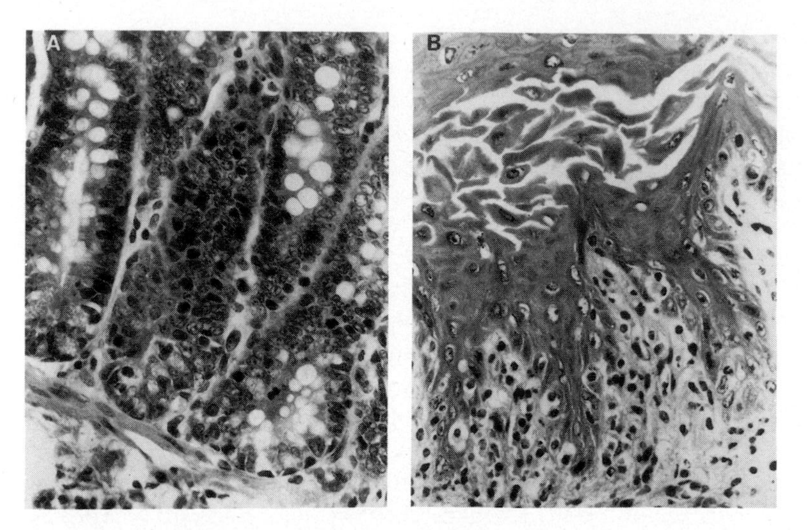

Figure 4 Photomicrographs showing GVHD in a bidirectional, fully allogeneic rat model. A. Host small bowel with lymphocytic cryptitis consistent with GVHD. (H&E, ×200.) B. Skin with florid GVHD (H&E, × 200.)

due to sepsis, with the source being the rejecting bowel. Deaths due to complications of rejection such as bowel necrosis, perforation, or peritonitis (7) or systemic infection and pneumonia (8,59) occur after 1 week. Fulminant rejection and graft necrosis have caused deaths in many series (7,8). Studies using immunosuppression with the standard regimens of CyA or azathioprine plus prednisone (2,8,51,59,60) achieve long-term survivals. In long-term survivors, deaths due to inanition are attributed to graft failure due to chronic rejection (7,8,59,60), pneumonia (59), or intestinal obstruction (8,59). Interestingly, although bacterial sepsis is common in animals, nonbacterial systemic infections are rare; Williams et al. reported two of their dogs with fatal systemic histoplasmosis (8).

The initial small bowel transplants in humans failed due to technical reasons, rejection, or sepsis (20). The first patient with small intestinal transplant under CyA immunosuppression reported by Goulet et al. (22) survived 205 days and died with hepatorenal failure and candidal sepsis. Two other children receiving small bowel transplants died with PTLD after surviving 4 to 6 months. Long-term survival (>405 days) after small bowel transplant in a 43-year-old woman was reported by Deltz et al. (29) using CyA and antilymphocyte globulin immunosuppression. Goulet et al. (30) reported survival from 5 months to 6 years after small intestine transplant in 5 children using CyA and predinone with ALG. Recently the results of the first clinical trial of intestinal transplant in humans using FK506 immunosuppression at the University of Pittsburgh were reported. Of the 23 patients transplanted, 4 patients died at 23, 70, 385, and 776 days, from sepsis (3 patients) or lymphoproliferative disorder (1 patient). The others were alive at intervals from 67 to >754 days (25,26).

V. SUMMARY

Over the past 40 years, the surgical methods and techniques for immunosuppression, monitoring graft function, and detecting rejection have been worked out in animal models. Considerable progress has been made in understanding the immunopathology of rejection reactions and the distribution of donor and host cells in the allograft. The histopathological changes characteristic of acute cellular rejection have been established, making mucosal biopsy an important means to monitor the allograft in the early posttransplant period. However, there are many important problems yet to be explored. The studies of Murase et al. (48), in which recipient cells were noted to be present in allografts without a rejection reaction, raise questions about tolerance of foreign cells and mechanisms for initiating rejection reactions. The clinical and pathophysiological aspects of chronic rejection, humoral rejection, and the role of host and graft lymph nodes in rejection and GVH reactions must be defined. Effects of therapeutic agents on the allograft have to be more fully explored. As human trials enlarge and experience with long-term survivors increases, these issues will be addressed.

REFERENCES

1. Lillehei RC, Goott B, Miller FA. The physiological response of the small bowel of the dog to ischemia including prolonged in vitro preservation of the bowel with successful replacement and survival. Ann Surg 1959; 150:543–560.
2. Lillehei RC, Goldberg S, Goott B, Longerbeam JK. The present status of intestinal transplantation. Am J Surg 1963; 105:58–72.
3. Cohen Z, MacGregor AB, Moore KTH, et al. Canine small bowel transplantation: A study of the immunological responses. Arch Surg 1976; 111:248–253.
4. Hardy MA, Quint J, State D. Effect of antilymphocyte serum and other immunosuppressive agents on canine jejunal allografts. Ann Surg 1970; 171:51–60.
5. Preston FW, Macalalad F, Wachowski TJ, et al. Survival of homografts of the intestine with and without immunosuppression. Surgery 1966; 60:1203–1210.
6. Taylor RMR, Watson JW, Walker FC, Watson AJ. Prolongation of survival of jejunal homografts in dogs treated with azathioprine (Imuran). Br J Surg 1966; 53:134–138.
7. Diliz-Perez HS, McClure J, Bedetti C, et al. Successful small bowel allotransplantation in dogs with cyclosporine and prednisone. Transplantation 1984; 37:126–129.
8. Williams JW, McClellan T, Peters TG, et al. Effect of pretreatment graft irradiation on canine intestinal transplantation. Surg Gynecol Obstet 1988; 167:197–204.
9. Monchik GJ, Russell PS. Transplantation of small bowel in the rat: Technical and immunological considerations. Surgery 1971; 70:693–702.
10. Brousse N, Canioni D, Rambaud C, et al. Intestinal transplantation in children: Contribution of immunohistochemistry. Transplant Proc 1990; 22:2495–2496.
11. Hansmann ML, Deltz E, Gundlach M, et al. Small bowel transplantation in a child: Morphologic, immunohistochemical, and clinical results. Am J Clin Pathol 1989; 92:686–692.
12. Hansmann ML, Hell K, Gundlach M, et al. Immunohistochemical investigation of biopsies in a successful small-bowel transplantation. Transplant Proc 1990; 22:2502–2503.
13. Schmid T, Oberhuber G, Koroszi G, et al. Major histocompatibility complex class II antigen expression on enterocytes during rejection of small-bowel allografts. Transplant Proc 1990; 22:2480.
14. Hurlbut D, Garcia B, Ohene-Fianko D, et al. Immunohistochemical assessment of mucosal biopsies following human intestinal transplantation. Transplant Proc 1992; 24:1195–1196.
15. Oberhuber G, Schmid T, Thaler W, et al. Increased number of intraepithelial lymphocytes in rejected small-bowel allografts: An analysis of subpopulations involved. Transplant Proc 1990; 22:2454–2455.
16. Garcia B, Zhong R, Wijsman J, et al. Pathological changes following intestinal transplantation in the rat. Transplant Proc 1990; 22:2469–2470.
17. Clark CL, Cunningham AJ, Crane PW, et al. Lymphocyte infiltration patterns in rat small-bowel transplants. Transplant Proc 1990; 22:2460.

18. Hell K, Gundlach M, Schmidt P, et al. Immunohistochemical analysis of immunocompetent cells involved in small-bowel rejection in the rat. Transplant Proc 1990; 22:2461–2462.
19. Iwaki Y, Starzl TE, Yagihashi A, et al. Replacement of donor lymphoid tissue in small-bowel transplants. Lancet 1991; 337:818–819.
20. Kirkman RL. Small bowel transplantation. Transplantation 1984; 37:429–433.
21. Cohen Z, Silverman RE, Wassef R, et al. Small intestinal transplantation using cyclosporine. Transplantation 1986; 42:613–621.
22. Goulet OJ, Revillon Y, Cerf-Bensussan N, et al. Small intestinal transplantation in a child using cyclosporine. Transplant Proc 1988; 20:288–296.
23. Starzl TE, Rowe MI, Todo S, et al. Transplantation of multiple abdominal viscera. JAMA 1989; 261:1449–1457.
24. Williams JW, Sankary HN, Foster PF, et al. Splanchnic transplantation: An approach to the infant dependent on parenteral nutrition who develops irreversible liver disease. JAMA 1989; 261:1458–1462.
25. Todo S, Tzakis AG, Abu-Elmagd K, et al. Cadaveric small bowel and small bowel-liver transplantation in humans. Transplantation 1992; 53:369–376.
26. Todo S, Tzakis A, Reyes J, et al. Intestinal transplantation in humans under FK506. Transplant Proc 1993; 25:1198–1199.
27. Grant D, Wall W, Zhong R, et al. Experimental clinical intestinal transplantation: Initial experience of a Canadian centre. Transplant Proc 1990; 22:2497–2498.
28. McAlister V, Wall W, Ghent C, et al. Successful small intestinal transplantation. Transplant Proc 1992; 24:1236–1237.
29. Deltz E, Schroeder P, Gundlach M, et al. Successful clinical small-bowel transplantation. Transplant Proc 1990; 22:2501.
30. Goulet O, Revillon D, Brousse JN, et al. Small-bowel transplantation in children. Transplant Proc 1990; 22:2499–2500.
31. Watson AJM, Lear PA. Current status of intestinal transplantation. Gut 1989; 30:1771–1782.
32. Banner B, Hoffman A, Cai X, et al. Transplantation of the small intestine: The pathologist's perspective. Am J Surg Pathol 1990; 14(suppl):109–116.
33. Tilney NL, Whitley WD, Diamond JR, et al. Chronic rejection-an undefined conundrum. Transplantation 1991; 52:389–398.
34. Clark CI. Recent progress in intestinal transplantation. Arch Dis Child 1992; 67:976–979.
35. Fenoglio-Preiser CM, Lantz PE, David M, et al. Gastrointestinal Pathology: An Atlas and Text. New York: Raven Press, 1989:225–244.
36. Schraut WH, Rosemurgy AS, Riddell RM. Prolongation of intestinal allograft survival without immunosuppressive drug therapy: Transplantation of small bowel allografts. J Surg Res 1983; 34:597–607.
37. Murase N, Demetris AJ, Furuya T, et al. Comparison of the small intestine after multivisceral transplantation with the small intestines transplanted with portal or caval drainage. Transplant Proc 1992; 24:1143–1144.
38. Goott B, Lillehei RC, Miller FA. Mesenteric lymphatic regeneration after autografts of small bowel in dogs. Surgery 1960; 48:571–575.
39. Schmid T, Korozsi G, Oberhuber G, et al. Lymphatic regeneration after small bowel transplantation. Transplant Proc 1990; 22:2446.
40. Heeckt PF, Halfter WM, Schraut WH, et al. Small bowel transplantation and chronic rejection alter rat intestinal smooth muscle structure and function. Surgery 1993; 114:449–457.
41. Schiller WR, Suriyapa C, Mutchler JHW, et al. Motility changes associated with canine intestinal allografting. J Surg Res 1973; 15:379–384.
42. Banner B, Dean P, Williams J, Morphologic features of rejection in long-surviving canine small bowel transplants. Transplantation 1988; 46:665–669.
43. Langrehr JM, Banner B, Lee KKW, Schraut WH. Clinical course, morphology, and treatment of chronically rejecting small bowel allografts. Transplantation 1993; 55:242–250.

44. Schraut WH, Lee KKW, Sitrin M. Recipient growth and nutritional status following transplantation of segmental small-bowel allografts. J Surg Res 1987; 43:1–9.
45. Banner BF, Sonmez-Alpan E, Yousem SA. An immunophenotypic study of the inflammatory cell populations in colon adenomas and carcinomas. Mod Pathol 1993; 6:295–301.
46. Brandtzaeg P, Halstensen TS, Kett K, et al. Immunobiology and immunopathology of human gut mucosa: Humoral immunity and intraepithelial lymphocytes. Gastroenterology 1989; 97: 1562–1584.
47. Murase N, Demetris AJ, Kim DG, et al. Rejection of multivisceral allografts in rats: A sequential analysis with comparison to isolated orthotopic small-bowel and liver grafts. Surgery 1990; 108:880–889.
48. Murase N, Demetris AJ, Matsuzaki T, et al. Long survival in rats after multivisceral versus isolated small-bowel allotransplantation under FK506. Surgery 1991; 110:87–98.
49. Nakamura K, Nalesnik M, Todo S, et al. Lymphocyte trafficking using in situ hybridization and physioanatomy of the intestinal immmune system after human small bowel transplantation. Transplant Proc 1992; 24:1197–1198.
50. Nakamura K, Nalesnik M, Jaffe R, et al. Morphological monitoring of human small bowel allografts. Transplant Proc 1993; 25:1212.
51. Holmes JT, Klein MS, Winawer SJ, Fortner JG. Morphological studies of rejection in canine jejunal allografts. Gastroenterology 1971; 61:693–706.
52. Zhong R, He G, Sakai Y, et al. Combined small bowel and liver transplantation in the rat: Possible role of the liver in preventing intestinal allograft rejection. Transplantation 1991; 52: 550–576.
53. Rosemurgy AS, Schraut WH. Small bowel allografts: Sequence of histologic changes in acute and chronic rejection. Am J Surg 1986; 151:470–475.
54. Schmid T, Oberhuber G, Korozsi G, et al. Histologic pattern of small bowel allograft rejection in the rat: Mucosal biopsies do not provide sufficient information. Gastroenterology 1989; 96: 1529–1532.
55. Madara JL, Kirkman RL. Structural and functional evolution of jejunal allograft rejection in rats and the ameliorating effects of cyclosporine therapy. J Clin Invest 1985; 75:502–512.
56. Yamataka A, Miyano T, Fukunaga K, et al. Patchy distribution of rejection changes in small intestinal transplantation. J Pediatr Surg 1992; 27:602–603.
57. Cohen A, Nordgren S, Lossing A, et al. Morphologic studies of intestinal allograft rejection: Immunosuppression with cyclosporine. Dis Colon Rectum 1984; 27:228–2344.
58. Stengl M, Schraut WH, Moynihan HL, Lee T. Rejection of ileal versus jejunal allografts. Transplantation 1989; 47:424–427.
59. Reznick RK, Craddock GN, Langer B, et al. Structure and function of small bowel allografts in the dog: Immunosuppression with cyclosporin A. Can J Surg 1982; 25:51–55.
60. Fujiwara H, Raju S, Grogan JB, et al. Total orthotopic small bowel allotransplantation in the dog. Transplantation 1987; 44:747–753.
61. Millard PR, Dennison AL, Hughes DA, et al. Morphology of intestinal allograft rejection and the inadequacy of mucosal biopsy in its recognition. Br J Exp Pathol 1986; 67:687–698.
62. Abu-Elmagd KM, Tzakis A, Todo S, et al. Monitoring and treatment of intestinal allograft rejection in humans. Transplant Proc 1993; 25:1202–1203.
63. Saat RE, Heineman E, DeBruin RWF, et al. Total orthotopic allogeneic small bowel transplantation in rats. Transplantation 1989; 47:451–453.
64. Hoffman AL, Makowka L, Banner B, et al. The use of FK506 for small intestine allotransplantation: Inhibition of acute rejection and prevention of fatal graft-versus-host disease. Transplantation 1990; 49:483–490.
65. Langrehr JM, Markus PM, Lee TK, et al. Lethal graft-versus-host disease after cyclosporine therapy in recipients of sensitized small bowel allografts. Transplant Proc 1992; 24:1138.
66. Diflo T, Maki T, Balogh K, Monaco AP. Graft-versus-host disease in fully allogeneic small bowel transplantation in the rat. Transplantation 1989; 47:7–11.

67. Deltz E, Ulrichs K, Schack T, et al. Graft-versus-host reaction in small bowel transplantation and possibilities for its circumvention. Am J Surg 1986; 151:379–386.
68. Langrehr JM, Hoffman RA, Banner B, et al. Induction of graft-versus-host disease and rejection by sensitized small bowel allografts. Transplantation 1991; 52:399–405.
69. Grant D, Zhong R, Gunn H, et al. Graft-versus-host disease associated with intestinal transplantation in the rat: Host immune function and general histology. Transplantation 1989; 48: 545–549.
70. Schraut WH, Lee KKW, Dawson PJ, Hurst RD. Graft-versus-host disease induced by small bowel allografts. Transplantation 1986; 41:286–290.
71. Sale GE, Shulman HM, eds. The Pathology of Bone Marrow Transplantation. New York: Masson, 1984.
72. Sale GE, Shulman HM, McDonald GB, Thomas ED. Gastrointestinal graft-versus-host disease in man: A clinicopathologic study of the rectal biopsy. Am J Surg Pathol 1979; 3:291–299.
73. Price B, Cumberland NS, Clark CL, et al. The effect of rejection and graft-versus-host disease on small intestinal microflora and bacterial translocation after rat small bowel transplantation. Transplantation 1993; 56:1072–1076.
74. Reyes J, Abu-Elmagd K, Tzakis A, et al. Infectious complications after human small bowel transplantation. Transplant Proc 1992; 24:1249–1250.
75. Crane PW, Clark C, Sowter C, et al. Cyclosporine toxicity in the small intestine. Transplant Proc 1990; 22:2432.

11

Pathology of Pancreatic Transplantation

Raouf E. Nakhleh
Henry Ford Hospital, Detroit, Michigan

I. OVERVIEW

Pancreatic transplantation is performed to alleviate signs and symptoms of diabetes mellitus and to prevent the development or progression of its chronic disabling effects (1–3). Multiple surgical procedures for pancreatic transplantation have been developed. The most common procedure today is the bladder-drained pancreaticoduodenal transplant (2,4–6). In this procedure, the exocrine graft is drained via the duodenum into the urinary bladder. This offers the opportunity to monitor exocrine function by measuring enzyme levels in the urine (3,7–9). Monitoring of urinary amylase level is the most common method of evaluating pancreatic function. Dysfunction produces a drop in the amylase levels. This test is not specific for rejection, which may be caused by cellular rejection, acute and chronic pancreatitis, necrosis, and infection (10). Normal morphology has also been documented in cases of hypoamylasuria, and may in some cases be due to a temporary physiological change.

Pancreatic and duodenal biopsies may be performed via a cystoscope (11–13). As in other endoscopic biopsy procedures, the duodenum is visualized and biopsied using forceps, whereas the pancreas is biopsied blindly using a long needle. Bladder-drained pancreaticoduodenal transplants in diabetic patients are typically performed simultaneously with a kidney transplant (4,5,9,14,15). Since it has been shown that the kidney is more likely to undergo rejection than the pancreas, the kidney is usually biopsied. Some institutions only rarely, if ever, biopsy the pancreas.

Pancreatic transplantation with intestinal anastomosis for exocrine drainage may also be performed (16). A segmental or whole organ can be transplanted by this method. Segmental transplants are used for living related pancreatic transplants, which are performed at only a few select institutions (2,6,16,17). From a tissue diagnosis perspective, biopsy can be performed percutaneously or at laparotomy (18–20). In some institutions, pancreas juice and urinary cytology is performed because open drainage is maintained for a period of time until the organ stabilizes (21–24). Serum amylase and blood glucose levels are monitored, but these parameters tend to be late markers of dysfunction (25). Bladder-drained procedures are often converted to intestinal drainage secondary to duodenal cuff problems (26,27).

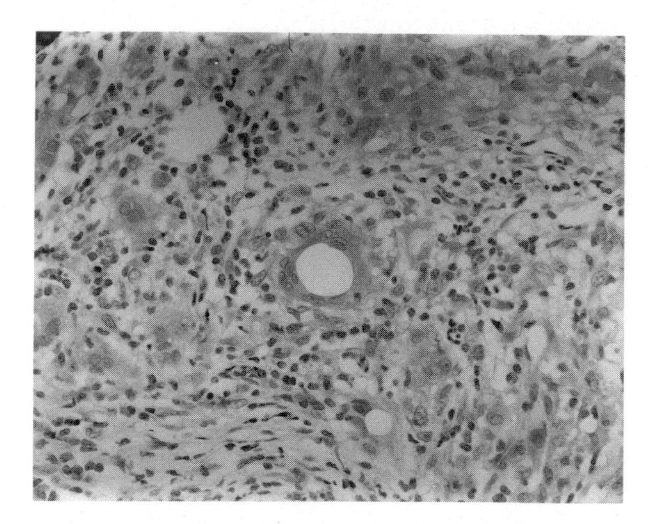

Figure 1 Duct-injected pancreas transplant. Chronic pancreatitis is seen with foreign-body giant cells present. Refractile material can occasionally be seen. (H&E.)

Duct-injected or duct-ligated procedures are still performed in some centers (2,6). In these procedures, the exocrine duct is either injected with synthetic material or is ligated (Fig. 1). The idea is to ablate the exocrine function, thus rendering an endocrine-only organ. Unfortunately, these procedures result in acute and chronic pancreatitis, which may lead to islet dysfunction as well (28–30). These organs may be biopsied via open laparotomy or percutaneously.

II. TECHNICAL PROBLEMS

Technical problems typically occur very early after transplantation. The most common technical problem is vascular thrombosis leading to necrosis of the transplanted organ (29,31–34). The high frequency of vascular thrombosis may be due to abnormal hemodynamics in the graft, with low flow in very large caliber vessels (splenic vein and artery) as compared with the small tributaries of the pancreatic parenchyma (33,34). The possibility of kinking or twisting of these very long vessels may also contribute to thrombosis.

Duodenal cuff problems are another major source of morbidity, although they less often lead to graft loss. In many cases duodenal dehiscence, ulceration and bleeding occurs (26). It is not clear why this occurs, but altered blood flow to the duodenum is a possibility, ultimately leading to ischemia and focal areas of necrosis. This may present as pain or hematuria and may be a source of intraabdominal leakage.

Clinical diagnosis of these problems is typically not the concern of the pathologist. Biopsy of the transplanted organ is rarely performed in these situations, although tissue may be removed during a corrective procedure.

In all cases of duodenal problems, cytomegalovirus infection should be investigated, since it may mimic some of these conditions.

III. REJECTION

Rejection in the pancreas is characterized in similar fashion to rejection of other transplanted solid organs as hyperacute, acute, and chronic.

A. Hyperacute Rejection

Hyperacute rejection is a difficult diagnosis to make because of the relatively high incidence of early organ failure due to vascular thrombosis. I am aware of only one case of probable hyperacute rejection (35). The patient had a negative crossmatch, but post-transplant panel-reactive antibody was 80%. Morphologically, extensive fibrin thrombosis of small and medium-sized arteries, veins, and capillaries was found.

B. Acute Rejection

Acute rejection is primarily a function of cell-mediated cytotoxicity. The cellular targets of rejection are the endothelial cells and the acinar and ductal epithelial cells. Islets and specifically beta cells (the main component of islets) are not primary targets of rejection (Fig. 2; see also color plate). This is fortuitous, since the beta cells are the primary reason for transplantation of the pancreas. Islets, however, may be involved late in rejection and may also stop functioning before becoming involved with inflammatory cells (29,36,37).

Rejection is usually described as two events: (1) rejection of the parenchymal tissues and (2) rejection of the vascular tissue. This separation may be accurate when one is considering an antibody-mediated rejection (hyperacute rejection). But in acute cellular rejection, the process is more dynamic, with probable intimate connection of the two processes.

We have had the opportunity to examine a large number of biopsy tissues and resection specimens of the pancreas and have found a relationship between interstitial inflammation and vascular lesions (37). It is exceedingly rare to find pancreatic transplants with cellular vascular rejection and without interstitial rejection. By the same token, when mild interstitial inflammation is present, endothelialitis may be found, but more advanced vascular lesions such as transmural vasculitis are not usually found. Vasculitis is usually seen with severe interstitial inflammation. From this kind of evidence we can conclude that a tem-

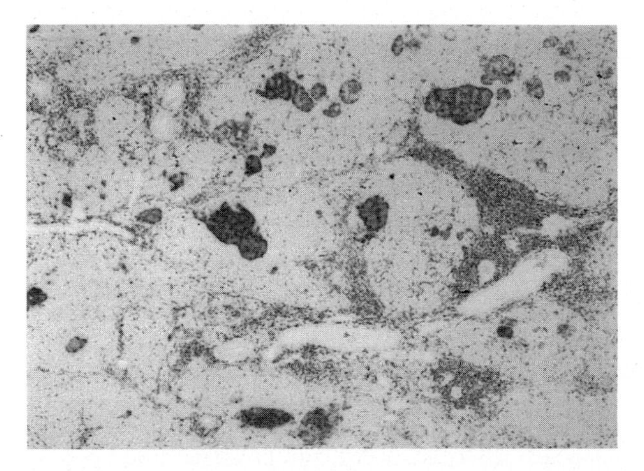

Figure 2 Acute pancreas rejection. This tissue is double-stained with antibodies to chromogranin A (red stain) and leukocyte common antigen (LCA) (brown stain). Chromogranin A demonstrates the islets while LCA shows the inflammatory infiltrates in rejection. Note that the islets are not involved by inflammation. The inflammation is primarily concentrated in fibrous septae but also infiltrates the pancreatic acinar tissue. [Double immunostains; chromogranin A (red) and leukocyte common antigen (brown), no counterstain.] (For optimal reproduction, see color plate.)

poral relationship exists between interstitial rejection and vascular cellular rejection. Interstitial rejection appears to occur first, with release of inflammatory mediators leading to upregulation of class II HLA antigens and other antigens on endothelial cells, resulting in cell-mediated injury or rejection.

Based on the above observations, morphological categories can be defined as stages or grades of rejection (Table 1). It is uniformly accepted that vasculitis and endothelialitis are the most specific findings in the diagnosis of rejection. Interstitial inflammation may be mimicked by other conditions, such as chronic pancreatitis and cytomegalovirus infection (12,36). The typical histomorphological appearance of rejection is that of a mixed inflammatory infiltrate with active necrosis of the acinar epithelial cells (Figs. 3 and 4). The infiltrate is predominantly lymphocytic, with plasma cells, eosinophils, neutrophils and monocytes. The inflammatory cells tend to be clustered in fibrous septae in a periductal and perivascular location (Figs. 5 and 6). The inflammatory cells involve the acinar tissue to a variable extent but are usually more dense in the septae. The inflammatory infiltrate will be composed of lymphocytes with mild episodes of rejection. As the severity of rejection progresses, the infiltrate becomes more mixed, to include plasma cells and eosinophils. Fibrosis occurs after destruction of the acinar tissue (Fig. 7). The islets are typically not involved, but we have seen islets overrun by inflammation in severe cases of rejection. If there is any question of isletitis and recurrence of diabetes, then insulin stains should be performed to verify the presence of sufficient numbers of beta cells (29,36,38) (Figs. 8 and 9). In rejection, the amount of beta cells should be normal (approximately 70 to 80%) in relationship to the total amount of islet tissue. The ratio of beta cells to total islet cells is emphasized because total islet mass may be diminished.

The mildest form of vascular rejection is endothelialitis. This is defined generally as inflammation of the endothelium, but morphologically a strict definition is applied. It is not sufficient to see lymphocytes adjacent or attached to the endothelium. The endothelial cells must also show evidence of damage, such as lifting of the endothelial cell from the basement membrane with undermining by lymphocytes. Vasculitis is defined as the transmural involvement of the artery by inflammatory cells. As this process progresses, fibrinoid necrosis of the muscular wall occurs. Hyperacute rejection is characterized by a neutrophilic vasculitis that is not accompanied by interstitial rejection. Vasculitis as a part of acute cellular vascular rejection usually shows a mixed inflammatory infiltrate with lymphocytes

Table 1 Classification Scheme of Pancreatic Rejection

Diagnosis	Features
No rejection	Normal tissue
Consistent with acute rejection	Patchy mononuclear or polymorphous infiltrates with possible acinar tissue damage without vascular lesions
Mild acute rejection	Patchy mononuclear or polymorphous infiltrates with possible acinar tissue damage and endothelialitis
Severe acute rejection	Patchy or diffuse polymorphous infiltrates with marked acinar tissue damage (individual cell necrosis and loss of acinar structure) and vasculitis with or without fibrinoid necrosis
Chronic rejection[a]	Fibrointimal vascular proliferation and/or intimal foam cell accumulation, which may be accompanied by infarctive tissue necrosis or fibrosis

[a]Chronic rejection may be seen in association with acute rejection.

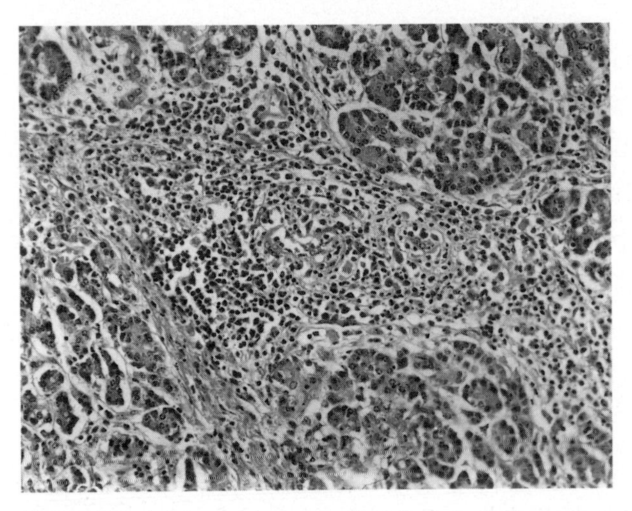

Figure 3 Acute pancreas rejection. A dense inflammatory infiltrate is present within septae and extends into acinar tissue. There are scattered necrotic cells within the acinar tissue. (H&E.)

and neutrophils predominantly and it is nearly always associated with severe interstitial rejection.

C. Chronic Rejection

Very little information is available regarding the pathogenic mechanism of chronic rejection of the pancreas. Research in chronic rejection has been primarily conducted on heart and kidney transplantation. A number of etiological agents have been suggested that may also apply to chronic rejection of the pancreas. The most notable possible contributing

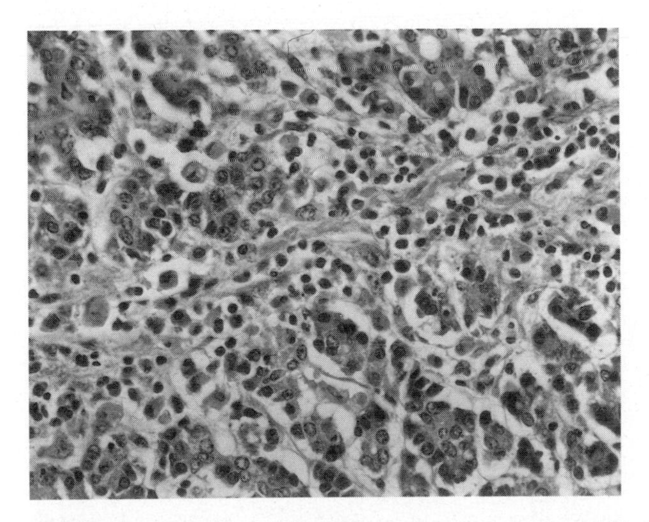

Figure 4 A higher magnification of acute rejection. This is a mixed inflammatory infiltrate predominantly composed of lymphocytes and plasma cells. (H&E.)

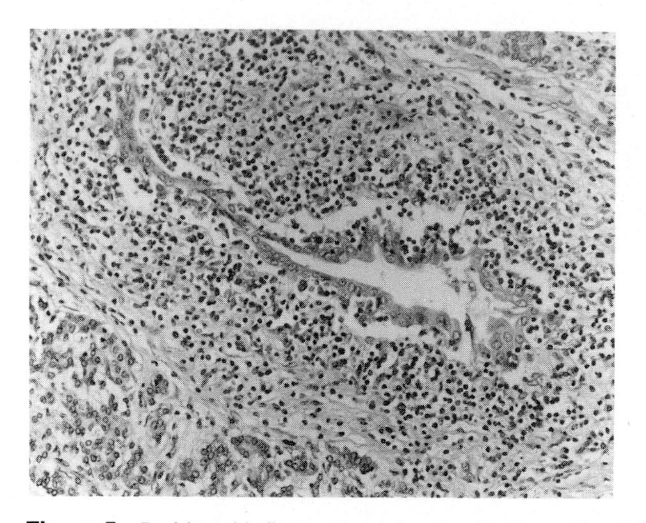

Figure 5 Periductal inflammation in acute rejection with epithelial damage. Ductal epithelial cells appear reactive with infiltration and destruction by lymphocytes. (H&E.)

factors include multiple acute rejection episodes, systemic or organ-specific infection, hyperlipidemia, and the toxic effects of cyclosporin A on vascular endothelial and smooth muscle cells (39).

Chronic rejection in the pancreas is characterized by arterial narrowing and interstitial fibrosis with variable loss of acinar and islet tissue (29,37) (Fig. 10). The arterial narrowing may have the appearance of fibrointimal proliferation or foam cell accumulation. This, in turn, will cause ischemic damage to the acinar and islet tissues. In combination with acute interstitial rejection, this will ultimately result in extensive fibrosis. It is very common to see chronic changes with ongoing acute rejection. The gross appearance of a pancreatec-

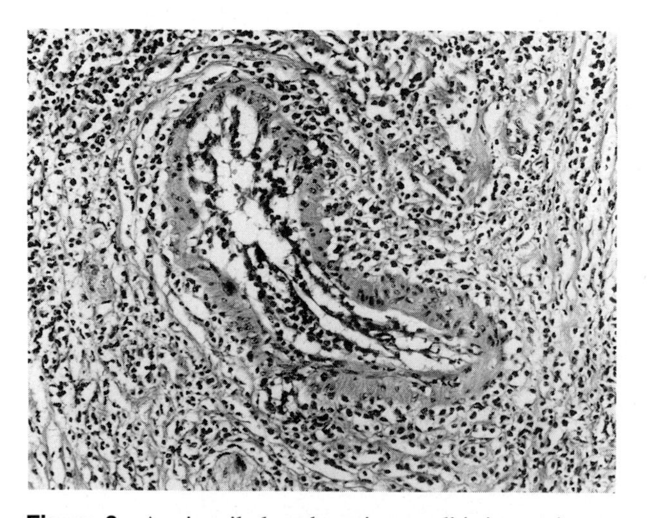

Figure 6 A primarily lymphocytic vasculitis is seen in a case of acute pancreas rejection. (H&E.)

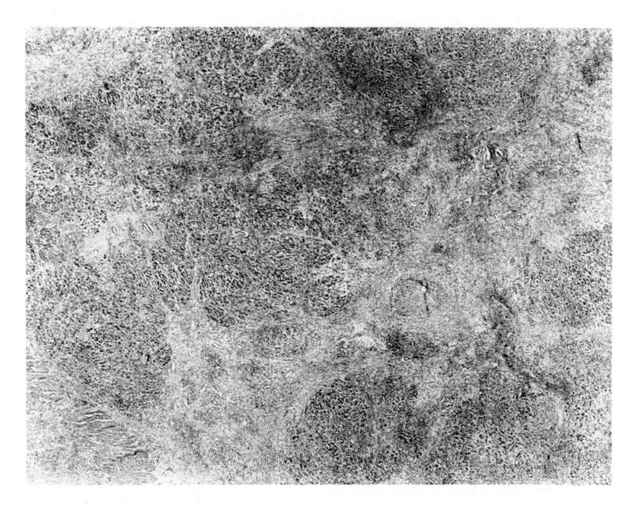

Figure 7 Severe rejection in a pancreas transplant which has resulted in extensive fibrosis. (H&E.)

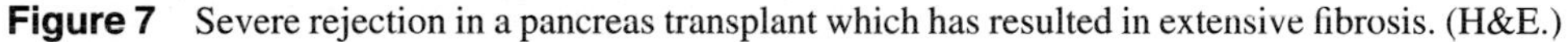

tomy specimen with chronic rejection can be very characteristic. The head of the pancreas usually has a normal appearance, with atrophy of the distal portion of the pancreas.

D. Other Chronic Changes

In some intestinally drained pancreas grafts, complete atrophy of the exocrine pancreas has been noted without any fibrosis (Fig. 11). Only the islets remain embedded in fibrofatty tissue. The mechanism by which this occurs is unclear.

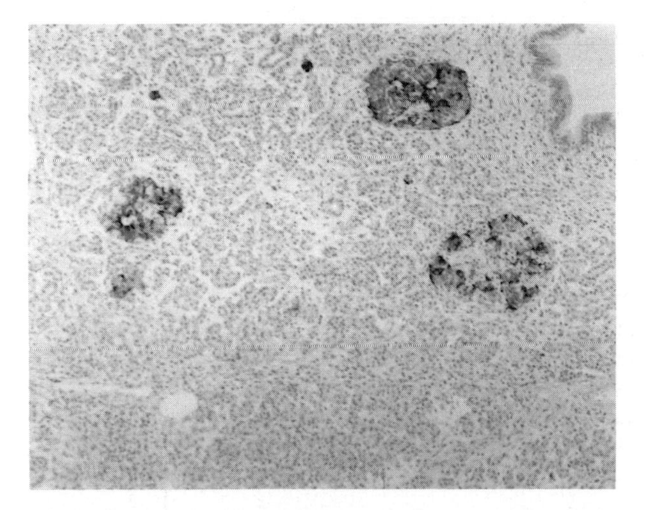

Figure 8 Insulin immunostain in a case of rejection. The majority of islet cells are positive for insulin. Compare this with Fig. 9. (Insulin immunostain with hematoxylin counterstain.)

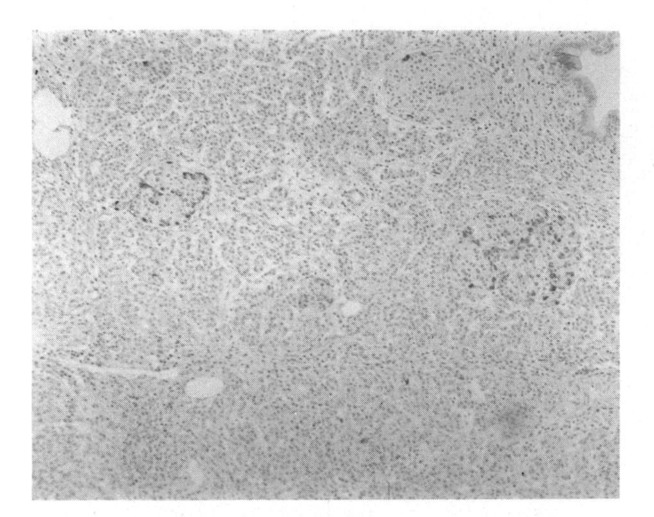

Figure 9 Serial section of the case shown in Fig. 8, now stained for glycogen. About 10% of islet cells are positive. (Glycogen immunostain with hematoxylin counterstain.)

IV. RECURRENT DISEASE

Recurrent disease is theoretically possible in any diabetic patient with a pancreas transplant. However, recurrent diabetes has been well documented only in identical twin and HLA-identical living related segmental transplants (36,38).

The early experience with identical twin-twin syngeneic transplants suggests that without immunosuppression, 100% of cases will have recurrence of disease. This experi-

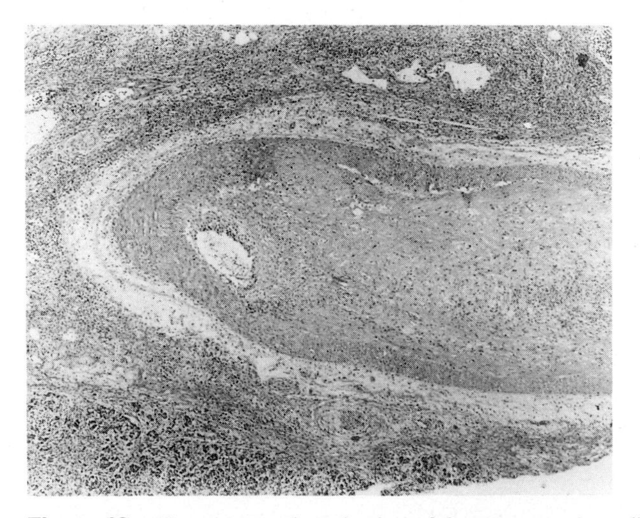

Figure 10 Chronic vascular rejection of the pancreas. A medium-size artery is shown with nearly complete occlusion by fibrointimal proliferation. A lymphocytic vasculitis persists with ongoing acute rejection. (H&E.)

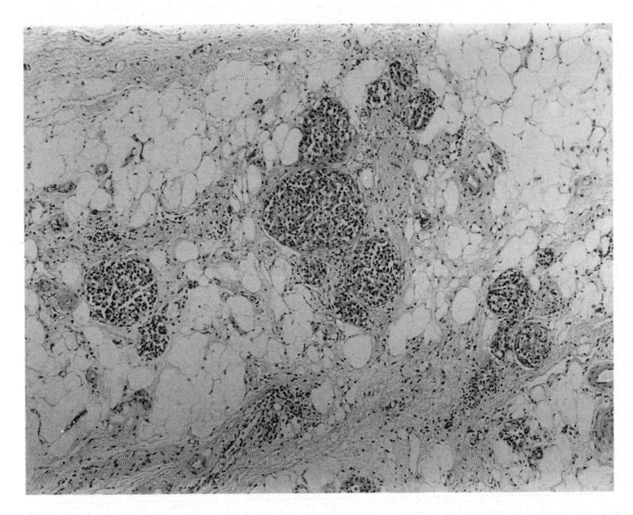

Figure 11 An intestinally drained segmental transplant with acinar atrophy. Only the islets remain with minimal fibrosis. (H&E.)

ence strongly reinforces the notion of a genetic predisposition for the development of diabetes mellitus. Immunosuppressive therapy has been shown to definitely delay the onset and progression of recurrent diabetes mellitus and may very well prevent recurrence (40).

Morphologically, recurrent diabetes mellitus is identical to the original disease (29,38). The earliest routine morphological finding is isletitis (inflammation of the islets) (Figs. 12 and 13; see also color plate). The inflammatory cells are mononuclear, with the majority being lymphocytes. Immunophenotyping has shown these to be predominantly

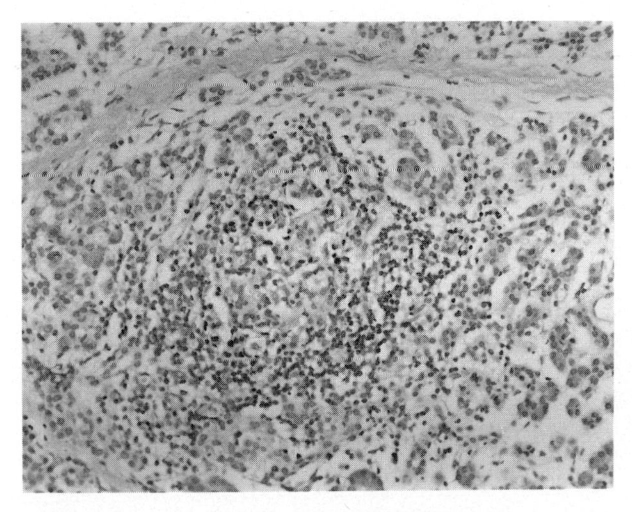

Figure 12 An identical twin segmental pancreas transplant with recurrent diabetes. Isletitis is shown with a predominantly lymphocytic infiltrate centered on an islet. (H&E.)

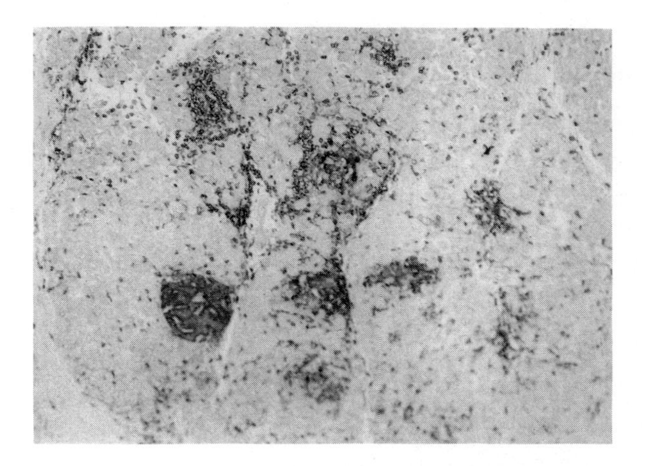

Figure 13 A pancreas with recurrent diabetes. The lymphocytes (brown) surround and involve islets (red) with destruction of beta cells. [Double immunostain chromogranin A (red) and leukocyte common antigen (brown), no counterstain.] (For optimal reproduction, see color plate.)

alpha-beta receptor + $CD8^{+}$/T lymphocytes with lesser numbers of CD4^{m}onocyte/ macrophages (41). Selective beta-cell loss also occurs. The best method to detect beta-cell loss presently is through immunohistochemistry. Monoclonal antibodies specific for insulin are applied to the tissues and detected by a chromogenic agent. Therefore the amount of insulin-producing cells can be estimated relative to the total amount of islet tissue and the amount of insulin-producing cells in normal tissues. Without special stains, recurrent diabetes can be diagnosed only if isletitis is found. But if isletitis is not present, the diagnosis of recurrent disease can be made only by documentation of beta-cell loss. Since the amount of beta (insulin-producing) cells can vary in different locations in the

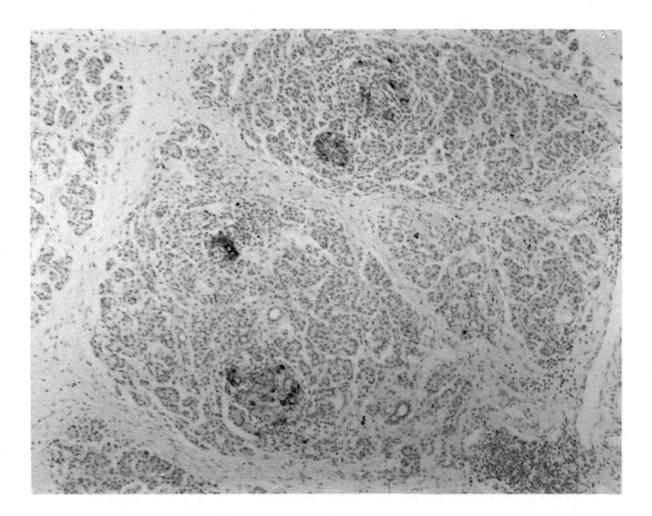

Figure 14 Insulin immunostain in a case of recurrent diabetes. Only a few insulin-producing cells remain in each islet, in contrast to Fig. 15. (Insulin immunostain with hematoxylin counterstain.)

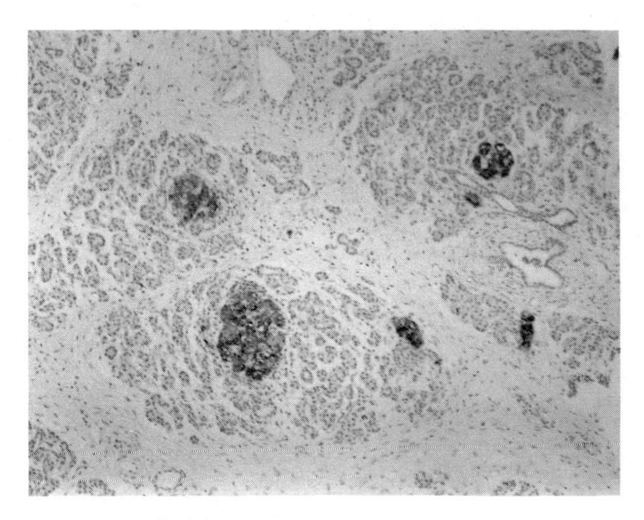

Figure 15 Serial section of the case shown in Fig. 14 stained for glycogen. The majority of cells within the islets are positive. (Glycogen immunostained with hematoxylin counterstain.)

pancreas, it is best to compare the amount of insulin-producing cells to the amount of glucagon-producing cells (Figs. 14 and 15). If the difference is dramatic, with the majority of islets containing predominantly glucagon-producing cells, a diagnosis of recurrent diabetes can be made. However, if the difference in the amount of the two types of cells cannot be easily distinguished and isletitis is not identified, semiquantitation may be appropriate. This is performed by estimating the approximate percentage of cells in the majority of islets for each cell type and then multiplying this number by the number of islets which stained for that cell type in a specified microscopic field or fields (this will vary depending on the size of the biopsy and the representative nature of a particular field). The product of this calculation for insulin is then compared with that for glucagon. If insulin is less than glucagon, the diagnosis of recurrent disease is likely (36).

V. INFECTION

As with other transplant patients, multiple infections can be a source of morbidity in the pancreatic transplant recipient. However, few infections affect the pancreas itself. Cytomegalovirus (CMV) is the organism most likely to cause diagnostic problems (42). Cytomegalovirus is just as likely to infect the pancreas and the duodenum as any other organ (Figs. 16 and 17). Cytomegalovirus inclusions may be seen in the pancreas but are more often noted in the duodenal tissues (26,29,43). In several instances, we have found CMV inclusions in the duodenal tissues but not the pancreatic tissue.

In the pancreas, CMV infection may be associated with a zonal area of inflammation and possible necrosis. The inflammatory cells consist of lymphocytes, plasma cells, neutrophils, and eosinophils. This infiltration is very similar to the infiltration seen in rejection. Cytomegalovirus inclusions can be seen in any cell type. In the duodenum, CMV inclusion can be seen in mucosal and submucosal epithelial cells as well as endothelial cells and myofibroblasts. In the pancreas, CMV can infect the ductal or acinar epithelial cells as well

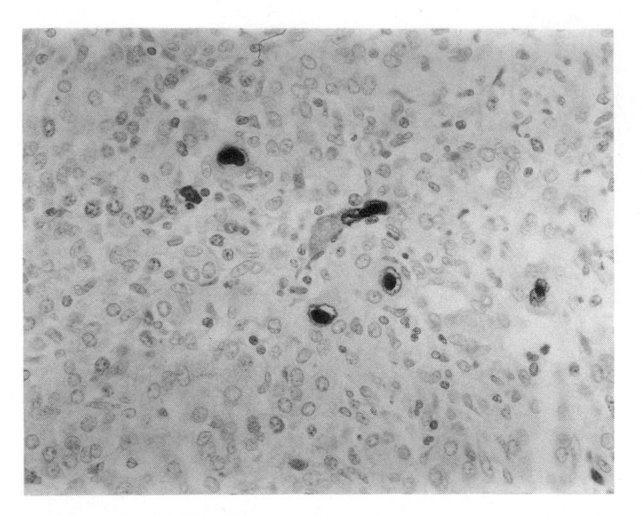

Figure 16 CMV infection of a pancreas transplant. (CMV immunostain with hematoxylin counterstain.)

as endothelial cells and myofibroblasts. On occasion, CMV inclusions may be seen with relatively little inflammation or cellular damage.

Bacterial and fungal organisms may also be found on rare occasions (usually in a resection specimen). Typically, tissue necrosis is present, with evidence of acute pancreatitis.

VI. PANCREATIC CYTOLOGY

Cytologic examination of the pancreatic exocrine drainage has been performed by at least two methods (21,22,24,44). In some institutions, segmental pancreatic transplants are

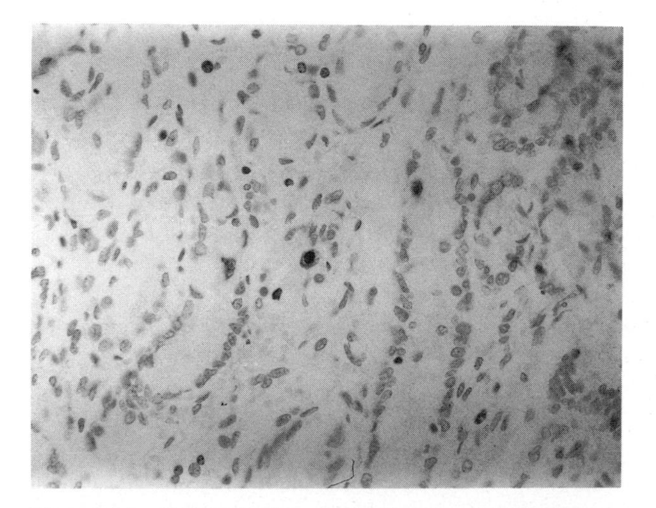

Figure 17 CMV infection of a duodenal cuff. (CMV immunostain with hematoxylin counterstain.)

drained externally until graft function stabilizes. In other institutions, urinary cytology is performed in patients with a pancreaticoduodenal cystostomy. Cytological monitoring is used as a screening tool for the detection of rejection. Features characteristic of acute rejection include increased overall cellularity, with >5% lymphocytes, eosinophil granules, and necrotic epithelial cells. The presence of a large number of neutrophils would, on the other hand, favor acute pancreatitis. Other pathological entities that can be evaluated by cytological examination include infectious organisms, bacterial and fungal, as well as viral nuclear inclusions. Advantages of monitoring urinary cytology or pancreatic drainage cytology is that rejection can be detected before clinical symptoms and before a decline in urine amylase occurs. On the other hand, cytological monitoring is not specific and should ideally be confirmed by biopsy (24,44).

VII. DUODENAL BIOPSIES

The duodenal tissue in bladder-drained pancreatic duodenal transplants can easily be biopsied with forceps using an ordinary cystoscope (11,13). Since this is transplanted tissue, it may be reflective of pancreatic pathology. Animal studies have shown that the duodenum is reflective of pancreatic pathology in two-thirds of the cases (45). More recently, we reviewed our experience of more than 80 cystoscopically obtained biopsies (46). Not surprisingly, duodenal tissue was obtained more frequently than pancreatic tissue. Of these biopsies, 25 cases contained both duodenal and pancreatic tissue. Of the cases in which rejection was present and both tissues were examined, over 80% were concordant regarding the presence of some form of rejection. However, the pancreatic tissues contained more specific findings (i.e., vascular changes) in a higher percentage of cases. Also in many of the duodenal biopsies, rejection could only be suggested. On the other hand, in one case, CMV was detected in the duodenum but not in the pancreas. A technical problem associated with duodenal biopsies is mucosal sloughing, which obscures some of the findings.

The findings most specific for rejection in the duodenum are vascular changes (endothelialitis and vasculitis) (13). Vascular changes are best and most frequently seen in the submucosa. Other changes characteristic of rejection include villous blunting, with epithe-

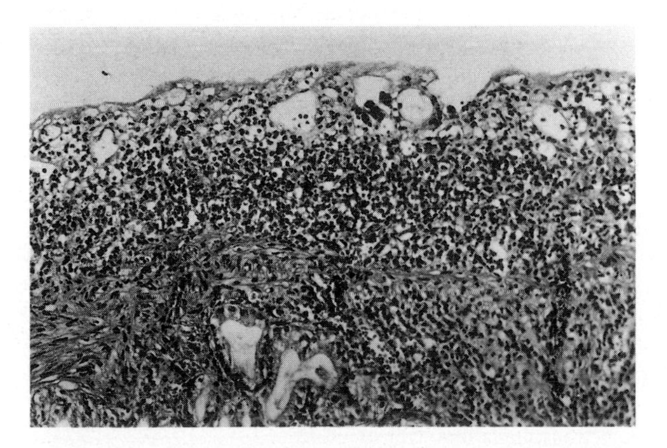

Figure 18 Duodenal rejection characterized by loss of villous architecture, epithelial necrosis, and lymphoplasmacellular infiltrates, with the lamina propria and extending to the submucosal tissues. (H&E.)

lial cell necrosis and an increased mixed inflammatory infiltrate in the lamina propria (Fig. 18). Mucosal sloughing occurs frequently during tissue processing and should be distinguished from epithelial necrosis. The inflammation typically extends into the submucosa and can involve submucosal glands with necrosis of individual cells. The presence of inflammation of the muscularis propria and perineural inflammation also support the diagnosis of rejection.

REFERENCES

1. Correy RJ, Zehr P. Quality of life in diabetic recipients of kidney transplants is better with the addition of the pancreas. Clin Transplant 1990; 4:238–241.
2. Sutherland DER, Mondry-Munns KC, Gillingham KJ. Report from the International Pancreas Transplant Registry. Diabetologia 1991; 34:S28–S29.
3. Stratta RJ, Sollinger HW, Perlman SB, et al. Early detection of rejection in pancreas transplantation. Diabetes 1989; 38:63–67.
4. Perkins JD, Fromme GA, Narr BJ, et al. Pancreas transplantation at Mayo: II. Operative and perioperative management. Mayo Clin Proc 1990; 65:483–495.
5. Sollinger HW, D'Alessandro AM, Stratta RJ, et al. Combined kidney-pancreas transplantation with pancreaticocystostomy. Transplant Proc 1989; 21:2837–2838.
6. Sutherland DER, Gillingham KJ, Mondry-Munn KC. Results of pancreas transplantation in the United States 1987–90 from the United Network for Organ Sharing (UNOS) Registry with comparison to 1984–87 results. Clin Transplant 1991; 5:330–341.
7. Brattstrom C, Tyden G, Reinholt FP, et al. Markers for pancreas-graft rejection in humans. Diabetes 1989; 38:57–62.
8. Brayman KL, Moss A, Morel PH, et al. Exocrine dysfunction evaluation of bladder-drained pancreaticoduodenal transplants using a transcystoscopic biopsy technique. Transplant 1992; 24:901–902.
9. Gruessner RWG, Nakhleh RE, Tzardis P, et al. Differences in rejection grading after simultaneous pancreas and kidney transplantation in pigs. Transplantation 1993; 56:1357–1364.
10. Munn SR, Engen DE, Barr D, et al. Differential diagnosis of hypoamylasuria in pancreas allograft recipients with urinary exocrine drainage. Transplantation 1990; 49:359–362.
11. Perkins JD, Munn SR, Marsh CL, et al. Safety and efficacy of cytoscopically directed biopsy in pancreas transplantation. Transplant Proc 1990; 22:665–666.
12. Carpenter HA, Engen DE, Munn SR, et al. Histologic diagnosis of rejection by using cystoscopically directed needle biopsy specimens from dysfunctional pancreatoduodenal allografts with exocrine drainage into the bladder. Am J Surg Pathol 1990; 14:837–846.
13. Marsh CL, Perkins JD, Barr D, et al. Cytoscopically directed biopsy technique in canine pancreaticoduodenal transplantation. Transplant Proc 1989; 21:2816–2817.
14. Nakache R, Mainetti L, Tyden G, Groth CG. Renal transplantation in diabetes mellitus: Influence of combined pancreas-kidney transplantation on outcome. Transplant Proc 1990; 22: 624–626.
15. Gruessner RW, Nakhleh R, Tzardis P, et al. Rejection in single versus combined pancreas and kidney transplantation in pigs. Transplantation 1993; 56:1053–1062.
16. Sutherland DER, Moudry KC, Goetz FC, Najarian JS. Long-term outcome of pancreas transplants functioning at one year. Transplant Proc 1989; 21:2845–2849.
17. Sutherland DER, Goetz FC, Glick BA, Najoria JS. Experience with 49 sequential pancreas transplants in 45 diabetic patients. Transplantation 1982; 34:330–338.
18. Sutherland DER, Casanova D, Sibley RK. Role of pancreas graft biopsies in the diagnosis and treatment of rejection after pancreas transplantation. Transplant Proc 1987; 19:2329–2331.
19. Gaber AO, Gaber LW, Shokouh-Amiri MH, Hathaway D. Percutaneous biopsy of pancreas transplants. Transplantation 1992; 54:548–550.

20. Allen RDM, Wilson TG, Grierson JM, et al. Percutaneous pancreas transplant fine needle aspiration and needle core biopsies are useful and safe. Transplant 1990; 22:663–664.
21. Klima G, Margreiter R, Konigsrainer A, et al. Pancreatic juice cytology (PJC) for early detection of pancreas allograft rejection. Transplant Proc 1989; 21:2782–2783.
22. Kubota K, Reinholt FP, Tyden G, et al. Findings in pancreatic juice cytology compared with histologic findings in the pancreatic graft. Transplant Proc 1990; 22:670.
23. Tyden G, Reinholt F, Bohman S-O, et al. Diagnosis of pancreatic graft rejection by pancreatic juice cytology. Transplant Proc 1989; 21:2780–2781.
24. Radio SJ, Stratta RJ, Taylor RJ, Linder J. The utility of urine cytology in the diagnosis of allograft rejection after combined pancreas-kidney transplantation. Transplantation 1993; 55: 509–516.
25. Morel P, Gillingham KJ, Mondry-Munn KC, et al. Factors influencing pancreas transplant outcome: Cox proportional hazard regression analysis of a single institutions experience in 357 cases. Transplant Proc 1991; 23:1630–1633.
26. Gruessner RWG, Dunn DS, Tzardis PJ, et al. Complications occurring after whole organ duodenopancreatic transplantation: Relation to the allograft duodenal segment. Transplant Proc 1990; 22:578–579.
27. D'Alessandro AM, Sollinger HW, Stratta RJ, et al. Comparison between duodenal button and duodenal segment in pancreas transplantation. Transplantation 1989; 47:120–122.
28. Kyriakides GK, Arora VK, Lifton J, et al. Porcupine pancreatic transplantation: 1. Autotransplantation of duct ligated segments. J Surg Res 1976; 20:451–460.
29. Sibley RK, Sutherland DER. Pancreas transplantation: An immunohistologic and histopathologic examination of 100 grafts. Am J Pathol 1987; 128:151–170.
30. Weinzierl G, Meister R, Schwille PO, Meister RH. Pancreas transplantation with and without duct occlusion by two glues in the diabetic rat. Transplantation 1990; 49:644–648.
31. Castoldi R, Staudacher C, Ferrari G, et al. Early postoperative surgical complications after combined segmental duct-occluded pancreas transplantation. Transplant Proc 1990; 22:582–584.
32. Frohnert PP, Velosa JA, Munn SR, et al. Morbidity during the first year after pancreas transplantation. Transplant Proc 1990; 22:577.
33. Paineau J, Cantarovich D, Couderc JP, et al. Human segmental pancreas transplantation with special reference to vascular thrombosis. Transplant Proc 1990; 22:586–587.
34. Ozaki CF, Stratta RJ, Taylor RJ, et al. Surgical complications in solitary pancreas and combined pancreas-kidney transplantations. Am J Surg 1992; 164:546–551.
35. Sibley RK: Pancreas transplantation. In: Sale GE, ed. The Pathology of Organ Transplantation. Boston, Massachusetts, 1990:179–215.
36. Nakhleh RE, Gruessner RWG, Swanson PE, et al. Pancreas transplant pathology: A morphologic immunohistochemical, and electron microscopic comparison of allogeneic grafts with rejection, syngeneic grafts, and chronic pancreatitis. Am J Surg Pathol 1991; 15:246–256.
37. Nakhleh RE, Sutherland DER. Pancreas rejection: Significance of histopathologic findings with implication of classification for rejection. Am J Surg Pathol 1992; 16:1098–1107.
38. Sibley RK, Sutherland DER, Goetz F, Michael AF. Recurrent diabetes mellitus in the pancreas iso- and allograft: A light and electron microscopic and immunohistochemical analysis of four cases. Lab Invest 1985; 53:132–144.
39. Paul LC, Fellstrom B. Overview: Chronic vascular rejection of the heart and the kidney—Have rational treatment options emerged? Transplantation 1992; 53:1169–1179.
40. Sutherland DER, Goetz FS, Sibley RK. Recurrence of disease in pancreas transplants. Diabetes 1989; 39:85–87.
41. Santamaria P, Nakhleh RE, Sutherland DE, Barbosa JJ. Characterization of T lymphocytes infiltrating human pancreas allograft affected by isletitis and recurrent diabetes. Diabetes 1992; 41:53–61.
42. Stratta RJ. Clinical patterns and treatment of cytomegalovirus infection after solid-organ transplantation. Transplant Proc 1993; 25:15–21.

43. Nakhleh RE, Gruessner RWG, Tzardis PJ, et al. Pathology of transplanted human duodenal tissue: A histologic study, with comparison to pancreatic pathology in resected pancreatico-duodenal transplants. Clin Transplant 1991; 5:241–247.
44. Kendall T, Radio SJ, Stratton RJ, et al. Confirmation of acute pancreas rejection by core biopsy in patients monitored by urine cytology. Mod Pathol 1994; 7:132A.
45. Nakhleh RE, Sutherland DER, Tzardis P, et al. Correlation of rejection of the duodenum with rejection of the pancreas in a pig model of pancreaticoduodenal transplantation. Transplantation 1993; 56:1353–1356.
46. Nakhleh RE, Sutherland DER, Benedetti E, et al. Diagnostic utility and correlation of pancreatic and duodenal cystoscopically directed biopsies of pancreaticoduodenal transplants. Mod Pathol 1994; 7:134A.

12

Pathology of Posttransplant Lymphoproliferative Disorders

Judith Ann Ferry and Nancy Lee Harris
Massachusetts General Hospital, Boston, Massachusetts

I. INTRODUCTION

Compared to the normal population, allograft recipients have a markedly increased risk of developing lymphoproliferative disorders. The clinical and pathological features of post-transplantation lymphoproliferative disorders (PTLDs) differ from those of lymphomas found in nonimmunosuppressed patients. They are characterized by unusual anatomical distribution, heterogeneous pathological features, variable, frequently unpredictable response to therapy, and, often, a rapidly fatal course. In recent years the increasing use of solid organ transplantation has markedly expanded the population at risk for PTLD. In this chapter, we will consider PTLDs to include lymphoid proliferations that occur as a result of immunosuppression, which will tend to progress unless immunosuppression is reduced or eliminated and are usually associated with Epstein-Barr virus (EBV). In this chapter we discuss the changing incidence and clinical features of PTLD in association with various immunosuppressive regimens; the histological, immunophenotypic, and genetic features of these disorders; their association with EBV; and the impact of these features and of available treatment modalities on the prognosis of patients with PTLD.

II. IMMUNOSUPPRESSIVE REGIMENS IN ALLOGRAFT RECIPIENTS

A. Conventional Immunosuppression

Regimens used for immunosuppression have changed over time, and this has resulted in variation in the features of PTLDs. In the early years of transplantation, azathioprine and less often cytoxan, in combination with steroids, formed the basis of the immunosuppressive regimen. Some patients were also subjected to lymphocyte depletion via thoracic duct cannulation, splenic ablation, irradiation of the allograft, and/or administration of anti-lymphocyte globulin. Patients treated in this way, almost all of whom were renal transplant recipients, had an estimated 60- to 350-fold increase in lymphoproliferative disorders compared to the normal population (1,2). These were usually diffuse large-cell lymphomas that arose several years after transplantation and frequently involved extranodal sites (Fig. 1), including the central nervous system and the allograft (3–5) (Table 1).

B. Cyclosporine

Cyclosporine has contributed to the widespread successful use of nonrenal solid-organ allografts, which require higher levels of immunosuppression. After the introduction of cyclosporine in 1979, many centers began to substitute this highly effective immunosuppressive agent for azathioprine. Cyclosporine, a cyclic endecapeptide of fungal origin, prevents allograft rejection by inhibiting the synthesis of interleukin 2 by T-helper cells, with resultant blockade of the activation of cytotoxic T lymphocytes (6). T-suppressor cells are relatively unaffected by cyclosporine (7). In addition, cyclosporine renders target cells resistant to all types of immune-mediated cytolysis, whether mediated by T cells, natural killer cells, or complement (8). Cyclosporine appears to inhibit the activation of EBV-specific cytotoxic T lymphocytes. In vitro, the growth of EBV–infected B cells is promoted by cyclosporine (9–11). Patients receiving cyclosporine may develop a severe primary or reactivation infection with EBV. They are at risk for uncontrolled proliferation of EBV-infected B lymphocytes, which may eventually give rise to a lymphoma (10,12).

When cyclosporine first became available, it was used at high doses, and was associated with an incidence of lymphoproliferative disorders of up to 10% (13,14). More experience with cyclosporine has shown that lower dosages provide effective immunosuppression; lowering the dosage and monitoring of serum levels has decreased the incidence

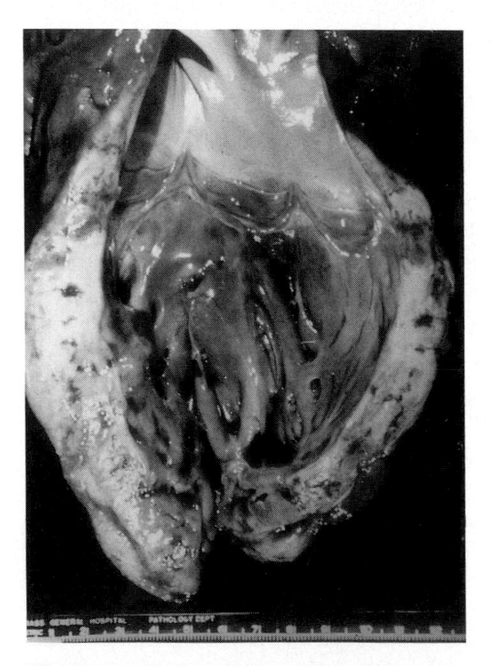

Figure 1 PTLD involving the heart of a conventionally immunosuppressed renal transplant recipient, with thickening and discoloration of the myocardium. The patient presented 40 months after transplantation with congestive heart failure. On microscopic examination, the PTLD was a centroblastic (diffuse large non-cleaved-cell) lymphoma.

Table 1 Incidence of PTLD: Review of the Literature[a]

Rx	All	Kidney	Heart	Liver	Lung or heart/lung	Interval (median)
CIT	n/a	0.38–1.2%	1.7%	n/a	n/a	6 months–4.5 years
CSA	0.3–1.2%	0–1.0%	0–11.9%	0.9–2.2%	0–7.9%	2–16 months
CSA+OKT3	n/a	0.6	11.4%	n/a	n/a	2 months
CSA+ >75mg OKT3	n/a	n/a	35.7%	n/a	n/a	1 month

[a]All series included multiple different types of allografts. CIT, conventional immunosuppressive therapy; CSA, any type of cyclosporine-based immunosuppression; n/a, not available; Rx, immunosuppressive regimen.
Source: From Refs. 1,4,14–20,22–25,34,35, and 47.

of PTLD to less than 2% overall. The relative incidence of PTLD has been estimated to be 20 times that found in the general population for renal allograft recipients and 120 times for cardiac allograft recipients during the first year posttransplantation, when the frequency of PTLD is highest (15). In general, patients with renal allografts have the lowest risk of PTLD, those with hepatic and cardiac grafts have an intermediate risk, and those with heart-lung transplants have the highest risk. In several recent large series, the incidence has ranged from 0 to 1% for renal transplants, from 0 to 11.9% for cardiac transplants, from 1.7 to 2.2% for hepatic transplants, and from 0 to 7.9% for lung or heart-lung transplants (15–25). In one review, the incidence of PTLD was 0.2% for renal, 0.9% for liver, and 1.5% for cardiac transplant recipients, with an incidence of 0.3% overall (14). This relatively low risk of PTLD is considered acceptable in light of the benefits of cyclosporine use (Table 1).

III. PTLD: CLINICAL FEATURES

Both cyclosporine-treated and conventionally immunosuppressed allograft recipients have an increased incidence of neoplasia of a variety of types; however, lymphomas make up a higher proportion in the cyclosporine group. Among cases recorded in the Cincinnati Transplant Tumor Registry (CTTR), which includes data on over 5000 tumors that have developed in allograft recipients worldwide, 26% of tumors in patients treated with cyclosporine, but only 11% of tumors in conventionally immunosuppressed patients, were PTLDs (26). In addition, PTLDs arising in patients treated with cyclosporine-based regimens occur at a shorter interval after transplantation. Cyclosporine-associated lymphomas reported to the CTTR occurred at a mean interval of 15 months after transplant, compared to 48 months in conventionally treated patients (26). The mean interval to the development of PTLD in cyclosporine-treated patients reported by individual medical centers has often been less than 6 months (7,18). Both cyclosporine and azathioprine-treated solid-organ transplant recipients who develop PTLD may present with either infectious mononucleosis-like symptoms or involvement of solid organs, sometimes with dysfunction of those organs (18,27); among cyclosporine-treated patients, gastrointestinal symptoms are frequent (18). Occasionally, the PTLD may be an incidental finding at autopsy, not directly contributing to the death of the patient (JAF/NLH, unpublished data) (13,28).

Lymphomas in allograft recipients are more likely to involve extranodal sites than lymphomas in the nonimmunosuppressed population (Fig. 1), although, compared to those in conventionally immunosuppressed patients, cyclosporine-associated PTLDs are more likely to involve lymph nodes and less likely to involve the central nervous system (CNS). Thirty-eight percent of lymphomas reported to the CTTR in conventionally immunosuppressed patients involved the CNS, as compared to 15% in cyclosporine-treated patients and 1% in the general population (26). There is a striking tendency for PTLDs in cyclosporine-treated patients to involve the gastrointestinal tract (13,18,29–31). In one series, 12 of 37 patients with PTLD presented with symptoms related to gastrointestinal disease, with involvement of the small intestine being more common than involvement of the colon or stomach (18).

Involvement of the allograft itself by PTLD is common, although the frequency varies with the type of graft. Cohen reviewed the literature and found that, while approximately one-third of renal and hepatic allografts were involved, there were no cases of cardiac allograft involvement by lymphoma (32). We have seen a case of PTLD in a cardiac allograft recipient in whom epicardium and residual native myocardium but not transplanted myocardium were involved by PTLD. We have not observed a case in which transplanted myocardium has been involved by PTLD (JAF/NLH, unpublished data). Cardiac involvement by PTLD in cardiac allograft recipients has been reported recently, although the distribution of tumor within the graft was not described (15). In 80% of heart-lung allograft recipients who developed a PTLD, the lungs were involved (32). It has been proposed that pulmonary allografts may be more commonly involved by PTLD than other grafts because oropharyngeal EBV can be aspirated into the graft, where it directly inoculates bronchial and alveolar epithelium and lymphocytes present locally, which may then give rise to PTLDs (33). In support of this, the presence of EBV can be demonstrated in transbronchial biopsies of a substantial number of pulmonary allograft recipients, using the polymerase chain reaction, in the absence of clinical or pathological evidence of PTLD (34).

IV. IMMUNOSUPPRESSION AND RISK OF PTLD

An increasing degree of immunosuppression results in an increased risk of developing a PTLD (15). Among both conventionally immunosuppressed and cyclosporine-treated patients, those who receive higher dosages of either cyclosporine or azathioprine or who are treated with the addition of other modalities—such as the monoclonal antibody OKT3 or antilymphocyte globulin—have a significantly greater risk of lymphoma (1,15,16,24,35). In a series of 5550 transplant recipients worldwide, PTLD developed in 0.4% of those receiving cyclosporine alone or in combination with steroids but in 8% of those treated with cyclosporine in combination with other agents (16). Investigators from Loyola University of Chicago recently described a striking example of such a trend. They studied a series of 154 cardiac allograft recipients, 79 of whom received OKT3 for prophylaxis or for treatment of rejection and 75 of whom did not. Only 1 patient in the group without OKT3 developed lymphoma, while 9, or 11.4%, of those who received OKT3 developed lymphoma ($p = 0.001$). The risk increased with a higher total dose of OKT3. Of patients who received more than a total of 75 mg of OKT3, 35.7% developed PTLD. Among those who received less than 75 mg of OKT3 and who developed lymphoma, the lymphomas occurred at a longer interval after transplantation, disease was more often localized, and the clinical course was less fulminant (24). Similarly, in a report of hepatic allograft recipients treated at Baylor University in Dallas, all patients who developed lymphoma within 3 months of transplantation had had rejection and additional large doses of immunosuppressive agents (21).

Although increasing dosage and increasing numbers of different immunosuppressive agents are associated with an increased risk of PTLD, there are occasional exceptions to this rule for which there is no clear explanation. In contrast to the situations just described, Olivari and coworkers, from Minneapolis, reported their experience with triple-drug immunosuppression including cyclosporine, azathioprine, and prednisone. They found that the addition of azathioprine to their cardiac and heart-lung recipients' immunosuppressive regimen allowed them to decrease the dose of cyclosporine, which was accompanied by a low frequency of PTLD. Only 2 of 134 cardiac allograft recipients and none of 7 heart-lung patients developed a PTLD (22). In contrast, renal allograft recipients at the University of Iowa, treated with a similar triple drug regimen, had a higher incidence of lymphoma than those treated with either cyclosporine and prednisone or azathioprine and prednisone (25). Some patients receiving relatively low doses of immunosuppression develop PTLDs (30), and some transplantation centers report no correlation between risk for PTLD and the type of maintenance or prophylactic immunosuppressive regimen used (19). Thus, the relationship between immunosuppression and PTLD is not straightforward, and it is possible that there are differences inherent in patient populations or as yet unrecognized factors that predispose to the development of PTLD.

It is also possible that a localized immune response provides the impetus for some cases of PTLD (15). In support of this interpretation is the fact that in both conventionally immunosuppressed and cyclosporine-treated patients, the allograft—frequently the site of rejection, an immune response—is often involved by PTLD. In addition, two cases of "reticulum cell sarcoma" developing at the site of equine antilymphocyte globulin injection have been reported (36,37). This foreign protein may evoke an immunological response associated with blast transformation of lymphocytes (36,37) that could conceivably evolve into lymphoma in an immunodeficient host unable to control lymphoid proliferation.

V. PTLD: HISTOLOGICAL FEATURES

Compared to lymphomas in the general population, PTLDs in transplant recipients often show distinctive histological, immunohistological, and genotypic features. The range of histological features seen in PTLDs includes infiltrates resembling infectious mononucleosis, atypical lymphoid infiltrates worrisome for lymphoma, and high-grade lymphomas. The infiltrates are often polymorphous and may be difficult to classify in the usual schemes for malignant lymphoma. This difficulty has led to the development of two different classifications for PTLDs, which are discussed below.

The classification of PTLD, based on observations of PTLD in azathioprine-treated renal transplant recipients and in allogeneic marrow recipients treated at the University of Minnesota, has included categories of atypical lymphoid hyperplasia, polymorphous diffuse B cell hyperplasia, atypical polymorphous B cell hyperplasia, polymorphous B cell lymphoma and immunoblastic sarcoma (38,39). Atypical lymphoid hyperplasia (ALH) is a nonspecific change that involves the paracortex of lymph nodes or the interstitial tissue of extranodal organs, without architectural obliteration. The infiltrate is composed of small lymphocytes, some with irregular nuclei, with admixed immunoblasts, lymphoplasmacytoid cells, and mature and immature plasma cells. Polymorphous diffuse B cell hyperplasia (PDBH) is characterized by an infiltrate of B cells at all stages of differentiation—lymphocytes, plasma cells, plasmablasts, centrocytes (cleaved cells), centroblasts (noncleaved cells) and immunoblasts—which obliterates the nodal architecture. There are no atypical immunoblasts and no necrosis (Fig. 2). Polymorphous B-cell lym-

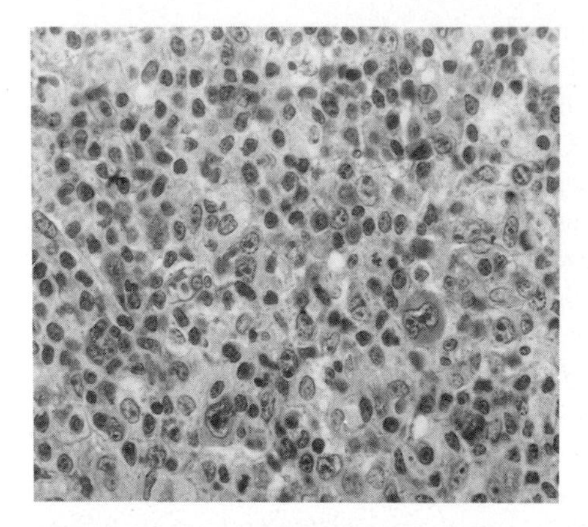

Figure 2 Polymorphous diffuse B-cell hyperplasia/PTLD, polymorphic, in the cervical lymph node of a cyclosporine-treated cardiac allograft recipient. Three months postoperatively, the patient had fever and cervical adenopathy. A biopsy showed diffuse obliteration of nodal architecture by a mixture of small lymphocytes, plasma cells, plasmablasts, small cleaved cells, and immunoblasts. The patient was treated with decreased immunosuppression and acyclovir, and the PTLD resolved.

phoma (PBL) has similar features, but atypical immunoblasts or necrosis or both are present, and plasmacytic differentiation is less prominent (Figs. 3 and 4). Atypical polymorphous B-cell hyperplasia (APBH), has features intermediate between PDBH and PBL, with atypical large cells, which may be multinucleated, and intense plasmacytic differentiation but no necrosis (38). The term "immunoblastic sarcoma" is used to designate diffuse high-grade lymphomas with numerous atypical large cells, often with prominent plasmacytic differentiation but without cleaved cells (39) (Fig. 5).

Using the University of Minnesota classification, PTLDs in 19 renal allograft recipients included 4 PDBH and 13 PBL. One patient had PDBH and PBL in separate sites and 1 had PBL and immunoblastic sarcoma in separate sites (4). In a series of 8 allogeneic marrow recipients with 22 different specimens involved by PTLDs, there were 4 showing atypical lymphoid hyperplasia (ALH), 4 with PDBH, 2 with atypical polymorphous B-cell hyperplasia (APBH), 9 with PBL, and 3 with immunoblastic sarcoma (38).

Recently, the University of Minnesota classification has been revised by Frizzera and Knowles and their coworkers. The new subtypes of PTLD include (a) plasmacytic hyperplasia, (2) PDBH/PBL, and (3) malignant lymphoma or multiple myeloma (40). In a study of 22 solid-organ recipients treated at Columbia University or New York University, presented in the form of an abstract, 7 patients had plasmacytic hyperplasia, 12 had PDBH or PBL, and only 4 had malignant lymphoma or multiple myeloma. Earlier studies from the University of Minnesota had suggested that the presence of atypical immunoblasts and necrosis correlated with the development of a PTLD with a more aggressive clinical course, so that these features were used to separate hyperplasias from lymphomas (39). In contrast, in the series of patients from New York City, the authors propose that PDBH, which by definition lacks these features, and PBL, which shows them, are characterized by overlapping clinical and pathological features and should be classified together as one distinct type of PTLD (40).

The second classification was produced by Nalesnik and coworkers at the University

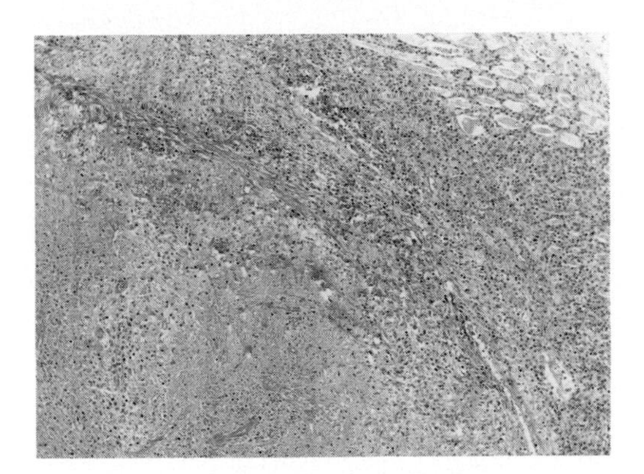

Figure 3 Polymorphous B-cell lymphoma/PTLD, polymorphic, involving the tonsils and adenoids of a cyclosporine-treated renal allograft recipient. There was extensive necrosis, and the lesion invaded skeletal muscle (upper left).

of Pittsburgh (18). Lymphoid proliferations are divided into polymorphic, monomorphic, and minimally polymorphic categories. In the polymorphic category, there is an infiltrate with a cellular composition similar to that seen in PDBH, APBH, and PBL. Atypical immunoblasts and necrosis may or may not be present (Figs. 2, 3, and 4). The monomorphic category includes obvious high-grade lymphomas (Figs. 5 and 6). In the minimally polymorphic category, the predominant cells are those of later stages of B-cell differentiation—i.e., plasma cells and plasmacytoid cells, with little polymorphism (Figs. 7 and 8). Using this classification, 83 specimens from 43 solid-organ recipients were grouped as follows: 47 were polymorphic, 24 were minimally polymorphic, and 12 were monomorphic. The minimally polymorphic category is not as common as these data imply, since 16 of the 24 specimens of this type were from a single patient (18). Specimens from different sites from

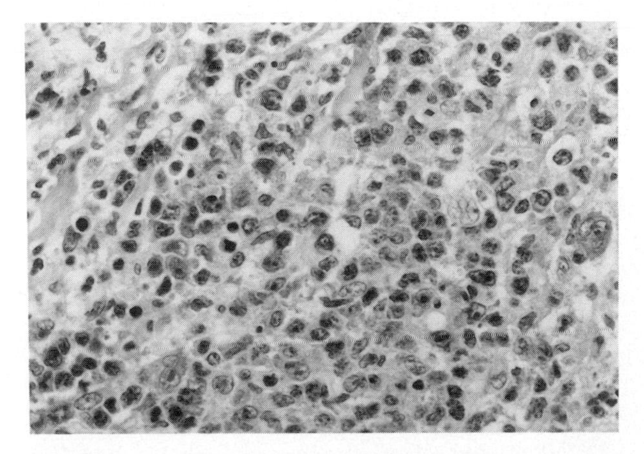

Figure 4 Polymorphous B-cell lymphoma/PTLD, polymorphic, involving the tonsils and adenoids of a cyclosporine-treated renal allograft recipient. Higher power shows a mixture of small and large cleaved cells, large noncleaved cells, plasma cells, and atypical immunoblasts.

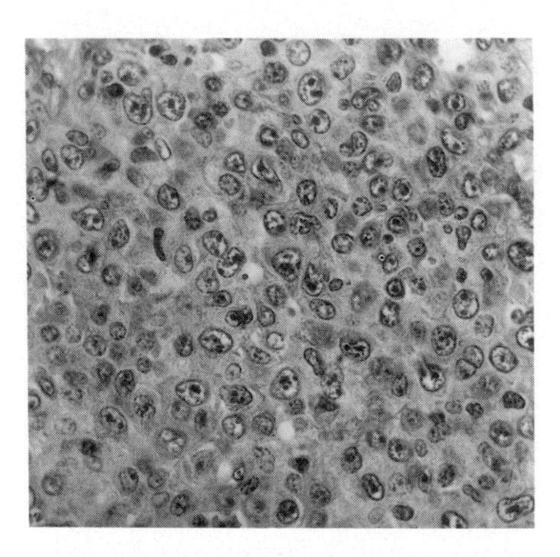

Figure 5 Malignant lymphoma, immunoblastic plasmacytoid/PTLD, monomorphic, in a cyclosporine-treated renal allograft recipient.

the same patient may show different patterns. Although necrosis and atypical immunoblasts have never been used in subclassifying PTLDs in the classification from the University of Pittsburgh, these features are found most frequently in cases in the polymorphic category (18).

A high proportion of the PTLDs seen at the medical centers where these classification systems were developed have been polymorphic lesions, with relatively few cases resembling the lymphomas found in the general population. Not all medical centers have reported such results, however. Ten cases of PTLD occurring in cardiac allograft recipients at Stanford were all described as diffuse large-cell lymphomas, including 8 immunoblastic, with no mention of polymorphism (41). In a series of PTLDs following bone marrow transplantation at the University of Washington, 14 of 15 were immunoblastic lymphoma

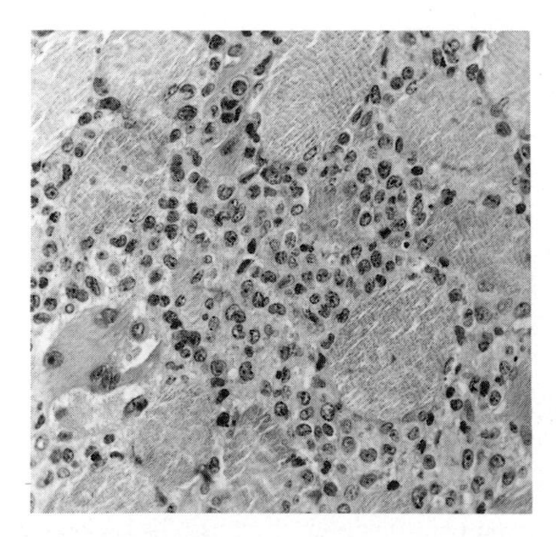

Figure 6 Malignant lymphoma, diffuse large cell, multilobated/PTLD, monomorphic, involving skeletal muscle from the chest wall in a patient who had received two hepatic allografts.

Figure 7 Polymorphous B cell lymphoma/PTLD, minimally polymorphic, involving a cervical lymph node in a cardiac allograft recipient. There is diffuse obliteration of the nodal architecture, and a "starry sky" pattern.

(42). In a total of 32 cases of PTLDs arising in solid-organ transplant recipients treated at Massachusetts General Hospital, 25 were diffuse high-grade lymphomas, including 15 immunoblastic (9 plasmacytoid), 2 centroblastic, 3 Burkitt's, 2 peripheral T-cell lymphomas, and 3 high-grade not otherwise specified (NOS). The remaining 7 cases included 3 diffuse mixed plasmacytoid, 1 low-grade B-cell lymphoma of mucosa-associated lymphoid tissue (MALT), 1 polymorphous B-cell hyperplasia, and 2 cases too necrotic or crushed to subclassify. Using the University of Minnesota classification, 25 of our cases were high-

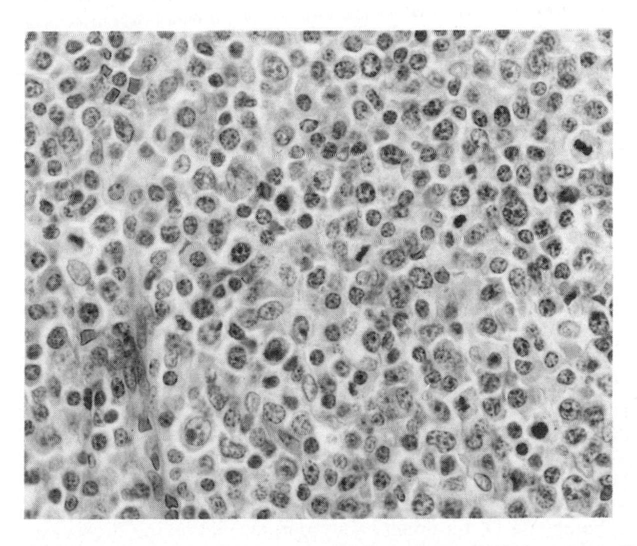

Figure 8 Polymorphous B cell lymphoma/PTLD, minimally polymorphic, involving a cervical lymph node in a cardiac allograft recipient. Higher power reveals plasma cells, plasmablasts, and a few large lymphoid cells, with numerous mitotic figures.

grade malignant lymphoma; only 5 were PBL, and 1 was PDBH (21,43) (JAF/NLH, unpublished data) (Figs. 2 to 10, Table 2). These findings suggest that there may be true variation in the types of PTLD encountered at different transplantation centers.

Several cases of CD30$^+$ anaplastic large-cell lymphoma of both B (44) and T (45,46) lineage have been described in renal transplant recipients. We have observed a case of gastric low-grade B-cell lymphoma of MALT in a renal transplant recipient (JAF/NLH, unpublished results) (Figs. 11 and 12). One case of angioimmunoblastic lymphadenopathy has been reported in a bone marrow transplant patient (42).

The incidence of Hodgkin's disease among allograft recipients is not increased (5). Only a few cases of Hodgkin's disease have been described in allograft recipients (47,48). In one of them, Hodgkin's disease involved a renal allograft and adjacent soft tissue, with ureteral obstruction and dysfunction of the allograft (49). Because PTLDs may be polymorphous—containing lymphocytes, plasma cells, and atypical immunoblasts that can resemble Reed-Sternberg cells—they may mimic Hodgkin's disease. A diagnosis of Hodg-

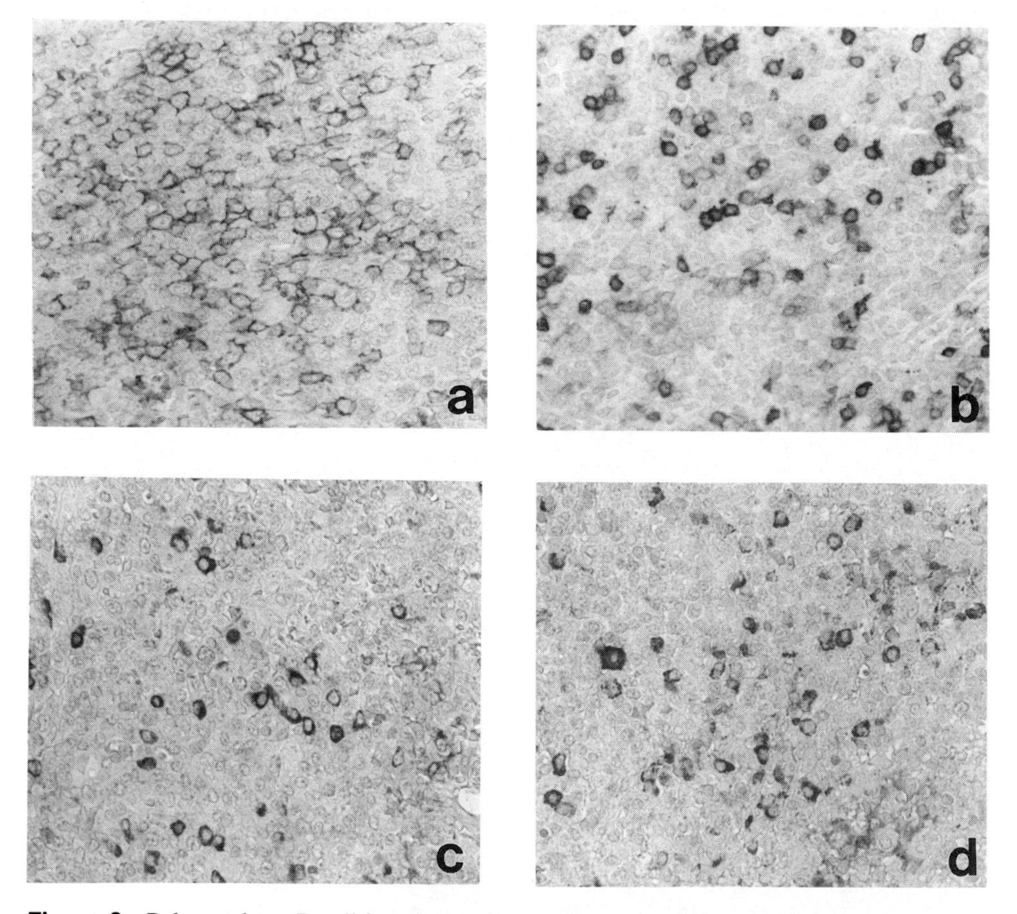

Figure 9 Polymorphous B cell lymphoma/PTLD, minimally polymorphic, involving a cervical lymph node in a cardiac allograft recipient. There is a mixture of B cells, CD20$^+$ (a), and T cells, CD3$^+$ (b), and of cells containing cytoplasmic κ (c) and λ (d) light chains. (Immunoperoxidase technique on paraffin sections.)

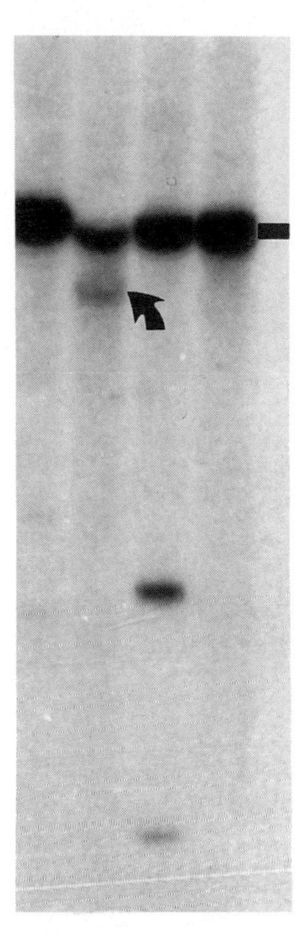

Figure 10 Polymorphous B cell lymphoma/PTLD, minimally polymorphic, involving a cervical lymph node in a cardiac allograft recipient. Genotyping reveals a clonal population of B cells (arrow), despite the apparent polytypic nature of the infiltrate on immunohistochemical analysis. (Lane 2, Southern blot hybridization using a J_h probe.) (Figures 7–10 represent the same case.)

Table 2 PTLD: Pathological Features of 32 Cases at MGH

Category	Number of cases
B-PTLD	25
Centroblastic	2
Immunoblastic (9 plasmacytoid)	12
Burkitt's	3
High grade, NOS	3
Mixed, plasmacytoid	3
MALT type	1
Polymorphous hyperplasia	1
T-PTLD (peripheral T-cell lymphoma)	2
Unknown (3 immunoblastic, 2 unclassified)	5

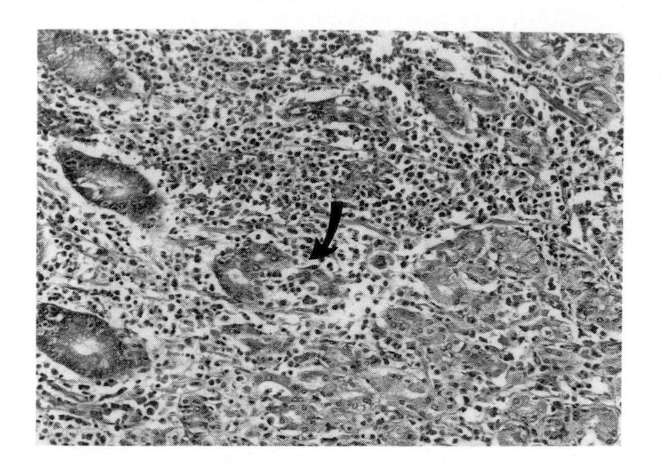

Figure 11 Low-grade B-cell lymphoma of mucosa-associated lymphoid tissue, involving the stomach and perigastric lymph node of an azathioprine-treated renal transplant recipient. The lamina propria of the stomach contains a dense infiltrate of small lymphoid cells and plasma cells. A lymphoepithelial lesion is present (arrow).

kin's disease in an allograft recipient should thus be made with caution; confirmation with immunophenotyping is recommended.

Based on our experience, lymphoid lesions in allograft recipients fall into three main groups: (a) ordinary, reactive hyperplasia (including rejection); (b) obvious high-grade lymphoma; and (c) atypical polymorphous infiltrates that cannot be classified confidently on histological grounds alone. Groups 2 and 3 are considered PTLD; group 2 includes the University of Minnesota's malignant lymphoma/multiple myeloma and some PBL as well as the University of Pittsburgh's monomorphic category. Group 3 includes most of Minne-

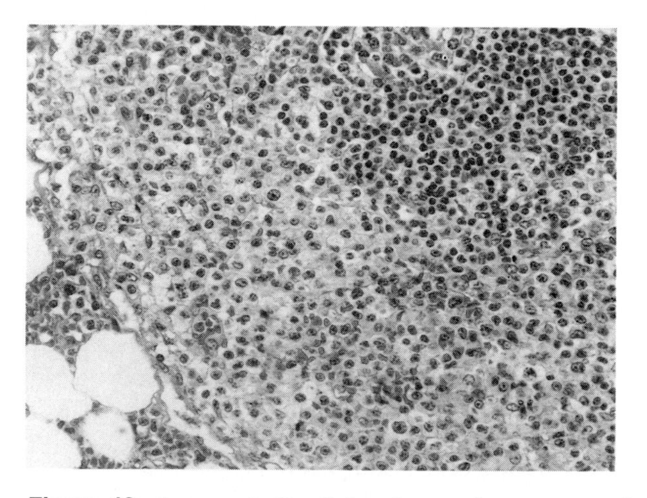

Figure 12 Low-grade B-cell lymphoma of mucosa-associated lymphoid tissue, involving the stomach and perigastric lymph node of an azathioprine-treated renal transplant recipient. The perigastric node contains a subcapsular infiltrate of lymphoid cells with abundant pale cytoplasm, consistent with marginal zone, or monocytoid B cells.

Table 3 Simplified Classification of PTLD

Proposed category	Features	University of Minnesota	University of Pittsburgh
Reactive lymphoid hyperplasia	Polyclonal	Some plasmacytic hyperplasia	
Atypical lymphoid proliferation[a]	Polymorphous, polyclonal	Plasmacytic hyperplasia	Some PTLD, polymorphic Some PTLD, minimally polymorphic
	Polymorphous, monoclonal	Rare plasmacytic hyperplasia, polymorphous diffuse B-cell hyperplasia, polymorphous B-cell lymphoma	Some PTLD, polymorphic Most PTLD, minimally polymorphic
Malignant lymphoma[b]	Monomorphous, monoclonal	Malignant lymphoma, multiple myeloma	PTLD, monomorphic

[a]Immunohistochemical and/or molecular genetic techniques required.
[b]Molecular studies are not required; subclassify by existing lymphoma classifications.

sota's PDBH/PBL and Pittsburgh's polymorphic and minimally polymorphic cases. Some cases in the Minnesota category of plasmacytic hyperplasia may represent reactive hyperplasia; others may represent true PTLDs. For those who see only occasional PTLDs, these broader categories may be simpler to use and more practical on a daily basis (Table 3).

VI. B-PTLDS: IMMUNOPHENOTYPIC AND GENOTYPIC FEATURES

B-cell proliferations account for the vast majority of PTLDs. In the Cincinnati Transplant Tumor Registry, 86% of cases recorded are B-cell lymphomas, while 14% are T-cell lymphomas and <1% null-cell (26). Of a total of 32 PTLDs seen at the Massachusetts General Hospital to date, 2 have been T-cell lymphomas, 25 have been B-cell infiltrates, and the remainder have not been phenotyped (20,43,50) (JAF/NLH, unpublished data) (Table 2).

In contrast to sporadic B-cell lymphoma, in which expression of monotypic immunoglobulin and/or clonal rearrangement of immunoglobulin heavy and light chain genes can nearly always be demonstrated, many reports of PTLD indicate that clonality often cannot be demonstrated (18). With respect to this feature, as for clinical and histological features, experiences at different institutions are often markedly different. However, the success of demonstrating clonality is highly dependent on the method used and variation in the type of analysis performed; i.e., immunophenotyping versus genotyping accounts for some of the differences reported.

A high frequency of apparently polyclonal PTLDs has been reported by those medical centers with a high frequency of polymorphic lesions. In a series of solid-organ transplant recipients treated at the University of Pittsburgh, 12 patients had clonal, 13 had nonclonal, and 5 had both clonal and nonclonal tumors by either immunohistologic techniques or molecular analysis of immunoglobulin genes (18). In this study, genotypic analysis was more sensitive in identifying clonal tumors than was immunophenotypic analysis, and immunophenotyping was, in turn, more sensitive than routine histological examination.

Monomorphous lesions were highly likely to be monoclonal (23/27), but only 17 of 31 specimens with a polymorphous appearance were polyclonal, while 14 were monoclonal. Similarly, applying molecular genetic analysis to cases studied using the revised University of Minnesota classification, 90% of plasmacytic hyperplasias were polyclonal lesions, while 100% of PDBH/PBL and malignant lymphomas or multiple myelomas were monoclonal tumors (51).

In contrast, institutions that have found a predominance of monomorphous PTLDs report a higher frequency of monoclonality. In the University of Washington series, in which 14 of 15 cases were immunoblastic lymphomas, although monoclonal immunoglobulin was detected in only 3 cases using immunohistologic techniques, 7 of 8 cases were found to be clonal by molecular techniques (42). All 18 monomorphous PTLDs reported in two series from Stanford and Massachusetts General Hospital showed clonally rearranged immunoglobulin heavy chain genes (41,43). Seven of them expressed monotypic immunoglobulin, and 11 were immunoglobulin-negative. Although the pathological features of PTLDs may differ from institution to institution, it seems clear that, for the high proportion of PTLDs that do not express monotypic immunoglobulin, genotypic analysis is the most reliable technique for assessing clonality (Figs. 7 to 10).

Genotypic analysis has disclosed that some patients with PTLDs appear to have multiclonal tumors. Just as the histological features may vary from site to site in the same patient, assessing the configuration of immunoglobulin genes by Southern blot hybridization may suggest the presence of more than one clonal population in a single site or distinct clonal populations in separate anatomic sites. In addition, in tumors with a single clonal population, the clonal band can vary in intensity, consistent with a clonal population of varying size arising in a background population of polyclonal cells. It has also been possible to find a clonal tumor involving one site and a polyclonal tumor involving another (18,20,43,52–55). However, studies assessing the configuration of Epstein-Barr viral genomes suggest that at least some cases of apparently "multiclonal lymphomas" may arise from the same clone of EBV-infected cells (see below).

Results of chromosomal analysis have been reported in only a small number of PTLDs; however, in the classification system from the University of Minnesota, chromosomal abnormalities have been found in PBL and immunoblastic sarcoma and not in lesions classified as hyperplasias (39). Compared to certain other high grade lymphomas, such as sporadic or endemic Burkitt's lymphomas, in which nearly 100% of cases have a c-*myc* rearrangement, and lymphomas in HIV-positive patients, in which approximately 40% have a c-*myc* rearrangement, c-*myc* alterations are infrequent in the posttransplant population (56) (Table 4). None of 13 patients with chromosomal analysis had a t (8;14) in 3 series of PTLD (4,38,57), and only 3 of 14 in another showed c-*myc* rearrangement, which was of the type found in sporadic Burkitt's lymphoma (54). All three cases were entirely or partially composed of a monomorphous population of large atypical lymphoid cells (54). Structural abnormalities of c-*myc* have been reported in cases of malignant lymphoma and multiple myeloma by Cesarman et al., although cases of plasmacytic hyperplasia and PDBH/PBL lacked these changes (51). C-*myc* rearrangements appear to occur only in monomorphic, monoclonal PTLDs. In cases with chromosomal analysis, no other recurring abnormalities have been found. Cesarman et al. have also reported abnormalities of p53 and N-*ras* in the malignant lymphoma/multiple myeloma group of PTLD (51). In contrast, however, other investigators have not demonstrated abnormalities of p53 genetic sequence or expression by polymerase chain reaction (58) or by immunohistochemical techniques (58–60).

Table 4 EBV-Related Lymphomas[a]

	PTLD	HIV NHL	Endemic BL	Sporadic BL
EBV	+	+/−	+	−/+
EBNA 1	+	+[a]	+	+[a]
EBNA 2	+	−/+[a]	−	−
LMP	+	+[a]	−	−
C-*myc* rearranged	−/+	+/−	+	+
Type of c-*myc* rearrangement	Sporadic pattern	Sporadic pattern	Endemic pattern	Sporadic pattern
EBV type	A	A or B[a]	A or B	A[a]

[a]Among EBV+ cases.
Abbreviations: BL, Burkitt's lymphoma; HIV NHL, non-Hodgkin's lymphoma in HIV-positive patients; EBV, Epstein Barr virus; PTLD, posttransplant lymphoproliferative disorder; EBNA, Epstein Barr nuclear antigen; LMP, latent membrane protein.
Source: From Refs. 43, 51, 54, 56, 59, 60, 71, 74, 75, 98, 103, and 104.

VII. PTLD: ASSOCIATION WITH EPSTEIN-BARR VIRUS

Lymphomas that develop in immunodeficient patients, including allograft recipients, are frequently associated with EBV (Table 4). Approximately 90% of patients with B-PTLDs have serological evidence of primary or reactivation EBV infection, with primary infection being slightly more common than reactivation; the remainder have evidence of long-past EBV infection (4,22,55,61–64). In one series of 142 solid-organ recipients, 9 previously seronegative patients developed a primary EBV infection. Of these patients, 6 developed a PTLD (57), suggesting that patients receiving immunosuppressive therapy may be at increased risk for lymphoma upon initial exposure to EBV.

In the overwhelming majority of B-PTLD there is evidence of EBV infection of the proliferating cells. In 14 to 100% of cases in different series (overall, 43%), the atypical lymphoid cells express Epstein-Barr nuclear antigen (25,57,63,65–67). Using more sensitive methods, Southern blot or in situ hybridization, the tumors are positive for EBV genomes in 95% of cases (20,24,30,38,42,44,54,55,57,66,68–70). Using probes to the fused termini of EBV to assess the clonality of the virus in these lesions has demonstrated that the virus has been present in a clonal, episomal form in 79% of cases. In 15%, an oligoclonal population is present, in 4% only linear replicating virus has been identified, and in 2%, no virus has been found (43,44,54,68,70). In a small portion of cases with monoclonally integrated EBV, additional small bands or smears, consistent with the presence of cells infected by an oligoclonal population of EBV or replicating EBV, have been found (54,70).

Nearly all tumors with clonally rearranged immunoglobulin genes contain EBV in a clonal, episomal form. In addition, occasional cases that appear to be polyclonal by immunoglobulin gene rearrangement may contain clonal EBV (44,54,68). This suggests that the methods for detection of EBV clonality may be more sensitive than that of immunoglobulin gene rearrangement, or, alternatively, that EBV can infect the B cells at a primitive stage, prior to immunoglobulin gene rearrangement. When patients have had multiple tumors in different sites, the tumors usually contain the same clone of EBV, even when distinct immunoglobulin gene rearrangements are found, indicating that the tumors share a common origin (43,54). Occasionally, the EBV clones in different tumors from the same patient may be different, consistent with true multiclonal lymphomas (43,68).

The pattern of EBV gene expression in PTLD is consistent with latent infection. The lymphoid cells characteristically express EBNA1, EBNA2, and latent membrane protein (LMP) (56,59,60,71). This pattern is distinct from other EBV-associated lymphomas. In endemic Burkitt's lymphoma and in the minority of sporadic Burkitt's lymphoma that contain EBV, EBNA2 and LMP are typically absent. In EBV-positive, HIV-related lymphomas, LMP is expressed, but EBNA2 may be absent (56). EBNA2 and LMP upregulate the expression of B-lymphocyte activation antigens (CD23) and adhesion molecules (LFA3 and ICAM-1) in vitro and in vivo and are thus considered to be effectors of lymphocyte growth (71). In in vitro studies using rodent fibroblasts, LMP has the capacity to induce transformation (72).

The frequent detection of EBV by serological, immunophenotypic, and genotypic studies supports the contention that PTLDs are associated with EBV. The pattern of latent gene expression and the finding of monoclonally integrated EBV in most cases suggest that the virus may have a primary role in the pathogenesis of PTLD. Some investigators have suggested that the rare EBV-negative lymphoma in transplant recipients may represent a sporadic lymphoma (73).

In the nonimmunosuppressed population, virtually all cases of EBV-positive lymphomas contain type A EBV (56,74). In patients infected with HIV, roughly equal numbers of lymphomas contain EBV of type A or type B (56,74). Type B EBV has a decreased capacity to transform B cells compared to type A, and it is possible that only immunodeficient individuals are at risk for spread of type B EBV beyond the oropharynx and for the development of type B EBV-positive lymphomas (74). These data suggest that PTLDs might also contain EBV of either strain; however, a recent study documented the exclusive presence of type A EBV in PTLD (75).

VIII. POSTTRANSPLANTATION T-CELL LYMPHOMA

Although the overwhelming majority of PTLDs have been B-cell proliferations, a handful of T-lineage lymphomas have also been described. Twenty cases of posttransplantation T-cell lymphoma have been reported (45,46,50,76–89). We have seen one additional case of T-cell lymphoma at Massachusetts General Hospital (JAF/NLH, unpublished data). Seventeen T-cell lymphomas have occurred in renal transplant recipients, 3 in marrow recipients (89), and one in a cardiac transplant recipient (81). The marrow transplant recipients were children; the solid-organ recipients were adults. The interval from transplantation to T-cell lymphoma ranged from 2 months to 19 years (median, 5 2/3 years). Patients typically presented with evidence of extranodal disease (cardiac or neurological dysfunction, vulvar mass, mediastinal mass, skin nodules, Sezary syndrome, pancytopenia, or hepatic mass) and sometimes with lymphadenopathy. One patient had involvement of the renal allograft (87). Four cases were classified as lymphoblastic lymphomas, including two of the cases occurring in allogeneic marrow recipients (83,84,89). The remainder have been peripheral T-cell lymphomas, usually of high-grade types, including immunoblastic (3 cases), anaplastic large cell (2), diffuse mixed (2), and others. In one case, the T-cell lymphoma was followed by development of a B-cell PTLD (77). One patient, a native of Trinidad/Tobago, was seropositive for HTLV-I (88). In only three cases, including the case of a patient who had celiac disease and developed intestinal lymphoma (76), were the tumors positive for EBV genomes (82,86). Follow-up of 21 patients with T-cell PTLD reveals 7 patients who remain alive and 14 who have died, 8 after very short intervals. Both of the T-cell lymphomas seen at Massachusetts General Hospital were associated with a systemic hemophagocytic syndrome and a rapidly fatal course. The longest survival reported, which was in the patient with celiac disease, has been 3 years (45,46,50,76–89; JAF/NLH, unpublished data). Of the remaining 6 survivors, 3 presented with cutaneous disease (85,88). Thus, in the case of patients presenting with extracutaneous disease, T-cell lymphomas appear to have a worse prognosis than B-cell PTLDs (see below). In contrast to the situation with B-cell PTLDs, T-cell lymphomas tend to occur at a longer interval after transplant and to be negative for EBV. The etiology of T-cell lymphomas in the post-transplantation setting is unclear, although reduced immune surveillance, chronic antigenic stimulation due to the presence of the graft, and the direct oncogenic effect of the immunosuppressive agents have all been suggested (82).

IX. PTLD: DONOR VERSUS RECIPIENT ORIGIN

The origin of the PTLD (donor versus recipient) has been investigated in a small number of cases, mostly in marrow allograft recipients. Of 25 analyzed tumors arising in marrow recipients, 18 have been of donor origin, 5 of recipient, and 2 of mixed donor-recipient origin (42,73,89,90). In 17 cases in solid-organ transplant recipients (12 renal, 3 hepatic, 2 heart-lung), 13 have been of recipient and 4 of donor origin (61,69,91–98). Theoretically, a solid-organ transplant recipient would be more likely to be able to recognize as foreign and mount an immune response to a tumor of donor origin if immunosuppressive therapy were decreased. Follow-up is only available in a limited number of cases (2 heart-lung, 2 liver, 8 renal), but 5 of 8 patients with tumors of recipient origin have died, while the 4 with tumors of donor origin are alive and well (2) or alive with disease (2) at last follow-up (61,69,91,92,94,96–98). One of those alive with disease at last published follow-up (97) was treated successfully for PTLD and later died of other causes with no evidence of PTLD at autopsy (unpublished data). Although at least some solid-organ recipients recover, when allogeneic marrow recipients develop a PTLD, it is nearly always fatal, regardless of its origin.

X. PTLD: TREATMENT AND OUTCOME

Therapeutic measures that have been used for treatment of PTLD include reduction of immunosuppression, surgery, acyclovir, radiotherapy, chemotherapy, and a combination of alpha-interferon and intravenous gamma globulin. Nevertheless, PTLD remains a leading cause of death among allograft recipients after the immediate postoperative period (19) (Table 5). Among published cases, B-cell PTLD is associated with 54% mortality in solid organ recipients (4,18,20–25,29,36,37,42–44,47,55,61,69,92,94,98). A better prognosis has been associated with a mononucleosis-like presentation, disease confined to lymph nodes, single-organ disease, resectable gastrointestinal tract disease, isolated pulmonary disease, polymorphous histology, polyclonality and response to decreased immunosuppression. A worse prognosis is associated with patients who present with organ dysfunction, central nervous system disease, disseminated disease, monomorphous or monoclonal tumors, or concurrent opportunistic infections (18,47,62).

Several medical centers have reported a correlation between histological, immunohistological, and genotypic features and outcome in PTLD. In a series of solid-organ transplant recipients treated at the University of Pittsburgh, the PTLD regressed with reduction in immunosuppression or resolved after treatment in 27 to 37 cases (18,62). Polymorphic lesions were slightly more likely to regress, although histological features alone were not strongly predictive of outcome. However, nearly all patients with nonclonal lesions and about half of patients with monoclonal lesions responded to decreased immunosuppression and surgery. Locker and Nalesnik subsequently expanded on these observations in their 1989 report. They found that most monomorphic monoclonal tumors would not regress with decreased immunosuppression alone. Among polymorphic tumors, those with no clonal population or with a small clonal population had a better chance of regression than did polymorphic tumors with a large clonal population (54).

Unfortunately, not all investigators have found results as favorable as those described at the University of Pittsburgh. Those medical centers reporting a high frequency of monomorphic, monoclonal PTLDs report a high mortality rate. Twenty-three of a total of 25 patients with PTLD from Stanford and Massachusetts General Hospital died; in at least 15 cases the immediate cause of death was PTLD. Only 2 of the 25 had polymorphous lesions (1 PDBH, 1 PBL); one of them is currently alive and well and the other died of other causes with no evidence of PTLD at autopsy (20,41,43).

Patients who respond to decreased immunosuppression clearly have a better prognosis than those who fail to respond. In devising treatment strategies for PTLD, it would be a great advantage to identify any features other than polyclonality that predict response to decreased immunosuppression. In one study of heart or lung allograft recipients, patients with early-onset disease (< 1 year) had significantly lower mortality than those with late-onset disease (36% versus 70%). Early-onset disease was associated with much greater likelihood of response to decreased immunosuppression (89% versus none) and much lower incidence of disseminated disease (23% versus 86%) (19). While it is accepted that patients who respond to a reduction in immunosuppressive therapy have a more favorable outcomc, not all studies have confirmed the finding of a relationship to the interval to developing PTLD. In a study of 19 PTLDs arising in cardiac transplant recipients, Chen and coworkers found no difference in outcome when they compared patients with early- and late-onset disease (47). The mortality of PTLD has been so high that, in cases of renal transplantation, it is recommended to decrease immunosuppressive therapy drastically, even if this results in rejection of the allograft (62). Accordingly, 4 of the 5 renal allograft recipients who recovered from PTLDs were on dialysis at last follow-up in one series (4).

Extent and location of disease are also important prognostic factors; localized disease is frequently more amenable to surgery or radiation, usually in combination with decreased immunosuppression. Surgical resection is especially useful in cases of gastrointestinal PTLD (18,32,47). Occasionally, radiation therapy is efficacious in cases of limited-stage disease (18,20,47,67). Central nervous system disease may respond to irradiation, although long-term survival is unusual (4).

Acyclovir is a synthetic purine nucleoside analogue with inhibitory activity against human herpesviruses. It blocks the replication of EBV in its linear form but is ineffective against EBV in its latent, episomal form. Because of its potential therapeutic effect in cases of EBV-associated disorders, it has been used to treat patients with PTLDs. In a series of 19 renal allograft recipients (18 treated with azathioprine-based regimens and 1 with cyclosporine), two distinct groups were identified: (a) young patients presenting with infectious mononucleosislike symptoms and widespread disease soon after transplantation and (b) older patients presenting with localized tumor masses at a longer interval after transplantation (4). Four of 8 patients in the first group had PTLDs that resolved with acyclovir, in 3 cases in combination with decreased immunosuppression. Only 1 of 11 patients in the second group recovered. The survivor was treated with decreased immunosuppression only. PTLDs in all patients who recovered expressed polytypic immunoglobulin. Ironically, patients in the first group who did not respond to therapy had a more rapidly fatal course than those in the second group. These results suggest that at least some patients in the first group had PTLDs containing linear replicating EBV which was inhibited by acyclovir. Although selected patients with PTLD may benefit from acyclovir therapy, Southern blot analysis has shown that most cases of PTLD have latent rather than replicating EBV (see above), which is unaffected by acyclovir. Thus, the majority of PTLDs would not be expected to respond to acyclovir.

Monomorphous monoclonal PTLDs tend not to respond to acyclovir or decreased immunosuppression alone. However, conventional lymphoma therapy may be effective in some of these cases. In a recent abstract, investigators reported 7 cases of "late onset" PTLD (> 4 months posttransplantation) in cardiac allograft recipients who were treated with combination chemotherapy, usually ProMACE-CytaBOM. Whenever the phenotype could be determined, the tumors were monoclonal. Five of 7 patients achieved a complete remission; however, neutropenic sepsis occurred in 5 of these patients, and 1 died of this complication (99). These results suggest that once a PTLD is overtly malignant, it requires therapy similar to that used for high-grade lymphomas arising in nonimmunosuppressed individuals, but that aggressive treatment of these iatrogenically immunosuppressed patients may be complicated by serious infections.

XI. EVALUATION OF CASES OF SUSPECTED PTLD

Biopsy of clinically abnormal tissue is an essential step in the diagnosis of PTLD. Tissue obtained from a possible case of PTLD should be sent fresh to the pathologist and should be accompanied by information on the clinical setting and the differential diagnosis. It should be divided—that is, a portion should be saved frozen for immunophenotyping and genotyping and a portion fixed for routine histological studies. Needle aspiration biopsies rarely yield sufficient tissue for these studies to be performed. Based on the features seen on light microscopic examination, the lesions are classified as reactive lymphoid hyperplasia, atypical lymphoid proliferation, or malignant lymphoma (see above, Table 3). Cases recognizable as lymphoma are classified according to one of the standard schemes—the working Formulation (100) or the Kiel Classification (101). In cases of histologically recognizable lymphoma, immunophenotyping studies are useful to confirm the lymphoid nature and to establish B- or T-cell origin. Since virtually all monomorphic lesions are monoclonal, studies to determine clonality may not be necessary in these cases. In atypical lymphoid proliferations, immunophenotyping studies are essential to determine clonality; lesions that are not clearly clonal by immunophenotyping should be subjected to molecular genetic analysis using probes to immunoglobulin and EBV genes to determine clonality (Table 3). Since the response to conservative therapy and the clinical outcome appear to correlate strongly with monoclonality, an attempt should be made in all cases to determine the presence or absence of a clonal population. In situ hybridization methods for detecting EBV genomes have been reported to be useful in distinguishing between PTLD and rejection, but they are not useful in distinguishing between monoclonal and polyclonal PTLD (102).

Because PTLDs typically grow rapidly and frequently present as disseminated disease and because of the immunosuppressed state of the patient, PTLDs are difficult to treat. Because experiences at different medical centers have varied and randomized clinical trials have not been performed, there is a certain lack of consensus concerning optimal treatment of these patients. It is generally agreed, however, that decreasing immunosuppression

Table 5 PTLD: Treatment Options

Treatment	Polymorphous polyclonal	Monomorphous monoclonal
Acyclovir	Effective	Not effective
Reduced immunosuppression	Effective	Necessary, not sufficient
Resection	Not required	Effective
Radiation	Not required	Effective
Chemotherapy	Not required	Effective, but infectious complications

should be part of the treatment approach to every patient with PTLD, regardless of histological type. Resectable lesions may be treated with surgery; in some of these cases, adjuvant therapy may not be necessary, sparing the patient the complications that may accompany chemotherapy. These two steps may result in complete remissions for many polyclonal and some monoclonal PTLDs. Acyclovir may be a useful adjunct to decreased immunosuppression for patients with polyclonal PTLD, but is not expected to be useful in lesions with clonally integrated, latent EBV. Patients with widespread monoclonal lesions frequently will not respond to a reduction in immunosuppression alone and will require treatment with cytotoxic chemotherapy (Table 5). At the present time, however, the mortality of PTLD remains unacceptably high. Improvement in the survival of allograft recipients will require the development of alternative methods of immunosuppression that do not impair the T-cell response to EBV, and thus do not predispose patients to PTLDs, and the availability of innovative, effective forms of therapy for those patients who do develop PTLD.

ACKNOWLEDGMENT

We are grateful to Bernadette Vijayakanthan for secretarial expertise and to Michelle Forrestall and Steve Conley for assistance with photography.

REFERENCES

1. Kinlen LJ, Sheil AGR, Peto J, et al. Collaborative United Kingdom-Australasian study of cancer in patients treated with immunosuppressive drugs. Br Med J 1979; 2:1461–1466.
2. Hoover R, Fraumeni JF. Risk of cancer in renal transplant recipients. Lancet 1973; 2:55.
3. Barnett LB, Schwartz E. Cerebral reticulum cell sarcoma after multiple renal transplants. J Neurol Neurosurg Psychiatry 1974; 37:966.
4. Hanto DW, Gajl-Peczalska KJ, Frizzera G, et al. Epstein-Barr virus (EBV) induced polyclonal and monoclonal B-cell lymphoproliferative diseases occurring after renal transplantation. Ann Surg 1983; 198:356–368.
5. Penn I. Depressed immunity and the development of cancer: Review. Clin Exp Immunol 1981; 46:459–474.
6. Orosz C, Fidelus D, Rooperian D, et al. Analysis of cloned T cell function: I. Dissection of cloned T cell proliferative responses using cyclosporin A. J Immunol 1982; 129:1865–1868.
7. Cohen DJ, Loertscher R, Rubin MF, et al. Cyclosporine: A new immunosuppressive agent for organ transplantation. Ann Intern Med 1984; 101:667–682.
8. Hudnall DS. Cyclosporin A renders target cells resistant to immune cytolysis. Eur J Immunol 1991; 21:221–226.

9. Bird AG, McLachlan SM, Britton S. Cyclosporin A promotes spontaneous outgrowth in vitro of Epstein-Barr virus-induced B-cell lines. Nature 1981; 289:300–301.
10. Crawford DH, Edwards JMB, Sweny P, et al. Studies on long-term T-cell-mediated immunity to Epstein-Barr virus in immunosuppressed renal allograft recipients. Int J Cancer 1981; 28:705–709.
11. York LJ, Qualtiere LF. Cyclosporine abrogates virus-specific T-cell control of EBV-induced B-cell lymphoproliferation. Viral Immunol 1990; 3:127–136.
12. Bejarano M, Masucci M, Ernberg I, et al. Effect of Cyclosporin-A (CsA) on the ability of T lymphocyte subsets to inhibit the proliferation of autologous EBV-transformed B cells. Int J Cancer 1985; 35:327–333.
13. Calne RY, Rolles K, White DJG, et al. Cyclosporin A as the only immunosuppressant in 34 recipients of cadaveric organs: 32 kidney, 2 pancreases and 2 livers. Lancet 1979; 2:1033.
14. Cockburn I. Assessment of the risks of malignancy and lymphomas developing in patients using Sandimmune. Transpl Proc 1987; 19:1804–1807.
15. Opelz G, Henderson R. Incidence of non-Hodgkin lymphoma in kidney and heart transplant recipients. Lancet 1993; 342:1514–1516.
16. Beveridge T, Krupp P, McKibbin C. Letter. Lancet 1984; 1:788.
17. Kahan BD, Flechner SM, Lorber MI, et al. Complications of cyclosporin therapy. World J Surg 1986; 10:348–360.
18. Nalesnik M, Jaffe R, Starzl TE, et al. The pathology of posttransplant lymphoproliferative disorders occurring in the setting of cyclosporine A-prednisone immunosuppression. Am J Pathol 1988; 133:173–192.
19. Armitage JM, Kormos RL, Stuart RS, et al. Posttransplant lymphoproliferative disease in thoracic organ transplant patients: 10 years of cyclosporine-based immunosuppression. J Heart Lung Transplant 1991; 10:877–887.
20. Ferry JA, Jacobson JO, Conti D, et al. Lymphoproliferative disorders and hematologic malignancies following organ transplantation. Mod Pathol 1989; 2:583–592.
21. Levy M, Backman L, Husberg B, et al. De novo malignancy following liver transplantation: A single center study. Transplant Proc 1993; 25:1397–1399.
22. Olivari M-T, Diekmann RA, Kubo SH, et al. Low incidence of neoplasia in heart and heart-lung transplant recipients receiving triple-drug immunosuppression. J Heart Transplant 1990; 9:618–621.
23. Pomerance A, Stovin PGI. Heart transplant pathology: The British experience. J Clin Pathol 1985; 38:146–159.
24. Swinnen LJ, Costanzo-Nordin MR, Fisher S, et al. Increased incidence of lymphoproliferative disorder after immunosuppression with the monoclonal antibody OKT3 in cardiac transplant recipients. N Engl J Med 1990; 323:1723–1728.
25. Wilkinson AH, Smith JL, Hansicker LG, et al. Increased frequency of posttransplant lymphomas in patients treated with cyclosporine, azathioprine and prednisone. Transplantation 1989; 47:293–296.
26. Penn I. The changing pattern of posttransplant malignancies. Transplant Proc 1991; 23:1101–1103.
27. Hanto DW, Najarian JS. Advances in the diagnosis and treatment of EBV-associated lymphoproliferative disorders in immunocompromised hosts. J Surg Oncol 1985; 30:215–220.
28. Oyer PE, Stinson EB, Jamieson SW, et al. Cyclosporine in cardiac transplantation: A 2½ year follow-up. Heart Lung Transplant 1983; 15(suppl 1):2546–2552.
29. Castro CJ, Klimo P, Worth A. Multifocal aggressive lymphoma of the gastrointestinal tract in a renal transplant patient treated with cyclosporin A and prednisone. Cancer 1985; 55:1665–1667.
30. Johnson M, Flye MW. Immunoblastic lymphoma in a cyclosporin-treated renal transplant recipient. Transplantation 1985; 39:673–674.
31. Rosenthal JT, Iwatsuki S, Starzl TE, et al. Histiocytic lymphoma in renal transplant patients receiving cyclosporine. Transplant Proc 1983; 15(suppl 1):2805–2807.

32. Cohen JI. Epstein-Barr virus lymphoproliferative disease associated with acquired immunodeficiency. Medicine 1991; 70:137–160.
33. Randhawa PS, Yousem SA, Paradis IL, et al. The clinical spectrum, pathology, and clonal analysis of Epstein-Barr virus–associated lymphoproliferative disorders in heart-lung transplant recipients. Am J Clin Pathol 1989; 92:177–185.
34. Hoffman DG, Gedebou M, Jimenez A, et al. Detection of Epstein-Barr virus by the polymerase chain reaction in transbronchial biopsies of lung transplant recipients: Evidence of infection? Mod Pathol 1993; 6:555–559.
35. Krueger TC, Tallent MB, Richie RE, et al. Neoplasia in immunosuppressed renal transplant patients: A 20-year experience. South Med J 1985; 78:501–506.
36. Cotton JR, Sarles HE, Remmers AR, et al. The appearance of reticulum cell sarcoma at the site of antilymphocyte globulin injection. Transplantation 1973; 16:154–157.
37. Deodhar S, Kuklinca AG, Vidt DG, et al. Development of reticulum cell sarcoma at the site of antilymphocyte globulin injection in a patient with renal transplant. N Engl J Med 1969; 280:1104–1106.
38. Shapiro RS, McClain K, Frizzera G, et al. Epstein-Barr virus associated B cell lymphoproliferative disorders following bone marrow transplantation. Blood 1988; 71:1234–1243.
39. Frizzera G, Hanto DW, Gajl-Peczalska KJ, et al. Polymorphic diffuse B cell hyperplasias and lymphomas in renal transplant recipients. Cancer Res 1981; 41:4262.
40. Chadburn A, Frizzera G, Chen J, et al. Clinico-pathologic analysis of 28 post-transplantation lymphoproliferative disorders (PT-LPDs). Mod Pathol 1994; 7:104A.
41. Cleary ML, Warnke R, Sklar J. Monoclonality of lymphoproliferative lesions in cardiac-transplant recipients: Clonal analysis based on immunoglobulin-gene rearrangements. N Engl J Med 1984; 310:477–482.
42. Zutter MM, Martin PJ, Sale GE, et al. Epstein-Barr virus lymphoproliferation after bone marrow transplantation. Blood 1988; 72:520–529.
43. Kaplan MA, Ferry JA, Harris NL, et al. Clonal analysis of post-transplant lymphoproliferative disorders, using both episomal EBV and immunoglobulin genes as markers. Am J Clin Pathol 1994; 101:590–596.
44. Borisch B, Gatter KC, Tobler A, et al. Epstein-Barr virus-associated anaplastic large cell lymphoma in renal transplant patients. Am J Clin Pathol 1992; 98:312–318.
45. Audouin J, Le Tourneau A, Diebold J, et al. Primary intestinal lymphoma of Ki-1 large cell anaplastic type with mesenteric lymph node and spleen involvement in a renal transplant recipient. Hematol Oncol 1989; 7:441–449.
46. Ng K, Trotter J, Metcalf C, et al. Extranodal Ki-1 lymphoma in a renal transplant patient. Aust NZ J Med 1992; 22:51–53.
47. Chen JM, Barr ML, Chadburn A, et al. Management of lymphoproliferative disorders after cardiac transplantation. Ann Thorac Surg 1993; 56:527–538.
48. Doyle TJ, Venkatachalam KK, Maeda K, et al. Hodgkin's disease in renal transplant recipients. Cancer 1983; 51:245–247.
49. Oldhafer KJ, Bunzendahl H, Frei V, et al. Primary Hodgkin's lymphoma: An unusual cause of graft dysfunction after kidney transplantation. Am J Med 1989; 87:218–220.
50. Kaplan MA, Jacobson JO, Ferry JA, et al. T-cell lymphoma of the vulva in a renal allograft recipient with associated hemophagocytosis. Am J Surg Pathol 1993; 17:842–849.
51. Cesarman E, Chadburn A, Frizzera G, et al. Molecular genetic analysis of post-transplantation lymphoproliferative disorders (PT-LPDs). Mod Pathol 1994; 7:104A.
52. Chadburn A, Cesarman E, Liu YF, Knowles DM. Multiple post-transplantation lymphoproliferative disorders (PT-LPD) in one anatomic site are multiclonal lymphomas. Mod Pathol 1994; 7:104A.
53. Cleary ML, Sklar J. Lymphoproliferative disorders in cardiac transplant recipients are multiclonal lymphomas. Lancet 1984; 2:489.

54. Locker J, Nalesnik M. Molecular genetic analysis of lymphoid tumors arising after organ transplantation. Am J Pathol 1993; 135:977–987.
55. Hanto DW, Birkenbach M, Frizzera G, et al. Confirmation of the heterogeneity of post transplant Epstein-Barr virus–associated B cell proliferations by immunoglobulin gene rearrangement analysis. Transplantation 1989; 47:458–464.
56. Shibata D, Weiss LM, Hernandez AM, et al. Epstein-Barr virus–associated non-Hodgkin's lymphoma in patients infected with the human immunodeficiency virus. Blood 1993; 81: 2102–2109.
57. Ho M, Miller G, Atchison RW, et al. Epstein-Barr virus infections and DNA hybridization studies in posttransplantation lymphoma and lymphoproliferative lesions: The role of the primary infection. J Infect Dis. 1985; 152:876–886.
58. O'Dowd JF, Dunne B, Willcocks TC, Parfrey NA. The p53 tumor-suppressor gene in the pathogenesis of post-transplant lymphoproliferative disease. Mod Pathol 1994; 7:117A.
59. Gascoyne R, Wolber R, McCarthy M, Keown P. P53 expression in post-transplant lymphoproliferative disorders. Mod Pathol 1994; 7:108A.
60. Kaplan MA, Harris NL. Expression of Epstein-Barr virus (EBV) gene products and related cellular proteins in post-transplant lymphoproliferative disorders (PTLD). Mod Pathol 1994; 7:112A.
61. Garnier JL, Berger F, Betuel H, Vuillaume M, et al. Epstein-Barr virus associated lymphoproliferative diseases (B cell lymphoma) after transplantation. Nephrol Dial Transplant 1989; 4:818–823.
62. Nalesnik MA, Makowka L, Starzl TE. The diagnosis and treatment of posttransplant lymphoproliferative disorders. Curr Probl Surg 1988; 25:365–472.
63. Thiru S, Calne RY, Nagington J. Lymphoma in renal allograft patients treated with cyclosporin A as one of the immunosuppressive agents. Transplant Proc 1981; 13:359–364.
64. Walker RJ, Tiller DJ, Horvath JS, et al. Malignant lymphoma in a renal transplant patient on cyclosporin A therapy. Aust NZ J Med 1989; 19:154–155.
65. Crawford DH, Thomas JA, Janossy G, et al. Epstein-Barr virus nuclear antigen positive lymphoma after cyclosporin A treatment in patient with renal allograft. Lancet 1980; 1:1355–1356.
66. Hanto DW, Frizzera G, Purtilo DT, et al. Clinical spectrum of lymphoproliferative disorders in renal transplant recipients and evidence for the role of the Epstein-Barr virus. Cancer Res 1981; 41:4253–4261.
67. Starzl TE, Nalesnik MA, Porter KA, et al. Reversibility of lymphomas and lymphoproliferative lesions developing under cyclosporin-steroid therapy. Lancet 1984; 1:583–587.
68. Cleary ML, Nalesnik MA, Shearer WT, et al. Clonal analysis of transplant-associated lymphoproliferations based on the structure of the genomic termini of the Epstein-Barr virus. Blood 1988; 72:349–352.
69. Hjelle B, Evans-Holm M, Yen T-S, et al. A poorly differentiated lymphoma of donor origin in a renal allograft recipient. Transplantation 1989; 47:945–948.
70. Katz BZ, Raab-Traub N, Miller G. Latent and replicating forms of Epstein-Barr virus DNA in lymphomas and lymphoproliferative diseases. J Infect Dis 1989; 160:589–598.
71. Young L, Alfiere C, Hennessy K, et al. Expression of Epstein-Barr virus transformation-associated genes in tissues of patients with EBV lymphoproliferative disease. N Engl J Med 1989; 321:1080–1085.
72. Wang D, Liebowitz D, Kieff E, et al. An EBV membrane protein expressed in immortalized lymphocytes transforms established rodent cells. Cell 1985; 43:831–840.
73. D'Amore ESG, Manivel JC, Gajl-Peczalska KJ, et al. B-cell lymphoproliferative disorders after bone marrow transplant: An analysis of ten cases with emphasis on Epstein-Barr virus detection by in situ hybridization. Cancer 1991; 68:1285–1295.
74. Boyle MJ, Sewell WA, Sculley TB, et al. Subtypes of Epstein-Barr virus in human immunodeficiency virus-associated non-Hodgkin lymphoma. Blood 1991; 78:3004–3011.

75. Frank D, Cesarman E, Knowles DM. Post-transplantation lymphoproliferative disorders (PT-LPDs) consistently contain type A and not type B Epstein-Barr virus (EBV). Mod Pathol 1994; 7:108A.
76. Borisch B, Hennig I, Horber F, et al. Enteropathy-associated T-cell lymphoma in a renal transplant patient with evidence of Epstein-Barr virus involvement. Virchows Arch A Pathol Anat Histopathol 1992; 421:443–447.
77. Euvrard S, Noble CP, Kanitakis J, et al. Brief report: Successive occurrence of T-cell and B-cell lymphomas after renal transplantation in a patient with multiple squamous cell carcinomas. N Engl J Med 1992; 327:1924–1926.
78. Garvin AJ, Self S, Sahovic EA, et al. The occurrence of a peripheral T-cell lymphoma in a chronically immunosuppressed renal transplant patient. Am J Surg Pathol 1988; 12:64–70.
79. Griffith RC, Saha BK, Janney CM, et al. Immunoblastic lymphoma of T-cell type in a chronically immunosuppressed renal transplant recipient. Am J Clin Pathol 1990; 93:280–285.
80. Hacker SM, Knight BP, Lunde NM, et al. A primary central nervous system T cell lymphoma in a renal transplant patient. Transplantation 1992; 53:691–692.
81. Kemnitz J, Cremer J, Gebel M, et al. T-cell lymphoma after heart transplantation. Am J Clin Pathol 1990; 94:95–101.
82. Kumar S, Kumar D, Kingma DW, et al. Epstein-Barr virus–associated T-cell lymphoma in a renal transplant patient. Am J Surg Pathol 1993; 17:1046–1053.
83. Lippman SM, Grogan TM, Carry P, et al. Post-transplantation T cell lymphoblastic lymphoma. Am J Med 1987; 82:814–816.
84. Maeda K, Bricker L, Ma CK, et al. T cell lymphoma in a renal transplant recipient. Henry Ford Hosp Med J 1987; 35:256–258.
85. Raftery MJ, Tidman MJ, Koffman G, et al. Post transplantation T cell lymphoma of the skin. Transplantation 1988; 46:475–477.
86. Shiong YS, Lian JD, Lin CY, et al. Epstein-Barr virus associated T-cell lymphoma of the maxillary sinus in a renal transplant recipient. Transplant Proc 1992; 24:1929–1931.
87. Ulrich W, Chott A, Watschinger B, et al. Primary peripheral T cell lymphoma in a kidney transplant under immunosuppression with cyclosporine A. Hum Pathol 20:1027–1030.
88. Zanke BW, Rush DN, Jeffery JR, et al. HTLV-1 T cell lymphoma in a cyclosporine-treated renal transplant patient. Transplantation 1989; 48:695–697.
89. Zutter MM, Durnam DM, Hackman RC, et al. Secondary T-cell lymphoproliferation after marrow transplantation. Am J Clin Pathol 1990; 94:714–721.
90. Gossett TC, Gale RP, Fleischman H, et al. Immunoblastic sarcoma in donor cells after bone marrow transplantation. N Engl J Med 1979; 300:904–907.
91. Barkholt L, Billing H, Juliusson G, et al. B-cell lymphoma in transplanted liver: Clinical, histological and radiological manifestations. Transplant Int 1991; 4:8–11.
92. Gassel AM, Westphal E, Hansmann ML, et al. Malignant lymphoma of donor origin after renal transplantation: A case report. Hum Pathol 1991; 22:1291–1293.
93. Maeda K, Hawkins ET, Oh HK, et al. Malignant lymphoma in transplanted renal pelvis. Arch Pathol Lab Med 1986; 110:626–629.
94. Meduri G, Fromentin L, Vieillefond A, et al. Donor-related non-Hodgkin's lymphoma in a renal allograft recipient. Transplant Proc 1991; 23:2649.
95. Penn I. Host origin of lymphomas in organ transplant recipients. Transplantation 1979; 27:214.
96. Randhawa PS, Yousem SA. Epstein-Barr virus–associated lymphoproliferative disease in a heart lung allograft: Demonstration of host origin by restriction fragment-length polymorphism analysis. Transplantation 1990; 49:126–130.
97. Spiro IJ, Yandell DW, Li C, et al. Brief report: Lymphoma of donor origin occurring in the porta hepatis of a transplanted liver. N Engl J Med 1993; 329:27–29.
98. Thomas JA, Hotchin NA, Allday MJ, et al. Immunohistology of Epstein-Barr virus–associated antigens in B cell disorders from immunocompromised individuals. Transplantation 1990; 49:944–953.

99. Swinnen LJ, Costanzo-Nordin MR, Fisher RI. Pro MACE-cyta BOM induces durable complete remissions in post cardiac transplant lymphoma. Proc Am Soc Clin Oncol 1992; 11:318A.
100. The non-Hodgkin's lymphoma pathologic classification project: National Cancer Institute sponsored study of classifications of non-Hodgkin's lymphomas: Summary and description of a working formulation for clinical usage. Cancer 1982; 49:2112–2135.
101. Lennert K, Feller AC. Histopathology of non-Hodgkin's lymphomas. 2nd ed. New York: Springer-Verlag, 1990.
102. Montone KT, Friedman H, Hodinka RL, et al. In situ hybridization for Epstein-Barr virus Not I repeats in posttransplant lymphoproliferative disorder. Mod Pathol 1992; 5:292–302.
103. Neri A, Barriga F, Knowles DM, et al. Different regions of the immunoglobulin heavy-chain locus are involved in chromosomal translocations in distinct pathogenetic forms of Burkitt lymphoma. Proc Natl Acad Sci USA 1988; 85:2748–2752.
104. Subar M, Neri A, Inghirami G, et al. Frequent c-myc oncogene activation and infrequent presence of Epstein-Barr virus genome in AIDS-associated lymphoma. Blood 1988; 72: 667–671.

13

Fine Needle Aspiration Cytology in Kidney, Liver, and Pancreas Allografts

Eeva von Willebrand and Irmeli Lautenschlager
Helsinki University Central Hospital, Helsinki, Finland

I. INTRODUCTION

Biopsy histology is considered as the "gold standard" in the diagnosis of allograft rejection and other intragraft complications. However, needle biopsy (NB) is a procedure that is associated with potential complications, such as bleeding or infections; therefore it is not used as a monitoring method. To develop a less traumatic method for the monitoring of the graft, fine needle aspiration biopsy (FNAB) has been introduced. The FNAB is an atraumatic procedure that enables frequent monitoring of the transplant. Transplant aspiration cytology (TAC) makes it possible to diagnose episodes of acute cellular rejection, to quantify the inflammation associated with the rejection, and to evaluate the effect of antirejection treatment on the transplant. The FNAB technique, developed for the monitoring of renal allografts more than 15 years ago (1–3), has also been used in liver transplantation for more than 10 years (4,5) and recently has also been applied to pancreatic transplantation (6,7).

Combined with FNAB cytology, additional immunohistological stainings may give more detailed information on the ongoing intragraft inflammatory process. Monoclonal antibodies against the most common immunological activation markers, such as MHC class II, IL-2-R, and ICAM-1, are commercially available, and their use makes it possible to demonstrate the immune activation associated with rejection. Although the diagnosis of rejection is mainly based on FNAB cytology, these additional markers of rejection may help the pathologist in decision making, especially in problem cases.

Additional important information is obtained from the parenchymal cell morphology in the FNAB. Acute tubular necrosis (ATN) in kidney, hepatocyte degeneration and cholestasis in liver, possibly also destruction of acinar or ductal tissue in pancreas or drug-induced toxic changes may be diagnosed from cytopreparations of FNAB.

In the following overview, the experience on kidney, liver, and pancreas FNAB is summarized. The correlations between transplant aspiration cytology, histology, biochemical graft function tests, and immunological markers of allograft rejection are discussed in detail. A composite color figure illustrating the types of cells and cellular changes that may be seen in FNAB is included with the text.

II. FINE NEEDLE ASPIRATION CYTOLOGY OF KIDNEY ALLOGRAFT

The aspiration biopsy technique was developed for modern clinical practice by Franzen et al. in 1960 (8) to diagnose urological malignancies and applied for the first time in 1968 by Pasternack for human renal transplants (9). The cytology of allograft rejection was at the time essentially unknown; during the following decade experimental work on rat and human kidney allografts (10–12) helped to clarify the immunological and cytological sequence of events in allograft rejection. The experimental work revealed that the inflammation, i.e., immunoactivation, associated with rejection is both earlier and more specific in the organ transplant than in the peripheral blood of the recipient. The advantage of FNAB is that the risk of complications to the graft or to the patient is minimal, the specimens can be obtained daily if necessary, and the method is also quick to perform. After experience of over 14,000 FNABs in kidney transplants, cytological analysis of aspiration biopsies has proven to be well suited for monitoring of the transplant during the early postoperative period, when the risk of acute rejection is highest. Regular follow-up of renal allografts with FNAB makes it possible to monitor the onset, type, intensity, and duration of the inflammatory episode of acute cellular rejection and also to monitor the effect of immunosuppressive treatment on the graft. Recent innovations and developments of the technique have been discussed in the bi-annual Transplant Aspiration Cytology Workshops held bi-annually since 1981.

A. Technical Aspects of Kidney FNAB

The biopsy is performed at the bedside without local anesthesia in aseptic conditions. The transplant is usually located easily by palpation, but when necessary, ultrasound guidance can be used. The aspiration biopsies are taken from the transplant using a 20- to 22-gauge spinal needle connected to a 20-mL syringe, containing 5 mL of RPMI-1640 tissue culture medium (supplemented with 5% human serum albumin, 50 IU/mL heparin, and 1% Hepes buffer). An aspiration biopsy pistol may be used but is not necessary for the procedure. The needle is inserted into the kidney cortex, full vacuum is applied, and the needle is moved back and forth three to four times. In this way the needle traverses through the entire cortex and reaches several periglomerular and perivascular areas. The vacuum is then let out, the needle is withdrawn, and a sample of 10 to 50 uL in volume is thus obtained. A blood specimen of similar size is taken from the fingertip into another syringe containing the same medium.

The FNAB and blood samples are processed in parallel. The cells are cytocentrifuged on to microscope slides, the smears are air-dried, and—for routine diagnostic use—stained with May-Grünwald-Giemsa (MGG). Parallel preparations can be stained either with other cytological stain or with immunocytological staining techniques.

B. Interpretation of the Cytological Specimens

The MGG-stained cytosmears of the graft and blood are examined microscopically and the findings reported on a standard report form (Table 1), derived from the First International Workshop on Transplant Aspiration Cytology in Munich in 1982. The three most important

Table 1 FNAB Report

INFLAMMATORY CELLS	FNAB	BLOOD	INCREMENT	CORRECTION FACTOR	CORRECTED INCREMENT
LYMPHOID BLAST CELLS	3	0	3	1.0	3.0
ACTIVATED LYMPHOCYTES	4	0	4	0.5	2.0
LGL LYMPHOCYTES	1	1		0.2	
LYMPHOCYTES	40	13	27	0.1	2.7
PMN:					
JUVENILE FORMS	0	0		0.1	
NEUTROPHILS	35	62		0.1	
BASOPHILS	0	2		0.1	
EOSINOPHILS	7	14		0.1	
MONOBLAST	0	0		1.0	
MONOCYTES	10	8	2	0.2	0.4
MACROPHAGES	0	0		1.0	
TOTAL CORRECTED INCREMENT					7.1
TOTAL BLAST CELLS/ CYTOPREP		22			

PARENCHYMAL CELLS	NORMAL	SWELLING	SWELLING VACUOLATION	NECROSIS
MORPHOLOGY SCORE	1	2	3	4
PARENCHYMAL CELLS		2		
PARENCHYMAL CELLS PER 100 INFLAMMATORY CELLS			20	
CONCLUSIONS:	CLEAR BLASTOGENIC REJECTION. SOME SWELLING AND DEGENERATION IN PARENCHYMAL CELLS			

features to be evaluated are (a) sample representativity, (b) the leukocyte differential, and (c) the morphological features of parenchymal cells.

1. *Sample Representativity*

Only representative FNABs can be evaluated; therefore, the FNAB representativity has to be assessed first. The cellular infiltration of acute rejection is always most pronounced in kidney cortex, which is why representative specimens should contain enough cortical structures. The representativity is assessed by calculating the ratio of tubular cells to inflammatory leukocytes. Cytological criteria for representativity and reproducibility of transplant aspirate specimens have been established by analyzing duplicate aspirates (13), where a correlation coefficient of 0.95 was obtained if both specimens contained at least 7 tubular cells per 100 inflammatory leucocytes. When the ratio of tubular cells to leukocytes in either sample was lower, the correlation coefficient fell accordingly. Similar results for double aspirate biopsy analysis have been published by other groups (14,15).

2. *Inflammatory Leukocytes*

Most of the inflammatory leukocytes in the cytological preparations can be identified according to standard hematologic criteria (1,3) in the routine MGG-stained smears; these include small lymphocytes, activated lymphocytes with increased cytoplasmic basophilia, and large granular lymphocytes (LGL), which are the morphological form of natural killer cells (16). Lymphoid blast cells are the most important cells at the onset of acute rejection. The blast cells are characterized by their large size, immature nuclei, and intense cytoplasmic basophilia. Different forms of monocyte-macrophage cells can also be seen in the specimens, including small monocytes, large monocytes with irregular, multilobulated nuclei, and macrophages with different stages of maturation. Appearance of large numbers of macrophages in the graft occurs in later phases of severe and irreversible rejections and also in acute vascular rejection in earlier phases. Some examples of inflammatory cells are demonstrated in Fig. 1.

Eosinophils are usually seen at the onset of immunoactivation, both in the aspirate and in the peripheral blood, indicating generalized immune response to the graft (17). Thrombocytes can be seen during rejection in the graft (18,19). Small thrombocyte aggregates disappear with successful rejection treatment, but large aggregates on endothelial cells are connected to worse prognosis (19). Neutrophil infiltration in the graft usually occurs only in irreversible rejections with necrotic changes.

3. *Morphology of Kidney Parenchymal Cells*

FNAB specimens consist mostly of single cells, although clusters of renal tubular cells or even parts of tubuli and whole glomeruli may be seen in the specimens. The major parenchymal cells in the aspirates are the proximal and distal tubular cells and endothelial cells from the kidney vascular endothelium, deriving mostly from capillary blood vessels.

The information received from epithelial cell morphology is useful in the differential diagnosis of acute rejection and other graft complications (Fig. 1). The parenchymal cells are examined and their morphology is scored from 1 to 4 (1 is normal and 4 represents necrosis) and recorded in the report (Table 1).

In acute tubular necrosis (ATN), tubular cells are swollen and there is cytoplasmic degeneration and irregular vacuolation. In very severe forms, necrotic tubular cells may also be seen. These changes are due to prolonged cold ischemia and normalize with improving graft function in 1 to 2 weeks. In pure ATN, there are no signs of immunoactivation.

Immunosuppressive drugs, especially cyclosporin A (CyA), can cause toxic changes in the graft epithelial cells. In acute CyA nephrotoxicity, the tubular cells are swollen, there is increased cytoplasmic basophilia, and prominent isometric vacuolation (20–22). The toxic isometric vacuolation is quite typical for acute CyA toxicity, although it is a nonspecific phenomenon. The deposits of CyA and its metabolites can be demonstrated by specific monoclonal antibodies and immunofluorescence techniques (20). After reduction of the CyA dose, the tubular cell morphology usually normalizes in 1 to 2 weeks. Isometric vacuolation is not seen in chronic CyA toxicity, where tubular atrophy and degeneration with interstitial fibrosis are the dominating features. Today, when most centers use triple-drug immunosuppressive treatment and lower CyA doses, acute CyA toxicity is not a very common complication.

At the onset of acute cellular rejection, the morphology of tubular and endothelial cells is usually normal and also remains normal in brief and mild rejections. In severe and prolonged rejections, on the other hand, there are progressive degenerative changes in tubular cells, and in irreversible rejections even necrosis may be seen.

Severe necrotic changes in tubular cells are seen in graft infarction (23), which is mostly due to vascular thrombosis.

C. Quantitation of Inflammation in the Transplant

1. Increment Method

The inflammation in the graft is evaluated with increment analysis: differential counts are performed of leukocytes from the aspirate and blood specimens and the blood values are subtracted from aspirate values to obtain the increment of inflammatory cells within the graft (Table 1). As all inflammatory cells in allograft rejection do not have equal diagnostic significance (10,11), correction factors are used in calculating corrected increment (3). The cells with greatest significance in acute rejection, the blast cells and macrophages, have a full correction factor of 1.0. The correction factors of all inflammatory cells are given in Table 1. The sum of the corrected increment values represents the total corrected increment (TCI), which describes the intensity of inflammation in the graft. Usually, a TCI higher than 3.0 and with a blast cell increment of 1.0 indicates acute rejection (24,25). No blast cells are seen in a stable graft, but during immunoactivation the number of blast cells rises up to 10 to 50 per cytopreparation and sometimes may be even higher (24). Helderman et al. demonstrated (26) that a total blast count of >6 cells per slide proved representative of rejection independent of the TCI score. With the increment method, it is possible to describe the aspirate findings with numerical grades instead of descriptive classifications only, and it is also possible to compare the patient results and perform computer analysis of the data.

2. FNAB Cytology in Monitoring of the Transplant

Monitoring of the transplant with regular FNABs makes it possible to define the course of intragraft events. In a stable graft, there is either no or minimal lymphocytic-monocytic infiltrate in the aspirates. When acute rejection begins, increasing amounts of lymphocytes and monocytes infiltrate the graft and blast cells are seen to appear in the aspirate. Lymphoid blast response is the hallmark of immune activation at the beginning of acute rejection and is mostly also associated with an elevated TCI and with impaired graft function. With successful rejection treatment, the inflammatory cells disappear from the graft and the graft function improves. In rejections not responding to treatment, macrophages infiltrate the graft, tubular cell degeneration increases, and graft necrosis ensues. The appearance of large numbers of macrophages in the graft usually indicates irreversible rejection.

In most cases of acute cellular rejection, the inflammatory episode follows this cytological pattern. In individual patients, however, different inflammatory profiles can be seen and different immunosuppressive treatment protocols clearly modify the aspiration cytology profiles. Today, when most centers use triple treatment—a combination with cyclosporine, azathioprine, and steroids—only approximately 30% of cadaver kidney grafts have any acute rejection episodes during the first postoperative month (27), compared to 70% in the older treatment protocols with azathioprine and steroids (28,29). The onset of rejection is also delayed and the inflammation milder, with fewer blast cells.

A major percentage of the rejections that do not respond to steroid treatment have histological features of acute vascular rejection (AVR) (30,31). Diagnosis of AVR is always based on histology. However characteristic cytological features seen in acute vascular rejection have been defined (32–34). There is early accumulation of monocytes and macrophages in the graft. Lymphocytic infiltrates and blast cells are not prominent in pure forms of AVR (35). Combinations of ACR and AVR are common (31,35) and often resistant to ordinary steroid rejection treatment. Monoclonal or polyclonal antibodies, OKT3 or ATG, are used in the treatment of these rejections (30,31).

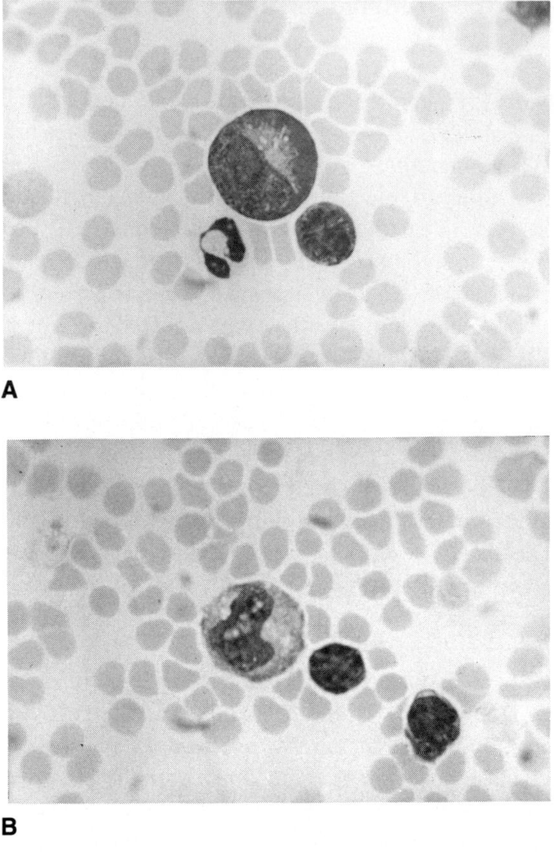

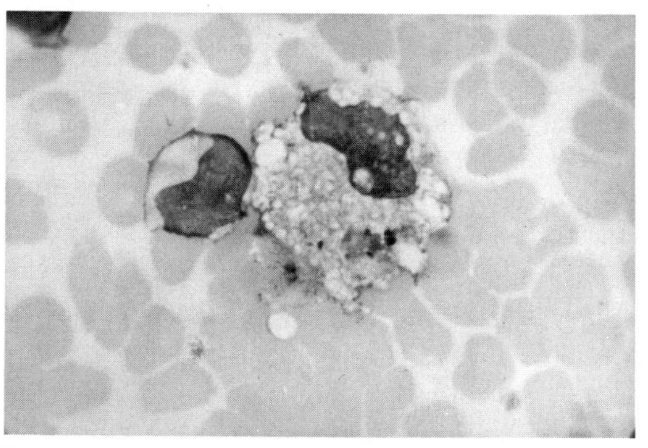

Figure 1 Inflammatory cells in MGG-stained cytocentrifuge preparations (A–C): A lymphoid blast cell with immature nucleus and cytoplasmic basophilia, a small lymphocyte and a neutrophil (A), a monocyte and two small lymphocytes (B), a macrophage and a lymphocyte (C). Kidney parenchymal cells in MGG-stained cytopreparations (D–F): A group of normal tubular cells (D), swelling, degeneration and vacuolation in tubular cells in ATN (E), isometric vacuolation and swelling in a tubular cell during CyA toxicity (F). Liver parenchymal cells in MGG-stained cytocentrifuge preparations (G–I): A group of normal hepatocytes (G), degenerative changes in hepatocytes (H), accumulation of bile in the hepatocytes indicating cholestasis (I). (For optimal reproduction, see color plate.)

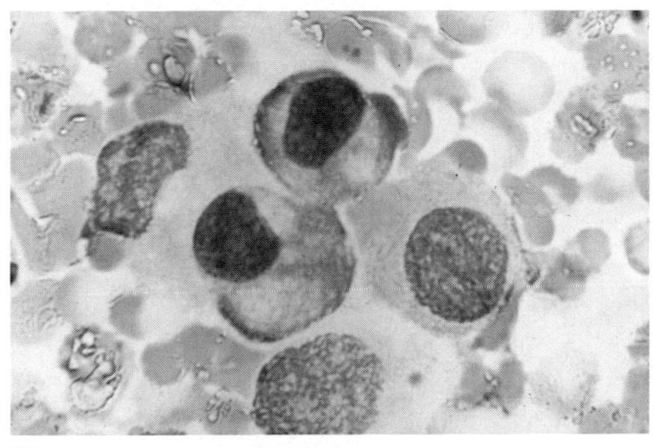

D

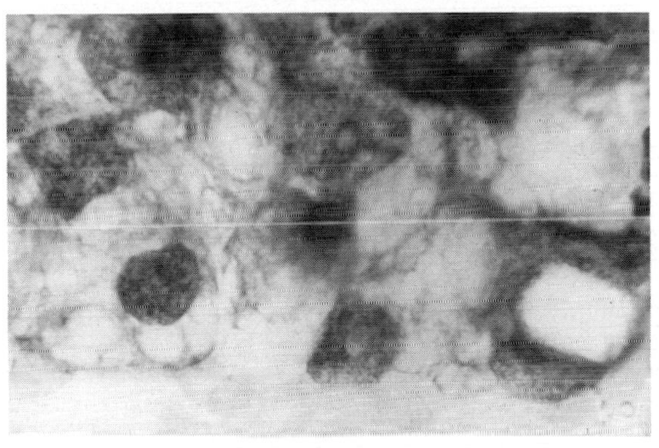

E

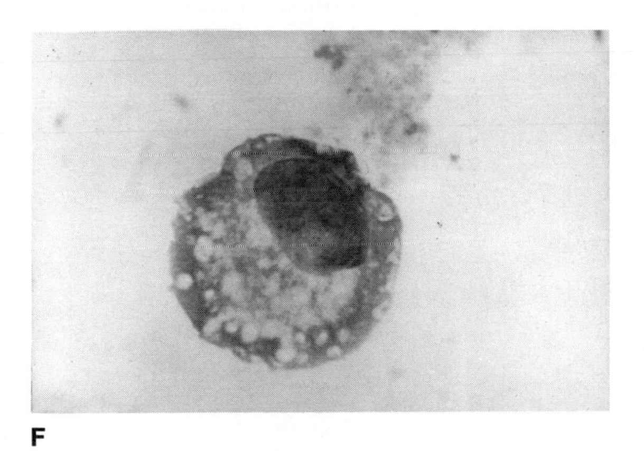

F

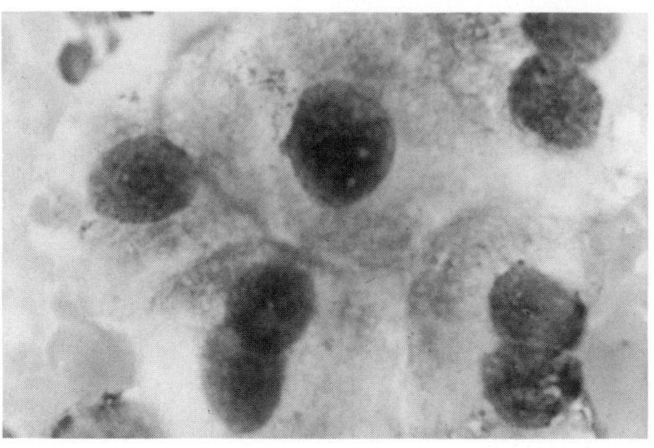

G

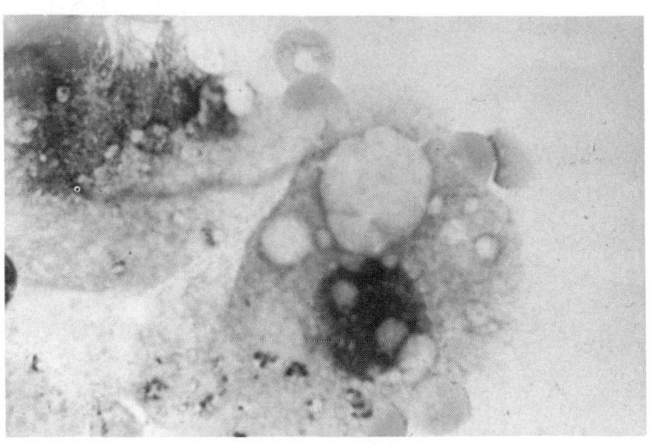

H

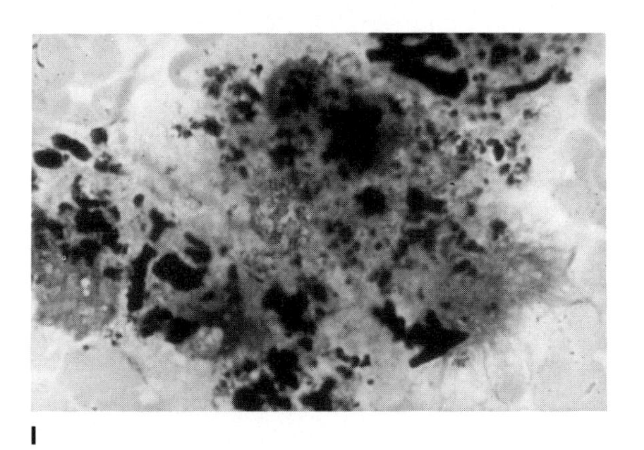

I

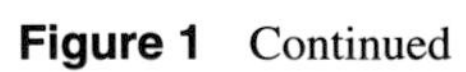

Figure 1 Continued

D. Immunocytology

1. Activation Markers and Adhesion Molecules in Acute Rejection

With immunocytological staining techniques and monoclonal antibodies, it is possible to evaluate in still more detail the transplant state and the nature of the inflammatory infiltrates in the graft (36–40). Analysis of activation markers and adhesion molecules of the graft-infiltrating inflammatory cells and parenchymal cells has proven to be useful in rejection diagnosis. In acute rejection, induction of interleukin-2 (IL-2) receptors (CD25) on activated lymphoid cells has been demonstrated (41,42), and HLA class II antigens are induced on the tubular cells (43–45). With successful rejection treatment, CD25-positive lymphoid cells disappear rapidly and class II expression diminishes to background level (42,46). In stable grafts, there is no induction of activation markers.

Adhesion molecules are also induced during rejection on different transplant components. Normal kidneys express constitutively several adhesion molecules on the endothelial cells of the vessels, for instance, intercellular adhesion molecule-1 (ICAM-1) and vascular cell adhesion molecule (VCAM-1) (47). Tubular cells do not normally express these molecules or express them only in small quantities on the luminal surfaces, but during rejection these adhesion molecules are induced also on tubular cells. The induction of ICAM-1 on tubular cells occurs early during rejection and disappears rapidly with successful rejection treatment (48,49). The role of the adhesion molecules in the rejection process is today under extensive investigation.

2. Lymphocyte Subsets in FNAB

With immunocytological techniques, it is also possible to analyze the different T- and B-lymphocyte subsets and also their state of activation. In most acute cellular rejections, the CD8 T lymphocytes dominate over the CD4 cells in the graft, although, at the beginning of the rejection episode, the CD4 T cells seem to be frequent (37,50,51). In severe and irreversible rejections, persistence of CD4 dominance in the graft has been seen (52).

Lymphocyte subpopulations in the graft are, however, variable both during different phases of rejection and also during viral infections and cannot as such be used as diagnostic findings. Analysis of the different inflammatory cell subsets does, however, give additional information on the transplant state.

E. Viral Infections

Viral infections, especially cytomegalovirus infections (CMV), often cause differential diagnostic problems in transplant patients. Cytomegalovirus infections can induce a generalized immunoactivation in the patient; lymphoid blast cells, activated lymphocytes, and large granular lymphocytes (LGL) are found in patients' blood and also in the FNAB (53–55). Cytomegalovirus infections are also often associated with rejections; patients with frequent and severe rejections have more CMV infections and, on the other hand, patients with CMV infection have more rejections. Cytomegalovirus infection has been shown to induce HLA class II antigens on kidney transplant tubular cells (57), and this could be the connection to the rejection process. Recent developments in CMV diagnostic techniques, especially the rapid immunological staining methods, have helped to solve this differential diagnostic problem (58,59).

F. Correlation Between FNAB Cytology and NB Histology

The correlation between aspiration cytology and histology in renal transplantation has been assessed in several studies (3,14,33), and a high concordance of simultaneous cytology and histology findings has been reported, particularly in acute cellular rejection, ATN, acute CyA toxicity, and also when the graft situation was stable (34,60–64).

In the first studies, the diagnostic value of FNAB was evaluated by correlating FNAB findings to the clinical course of rejection and response to treatment (1,2). The cytology findings were also correlated to histology of nephrectomy specimens in irreversible rejections and to the cytology of the inflammatory infiltrates after enzymatic digestion of the removed kidneys (10). Since then, several centers have reported a high concordance of simultaneous FNAB and core biopsy findings in different clinical situations, but particularly in acute cellular blastogenic rejection, ATN, acute CyA toxicity, and when the graft situation was stable (60–64).

FNAB and histology were compared in the monitoring of acute cellular rejection by Belitsky et al. (14,64) in a study with dog renal allografts, where a high concordance between serial FNAB and NB specimens was demonstrated over the entire course of rejection. It has also been shown that there is a relation between the severity of acute rejection (i.e., mild, moderate, severe) in histological sections and the level of inflammation in cytology (65). Diagnostic sensitivities and specificities of >90% have been reported in a prospective study comparing cytology and histology in monitoring of kidney transplant patients (26). In a blind study comparing cytology and histology in 200 consecutive patients (25), a high sensitivity and specificity both in acute cellular rejection (81 and 92%, respectively) and in stable kidney grafts (78 and 82%) was reported.

Recently, a prospective, randomized study (66) compared cytology, histology, and immunohistology in rejection diagnosis, using clinical evaluation of rejection as the "gold standard." The respective specificities were 96, 87, and 80%; sensitivities were 59, 75, and 77%. Cytology in this analysis had an increased tendency to miss clinical rejection episodes but proved most reliable in the monitoring of nonfunctioning or stable grafts.

G. Cytology in the Differential Diagnosis of Organ Transplant Failure

The cytology patterns in the different diagnostic groups based on histology (24) are presented in Table 2. In normal grafts with good function, the cytology findings are also normal, with the TCI values low (from 0 to 3), no blast cells, and normal tubular cell morphology score (GCC). In acute cellular rejection, TCI is high (4 to 15), with blast cells

Table 2 Correlation Between Cytology and Histology

	FNAB cytology			
NB histology	TCI	Bl%	Mp%	GCC
Normal graft	0–3	0%	0%	1, −2
Acute cellular rejection	>3–15	>1%	0%	1, −3
Irreversible rejection	>3	>1%	>1%	3, −4
Acute vascular rejection	>3–15	0–1%	>1%	1, −4
Chronic rejection	>3–5	0%	0–1%	2, −3
Acute tubular necrosis	0–3	0%	≤1%	2, −4
Acute CyA toxicity	0–3	0%	0%	2, −3

Abbreviations: TCI, total corrected increment; Bl, blast cells; Mp, macrophages; GCC, graft tubular cell morphology score, 1–4 (1 = normal, 4 = necrosis).

and lymphocytic infiltration and activation. In irreversible rejection, TCI values are often even higher, with macrophages present and GCC score showing tubular cell degeneration. In acute vascular rejection, the cell infiltrate is dominated by mononuclear phagocytes, with only a few blast cells, and the GCC score demonstrates tubular degeneration. Typical for cytology of chronic rejection is lymphocytic-monocytic inflammation with no blast cells and degeneration in the parenchymal cells. In acute CyA toxicity, there is no inflammation in the graft and no blast cells, only morphological alterations in the tubular cells, consisting mostly of swelling, degeneration, and isometric vacuolation.

The most reliable way to evaluate events in a transplanted kidney is to take specimens of the graft itself, and the method most often used is the classic needle biopsy (NB). The NB histology gives an excellent picture of the situation at the biopsy site and is usually representative of the whole transplant. However, because of the bleeding complications related to the NB needle, it is not often used for monitoring of the graft.

FNAB cytology is a method developed for regular monitoring of intragraft events in clinical transplantation. The advantage of FNAB is that it can be performed daily, if necessary, on human renal transplants without risk to the graft or the patient. Repeated aspiration biopsies give a dynamic picture of the process in the graft and enable one to evaluate the effect of changes in immunosuppressive treatment on the process. The main drawback of the method is that the information gained from the FNAB is limited in certain respects when compared to core needle biopsies. The diagnostic categories for renal allograft FNABs are presented in Table 3. FNAB is good for diagnosing a stable normal graft, acute cellular rejection, acute tubular necrosis, acute CyA toxicity, and graft necrosis but much poorer in the diagnosis of acute or chronic vascular rejection. Vascular changes in a kidney graft cannot be evaluated without a NB. Therefore the two procedures should be used together, with FNAB as the monitoring method.

III. FNAB IN THE MONITORING OF LIVER ALLOGRAFTS

Acute rejections have been reported to appear in about 60% of liver transplant patients, and approximately 10% develop chronic rejection (67–70). Acute liver allograft rejection occurs usually during the first month after transplantation but may also appear later. Of first rejection episodes, 95% are seen between days 4 and 21 after transplantation (69), and impaired liver function occurring between the fourth and tenth day is considered to be rejection unless proven otherwise (71).

Diagnosis of acute liver allograft rejection is difficult, since the clinical signs and laboratory parameters (i.e., levels of transaminases, alkaline phosphatase and bilirubin) reflecting pathological processes of the graft may also be associated with multiple other causes of liver dysfunction during the postoperative course. Until recent years, the only reliable method to diagnose liver rejection has been a histological examination of a core needle biopsy specimen. However, the conventional core needle biopsy always carries some risk of complications, such as bleeding or infections. FNAB has provided a reliable diagnostic tool for the monitoring of hepatic transplants, as it has in kidney grafts.

Based on experience with FNAB in the monitoring of kidney allografts and on our experimental work in the pig liver transplantation model (4,72,73), the method was applied to clinical liver transplantation in Helsinki in 1982 (5,74). The liver FNAB and transplant aspiration cytology were rapidly adapted by many liver transplant centers, especially in Europe, and various groups have reported their experiences (75–83). The atraumatic procedure, which can be safely repeated even daily, makes it possible to monitor the liver

Table 3 Diagnostic Categories for Renal Allograft Fine Needle Biopsies

1. Normal
2. Borderline immune activation
3. Acute cellular rejection
4. Acute vascular rejection
5. Chronic rejection
Differential diagnosis
1. Acute tubular necrosis
2. Acute cyclosporin toxicity
3. Graft necrosis
4. Other:
Lymphocele
Hematoma
Viral infection
Bacterial infection

transplant in situ, to visualize the onset and intensity of inflammation associated with rejection, and the response of inflammation to immunosuppressive therapy. Morphological changes in the liver parenchymal cells, or bile droplets in the hepatocytes, are findings that provide additional information on the extent of graft damage or cholestasis.

A. Technical Aspects of Liver FNAB

Liver allografts are monitored with FNAB from the day of transplantation at 1- to 3-day intervals. The skin is punctured preferably at the medial part of the right costal margin to minimize the risk of complications or contamination from the intraperitoneal cavity (84). In some patients, the liver is best found through the right medial axillary line, especially if the graft is small. Ultrasound guidance is advisable only if the patient has major ascites and the liver is small; ultrasound is needed in less than 2% of the cases. FNABs are also taken from patients with severe liver insufficiency or with low platelet counts and coagulation factors (84). In our material consisting of 3000 liver FNABs, no complications have occurred. A similar experience with more than 3000 liver FNABs without complications has also been reported by others (85). These findings compare favorably with the complications reported on normal core NB which include bleeding, sepsis, lung empyema, and even death of the patient (67,68).

The technique obtaining and processing the aspirates and the corresponding blood specimens is the same as that used in renal allografts. The quantitation of inflammation by the "increment" method is also similar (74). The FNAB is considered representative if the specimen contains at least 7 hepatocytes per 100 inflammatory cells and no contamination—e.g., from the intraperitoneal cavity—is recorded. In our material, when the liver FNABs are obtained as described above, 87% of the specimens are representative (84).

B. Inflammation Associated with Rejection

In biopsy histology, the hallmark of acute liver allograft rejection is infiltration of mononuclear cells in the portal areas. The inflammatory infiltrate consists mainly of lymphoid cells, but neutrophils, eosinophils, and mononuclear phagocytes are also usually seen. Inflammation together with bile duct and vascular involvement, as well as cholestasis, are characteristic histological findings of acute rejection (86–88).

In FNAB, the hallmark of acute liver rejection is the appearance of lymphoid blasts and increase of lymphocytes in the graft (4,73,74,84). The inflammatory profile of acute liver rejection monitored with FNAB is very typical and usually easy to diagnose with TAC. At the beginning of an acute cellular rejection, the inflammatory infiltrate consists mainly of lymphocytes, lymphoid blast cells, activated lymphocytes, and some monocytes (4, 73,74,84). The neutrophil or eosinophil infiltration of the graft, described in biopsy histology, is not usually possible to evaluate over the blood background. However, blood eosinophilia correlates with the peak of immune response in the graft (74). At more advanced stages of rejection, the cellular infiltrate becomes dominated by mononuclear phagocytes, and large numbers of macrophages are usually associated with irreversible rejection and parenchymal necrosis (4,73). With successful antirejection treatment, the episode is usually interrupted at the stage of lymphoid response before severe tissue damage and the appearance of macrophages occurs.

The clinical diagnosis of rejection is never based on the FNAB findings only but also on other laboratory parameters and clinical signs (89). The inflammation of ⩾3.0 corrected increment units (CIU) together with lymphoid blasts in the FNAB differential count is considered as the beginning of immune activation in the graft (84). It is known from biopsy histology and FNAB cytology that a few days after transplantation some inflammatory infiltrate may appear in the portal areas without any tissue damage and may disappear without any clinical signs of rejection or additional immunosuppression (88,90). This type of immune activation may be initiated by donor cells in the liver allograft or represent "subclinical" forms of the alloresponse under certain immunosuppressive conditions (82). Thus, the FNAB findings, like the NB histology, should always be evaluated and correlated with the clinical picture and graft function tests before the clinical diagnosis of rejection can be established. Graft dysfunction together with typical cytological findings are needed for the clinical diagnosis of acute liver allograft rejection. FNAB is used not only in diagnosing of acute cellular rejection but also in the monitoring of response to antirejection therapy (74,84,89). Usually, in specimens obtained before rejection, the TCI is low (<2.0 CIU) and peaks rapidly to a significant level (>3.0 CIU), when the lymphoid activation and blast response begin in the graft. Depending on the activation level, very high TCI values can be recorded (10.0 to 15.0 CIU, even up to 30.0 CIU). With successful antirejection treatment, the inflammation of rejection usually subsides within 5 to 7 days, and the CIU values normalize (<3.0 CIU). Although, our experience on FNAB in the monitoring of response to antirejection therapy is mainly based on steroid-treated rejections, the reliability of the method during steroid-resistant and OKT3-treated rejections has been proven by others (91).

C. FNAB Cytology and Infections

Differential diagnostic problems in FNAB monitoring may be caused by any intragraft processes, especially by infections, which induce inflammation in the graft. Systemic infections in general have no effect on the inflammatory profile in the FNAB (92). The total inflammation in the liver transplants of recipients undergoing bacteremia or viral infections seldom exceeds 3.0 CIU (92), and the cellular changes associated with the immune response against the infections are mainly recorded in peripheral blood. Bacterial infections usually cause granulocytosis, but the immune response against viral agents is lymphocyte-dominated. When the blood background is subtracted from the FNAB differential, the changes recorded in blood have practically no effect on increment. However, infections located in the allograft are recorded in FNAB. The cellular changes associated with bacterial, fungal, and various viral infections may cause differential diagnostic problems in the FNAB but may also be helpful in the diagnosis of these complications in the graft.

Presence of large numbers of granulocytes together with bacteria in the FNAB indicates a bacterial infection in the graft. Liver abcesses or cholangitis are the usual causes of a granulocyte-dominated cellular picture in FNAB specimens. Large numbers of neutrophils together with macrophages in the aspirates may indicate a contamination from hematoma or wound infection. Contamination of the aspirate from intraperitoneal cavity and ascites is characterized by large numbers of macrophages accompanied with a few mast cells and often groups mesothelial cells. If there is any doubt of contamination, the specimen should not be considered representative and a new aspiration should be performed.

Viral infections affecting liver allografts are the most dangerous findings to interpret falsely. Although hepatitis A or B are quite easily diagnosed by virological methods, other viral infections of the liver, e.g., cytomegalovirus (CMV) infection, are a common complication and may cause problems. Depending on the material, 40 to 60% of liver transplant recipients undergo a CMV infection during the first postoperative year (93,94). The clinical signs of CMV infection, including fever and elevation of liver enzymes, cannot be distinguished from rejection (95). The conventional virological methods, like serology or virus culture, are not of help in an acute situation, as they give the diagnosis only retrospectively. The new rapid methods based on the shell vial culture and direct detection of viral antigens or DNA in the cells or tissues are of great value in diagnosing of CMV infection in liver transplant patients.

The immune response against CMV is lymphocyte-mediated and is seen as lymphoid activation and presence of atypical lymphocytes (blasts) in blood and as an increase in number of large granular lymphocytes (LGL) (95). In a detailed cellular analysis, we compared the inflammatory picture of rejection to that of severe CMV infection (95). All patients had fever, and elevated liver enzymes indicated graft dysfunction. The diagnosis of CMV infection was based on rapid antigen detection directly from blood, and confirmed with shell vial culture. During CMV infection, a mild lymphoid activation with a few blast cells was seen in both FNAB and blood. The blast response was followed by elevation of LGLs in the blood. Inflammation associated with CMV subsided with successful antiviral therapy, indicating that it was due to viral infection and not to rejection. Inflammation in the FNAB caused by viral infection has also been reported by others (96). The CMV-associated inflammation was usually seen as mild lymphocytosis in the graft, and only a minor lymphoid activation was recorded both in the FNAB and in the blood (96).

Hepatitis C virus (HCV) infection also causes lymphocytosis in the graft, but this cell infiltration is dominated by small lymphocytes and practically no activation or lymphoid blasts are seen (Lautenschlager, unpublished data). Hepatitis B reactivation usually occurs several weeks after transplantation and not during the first weeks of FNAB monitoring, when most acute rejection occur. However, a differential diagnosis may be very difficult in the case with a combined viral infection and rejection. The diagnosis of viral infection is always virological, and one should not try to guess it from any cellular or morphological changes. The specific and rapid diagnostic methods—like direct antigen detection or DNA-hybridization methods and PCR techniques to diagnose various viral infections—are nowadays available in every modern transplant center.

D. Liver Parenchymal Cell Morphology and Cholestasis

Normal liver FNAB contains hepatocytes in clusters and in single-cell form. Liver tissue damage is recorded as degenerative changes in the liver parenchymal cells. Degenerative changes, mainly irregular vacuolation and sometimes necrosis of hepatocytes, are recorded together with inflammation during acute rejection. Necrotic cells in the FNAB indicate severe tissue damage. If no inflammation is seen in the FNAB, these changes indicate graft damage due to other reasons, such as drug toxicity or vascular complications, e.g., thrombosis or obstructive processes. The hepatocyte morphology is semiquantitatively scored from 1 (slight changes) to 4 (necrosis) (84).

Hepatotoxic drugs may cause morphological changes of liver cells. The most common in transplant patients is cyclosporine A (CyA) induced hepatotoxicity. The typical morphological change associated with CyA toxicity is the isometric vacuolation of hepatocytes (74,97), quite similar to that described previously for kidney tubular epithelial cells. Deposits of CyA in the cells can be demonstrated by immunofluorescence or immunoperoxidase stainings and monoclonal antibodies (74). The typical, though not specific, morphological changes of CyA toxicity correlate well with the immunological demonstration of CyA in the cells. CyA deposits correlate to some extent with high dose of CyA, but not always with CyA blood levels (74,89). Nowadays, however, CyA toxicity is rarely seen, since the doses used are low, and CyA is mainly used in combination therapy together with azathioprine and steroids.

As bile ducts or vascular endothelial cells are seldom recorded in the FNAB specimens, the information of tissue damage is based mainly on hepatocyte changes. The degree of tissue damage, e.g., liver necrosis, due to rejection is also difficult to assess from FNAB. Needle biopsy histology has ben found more sensitive for diagnosing hepatocyte necrosis, especially focal necrosis of the liver, than FNAB cytology (83). To assess the degree of graft necrosis as well as bile duct or vascular changes, NB histology is necessary

Cholestasis is often recorded in association with inflammatory episodes of rejection (74). Bile droplets in the hepatocytes or between them indicate either impaired graft function or extracellular cholestasis during acute rejection. Cholestasis may also indicate biliary complications or impaired graft function for other reasons. Evidence of cholestasis without inflammation in the FNAB is an important finding in the differential diagnosis between rejection and other biliary processes. Cholestasis is semiquantitatively scored from 1 to 3 according to the amount of bile recorded in the FNAB specimen (84). Cholestasis is also seen as an elevation in serum bilirubin levels (74,89). FNAB has been reported to be even more sensitive than NB histology for diagnosing cholestasis (83).

Posttransplant cholestasis, often recorded about 1 week after transplantation, is sometimes falsely interpreted as rejection (89). However, the posttransplant cholestasis is not associated with inflammation and can easily be distinguished from rejection. The FNAB monitoring is also helpful in demonstrating this process in the graft and avoiding unnecessary additional immunosuppressive therapy.

E. Correlation of FNAB Findings with Biochemical Markers of Liver Dysfunction

Biochemical parameters reflecting hepatic dysfunction are nonspecific, and elevated serum levels are seen due to any cause of tissue damage. Immediately after transplantation, increased levels of serum transaminases and other liver function markers are due to surgery. Alkaline phosphatase and bilirubin increases may reflect cholangitis, obstruction or infections as well. A rapid increase of serum transaminases, gamma-GT, alkaline phosphatase, and bilirubin is usually associated with acute rejection. All those biochemical parameters correlate with the inflammatory episodes of acute rejection, but the evidence of rejection with typical lymphoid activation and blast response in FNAB is recorded 1 to 3 days earlier in the graft (74,89). After successful antirejection therapy, elevated levels of biochemical markers last somewhat longer in the circulation than the inflammation in the graft, indicating that the graft dysfunction still exists a few days after the immunological antiallograft reaction has subsided.

F. Correlation Between FNAB and NB Histology

A close correlation between FNAB and NB was recorded in our experimental model of pig liver rejection (3,73). In human liver allografts, a good correlation of FNAB and NB has been reported by several groups (77,79,81,83,98). When FNAB and NB were performed in parallel and correlated with clinical situation, the positive predictive value of cytological diagnosis was 86.3%, the sensitivity 76.7%, and the specificity 86.9% in the diagnosis of acute cellular rejection (77). In another study of 24 patients, when FNAB was correlated with NB histology only, a specificity of 69% and sensitivity of 95% was reached (83). When the results of 865 aspiration biopsies and 155 core biopsies in 141 patients were correlated with the retrospective clinical diagnosis of the presence or absence of acute rejection (98), there were almost no false-negative findings either in cytology or histology (<0.1%). However, with both methods, a large number of positive results were obtained without any clinical sign of rejection. Thus, in the diagnosis of acute rejection, both FNAB and NB findings should always be evaluated and correlated with the clinical picture and graft function, as stressed previously.

The diagnostic value of FNAB decreases after some months postoperatively (77), when chronic pathology of the graft begins to dominate and acute rejections seldom occur. The diagnosis of chronic rejection is mainly based on bile duct and vascular changes, and only minor inflammatory infiltrate is seen in the graft (70,87). The changes typical for chronic rejection, e.g., vanishing bile ducts, can be recorded only in NB histology. Although FNAB is useful in the monitoring of liver grafts during the first weeks postoperatively, NB is the only reliable method to diagnose chronic rejection and other late complications.

It should be emphasized that the FNAB is not intended to replace NB histology. The optimal diagnostic procedure would be to use both of these methods concomitantly. For the first weeks after transplantation, when most rejections occur, the FNAB is a most suitable, reliable, and atraumatic method for frequent, even daily, monitoring of liver grafts. The FNAB is sufficient to diagnose inflammatory episodes of acute cellular rejection, and to follow up the response to antirejection therapy. Although a disadvantage of FNAB is that no information about bile duct lesions and vascular changes is obtained, the lymphoid activation and inflammatory response are the major components of acute cellular rejection and can be monitored in detail by FNAB. During the early posttransplant period, NB may be obtained, if necessary, to confirm the diagnosis, or in order to assess the degree of parenchymal damage and the need for retransplantation. Also, if the FNAB findings indicate that graft dysfunction, cholestasis or hepatocyte necrosis is due to reasons other than rejection, NB is recommended. In late pathological processes, especially if there is any doubt of chronic rejection, NB is the only reliable diagnostic method.

G. Immunocytology of Liver FNAB

FNAB can be used for more detailed analysis of intragraft events. Inflammatory cell subtypes or activation markers indicating rejection may be demonstrated by immunocytological techniques and monoclonal antibodies to confirm the cytological findings of rejection. The demonstration of increased expression of MHC antigens on the parenchymal cells, also considered as markers of rejection, may be added to the diagnostic procedure. Recently, induction of adhesion molecules (or their ligands) has been added to the classic activation markers. Especially, the induction of intercellular adhesion molecule-1 (ICAM-1) on hepatocytes has been demonstrated to be an early though rather nonspecific marker of immunoactivation associated with rejection (99).

Lymphocyte subpopulations have been analyzed in FNAB in the experimental model and in clinical transplantation (73,74). At the very beginning of immune activation, a CD4 lymphocyte predominance is seen in the inflammatory infiltrate, but in a later phase of the immunological cascade, when the clinical rejection is usually recorded, there is a CD8 predominance. B cells are also involved in inflammation. However, lymphocyte subpopulations vary greatly depending on the immunosuppression used and are present in various infections; they cannot be used as a specific diagnostic tool.

Expression of activation markers on the surface of lymphoid cells in the graft has been demonstrated to correlate with the blast response and the inflammatory peak of rejection (84,100). Increase of MHC class II positive lymphocytes and appearance of IL-2 receptor (IL-2-R) expressing lymphoid cells in the graft are the most common markers of immune activation. However, the routine FNAB cytology, without immunohistochemistry of lymphoid activation markers, is usually informative enough to diagnose graft rejection and to follow the response of antirejection therapy.

Expression of transplantation antigens, especially class II antigens, and certain adhesion molecules are induced on the parenchymal cells during liver rejection. Although, the parenchymal cells of a normal liver do not express MHC class II antigens in a significant amount, they are induced on the surface of hepatocytes during rejection episodes. Several groups have also demonstrated the presence of class II on the parenchymal cells of the grafts undergoing acute cellular rejection monitored by FNAB (76,100,101). In our series, hepatocyte class II expression was seen only in livers with a very strong immune activation, but bile duct cells were always strongly class II–positive in the FNAB during rejection (100). The problem is that the upregulation of MHC antigens is also associated with viral infections—e.g., viral hepatitis and CMV—and cannot be considered as a specific marker of rejection (95,102). In our study on cellular findings in CMV infection, a strong class II expression on hepatocytes was seen during systemic CMV infections without evidence of graft rejection or typical CMV hepatitis (95).

Hepatocytes do not normally express ICAM-1, but induction of ICAM-1 on hepatocytes is seen in association with rejection, and it may also be used as an activation marker (99). The induction of ICAM-1 in liver allografts is a very early marker of immune activation and can be recorded even before the lymphoid activation and blast response in the FNAB monitoring. The ICAM-1 is upregulated as well in association with rejection or infections. It is induced during bacterial sepsis and especially strongly expressed on hepatocytes during CMV infections (99). Thus, the induction of class II antigens or ICAM-1 can be considered rather unspecific markers of immune activation in the graft.

IV. FNAB IN THE MONITORING OF PANCREATIC ALLOGRAFTS

The most reliable method to diagnose pancreatic allograft rejection is biopsy histology (103). However, pancreatic allograft biopsies are associated with high risk of complications, although various techniques to obtain histological specimens have been described. The clinical diagnosis of pancreas rejection is difficult, since these noninvasive methods do not necessarily reflect the intragraft events. Elevated serum glucose and amylase levels are not yet seen at the beginning of a rejection episode (104). Measurement of urinary amylase is somewhat more helpful, and a decrease in urinary amylase has been seen to precede clinical signs of pancreas rejection (105). The high postbiopsy complication risk has increased the interest in developing less traumatic methods to monitor pancreatic allografts and the FNAB method has also been introduced in pancreatic transplantation.

Based on an experimental study of dog pancreas allografts (6), the FNAB was also applied to clinical pancreatic transplantation a few years ago (7,106). A good correlation between pancreas FNAB findings and NB histology in the diagnosis of acute rejection has been demonstrated (6,7). Although the experience of FNAB in pancreatic transplantation is still quite limited, the results are encouraging.

The cytological diagnosis of pancreas rejection is made when the total corrected increment (TCI) of immune activated cells is >2.6, with at least 50% of the score produced by lymphoid blast cells (7). FNAB may be used safely for frequent monitoring of pancreas allografts, but it is more difficult to get representative aspiration specimens from the pancreas then kidney or liver grafts. Ultrasound location of the pancreas allograft is recommended at all times.

V. SUMMARY

Histological examination of needle biopsy remains the "gold standard" to diagnose rejection and other intragraft complications after organ transplantation, but conventional biopsies always carry some risks of complications and cannot be used for frequent monitoring of the graft. FNAB is an atraumatic method that makes it possible to obtain aspiration material from the graft, even daily, to evaluate the onset, type, intensity, and duration of inflammatory episodes of rejection. Parenchymal changes in the FNAB specimen give some additional information on intragraft events and possible complications. FNAB is a reliable method to diagnose acute cellular rejection, and it can be used for monitoring of organ grafts during the immediate postoperative period, when most acute rejections occur. The FNAB diagnosis may be confirmed by biopsy histology, if necessary. The diagnosis of vascular rejection or chronic rejection and other chronic complications are established only by biopsy histology.

REFERENCES

1. von Willebrand E. Fine needle aspiration cytology of human renal transplants. Clin Immunol Immunopathol 1980; 17:309–322.
2. Häyry P, von Willebrand E. Monitoring of human renal allograft rejection with fine-needle aspiration cytology. Scand J Immunol 1981; 13:87–97.
3. Häyry P, von Willebrand E. Practical guidelines for fine needle aspiration biopsy of human renal allografts. Ann Clin Res 1981; 13:288–306.

4. Lautenschlager I, Höckerstedt K, Taskinen E, et al. Fine-needle aspiration cytology of liver allografts in pig. Transplantation 1984; 38:330–334.
5. Lautenschlager I, Höckerstedt K, von Willebrand E, et al. Aspiration cytology of a human liver allograft. Transplant Proc 1984; 16;1243–1246.
6. Ekberg H, Allen RDM, Greenberg ML, et al. Early diagnosis of rejection of canine pancreas allografts by fine-needle aspiration biopsy. Transplantation 1988; 46:485–489.
7. Allen RDM, Wilson TG, Grierson JM, et al. Percutaneous pancreas transplant fine needle aspiration and needle core biopsies are useful and safe. Transplant Proc 1990; 22:663–664.
8. Franzen S, Giertz G, Zaijcek J. Cytological diagnosis of prostatic tumors by transrectal aspiration biopsy. Br J Urol 1960; 32: 193–196.
9. Pasternack A. Fine-needle aspiration biopsy of human renal homografts. Lancet 1968; 2: 82–84.
10. von Willebrand E, Häyry P. Composition and in vitro cytotoxicity of cellular infiltrates in rejecting human kidney allografts. Cell Immunol 1978; 41:358–372.
11. von Willebrand E, Soots A, Häyry P. In situ effector mechanisms in rat kidney allograft rejection: I. Characterization of the host cellular infiltrate in rejecting allograft parenchyma. Cell Immunol 1979; 46:309–326.
12. Häyry P, von Willebrand E, Soots A. In situ effector mechanisms in rat kidney allograft rejection: III. Kinetics of the inflammatory response and generation of donor-directed killer cells. Scand J Immunol 1979; 10:95–108.
13. von Willebrand E, Häyry P. Reproducibility of the fine needle aspiration biopsy. Analysis of 93 double biopsies. Transplantation 1984; 38:314–316.
14. Belitsky P, Campbell J, Gupta R. Serial biopsy controlled evaluation of fine needle aspiration in renal allograft rejection. Lab Invest 1985; 53:580–585.
15. Vereerstraeten P, Romasco F, Monsieru R, et al. Representativeness and reproducibility of WBC counts in fine needle aspiration specimens from kidney transplants. Transplant Proc 1985; 17:2106–2107.
16. Saksela E, Timonen T, Ranki A, Häyry P. Morphological and functional characterization of isolated effector cells responsible for human natural killer cell activity to fetal fibroblasts and to cultured cell line targets. Immunol Rev 1979; 44:71–123.
17. Lautenschlager I, von Willebrand E, Häyry P. Blood eosinophilia, steroids and rejection. Transplantation 1985; 40:354–357.
18. Smith N, Chandler S, Hawker RJ, et al. Indium-labelled autologous platelets as diagnostic aid after renal transplantation. Lancet 1979; 2:1241–1242.
19. von Willebrand E, Zola H, Häyry P. Thrombocyte aggregates in renal allografts: Analysis by the fine needle aspiration biopsy and monoclonal anti-thrombocyte antibodies. Transplantation 1985; 39:258–262.
20. von Willebrand E, Häyry P. Cyclosporin A deposits in renal allografts. Lancet 1983; 2: 189–192.
21. Egidi F, De Vecchi A, Pagliari B, et al. Lack of relationship between blood cyclosporine levels and nephrotoxicity as assessed by fine needle aspiration biopsy of renal allografts. Transplant Proc 1985; 17:2096–2097.
22. Santelli G, Ouziala M, Charpentier B, Fries D. Predictive value of fine needle aspiration biopsy for cyclosporine nephrotoxicity. Transplant Proc 1985; 17:2094–2095.
23. Hughes DA, Rapoport J, Roake JA, et al. Confirmation of renal allograft infarction using fine-needle aspiration cytology. In: Yussim A, Hammer C, eds. Contributions to Transplantation Medicine: Transplant Monitoring. Wolfgang Pabst Verlag, Lengerich, Germany 1992.
24. von Willebrand E. Long-term experience with fine needle aspiration in kidney transplant patients. Transplant Proc 1989; 21:3568–3570.
25. Reinholt FP, Bohman S-O, Wilczek H, et al. Fine needle aspiration cytology and conventional histology in 200 renal allografts. Transplantation 1990; 49:910–912.

26. Helderman JH, Hernandez J, Sagalowsky A, et al. Confirmation of the utility of fine needle aspiration biopsy of the renal allograft. Kidney Int 1988; 34:376–381.
27. Isoniemi H, Ahonen J, Eklund B, et al. Renal allograft immunosuppression: Early inflammatory and rejection episodes in triple drug treatment compared to double drug combinations or cyclosporin monotherapy. Transplant Int 1990; 3:92–97.
28. Häyry P, von Willebrand E, Ahonen J, Eklund B. Glucocorticosteroids in renal transplantation: I. Impact of high vs. low dose postoperative methyl-prednisolone administration on the first episode(s) of rejection. Scand J Immunol 1982; 16:39–49.
29. Häyry P, von Willebrand E, Ahonen J, et al. Effects of cyclosporine, azathioprine and steroids on the renal transplant, on the cytological patterns of intragraft inflammation and on concomitant rejection-associated changes in the recipient blood. Transplant Proc 1988; 20: 153–162.
30. Salmela K, von Willebrand E, Kyllönen L, et al. The association of HLA-DR antigens with acute steroid resistant rejection and poor kidney graft survival. Transplantation 1991; 51: 768–771.
31. Salmela K, von Willebrand E, Kyllönen L, et al. Acute vascular rejection in renal transplantation—Diagnosis and outcome. Transplantation 1992; 54:858–862.
32. von Willebrand E, Taskinen E, Ahonen J, Häyry P. Recent modifications in the fine needle aspiration biopsy of human renal allografts. Transplant Proc 1983; 15:1195–1197.
33. Cooksey G, Reeve RS, Wenham PW, et al. Comparison of fine needle aspiration cytology with histology in the diagnosis of renal allograft rejection. In: Kreis H, Droz D, eds. Renal Transplant Cytology. Milan: Wichtig Editore, 1984:73–78.
34. Reeve RS, Cooksey G, Wenham PW, et al. A comparison of fine needle aspiration cytology and tru-cut tissue biopsy in the diagnosis of acute renal allograft rejection. Nephron 1986; 42: 68–71.
35. von Willebrand E, Salmela K, Isoniemi H, et al. Induction of HLA Class II antigen and interleukin 2 receptor expression in acute vascular rejection of human kidney allografts. Transplantation 1992; 53:1077–1081.
36. Wood RFM, Bolton EM, Thompson JF, Morris PJ. Monoclonal antibodies and fine needle aspiration cytology in detecting renal allograft rejection. Lancet 1982; 2:278.
37. von Willebrand E. OKT 4/8 ratio in the blood and in the graft during episodes of human allograft rejection. Cell Immunol 1983; 77:196–201.
38. Bolton EM, Thompson JF, Wood RF, Morris PJ. Immunoperoxidase staining of fine needle aspiration biopsies and needle core biopsies from renal allografts. Transplantation 1983; 36:728–731.
39. Cooksey G, Reeve RS, Paterson AD, et al. Lymphocyte subpopulations in cytologic aspirates from human renal allografts. Transplant Proc 1985; 17:630–632.
40. Hughes DA, Kempson MG, Carter NP, Morris PJ. Immunogold-silver/Romanowsky staining: Simultaneous immunocytochemical and morphological analysis of fine-needle aspirate biopsies. Transplant Proc 1988; 20:575–576.
41. Hancock WW, Gee D, De Moerloose P, et al. Immunohistological analysis of serial biopsies taken during human renal allograft rejection. Changing profile of infiltrating cells and activation of the coagulation system. Transplantation 1985; 39:430–438.
42. von Willebrand E, Häyry P. Relationship between cellular and molecular markers of inflammation in human kidney allograft rejection. Transplant Proc 1987; 19:1644–1645.
43. Häyry P, von Willebrand E, Ahonen J, Eklund B. Do well-to-do and repeatedly rejecting renal allografts express the transplantation antigens similarly on their surface? Scand J Urol Nephrol 1981; 64(suppl):52–55.
44. Hall BM, Duggin GG, Philips J, et al. Increased expression of HLA-DR antigens on renal tubular cells in renal transplants: Relevance to the rejection response. Lancet 1984; 2:247–251.
45. Fuggle SV, McWhinnie DL, Chapman JR, et al. Sequential analysis of HLA-class II antigen

expression in human renal allografts: Induction of tubular class II antigens and correlation with clinical parameters. Transplantation 1986; 42:144–150.
46. Häyry P, von Willebrand E. The influence of the pattern of inflammation and administration of steroids on class II MHC antigen expression in renal transplants. Transplantation 1986; 42:358–363.
47. Bishop GA, Hall BM. Expression of leucocyte and lymphocyte adhesion molecules in the human kidney. Kidney Int 1989; 36:1078–1085.
48. von Willebrand E, Loginov R, Salmela K, et al. Relationship between intercellular adhesion molecule-1 and HLA class II expression in acute cellular rejection of human kidney allografts. Transplant Proc 1993; 25:870–871.
49. von Willebrand E, Sandberg M, Salmela K, Isoniemi H, Häyry P. Expression of ICAM-1 and HLA class II in acute cellular and vascular rejection of human kidney allografts. Transplant Int, 1994; 7:308–310.
50. Vereerstraeten P, Romasco F, Kinnaert P. T cell subset patterns in peripheral blood and in fine needle aspiration lymphocytes after kidney transplantation. Transplant Proc 1985; 17:2115–2116.
51. Waugh J, Bishop GA, Hall B, et al. T cell subsets in fine needle aspiration biopsies from renal transplant recipients. Transplant Proc 1985; 17:1701–1703.
52. Lautenschlager I, von Willebrand E, Häyry P. Does T4 predominance in the graft signify severe rejection? Transplant Proc 1986; 18:1311–1313.
53. Nguyen L, Hammer C, Dendorfer U, et al. Changes in large granular lymphocyte size and number in kidney transplant patients during rejection and viral infection. Transplant Proc 1985; 17:2110–2111.
54. Ouziala M, Santelli G, Charpentier B, Fries D. Diagnostic value of fine needle aspiration biopsy during viral infections in renal transplant recipients. Transplant Proc 1985; 17:2098–2099.
55. Hammer C. Diagnosis of inflammatory events. In: Hammer C: Cytology in Transplantation. Verlag RS Schulz, West Germany, 1989; p 127–154.
56. von Willebrand E, Lautenschlager I, Ahonen J. Cellular activation in the graft and in the blood during CMV disease. Transplant Proc 1989; 21:2080–2081.
57. von Willebrand E, Pettersson E, Ahonen J, Häyry P. CMV infection, class II antigen expression, and human kidney allograft rejection. Transplantation 1986; 42:364–367.
58. Smith TF. Rapid methods for diagnosis of viral infections. Lab Med 1987; 18:16–20.
59. Van der Bij W, Toresma R, van Son WJ, et al. Rapid immunodiagnosis of active cytomegalovirus infection by monoclonal antibody staining of blood leucocytes. J Med Virol 1988; 25:179–188.
60. Droz D, Campos H, Noel LH, et al. Renal transplant fine needle aspiration cytology: correlations to renal histology. In: Renal Transplant Cytology, (H. Kreis and D. Droz, eds), 1984, p 59–65. Wichtig Editore, Milan.
61. De Vecchi A, Egidi F, Banfi G, et al. Comparison of fine needle aspiration biopsy and needle biopsy in renal transplantation. In: Kreis H, Droz D, eds. Renal Transplant Cytology. 1984: 67–72. Milan: Wichtig Editore.
62. Koller C, Hammer C, Gokel JM, et al. Correlation between core biopsy and aspiration cytology. Transplant Proc 1984; 16:1298–1300.
63. Egidi F, De Vecchi A, Banfi G, et al. Comparison of renal biopsy and fine needle aspiration biopsy in renal transplantation. Transplant Proc 1985; 17:61–63.
64. Gupta R, Campbell J, Om A, Belitsky P. Serial monitoring of cellular rejection by simultaneous histology and fine needle aspiration cytology. Transplant Proc 1985; 17:2123–2124.
65. Hughes DA, McWhinnie DL, Sutton R, et al. Can incremental scoring of fine-needle aspirates predict histopathologic renal allograft rejection? Transplant Proc 1988; 20:690–691.
66. Gray DWR, Richardson A, Hughes D, Fuggle S, et al. A prospective, randomized, blind

comparison of three biopsy techniques in the management of patients after renal transplantation. Transplantation 1992; 53:1226–1232.
67. Saliba F, Gegenheim J, Samuel D, et al. Orthotopic liver transplantation in humans: Monitoring by serial graft biopsies. Transplant Proc 1989; 1987:2454–2456.
68. Ascher NL, Stock PG, Bumgardner GL, et al. Infection and rejection of primary hepatic transplantation in 93 consecutive patients treated with triple immunosuppressive therapy. Surg Gynecol Obstet 1988; 167:474–484.
69. Klintmalm GBM, Nery JR, Husberg BS, et al. Rejection in liver transplantation. Hepatology 1989; 10:978–985.
70. Freese DK, Snover DC, Sharp HL, et al. Chronic rejection after liver transplantation: A study of clinical, histolopathological and immunological features. Hepatology 1991; 13:882–891.
71. Calne RY. Diagnosis of rejection. In: Calne RY, ed. Liver Transplantation. London: Grune & Stratton, 1987:301.
72. Häyry P, von Willebrand E, Ahonen J, et al. Monitoring of organ allograft rejection by transplant aspiration cytology. Ann Clin Res 1981; 13:264–287.
73. Lautenschlager I, Höckerstedt K, Taskinen E, et al. Fine-needle aspiration biopsy in the monitoring of liver allografts: I. Correlation between aspiration biopsy and core biopsy in experimental pig liver allografts. Transplantation 1988; 46:41–46.
74. Lautenschlager I, Höckerstedt K, Ahonen J, et al. Fine-needle aspiration biopsy in the monitoring of liver allografts: II. Applications to human allografts. Transplantation 1988; 46:47–52.
75. Vogel W, Margreiter R, Schmalzl F, Judmaier G. Preliminary results with fine needle aspiration biopsy in liver grafts. Transplant Proc 1984; 16:1240–1242.
76. Zannier A, Faure JL, Neidecker J, et al. Monitoring of liver allografts using fine-needle aspiration biopsy: Value of hepatocyte MHC-DR expression in the diagnosis of acute rejection. Transplant Proc 1987; 19:3810–3811.
77. Kirby RM, Young JA, Hubscher SG, et al. The accuracy of aspiration cytology in the diagnosis of rejection following orthotopic liver transplantation. Transplant Int 1988; 1:119–126.
78. Hammerer P, Kraemer-Hansen H, Kremer B, et al. Aspiration cytology of liver transplants. Transplant Proc 1988; 20:640–641.
79. Greene CL, Fehrman I, Tillery GW, et al. Liver transplant aspiration cytology is a useful tool for identifying and monitoring allograft rejection. Transplant Proc 1988; 20:657–658.
80. Di Tondo U, Ciardi A, Pecorella I, et al. Postoperative liver transplant monitoring with fine-needle aspiration biopsy. Transplant Proc 1989; 21:2311–2312.
81. Carbonel F, Samuel D, Reynes M, et al. Fine needle aspiration biopsy of human liver allografts: Correlation with liver histology for the diagnosis of acute rejection. Transplantation 1990; 50:704–707.
82. Schlitt HJ, Nashan B, Ringe B, et al. Differentiation of liver graft dysfunction by transplant aspiration cytology. Transplantation 1991; 51:786–792.
83. Kubota K, Ericzon BJ, Reinholt FP. Comparison of fine-needle aspiration biopsy and histology in human liver transplants. Transplantation 1991; 51:1010–1013.
84. Lautenschlager I, Höckerstedt K, Häyry P. Fine-needle aspiration biopsy in the monitoring of liver allografts. Transplant Int 1991; 4:54–61.
85. Schlitt HJ, Nashan B, Ringe B, et al. Routine monitoring of liver allografts by transplant aspiration cytology (TAC)—Clinical experience with 3000 TACs. Transplant Proc 1993; 251:1970–1972.
86. Porter KA. Pathology of liver transplantation. Transplant Rev 1969; 2:129–170.
87. Wight DGD, Portman B. Pathology of rejection. In: Calne RY, ed. Liver transplantation. London: Grune & Stratton, 1987:385–410.
88. Snover DC, Freese DK, Sharp HL, et al. Liver allograft rejection. An analysis of the use of biopsy determining outcome of rejection. Am J Surg Pathol 1987; 11:1–10.
89. Höckerstedt K, Lautenschlager I, Ahonen J, et al. Diagnosis of rejection in liver transplantation. J Hepatol 1988; 2:217–221.

90. Nashan B, Schlitt HJ, Wittekind CW, et al. Patterns of immune activation during the first four weeks in liver transplant patients. Transplant Proc 1989; 21:3623–3624.
91. Nashan B, Schlitt HJ, Ringe B, et al. Transplantation aspiration cytology in the diagnosis of steroid resistant rejection in liver allograft patients. Transplant Proc 1990; 22:2297–2298.
92. Höckerstedt K, Lautenschlager I, Ahonen J, et al. Differentiation between acute rejection and infection in liver transplant patients. Transplant Proc 1989; 21:2317–2318.
93. Sayage LH, Gonwa TA, Goldstein RM, et al. Cytomegalovirus in orthotopic liver transplantation. Transplant Int 1989; 2:96–101.
94. Paya CV, Hermans PE, Wiesner RH, et al. Cytomegalovirus hepatitis in liver transplantation: Prospective analysis of 93 consecutive orthotopic liver transplantations. J Infect Dis 1989; 160:752–758.
95. Lautenschlager I, Höckerstedt K, Salmela K, et al. Fine-needle aspiration biopsy (FNAB) in the monitoring of liver allografts: Different cellular findings during rejection and CMV infection. Transplantation 1990; 50:798–803.
96. Nashan B, Schlitt HJ, Ringe B, et al. Differential diagnosis of viral infections and acute rejection episodes in liver allograft patients by transplant aspiration cytology. Transplant Proc 1991; 23:1507–1508.
97. Ciardi A, Pecorella I, Rossi M, et al. Morphologic features in liver transplantation. Transplant Proc 1988; 20:637–639.
98. Schlitt J, Nashan B, Krick P, et al. Intragraft immune events after human liver transplantation: Correlation with clinical signs of acute rejection and influence of immunosuppression. Transplantation 1992; 54:273–278.
99. Lautenschlager I, Höckerstedt K. ICAM-1 induction on hepatocytes as a marker for immune activation of acute liver allograft rejection. Transplantation 1993; 56:1495–1499.
100. Lautenschlager I, Höckerstedt K, Häyry P. Activation markers in acute liver allograft rejection. Transplant Proc 1988; 20:646–647.
101. Vogel W, Wohlfahrter P, Then P, et al. Longitudinal study of major histocompatibility complex antigen expression on hepatocytes in fine-needle aspiration biopsies from human liver grafts. Transplant Proc 1988; 20:648–649.
102. Zannier A, Pujol D, Berger F, Pallard P. Characterization of cellular infiltrate and HLA-DR expression in chronic hepatitis B-virus infection using fine-needle aspiration cytology. Transplant Proc 1988; 20:652–653.
103. Sibley RK, Sutherland DER. Pancreas transplantation: An immunohistologic and histopathologic examination of 100 grafts. Am J Pathol 1987; 128:151–170.
104. Brattström C, Tyden G, Reinholt F, et al. Markers for pancreas graft rejection in humans. Diabetes 1989; 38(suppl 1):57–60.
105. Prieto M, Sutherland DER, Fernandez-Cruz L, et al. Experimental and clinical experience with urine amylase monitoring for early diagnosis of rejection in pancreas transplantation. Transplantation 1987; 43:73–79.
106. Wang SE, Nghiem DD. Initial evaluation of pancreatic cellular subpopulations by fine needle aspiration in clinical pancreas transplantation. Transplant Proc 1990; 22:616–618.

14

Clinical Diagnosis in Heart and Lung Allograft Rejection

Vincent G. Valentine
Ochsner Transplant Center and Louisiana State University School of Medicine, New Orleans, Louisiana

Robert C. Robbins and James Theodore
Stanford University School of Medicine, Stanford, California

I. INTRODUCTION

Heart, lung, and heart-lung transplantation have become established as effective forms of therapy for selected patients with irreversible end-stage cardiac, cardiopulmonary, and pulmonary diseases. The modification of numerous factors has resulted in improved long-term survival. Improved patient selection, advancements in donor organ procurement and preservation, refinements in surgical techniques, improved immunosuppression, and more effective overall patient management represent some of the changes that have occurred in the last 15 years. Acute and chronic rejection, in addition to infection, remain the major barriers to further improvement in the long-term results of thoracic organ transplantation.

A. General Overview

Sufficient experience with heart, heart-lung, and lung transplantation has been achieved to permit definition of the long-term clinical course. The nature and frequency of complications that arise with these procedures can often be related to specific periods of time following transplantation. Primary graft dysfunction resulting from prolonged ischemia and/or inadequate preservation, nosocomial or donor-transmitted infection, multisystem organ dysfunction, and errors in surgical technique are the major early complications. The most devastating complication is immediate graft loss secondary to hyperacute rejection; although this is an extremely rare occurrence, it is invariably fatal. Hyperacute rejection is mediated by recipient preformed antibodies to donor antigen. Investigation for preformed recipient antibodies is performed against a wide panel of reactive antigens during the potential recipient's pretransplant evaluation. Donors and recipients are matched by ABO blood group, and lymphocytotoxic cross-matching is prospectively done for potential recipients with high levels of preformed antibodies.

T-cell–mediated acute rejection is the most common form of rejection and has a wide spectrum of severity. Chronic rejection is more indolent and poorly understood. This chapter emphasizes the diagnosis and management of acute rejection in heart and lung allografts. Graft coronary artery disease and obliterative bronchiolitis (OB), both of which may be the result of chronic rejection, are also discussed.

The majority of acute rejection events occur in the first 3 months following transplantation. Keenan et al. reported that approximately 90% of acute lung rejection events occurred within the first 6 weeks following heart-lung and double lung transplantation (1). A similar experience has also been reported following single-lung transplantation (2). Although most deaths are not directly related to acute rejection, multiple acute rejection episodes may lead to the development of chronic rejection, with its attendant morbidity and mortality. Because each rejection episode may progressively injure the allograft, long-term graft function and patient survival rely on early recognition and prompt treatment of acute rejection. Cyclosporine-based immunosuppression has made the clinical findings of rejection less sensitive, and allograft biopsy is the "gold standard" for the diagnosis of rejection. Consequently, proper surveillance for the earliest detection of rejection requires a multidisciplinary approach for assessing the status of the allograft. Routinely, these diagnostic procedures involve chest radiography, electrocardiography, echocardiography, and right ventricular endomyocardial biopsies for monitoring the heart; for assessing the lung, these procedures include chest radiography, pulmonary function studies with arterial blood gases, and bronchoscopy with transbronchial lung biopsies. The diagnosis of rejection by analysis of blood and bronchoalveolar lavage (BAL) fluid are under investigation but are not currently accurate enough for clinical application.

II. CARDIAC TRANSPLANTATION

A. Acute Cardiac Rejection

1. Clinical Manifestations

Acute cardiac rejection can occur in totally asymptomatic patients or may present with signs and symptoms of severe cardiac failure. There are no clinical signs or symptoms unique to rejection episodes. Angina pectoris, even in the presence of severe myocardial ischemia, is rare following cardiac transplantation because of denervation, which occurs with excision of the native heart. This denervation is generally thought to be permanent. There is controversial evidence suggesting that cardiac reinnervation may occur over time following transplantation (3). Approximately 5% of long-term survivors with documented ischemic graft coronary disease have reported anginal-type chest pain. (S. Hunt, personal communication).

Palpitations, malaise, presyncope, or syncope can result from rejection-related graft dysfunction. Severe episodes of acute rejection may produce overt signs of congestive heart failure resulting from left or right ventricular dysfunction. Symptoms of fatigue, dyspnea, and orthopnea result from decreased cardiac output. Deterioration in cardiac function may be due to an inappropriate heart rate response, inadequate stroke volume, or a combination of both. The physical signs are nonspecific and may include fever, irregular amplitudes and/or rhythms of the pulse, distended neck veins, poor carotid upstrokes, displaced or attenuated point of maximal impulse, S3 or S4 gallop rhythms, pericardial friction rub, peripheral edema, and hepatomegaly, particularly in children. Routine laboratory data may demonstrate a leukocytosis, elevated serum LDH isoenzymes, and evidence of end-organ congestion and hypoperfusion with liver enzyme abnormalities and azotemia. The chest radiograph may show an increase in the cardiothoracic ratio with or without the development of pleural effusions and/or pulmonary edema.

The institution of routine surveillance biopsies for cardiac rejection in the cyclosporine era has demonstrated that most mild to moderate forms of acute rejection are clinically silent. The majority of rejection events are clinically insignificant, are frequently discovered on routine surveillance biopsies, and are commonly of a mild or moderate histologic grade. Yeoh et al. reported that 62% of mild rejection episodes produced no evidence of allograft dysfunction, 29 percent had mild allograft dysfunction, and 9 percent had severe dysfunction (4). The most common clinical findings were sinus tachycardia (heart rate > 120 beats per minute), elevated jugular venous distention, and appearance of an S3 gallop. Furthermore, they observed that mild rejection episodes with allograft dysfunction progressed to moderate rejection more frequently than those without allograft dysfunction. The assessment of acute cardiac rejection should not be based solely on the histopathologic findings but should be integrated with data from the history and physical examination, electrocardiogram, and echocardiogram.

2. Electrocardiogram and Electrophysiology

Twelve-lead surface electrocardiogram (ECG) patterns are not specific for cardiac rejection. Gao et al. reported that in the first year following heart transplantation, an incomplete or complete right bundle branch block was the most common abnormality and that repolarization abnormalities did not correlate with rejection episodes. In the precyclosporine era, a greater than 20% fall in the summation of the QRS complex voltage on leads I, II, III, V_1, and V_6 in serial ECGs was felt to be indicative of heart rejection and required tissue confirmation (5). Since the advent of cyclosporine, the summation of QRS complex voltage is no longer considered valid for detecting rejection. Scott et al. demonstrated an association between cardiac rejection and frequent atrial premature complexes recorded on ambulatory 24-hr ECG monitoring. The presence of atrial flutter was closely associated with rejection and regarded as an indication for a heart biopsy (6). In addition, they confirmed other reports that ventricular dysrhythmias were not associated with rejection (7,8). Expanded applications of ECG have been utilized in attempting to detect early rejection (9). These have included, among others, ECG signal averaging (10), fast-Fourier-transformed electrocardiography (11), and intramyocardial ECG utilizing intramyocardial electrograms (IMEG) (12–14).

Electrocardiographic signal averaging is a technique that averages together multiple samples of a repeating waveform, permitting the detection of signals that are otherwise masked by random noise. Although this approach increased the overall sensitivity (82%) for detecting cardiac rejection over that of the standard ECG (37%), it is considered to be unreliable in the early postoperative period (9,10,15). The frequency analysis of the electrocardiogram by fast-Fourier transformations (FFT-ECG) represented a new approach initially tested by Haberl et al. (11). Fast-Fourier transform is an algorithm that analyzes frequencies not otherwise detected in the surface ECG. It was shown that changes in the frequency content of the QRS complex and ST segment occur with rejection and that these changes normalize 1 to 2 weeks following treatment. The sensitivity of FFT-ECG is approximately 80% for rejection, with a specificity of only 42% (9,11,15). Recent experimental results obtained on the QRS frequency content after heterotopic heart transplantation indicate that the usefulness of these alterations may be limited to diagnosis at the onset of rejection. Furthermore, it appears that FFT-ECG does not describe the later stages of the rejection reaction (15,16). With further study and reproducible results, this method may hold promise as an adjunct to the heart biopsy to determine the timing and reduce the number of biopsy procedures. At present, however, it is not sensitive enough to replace the heart biopsy (9).

The IMEG is an ECG technique that has been used for detecting cardiac rejection. The IMEG measurements, obtained directly from the myocardium, are used to monitor changes in myocardial voltage amplitudes. Acute rejection causes decreases in ECG voltage, and early detection of these changes may be beneficial (12–14). Cyclosporine has made the change in the surface electrocardiogram QRS voltage less sensitive and more unreliable as an index of rejection. Because it requires an implantable pacemaker and epicardial lead system for telemetric monitoring to obtain a more direct measure of myocardial voltage change, IMEG may enhance the sensitivity for detecting rejection even with cyclosporine therapy.

Warnecke et al. reported the use of IMEG in heart recipients receiving cyclosporine and prednisone therapy and observed a significant correlation between voltage drop (greater than 15%) and biopsy-proven rejection (12). The same group later reported that no false-negative results were obtained with IMEG and that with retrospective analysis, IMEG showed a 100% negative predictive value in biopsy-proven rejection (17). It was suggested that a normal IMEG, together with a completely normal echocardiographic assessment of cardiac function, would preclude the need for endomyocardial biopsy to rule out rejection. On the other hand, however, false-positive results with IMEG were observed with dysrhythmias and infections.

A major disadvantage of IMEG is the necessity for implanting a pacemaker and an epicardial lead system (15). Additionally, cyclical changes in IMEG patterns during the day (18), insufficient information on its long-term usefulness, and its inability to distinguish irreparable myocardial damage after rejection from an ongoing rejection process if depressed intramyocardial voltage amplitude persists all represent limitations of this method (9). The other major problem is the lack of confirmation of IMEG results by other groups (19).

3. *Echocardiography*

A number of echocardiographic findings are commonly present in the heart allograft, some unique, which generally appear to be of little or no clinical consequence with respect to rejection. These include the "snowman" atria, created by the surgical anastomoses of the donor atria to the recipient atria (20); decreased left ventricular size in comparison to normal (20); trace to minimal mitral regurgitation (20); and small pericardial effusions, particularly within the first 10 days following transplantation (21).

Early studies with ultrasound and with M-mode and 2D echocardiography demonstrated significant increases in left ventricular wall thickness and myocardial mass with acute rejection as a result of the myocardial interstitial edema that was associated with it (22–24). Although these findings are still significant if present, the introduction of cyclosporine therapy has made such changes much less apparent for the early detection of rejection by echocardiographic techniques.

Earlier studies with echophonocardiograms (25) and more recent quantitative studies with Doppler echocardiography (26,27), have demonstrated changes in early diastolic function with acute rejection that could be associated with decreases in left ventricular diastolic compliance. Rejection of increasing magnitude was associated with progressive shortening of isovolumic relaxation time (IVRT) and with increases in peak early mitral flow velocity (M1). These results, however, have not gone unchallenged, and further studies are warranted.

The detection of significant reductions in ventricular systolic function by echocardiography warrants endomyocardial biopsy to rule out rejection as an important first step in the clinical evaluation. Ventricular systolic dysfunction is generally associated with more advanced stages of rejection, and echocardiographic techniques are still relatively insensitive in detecting milder stages of rejection.

Utilizing computer-assisted 2D echocardiographic measurements of left ventricular volume and global ejection fraction, Moriguchi et al. found that 10% decreases in left ventricular ejection fraction or 30% increases in end-systolic volume identified 76% of moderate acute rejection episodes with a specificity of 96% in biopsy-proven rejection (28). Angermann et al. showed functional changes indicative of a diminished cardiac output during acute rejection using an analysis of ventricular cross-sectional area velocity changes in a computerized evaluation of the endomyocardial border throughout the cardiac cycle with 2D echocardiographic short-axis views (29,30).

In studies on the clinical consequences of mild cardiac rejection. Yeoh et al. found ventricular systolic dysfunction in 25% of biopsy-proven episodes of mild acute rejection (4). Moreover, untreated cases of mild rejection with systolic dysfunction were more likely to progress to moderate rejection than those untreated cases with normal function (30% vs. 10% of the respective cases). These data further emphasize the usefulness of echocardiographic monitoring of cardiac function with rejection for both diagnostic and therapeutic purposes. The untreated allograft dysfunction during mild rejection forecasts a greater risk for the progression of rejection to more advanced stages. Warnecke et al. utilized echocardiographic monitoring of diastolic function in their noninvasive surveillance for heart rejection with IMEG. They suggested that treatment of rejection episodes detected by IMEG can be withheld until early signs of left ventricular diastolic dysfunction were present, provided that infection, which could affect IMEG measurements, was excluded (17). It would seem more likely, however, that only the more advanced forms of rejection would be detected under these circumstances, due to the relative insensitivities of the methods, and cause unnecessary delays in treatment. As a general rule, where possible, endomyocardial biopsy should be obtained to direct therapy.

Serial estimates of left ventricular fractional shortening have been useful in suggesting rejection in pediatric heart transplantation where practical considerations have constrained the use of serial endomyocardial biopsies for monitoring rejection in infants and small children (31). Significant reductions in left ventricular fractional shortening on serial measurements warrant biopsy to rule out rejection.

Boucek et al. (32) recently suggested that echocardiography can be used successfully for primary rejection surveillance in infants, thus making the need for heart biopsies infrequent. The use of a rejection grading system that reflects the degree of echocardiographic abnormality of left ventricular performance is used. Rejection grade, determined from the summation of weighted scores for functional variables derived from assessments of left ventricular systolic and diastolic dynamic functions, diastolic static properties, and degrees of mitral regurgitation have been shown to correlate with rejection. Echocardiography was 98% accurate in predicting biopsy results, with a sensitivity of 92% and specificity of 98%. These highly favorable results await confirmation from other groups.

Valantine et al. (21) showed that increasing pericardial effusions may be temporally related to rejection episodes. Pericardial effusions following cardiac surgery generally maximize by the tenth postoperative day and usually resolve without complications.

Increasing, persisting, or newly forming pericardial effusions beyond 2 weeks after transplantation should alert one to the possibility of rejection.

Although the echocardiographic demonstration of diffuse ventricular wall motion abnormalities can be related to rejection, the presence of regional ventricular wall motion abnormalities cannot. The latter findings, more in keeping with ischemic heart disease, are usually the consequence of graft coronary artery disease, which requires coronary arteriography for confirmation. This will be further discussed below under "Chronic Heart Rejection."

Among noninvasive techniques, echocardiography is the most useful for assessing the long-term functional status of the allograft in heart transplant recipients. It is ideally suited for the performance of serial studies, for possibly detecting changes in cardiac function and structure that can be associated with rejection, or in the case of known rejection for making management decisions regarding therapy. However, although it is of value as an aid for the detection of rejection and of importance in the long-term management of heart transplant patients, echocardiography is still inadequate in its present form to replace endomyocardial biopsy in the diagnosis of acute rejection. Echocardiography does have merit as an adjunct to endomyocardial biopsy in the surveillance for rejection. The development of significant decreases in ventricular function detected by echocardiography requires an endomyocardial biopsy to rule out rejection.

4. *Other Noninvasive Methods*

Other methods that have been used for the noninvasive diagnosis of acute rejection fall into two general categories: (1) the assessment of peripheral blood for indices of an activated immune system during rejection and (2) the use of imaging techniques. Peripheral blood assessment includes the use of cytoimmunologic monitoring (CIM) and measurements of immunologic and biochemical markers, most often representing derived products of lymphocyte activation. The newer imaging techniques include magnetic resonance imaging and nuclear radionuclide imaging. Although these methods are of interest and, to a large extent, are still under investigation, none have been generally accepted as a reliable means for diagnosing rejection.

a. Cytoimmunologic Monitoring. The cellular immune response during rejection involves the activation of T lymphocytes, which can also be reflected by changes in the composition of lymphocytes populating peripheral blood. The unique ability of T lymphocytes to bind sheep erythrocytes led to the development of the E-rosette assay. This permitted the separation and quantitation of T cells from other mononuclear cell populations in blood. Measurements of circulating T lymphocytes and use of the E-rosette assay to detect effector circulating lymphocytes were found to be helpful in predicting impending rejection in the precyclosporine era (33,34). In cyclosporine-treated recipients, however, the quantitative measurements of circulating T lymphocytes became unreliable, curtailing the ability to predict rejection (35,36).

Since the introduction of cyclosporine, quantitative assessments of peripheral lymphocytes and their subsets have been utilized as a method to monitor for rejection on the basis of techniques originally developed by Hammer et al. in Munich (37). Through the quantitation of peripheral lymphoblasts and prelymphoblasts as measures of lymphocyte activation in mononuclear concentrates from recipients' blood, increases in activated lymphocytes to levels greater than 5% of the lymphoid population in blood was considered to be suggestive of acute rejection. Similar results, however, could also be seen with infections, particularly those that were viral in nature. Whereas early reports revealed good correlations between increases in peripheral activated lymphocytes and biopsy-proven rejection, with sensitivities and specificities of up to 93% and 70% respectively (38–42), later studies attempting to confirm the earlier results demonstrated lower sensitivities (43–48). The latter studies also suggested that CIM may be more sensitive when performed frequently within the first 90 days following transplantation, with sensitivity thereafter falling to less than 70% (9,46–48).

Other attempts to discriminate between infection and rejection with CIM have included determinations of CD4/CD8 lymphocyte ratios. Results of these studies suggested that decreases in the CD4/CD8 ratio to less than 1.0 could be indicative of viral or fungal infections, and increases in the ratio to values greater than 1.0 could be correlated with rejection within 3 months following transplantation. The overall sensitivity for detecting rejection, however, was less than 70% (49–51).

Despite the early favorable reports, CIM has not been widely accepted as an effective method for detecting rejection in its present form. It is still plagued to some extent by the inability to discriminate between infection and rejection and is lacking in sensitivity beyond the third month of transplantation. Although additional study is still warranted, it does not preclude the need for endomyocardial biopsy to rule out rejection.

b. Immunologic and Biochemical Markers. A variety of assays have been developed for the detection of immunologic and biochemical products in blood or urine. These assays could be used as possible markers of an activated immune system in association with acute rejection. These include measures of transferrin receptors and interleukin-2 (IL-2) receptors on lymphocytes (52–56), soluble IL-2 receptors (57–59), prolactin (60,61), and beta$_2$-microglobulins (62) in serum, neopterin levels in serum and urine (63–65), and polyamines and thromboxane B2 in urine (66–68). Most of these, in some degree, are associated with lymphocyte activation and proliferation with the possible exception of prolactin, a pituitary hormone, which also has a role in the regulation of humorally mediated immune responses.

These methods may have some limited adjunctive role in monitoring for acute rejection. However, as the sole means of diagnosing rejection, their sensitivity and specificity is insufficient. Discrimination between infection and rejection remains a problem, and additional studies are needed to validate these approaches.

c. Magnetic Resonance Imaging. Magnetic resonance imaging (MRI) and ECG-gated MRI have been used as a noninvasive means for detecting cardiac rejection. Image contrast with MRI is dependent upon tissue differences in proton concentration, flow and diffusion characteristics, and proton relaxation times—i.e., T1 (spin-lattice relaxation time) and T2 (spin-spin relaxation time) (69,70). Prolonged proton relaxation times have been correlated with acute rejection, particularly T2, as a result of increases in tissue water (myocardial edema) accompanying the rejection reaction (70–74). Additionally, increases in left ventricular wall thickness have also been detected by MRI and correlated with rejection, observations similar to those noted with echocardiography.

Initial studies indicate that MRI is only sensitive for detecting moderate to severe grades of acute rejection. It appears to be inadequate for detecting mild rejection or any pattern of rejection within the first month following transplantation (73). During this time period, prolonged T2 relaxation times are nonspecific, since myocardial edema is commonly present in the early postoperative period (72). Beyond the first month, prolonged T2 relaxation times appear to correlate with biopsy-proven rejection, particularly those of advanced grade. Moreover, in recent studies reported by Smart et al. (74), changes in myocardial/skeletal muscle signal intensity as detected by serial MRIs may be more sensitive but less specific than endomyocardial biopsy.

Some question has been raised regarding the feasibility of detecting acute rejection events by alterations of proton relaxation times and signal intensity, since the degree of myocardial edema accompanying rejection is considered to be less with the use of cyclosporine (75). Detection may be improved with the use of contrast materials. Mousseaux et al. showed that gadolinium-DOTA produced an increase in signal intensity in rejecting orthotopic hearts, indicating that MRI contrast agents may be useful for the detection of rejection (76).

Using P^{31} nuclear magnetic resonance (NMR) spectroscopy, Hall et al. performed studies that revealed decreases in phosphate metabolites during rejection, indicative of changes in myocardial high-energy phosphate metabolism (77). Although it may be of some value in the future, the major limitations to MRI at present include issues such as cost, resolution of some of the inherent technicalities with its use, and the need for further clinical validation in a larger number of cardiac transplant recipients.

d. Radionuclide Imaging. A number of radionuclide imaging techniques have been utilized to assess cardiac rejection noninvasively. In general, two basic strategies have been employed for evaluating cardiac allografts for rejection with radionuclides. One approach involves the use of radionuclides for quantitative measures of global or regional ventricular function, where alterations in functions can be indirectly associated with rejection. The other assesses the myocardial uptake of radionuclide labels as indicators of tissue injury in the myocardium, which, in turn, can be directly related to rejection.

Quantitative assessments of left ventricular function can be made by radionuclide ventriculography utilizing technetium-99m-labeled red cells or some other technetium-99m radiopharmaceutical, depending upon the specific nature of the technique used (78). In early reports on cardiac recipients evaluated with radionuclide ventriculograms, moderate to severe rejection episodes correlated strongly with decreases in stroke volume and end-diastolic volume, with a less significant relationship between rejection and ejection fraction or end-systolic volume (79–82). In recent studies by Latre et al. (83), alterations in diastolic parameters of ventricular function (decreases in peak filling and average filling rates) were shown to correlate well with increasing severity of rejection by biopsy, whereas decreases in global ejection fraction occurred only with more severe episodes of rejection. This suggests that abnormalities of ventricular diastolic function (filling rates) may be a more sensitive index for detecting milder forms of rejection by these methods.

Radionuclide imaging scans of myocardium were found to be useful for detecting acute cardiac rejection in animal studies (84). The radionuclides most commonly used in these studies, and their respective "targeting" properties, are as follows: technetium-99m pyrophosphate (specific for ischemic myocardial necrosis), gallium 67 (nonspecific for inflammation), thallium 201 (specific for organ perfusion and vascular integrity), indium-111-labeled antimyosin monoclonal antibodies (AMAs) (specific for myosin, exposed following myocardial cell injury and necrosis), and indium-111-labeled hematologic elements (nonspecific for inflammation) (9,75,78). In a predominantly nonimmunosuppressed rat heterotopic cardiac transplant model, all, except for thallium, showed enhanced myocardial uptake with rejection, with a positive correlation between increases in myocardial uptake and the degrees of histologic rejection. Thallium showed an inverse relationship and a negative correlation with increasing rejection as a result of decreased myocardial uptake due to the loss of perfusion as a consequence of tissue injury and vascular stasis.

Although the animal results would seem to indicate the potential usefulness of these techniques for "diagnosing" acute rejection, their use in human cardiac transplant recipients has not been widely accepted. In one study in human cardiac transplant recipients, the myocardial uptakes of technetium-99m pyrophosphate were not significantly different in those with acute cardiac rejection in comparison to those without rejection (85). In another study, gallium 67 was reported to be sensitive for detecting acute cardiac rejection (86). However, criticisms raised regarding the use of gallium 67 include the marked accumulation in the sternum and high radiation exposure (75).

The most extensive clinical experience for detecting rejection by these methods has been with indium-111-labeled antimyosin monoclonal antibodies (AMA). As noted earlier, the AMAs are directed against myosin that becomes exposed following ischemic or rejection-mediated cellular membrane injury. Their use was initially established in patients with coronary artery disease to localize areas of myocardial necrosis (87). Increases in the myocardial uptake of indium-111 AMA have been correlated with acute rejection in a number of studies (77,88,89). In one study, AMA uptake was frequent in the early period following cardiac transplantation and could not distinguish mild from moderate acute rejection (90). Frist et al. (91) reported an 80% sensitivity and specificity for detecting moderate rejection with AMA. In recent studies, where measurements of myocardial uptakes for AMA were done in conjunction with measures of ventricular diastolic function by radionuclide ventriculography, Latre et al. were able to distinguish accurately between treatable and nontreatable episodes of acute cardiac rejection (83).

Despite these results, the general clinical use of indium-111-labeled AMA for the detection and management of acute rejection in cardiac transplantation is limited by a number of factors. These include a 48-hr delay for optimal imaging from the time of injection, the development of antimurine antibodies by the host against the injected AMA, limitations in the number of scans that can be performed due to radiation burden from the indium 111, which clears slowly, and the possibility of negative imaging from high-dosage steroid therapy given during rejection (75).

Although radionuclide imaging techniques still hold some promise for monitoring cardiac rejection in the future with further developments, some of the concerns raised previously still hold true. As was pointed out by Baughman, even though a number of radionuclide agents have shown the capacity for demonstrating cardiac rejection in experimental animals, these agents would, as a rule, be less sensitive in human cardiac transplant recipients, in whom the gradations and severity of histologic rejection are less than those seen in untreated animals (92).

In general, even though none of the currently available noninvasive techniques have the sensitivity or specificity to replace endomyocardial biopsy for diagnosing cardiac rejection, they do, nonetheless, have some importance in the overall management of cardiac transplant recipients. These techniques can be of use in the surveillance for rejection, particularly as adjuncts to the endomyocardial biopsy to assist in the timing of biopsy, and in the monitoring of allograft function during various stages of rejection to assist in management decisions regarding therapy.

An obvious aim of noninvasive methodology has been the desire to minimize the need for invasive biopsy procedures. Towards this end, Kemkes et al. (75) recently suggested that CIM and fast-Fourier transformation-ECG could be used for the daily monitoring of rejection during the early postoperative period following transplantation. If both methods suggested rejection, AMA scintigraphy would then be done in follow-up to confirm and establish the grade of rejection, thus reducing the number of biopsies that might be needed. This approach would require a prospective study for confirmation. In other situations, some of the noninvasive changes, particularly those found by echocardiography, MRI, and radionuclide imaging in association with negative biopsies, may be related to the development of graft arteriosclerosis. Additional research and refinements of technique are needed to further advance the use of noninvasive methodology for the diagnosis of cardiac rejection.

5. Heart Biopsy

The successful clinical development of heart transplantation was critically dependent upon an accurate means for monitoring rejection in the cardiac allograft. Caves et al. reported the use of transjugular endomyocardial biopsy as a direct and effective method for detecting cardiac rejection in heart transplant recipients (93). Through modifications of a bioptome originated by Sakakibara and Konno (94), which permitted percutaneous insertion through the right internal jugular vein, it was shown that multiple endomyocardial biopsies could be performed serially in these patients to monitor for rejection as part of routine surveillance or as clinically indicated.

As has been suggested in previous sections, there are no satisfactory alternatives to endomyocardial biopsy in the routine surveillance for cardiac rejection, since other methods currently available lack the necessary sensitivity and/or specificity for diagnosis. Although invasive, the procedure is considered to be safe and associated with minimal patient discomfort, can be repeated at frequent intervals without significant long-term untoward effects, and can be performed as an outpatient procedure on a routine basis. The histology of the myocardial tissue obtained at biopsy can be assessed promptly and with accuracy, permitting the diagnosis of rejection (and grades), if present, to be made in less than 24 hr. In urgent cases, a diagnosis can be obtained within several hours by frozen sections obtained at biopsy. It is uniformly accepted as the definitive means for detecting rejection and represents the "gold standard" with which all other methods are compared (95). The transvascular technique for obtaining endomyocardial biopsies is well standardized and will not be a point of discussion here (96,97).

Endomyocardial biopsy is a safe, reproducible procedure but has some associated risks. Complications that can be related to endomyocardial biopsy usually occur during the course of the procedure itself (97). Complications that may arise, in rank order of importance, include: *right ventricular perforation* and *pericardial tamponade*; *malignant ventricular dysrhythmias*, which may require cardioversion; *transient complete heart block*, which may require the temporary use of a transvenous pacemaker; *pneumothorax*, particularly of the right lung, because of the use of the right internal jugular or right subclavian vein as a venous access site; *inadvertent puncture of carotid or subclavian artery*; *supraventricular dysrhythmias*, which may require medical therapy if sustained; nerve paresis, in particular the development of transient Horner's syndrome, vocal cord paralysis, or, more rarely, temporary diaphragmatic weakness from the infiltration of local anesthetic agents into the area of the internal jugular vein and carotid sheath; and *venous hematomas* at the access sites (97).

Surveillance for rejection is a critical facet of transplant management, as patients are often asymptomatic and show no signs of graft dysfunction during the milder stages of rejection. Since early detection to preserve allograft function is the primary aim and noninvasive techniques are considered to be unreliable, proper surveillance for rejection requires a schedule of endomyocardial biopsies to be performed at fixed intervals following transplantation, or more often if need be, as dictated by the rejection history of the individual patient. Most programs follow standard surveillance protocol schedules for cardiac rejection. Currently at Stanford, postoperative endomyocardial biopsies in cardiac recipients are performed weekly for the first month, biweekly for the second month, monthly for the next 4 months (months 3 through 6), and every 3 months thereafter.

As indicated previously, biopsies may need to be done more frequently depending upon the status of the cardiac allograft and the clinical circumstances encountered. Detection of mild heart rejection by routine surveillance biopsy usually goes without acute immunosuppressive therapy provided that cardiac function is well preserved, and a repeat biopsy is usually performed in 1 week to determine if progression/regression of rejection has occurred. It should be noted that cytomegalovirus (CMV) infections can produce histologic changes that are difficult to discriminate from acute rejection. Cytomegalovirus should be carefully looked for and ruled out, in view of the serious consequences that may arise if rejection dosages of steroids are administered to someone with active CMV disease. In more advanced grades of rejection that require full-dosage antirejection therapy with corticosteroids, repeat biopsies are usually performed at 1 week and 1 month following the completion of therapy. If evidence of graft dysfunction persists or worsening of function becomes apparent, biopsies may be obtained sooner or more frequently, as dictated by the clinical course. Even though it is considered to be the gold standard, it is possible to have a negative endomyocardial biopsy with an episode of acute cardiac rejection, even in the presence of hemodynamic instability. This may occur with the "atypical" picture that can be associated with humoral mediated rejection where the typical lymphocytic infiltrates, usually expected in the myocardium, are absent or as a result of tissue sampling errors or difficulties in histologic interpretation. Repeat biopsy is usually warranted with the continuation of graft dysfunction.

Endomyocardial biopsy continues to be one of the mainstays of clinical management in heart transplantation. The grades of acute cardiac rejection are now well standardized and are discussed in Chap. 6. The pathophysiologic course of the various grades of acute rejection and their effect on cardiac function are reasonably well understood, and this is of use for guiding therapeutic decisions through the serial use of endomyocardial biopsies over fixed intervals of time. It is possible to detect rejection before the development of abnormal graft function. In the grand scheme of posttransplant management, the primary goals are proper surveillance, accurate diagnosis, and timely treatment of rejection in order to preserve long-term function of the cardiac allograft.

B. Chronic Heart Rejection (Graft Atherosclerosis)

In cardiac transplant recipients surviving more than a year following operation, the major limitation for extended survival has been the development of graft atherosclerosis (98–101). Posttransplant graft atherosclerosis is an unusual form of accelerated coronary artery disease; it is believed to be the result of chronic rejection and is analogous to the chronic vascular injury seen in renal allografts (102). Unlike naturally occurring coronary artery disease, the histologic changes are diffuse, with concentric intimal proliferation involving the entire length of the coronary artery and frequently extending into smaller vessels, preventing the development of an adequate collateral circulation (103). Discussed briefly here, graft atherosclerosis is discussed at greater length in Chap. 5.

Even though generally held as the mechanism involved, chronic rejection has never been unequivocally proven to be the cause of graft atherosclerosis in humans. Immune-mediated injury to endothelium, with progression to the more advanced intimal proliferative lesions, appears to be in keeping with experimental findings (104,105) and a "response to injury" thesis proposed by Ross for atherosclerosis (106). In an experimental heterotopic heart transplant model in rats, the degree of vascular disease arising in nonsyngeneic allografts correlated with the degree of histocompatibility (107). In limited human studies, graft coronary artery disease has been associated with mismatches at the HLA-A2 focus (108), the detection of cytotoxic B-cell antibodies (109), and episodes of acute rejection (100). Regarding the latter, however, studies at Stanford failed to show a correlation between episodes of acute rejection and graft coronary disease (110). More recent studies have shown a correlation between CMV infections and graft atherosclerosis (111,112). Cytomegalovirus infection has also been associated with increased rejection in kidney (113,114) and liver transplantation (115). Cytomegalovirus is believed to promote rejection reactions through the upregulation of major histocompatibility complex (MHC) class I and II antigen expression on cell surfaces (116,117).

The incidence and severity of graft atherosclerosis varies and appears to be directly related to the duration of allograft survival. It has occurred as early as 3 months following surgery, with reported incidences of 1 to 4% at 1 year and between 40 to 50% at 5 years posttransplantation (100,103,118). The clinical introduction of cyclosporine has made no significant impact on the occurrence of graft coronary disease, and its incidence remains similar to that seen during the precyclosporine era (110). This finding dampened hopes that more effective immunosuppression might prevent the development of atherosclerosis in the allograft.

The identification of risk factors that predispose to the development of graft atherosclerosis has not been fruitful. Patient age, lipid profiles, and blood glucose levels—common associated risk factors for ordinary coronary disease—do not correlate with graft atherogenesis. It occurs just as frequently in recipients transplanted for cardiomyopathy as it does in those transplanted for coronary arteriosclerosis (102). This tends to place greater emphasis on immune-related mechanisms rather than metabolic ones for the development of graft coronary disease in the heart transplant in comparison to that acquired in the nontransplant population.

Whether manifested gradually or abruptly, the clinical consequences of graft atherosclerosis are all quite serious and may include impaired left ventricular function, congestive heart failure, dysrhythmias, myocardial infarction, and sudden death. Although rapidly progressive and ischemic in nature, anginal-type symptoms are usually absent with graft coronary disease as a result of cardiac denervation. Typically, myocardial infarction is silent and is often discovered for the first time at autopsy. Recently, however, as noted earlier, chest pain has been reported in recipients with acute ischemic cardiac events, suggesting the possibility of cardiac reinnervation.

Since the initial clinical manifestations of graft coronary artery disease are most often associated with advanced disease, in the absence of angina pectoris as an early warning sign, the serial use of coronary angiography is required as a method of surveillance for the early detection of graft atherosclerosis. Diagnosis relies on inspection and careful comparisons of coronary angiograms that are obtained at regular intervals, or for clinical indications, following heart transplantation. As a matter of routine, coronary angiograms are performed within 2 to 4 weeks of transplantation in order to obtain qualitative/quantitative assessments of arterial luminal diameters as baseline points of reference that can later be comparatively followed with serial studies for changes in luminal size.

Diffuse concentric narrowing of epicardial coronary arteries that extends into smaller branches, and the lack of coronary collaterals are distinctive morphological features of graft coronary artery disease. While focal discrete epicardial stenosis, seen with ordinary coronary artery disease, is more readily detected by coronary angiography, the diffuse and concentric nature of graft atherosclerosis can make angiographic detection more difficult and may underestimate the degree of coronary artery disease (102,119). This problem can readily be overcome by careful comparisons of serially obtained angiograms. On very rare occasions, graft coronary disease may affect only intramyocardial arterioles, and endomyocardial biopsy is usually normal unless it happens to contain a section of involved arterioles. Although rare, this should be suspected in unexplained graft failure where rejection has been ruled out and the coronary angiogram is normal (102).

Advances in ultrasound imaging technology have led to the development of intravascular ultrasound imaging probes that can be used to measure the intraluminal diameters of vessels directly in addition to providing intravascular images. Intravascular ultrasound has recently been used to assess the coronary arteries of heart transplant recipients (120). This technique shows the potential for earlier detection of the concentric intraluminal narrowing of graft atherosclerosis than coronary angiography. Studies are currently in progress to determine whether intracoronary ultrasonography imaging is more sensitive than coronary angiography for detecting the early lesions of graft coronary artery disease.

Other methods have been used to monitor for graft coronary artery disease. Serial electrocardiograms can be useful for detecting silent myocardial infarction or ventricular ectopy. In the latter case, the demonstration of LOWN type III ventricular dysrhythmias by Holter monitoring has been correlated with a poor prognosis and a high incidence of graft coronary artery disease (121). Abnormalities in systolic and diastolic ventricular function and, in particular, the detection of segmental wall motion abnormalities by 2D echocardiography or radionuclide ventriculography may be indicative of graft coronary artery disease. Global wall motion dysfunction may be seen with diffuse coronary disease as well. However with global, systolic, or diastolic ventricular dysfunction, acute rejection should also be given serious consideration and be excluded. Although exercise and thallium-201 dipyridamole scanning are utilized to screen for myocardial ischemic disease (122), they have not been shown to be sensitive or specific enough for detecting graft atherosclerosis in cardiac transplants given the propensity of these patients to develop diffuse concentric disease (121). Since similar changes can be seen with acute rejection events, these events again would have to be ruled out. Under most circumstances, noninvasive methods would have a greater tendency to detect the abnormalities associated with graft coronary artery disease at the later stages of disease and require exclusion of acute rejection. In general, they can be considered as useful adjuncts and complementary to coronary angiography for making the diagnosis of graft atherosclerosis. As more experience is accrued with intracoronary ultrasonography, it has the potential to replace coronary angiography for the diagnosis of graft atherosclerosis.

Cardiac retransplantation offers the only definitive therapy for severe graft atherosclerosis. Although angioplasty may be of some benefit on occasion, where focal stenosis exists, it should be considered only palliative at best, given the diffuse nature of the coronary artery disease usually present. Despite inferior long-term results with retransplantation as compared to primary cardiac transplantation (123), it still offers the best chance for extended survival in carefully selected recipients with graft atherosclerosis. In this context, the early diagnosis of graft coronary artery disease takes on greater importance if the cardiac recipient is to have every opportunity for extended life. In cases of allograft dysfunction in which acute rejection has been excluded by endomyocardial biopsy and cannot be accounted for otherwise, the diagnosis of graft atherosclerosis should be given serious consideration in recipients surviving for more than 6 months and, in particular, in those who have survived for more than a year following transplantation.

III. REJECTION IN LUNG ALLOGRAFTS

In lung transplantation more than in heart transplantation, the clinical manifestations of rejection can be affected by a variety of factors that are unrelated to rejection per se. Whereas orthotopic heart transplantation involves the same procedure for all indications, lung transplantation, in comparison, encompasses a variety of transplant procedures that are selected on an individual basis to meet specific sets of clinical indications for a variety of pulmonary and cardiopulmonary disorders. As a result of this diversity, for both procedure and disease, the type of transplant operation, the nature of complications that may arise, and the clinical disorder for which transplantation is undertaken may all have some bearing on how rejection of the lung allograft becomes clinically manifest.

The various lung transplant procedures include en bloc combined heart-lung transplantation and en bloc double-lung transplantation with tracheal anastomosis; bilateral sequential single-lung transplantation utilizing bronchial anastomosis for replacement of both lungs; and unilateral single-lung transplantation. Currently among these procedures, the en bloc double lung transplant is the least used clinically, as a result of frequent complications at the tracheal anastomotic site (124). On rare occasions, combined heart-single lung transplants have also been performed (125). More recently, lung lobes derived from living related donors have been successfully transplanted, both unilaterally and bilaterally, as replacements for whole lung (126).

Despite differences in the clinical course that may arise with the various procedures, in general the clinical manifestations, consequences, and diagnosis of lung rejection are similar enough for all forms of lung transplantation to permit a common discussion of all. Where important differences may exist, these are addressed and discussed accordingly.

A. Acute Lung Rejection

1. Clinical Manifestations

There are no unique clinical features that readily distinguish the early manifestations of acute lung rejection from other disorders that can affect the allograft. Although the history and physical examination are of value for detecting abnormalities that warrant further clinical investigation, in particular to rule out infection, the findings are usually nonspecific and often irrelevant with respect to rejection.

Modifications of the allograft incurred at the time of harvesting and transplantation may also contribute to some of the early pulmonary changes that can be seen. Disruption of the bronchial circulation and pulmonary lymphatic system, denervation, impairment of mucociliary clearance, possible alterations of local immune responses to inhaled antigens or pathogens aspirated from the upper respiratory tracts (e.g., infected sinuses, as in cystic fibrosis and bronchiectasis), or inadequate preservation can make the allograft more vulnerable to the development of pulmonary infections, interstitial edema, or diffuse alveolar damage (DAD), which in turn, can further obscure the early recognition of acute rejection.

The clinical manifestations of acute rejection can be either insidious or dramatic at onset, and patients may present with a variety of signs and symptoms that may include malaise, fever, dyspnea, cough, leukocytosis, oxygen desaturation, tachypnea, tachycardia, adventitial breath sounds on chest auscultation, dullness to percussion, and pulmonary infiltrates with or without pleural effusions by chest radiography. These findings can fit equally well with infection, and in some cases in the absence of infection, with DAD or the various forms of pulmonary edema that can arise. Even though these findings are not pathognomonic for acute rejection or infection, knowing the time of occurrence since transplantation can be useful in considering the likelihood of rejection in a given patient.

Complications arising in the early posttransplant period are usually those associated with surgery, inadequate graft preservation, covert donor-organ complications, infection, and acute rejection. Intrathoracic hemorrhage, anastomotic breakdowns, primary graft failure or the "reimplantation response," as well as episodes of acute rejection and infection are most likely to occur within the first 2 weeks following transplantation. In addition, pulmonary edema may also arise during this period from volume overload associated with excessive fluid administration and/or renal insufficiency.

In an analysis of 144 lung transplants (heart-lung, single lung, double lung) performed over a 9 year period, the Pittsburgh group documented the temporal sequence of postoperative complications that occurred following transplantation (127). Excluding surgical complications, the adult respiratory distress syndrome (ARDS), resulting from graft ischemic/ preservation injury, tended to occur in the immediate postoperative period. Bacterial pneumonia and acute rejection appeared in the first few weeks following transplantation. Cytomegalovirus infection and/or pneumonitis as well as fungal, other viral, and *Pneumocystis carinii* infections occurred later in the posttransplant course. The recognition of temporal relationships, although not absolute, permits anticipation of the possible disorders that might occur at various times from transplantation.

Acute lung rejection is distinctly uncommon in the first postoperative week. Adult respiratory distress syndrome from severe pneumonia, preservation injury, or pulmonary edema are the complications most frequently observed in the first postoperative week. Pneumonia, though somewhat uncommon, is more likely to be due to aerobic gram-negative rods and less often to gram-positive bacteria; rarely, other nosocomial pathogens such as *Legionella* species may be involved. Preservation injury or acute rejection may be confirmed histopathologically by transbronchial lung biopsy once infection is ruled out by blood cultures and/or special stains and cultures performed on airway secretions or BAL fluid obtained by fiberoptic bronchoscopy. Pulmonary edema as a result of disrupted pulmonary lymphatics, in conjunction with fluctuations in volume, instabilities of the early postoperative state, and varying degrees of renal impairment may also occur during this period and remains as a diagnosis of exclusion. However, the aggressive use of diuretics, intravascular volume restriction, and the heightened awareness of altered pulmonary fluid dynamics lessens the likelihood of pulmonary edema during this time.

The incidence of acute lung rejection is at its peak between the second and sixth postoperative week. The potential for rejection remains elevated until the fourth postoperative month, at which time rejection episodes begin to decline provided that immunosuppressive therapy remains adequate. A large part of the clinical effort during this period is devoted to the early detection of rejection and infection and the management of complications that may arise. This primarily involves close clinical observation, serial chest radiographs, pulmonary function studies, and surveillance transbronchial lung biopsies with BAL to monitor for rejection and infections in the allografts of lung transplant recipients. In the case of heart-lung transplant recipients, this would also include endomyocardial biopsy to monitor for asynchronous heart rejection. Along with routine surveillance, additional bronchoscopies with biopsy and BAL are performed as dictated by clinical indications. Asymptomatic acute lung rejection that may be suspected by leukocytosis, abnormal chest radiographs, and deteriorating pulmonary function and arterial blood gas measurements can be confirmed by transbronchial biopsy with the exclusion of infection.

The "reimplantation response," most likely a less severe form of preservation injury, may also arise in the second postoperative week and can be confused with rejection and infection on chest film or clinical grounds alone. Even though the tendency for acute rejection is at its highest during the early posttransplant period, the risk for infection in the lung allograft is ever-present. This risk for infection is further enhanced when acute rejection is treated with high-dose corticosteroid therapy, or, in cases of persistent or recurrent rejection, with the use of cytolytic therapy with monoclonal or polyclonal antibodies. Susceptibilities to opportunistic and latent infections are particularly enhanced with augmented levels of immunosuppression. All of these factors further emphasize the need for diagnostic precision before embarking on a course of aggressive immunosuppressive therapy.

2. *Chest Radiography*

The chest radiograph has played an important surveillance role in monitoring for complications that may arise in the lung allograft following transplantation. Although valuable for early detection of abnormal changes in the lung, the chest radiograph lacks the sensitivity and specificity for discriminating between acute rejection, infection, and pulmonary edema in the allograft. Most of thc radiographic changes seen in the early postoperative period following heart-lung and lung transplantation are similar to those radiographic changes seen following other major thoracic or cardiac surgery. The changes observed in the transplanted population, however, may differ as a result of a number of factors, which include the physical trauma associated with procurement and implantation of the allograft; alterations that may arise from the surgical disruption of the bronchial circulation, pulmonary neural supply, or pulmonary lymphatic system; potential leaks or dehiscence of the various anastomotic sites; and the sequelae of acute allograft rejection. Additionally, the risk of infection is greater in transplant recipients because of the immunosuppressive therapy required to maintain their allografts. The ability to distinguish rejection from opportunistic infections and other pulmonary complications is critical to the successful long-term management of lung transplant recipients.

Radiographic abnormalities most frequently seen with acute rejection have included hilar flare, ill-defined opacities or infiltrates, "airspace" disease, peribronchial cuffing, subpleural effusions, prominent septal lines, and pleural effusions (128,129). Although generally considered to be nonspecific, some of these changes are more likely than others to be associated with rejection. Pleural effusion is reportedly found in 65% of acute rejection episodes and is probably the most common abnormality present in the early posttransplant period (129). Among all abnormalities, the combination of prominent septal lines with pleural effusion has been reported to be the radiographic finding most suggestive of acute rejection (129). Bergin et al., in a study that correlated radiographic findings with transbronchial lung biopsy results in heart-lung transplant recipients, found that the combination of septal lines and new or increasing pleural effusions without a concomitant increase in cardiac size or vascular pedicle width or evidence of vascular redistribution indicated acute lung rejection with a sensitivity of 68%, specificity of 90%, and overall accuracy of 83% (129).

The likelihood of an abnormal chest radiograph with acute lung rejection tends to be greater in the early posttransplant period. Millet et al. reported the chest radiograph to be abnormal in 74% of the acute lung rejection episodes that occurred in the first month following heart-lung transplantation but abnormal in only 23% of acute rejection episodes that occurred thereafter (128). Since these radiographic abnormalities may not readily distinguish rejection from infection, transbronchial lung biopsy with BAL is warranted to confirm rejection and to rule out infection. Millet et al. concluded from their studies that the chest radiograph provides a useful indication for transbronchial biopsy and BAL during the first postoperative month. Reductions in the forced expiratory volume in the first second (FEV_1) and vital capacity (VC), together with symptoms and an abnormal chest exam, provided a more reliable indication for bronchoscopy for ruling out rejection or infection beyond the first month (128).

Despite the nonspecific nature of the chest radiograph, the "clinical diagnosis" of acute lung rejection has been made on the basis of radiographic criteria alone. This represents a presumptive diagnosis of acute rejection based upon the clearance of radiographic abnormalities following a course of antirejection therapy with high-dosage corticosteroids following the exclusion of infection (130). Although biopsy confirmation of rejection is preferable before the commencement of therapy, this approach has been used in situations where the risks of lung biopsy were considered to be excessive. In this situation, however, some caution is warranted, since the misdiagnosis of infection for rejection with the institution of "blind" antirejection therapy also carries with it considerable risk. In general, with the possible exception of the first postoperative week, the development of asymptomatic pulmonary infiltrates on the chest radiograph mandates bronchoscopy with transbronchial lung biopsy and BAL for proper diagnosis and, in particular, to rule out acute lung rejection and infection.

3. Pulmonary Function

Pulmonary function tests are important for assessing the long-term functional integrity of the lung allografts following transplantation. In this capacity, they also play a major role in the long-term surveillance of the allografts for the development of complications. Functional abnormalities as a consequence of complicating disease can be readily detected by serial measurements of pulmonary function performed at frequent intervals. Even though they are sensitive for detecting and accurately defining the underlying physiologic abnormalities present in the lungs, pulmonary function tests, in and of themselves, do not provide specific diagnoses with respect to etiology. In this regard they are similar to the chest radiograph in their inability to clearly distinguish between acute rejection, infection, and pulmonary edema, particularly in the earlier phases of the posttransplant period. After the first few months, however, the assessment of pulmonary function is more useful than the chest radiograph in providing indications for transbronchial lung biopsy with BAL to rule out acute rejection and exclude infection, since radiographic abnormalities tend to be less prevalent with acute rejection beyond that point (128). Despite the fact that these tests do not identify specific disease, there are some specific changes found on pulmonary function testing that may tend to favor rejection over infection in some circumstances.

Although comprehensive pulmonary function testing provides more information, spirometry has been an effective means of monitoring pulmonary function in heart-lung and lung-transplanted patients. It can be done frequently and expeditiously with minimal discomfort to patients. It is more than sufficient for detecting significant functional changes that may occur with complications. As part of the spirometric measurement, the flow volume relationships for the lungs ("flow-volume loop") can also be determined from the forced expiratory and inspiratory vital capacity maneuvers. This permits measurements of the forced expiratory flow rates at 25% (FEF_{25}), 50% (FEF_{50}), 75% (FEF_{75}) and the determination of the slope of the line between the forced expiratory flow rate at 25% and 75% (FEF_{25-75}) of the forced vital capacity (FVC). At Stanford, in addition to spirometry, we also include measurements of diffusing capacity for carbon monoxide (DLCO) and arterial blood gases as part of routine surveillance. The more comprehensive studies in our program are usually performed at 3 to 6 months and 12 months posttransplant and then annually thereafter.

In uncomplicated cases, the early postoperative functional abnormalities in heart-lung and lung transplantation are those usually associated with major cardiac or thoracic surgery. These primarily involve reductions in lung volumes [total lung capacity (TLC), inspiratory capacity (IC), vital capacity (VC), forced vital capacity (FVC)], and timed volumes [e.g., forced expiratory volume in 1 sec (FEV_1)] as a result of a moderately severe restrictive defect (131). Alterations of the chest wall from surgery and disparities in volume, where the lung allograft may be smaller with respect to the thoracic cavity, are the principal causes of the restriction. These tend to improve with time and usually are of little consequence to long-term function in heart-lung and bilateral lung-transplanted patients (132,133). In single-lung transplantation however, some of these functional abnormalities may persist, depending upon the mechanical properties of the nontransplanted lung. Despite this, nonetheless, overall function is still significantly improved when compared to overall function prior to transplantation. Although some impairment in gas exchange may also be present in the immediate postoperative period, this tends to resolve within the first few weeks, and gas exchange becomes essentially normal by the first month following transplantation with an uncomplicated postoperative course.

Changes in baseline airway function and gas exchange (arterial blood gases) appear to be of greater importance than changes associated with restriction in monitoring pulmonary function for complications, most notably rejection and infection. Among these, even though not diagnostic, significant reductions in mid-expiratory flow rates (FEF_{25-75}) and FEV_1 tend to favor rejection over other causes, warranting follow-up transbronchial lung biopsy with BAL for confirmation. Not infrequently, however, mild acute rejection may be found by transbronchial lung biopsy without concomitant changes in baseline function, both in the presence or absence of chest radiographic abnormalities. This further emphasizes the need for surveillance lung biopsies for the detection of acute lung rejection, particularly in the early posttransplant period.

In separate studies, the Papworth and Stanford groups demonstrated the development of obstructive airway dynamics as a manifestation of lung rejection in heart-lung transplant recipients (134,135). In the reports from Papworth, a significant fall in the FEV_1 was emphasized and used as an indication for lung biopsy to confirm rejection and rule out infection. In a prospective study at Stanford, in which transbronchial lung biopsy and BAL results were compared with measurements of pulmonary function 16 heart-lung transplant recipients, Starnes et al. demonstrated significant reductions in FEV_1, FEF_{25-75}, and arterial oxygen tension from baseline values during episodes of acute lung rejection, with no change in the FVC (135). Computed as mean values (±SD), FEV_1 fell from 75.7 ± 20.1% to 52.7 ± 18.3% of predicted, FEF_{25-75} from 97.6 ± 30.5% to 49.8 ± 22.3% of predicted, and

Pa_{O_2} from 92.1 ± 8.8 mmHg to 71.4 ± 18.8 mmHg during rejection, with all changes significant at *p* values less than 0.05 (ANOVA). The most dramatic fall was in the FEF_{25-75}. In comparison, pulmonary infection, including CMV and *Pneumocystis carinii*, produced a significant fall in Pa_{O_2} from baseline values with less dramatic changes in FVC, FEV_1, and FEF_{25-75}, which were not statistically significant. Although some decline in FEV_1 and FEF_{25-75} did occur with infection, these changes were less than those associated with rejection. In comparing deterioration of pulmonary function between patients with rejection and infection, the best discriminating parameter was the fall in FEF_{25-75}. The FEF_{25-75} during rejection was significantly lower than the FEF_{25-75} during infection (135).

Similar obstructive changes in heart-lung recipients with acute lung rejection were also reported by the Hanover Transplant Group, who found significant reductions in FEV_1, the FEV_1/inspiratory vital capacity (IVC) ratio, and FEF_{50} along with an increase in the $P(A\text{-}a)_{O_2}$ gradient (136). They further suggested that changes in pulmonary function might discriminate between rejection and infection, particularly if the latter is divided into viral and bacterial infection. In viral infections, particularly with CMV the most impressive finding was a significant decrease in DLCO without any significant obstructive or restrictive changes or change in the $P(A\text{-}a)_{O_2}$ gradient. In bacterial pneumonia, on the other hand, decreases in IVC and FEV_1 were found in conjunction with an increase in the $P(A\text{-}a)_{O_2}$ gradient. There were no significant changes in the FEV_1/IVC ratio and FEF_{50}. These functional changes are consistent with increasing restriction without significant airway obstruction, since the decreases in IVC and FEV_1 are in proportion to one another as reflected by the lack of change in the FEV_1/IVC ratio and FEF_{50}. One drawback in these studies, however, is the small size of the study population.

In a larger study reported from Papworth, the ability of pulmonary function tests to distinguish between rejection and infection was not readily apparent (134). In measurements of VC, FEV_1, DLCO, and total lung capacity (TLC) that were correlated with lung biopsy results, all parameters except TLC were significantly reduced for both rejection and infection, with the decrease in TLC occurring only with rejection. The latter finding indicates the development of a restrictive component with rejection, along with obstruction, which differs from the Hanover study where an increase in restriction was associated with bacterial pneumonia (136). Although the FEV_1 was significantly reduced with both rejection and infection in the Papworth study, the reduction in FEV_1 was greater during rejection. However, no measurements of the midexpiratory flow rates, which may be more sensitive for detecting early changes in small airway dynamics, were reported by the Papworth group.

The sensitivity of pulmonary function tests for detecting rejection and infection was also analyzed by the Papworth group from their results (134). Pulmonary function testing showed a sensitivity of 86% for detecting rejection within the first 3 months following transplantation and a 75% sensitivity in the period thereafter. The sensitivity for detecting infection was 75%. Although these two complications could not be distinguished, assessment of pulmonary function had a sensitivity of 84% for detecting the occurrence of acute lung complications following transplantation.

The interpretation of pulmonary function in single-lung transplant recipients is more complex. These recipients are not the physiologic equivalents of heart-lung or double-lung transplant recipients. The single-lung recipients have a lung allograft that functions in parallel with their native lung, which retains its pathology. Thus, the allograft and native lung, depending on the original disease, make different contributions to subsequent lung function. It is not possible to separate the effect of each lung on pulmonary function without highly invasive split function studies requiring double-lumen intubation. Such studies seem impractical on a surveillance basis. Therefore, conventional pulmonary function tests have been employed to monitor function in these patients as well (137). Despite limitations and their lack of specificity, serial spirometry and arterial blood gas measurements have been found useful and reasonably sensitive as screening tests for detecting acute complications in single-lung transplant recipients provided that each patient serves as his or her own baseline control (138,139).

In an early study, serial measurements of pulmonary function were compared prospectively with transbronchial lung biopsy and BAL results in 6 patients following single-lung transplantation for either pulmonary fibrosis or pulmonary hypertension. Marshall et al. found that the presence of significant disease in the allograft was reflected by acute decrements in function (139). Some 85% of the episodes of acute rejection or significant infection were associated with falls in the FEF_{25-75} or Pa_{O_2} of more than 10% from baseline values. Although these functional changes demonstrated a sensitivity of 85% for detecting these acute complications, the specificity was only 50%. It should be noted, however, that changes in Pa_{O_2} and FEF_{25-75} frequently occurred after the diagnosis of significant disease and had later returned to baseline before resolution of the histological process. This suggests that pathological changes may either appear earlier than physiological disruption in the single-lung recipients or that such changes are masked by the function of the native lung. Nevertheless, the positive predictive value of these changes was high, with 74% for falls in FEF_{25-75} and 82% for falls in Pa_{O_2}. These changes were associated with significant morphological or BAL abnormalities.

In a larger study by Becker et al. on pulmonary functional changes associated with acute complicating events in single-lung transplantation, the pathology of the native lung was found to be a key determinant in limiting the detection of rejection in single-lung transplant recipients (SLT) by spirometry (140). In their study, the effects of acute episodes of rejection, infection, and bronchiolitis on the pulmonary function of 30 SLT patients with varying underlying disease states were prospectively analyzed. The study population included 17 patients with obstructive pulmonary disease (SLT-OBS), 6 with pulmonary fibrosis (SLT-IPF), and 7 with pulmonary vascular disease (SLT-PVD). This well-done study clearly defined the diagnostic limitations of spirometry in this patient population and demonstrated that the sensitivity, specificity, and positive predictive value of an abnormal spirogram in SLT is limited by the pathological nature of the remaining native lung, the function of which also greatly influences overall pulmonary function. In these studies, rejection was associated with significant reductions in FVC for all patient groups. Rejection was associated with significant decreases in FEV_1 in SLT-OBS and SLT-PVD but not in SLT-IPF. A significant fall in FEF_{25-75} during rejection was seen only in the SLT-PVD group. The greatest falls in FVC, FEV_1, and FEF_{25-75} were most often seen with acute bronchiolitis, followed by acute rejection. The sensitivity and specificity of spirometry as a predictor of rejection/infection is significantly lower in SLT than it is for heart-lung transplantation, with SLT-PVD having the most and SLT-OBS the least useful prognostic values spirometrically. The most accurate spirometric parameters for predicting acute pulmonary events also varied among the different patient populations (140). In SLT-OBS, although results were uniformly poor, the best parameter for predicting an acute event appeared to be a 10% fall in FEF_{25-75}, which showed a sensitivity of 48%, specificity of 56%, and a positive predictive value of 65%. In SLT-IPF, a drop in FVC of 15% appeared to be more useful clinically, with a sensitivity of 69%, specificity of 76%, and positive predictive value of 64%. In SLT-PVD, a 10% decrease in FVC showed a sensitivity of 61%, specificity of 82%, and positive predictive value of 85%. Thus, from these results, the nature of the underlying pulmonary disease for which SLT is performed appears to dictate which spirometric parameter will be the most useful for predicting acute events in the allograft.

Becker et al. concluded that the lack of specificity of spirometry in predicting rejection does not mean that it lacks clinical utility, only that changes in spirometry cannot be unequivocally attributed to changes in graft function (140). In this case, there may still be active disease in the native lung, which will also effect function. As such, a change in spirometry remains significant in that it may indicate an alteration in either the allograft or the native lung which will require attention.

In summary, even though pulmonary function tests are lacking in specificity, the close monitoring of pulmonary function permits the early detection of rejection and infection in SLT, often prior to the onset of clinical symptoms. Any significant alteration in pulmonary mechanics or gas exchange, even in the absence of clinical signs or symptoms, should prompt bronchoscopy with transbronchial lung biopsy and bronchoalveolar lavage to rule out rejection and/or infection.

4. *Radionuclide Ventilation:Perfusion ($\dot{V}/\dot{Q}$) Scans*

Serial quantitative radionuclide ventilation:perfusion ($\dot{V}/\dot{Q}$) scans can be useful for the detection of acute lung rejection in single-lung transplants (SLT). Although there are no characteristic $\dot{V}/\dot{Q}$ patterns that are diagnostic of rejection, serial scans permit the detection and comparison of $\dot{V}/\dot{Q}$ changes in the lung allograft with those in the recipient's native lung, which may be an index of rejection. The respective distributions of ventilation and perfusion are dependent upon the mechanical properties of the lung (i.e., elastic properties, or compliance, and airway resistance) and pulmonary vascular resistances. Early changes in $\dot{V}/\dot{Q}$ patterns that develop in the allograft during acute rejection are more likely to be seen in SLT because of the differences in lung mechanics and vascular resistance that exist between the allograft and native diseased lung. In double-lung (DLT) and heart-lung (HLT) transplants, however, it would not be particularly useful to monitor for rejection with $\dot{V}/\dot{Q}$ scans, since the mechanical and vascular properties are the same for both lungs; as a result, the changes in $\dot{V}$ and $\dot{Q}$ during acute rejection would be essentially the same in both lungs and difficult to distinguish.

At Stanford, quantitative $\dot{V}/\dot{Q}$ scans are performed utilizing ^{99m}Tc-labeled macroaggregated albumin to assess perfusion and krypton-81m gas for assessing ventilation, with the relative ventilation and perfusion calculated for each lung. Following SLT, $\dot{V}$ and $\dot{Q}$ to the allograft increases progressively postoperatively, with the differences in $\dot{V}$ and $\dot{Q}$ between the native recipient lung and allograft reflecting differences in their dynamic properties.

In SLT for pulmonary fibrosis, or emphysema/COPD, both $\dot{V}$ and $\dot{Q}$ tend to divert gradually toward the transplanted lung with the passage of time (141–143), whereas in SLT for pulmonary hypertension, the entire $\dot{Q}$ is essentially diverted to the allograft in the immediate postoperative period with only minor shifts in $\dot{V}$ because of the high pulmonary vascular resistance in the native lung (141). These factors must be taken into account in assessing $\dot{V}/\dot{Q}$ changes that may be associated with acute rejection.

Early reports noted shifts in $\dot{Q}$ away from the allograft toward the nontransplanted lung during acute episodes of rejection and infection in SLT for emphysema (144,145). Later, similar results were also reported by the St. Louis group (Barnes) for episodes of acute rejections in SLT for emphysema (143). Rejection events in these studies, however, were defined by the patient's clinical response to pulsed methylprednisolone, without tissue confirmation of rejection by transbronchial lung biopsy.

In SLT for pulmonary fibrosis and pulmonary hypertension, Kramer et al. showed that, during acute episodes of biopsy-proven lung rejection, there was a shift of $\dot{V}$ away from the transplanted lung without any changes in perfusion (141). The latter finding is not surprising in SLT for pulmonary hypertension since most or all of the $\dot{Q}$ goes to the allograft because of the large difference in pulmonary vascular resistance found between the two lungs. There are no recent data regarding the changes in $\dot{V}/\dot{Q}$ during infection or pulmonary edema. It is highly unlikely that $\dot{V}/\dot{Q}$ scanning in this form would be specific in this regard.

In summary, although quantitative radionuclide ventilation:perfusion scans appear to be of some use in monitoring for acute rejection in SLT, they lack specificity for making the diagnosis. If $\dot{V}/\dot{Q}$ changes arise that warrant further consideration, transbronchial lung biopsy and bronchoalveolar lavage are indicated to rule out rejection and/or infection. Surveillance transbronchial lung biopsies and bronchoalveolar lavage are also needed in SLT, DLT, and HLT to effectively manage patients in monitoring for lung rejection and infections and other complications with the goal of preventing chronic allograft dysfunction.

5. *Bronchoalveolar Lavage*

So as to fully explain some of the recent findings obtained from BAL in lung allograft recipients, a brief review of the basic immunology of lung rejection is in order. The immune response to an alloantigen, such as a lung allograft or any foreign agent from the atmosphere that is uniquely in direct contact with the lung, is diversified. Donor cells (DC) appear to initiate this immune response by expressing different MHC from the recipient. These DC, in turn, trigger cellular and humoral immunity from recipient lymphocytes, which are crucial in the generation of the rejection response (147). Unregulated cellular immunity relies on the activation of T-helper lymphocytes. Recently, T-helper lymphocytes have been divided into two types, Th-1 and Th-2, based primarily on the cytokines they produce (148,149). Some of these cytokines have been shown to stimulate B lymphocytes to yield specific IgG subtypes. Analysis of these specific IgG subtypes may provide markers of Th-1 and Th-2 activity. For example, Th-1 helper T-cell clones release gamma interferon (IFN), which, in turn, stimulates the production of IgG2; whereas Th-2 lymphocytes produce IL-4, which, in turn, stimulates the production of IgG1 from B lymphocytes (150,151). Wilkes et al. (152) have recently demonstrated the differential effects of accessory cell populations on IgG synthesis by demonstrating that B lymphocytes in the peripheral blood produce IgG1 and IgG2 in response to the lung allograft. In their human lung model, they found that IgG2 production was dependent solely on gamma IFN production from T lymphocytes, suggesting that IgG2 production in response to the lung alloantigen relies primarily on the activation of Th-1 lymphocytes. During acute allograft rejection, infiltrating lymphocytes preferentially produce gamma IFN. In this regard, the lung allograft is an immunological reservoir where many immunocompetent cells can be a source of alloantigen (153). When activated recipient T lymphocytes accumulate into and infiltrate the lung allograft, the result is believed to be acute lung rejection.

Especially when compared to open lung biopsy, BAL is a benign procedure. Fortunately, BAL provides an opportunity to retrieve large numbers of cells from the lung allograft. Therefore, sampling this immunologic environment with BAL may be valuable in diagnosing the pulmonary complications following heart-lung or lung transplantation (154,155). Moreover, it would appear to be a sensitive means to detect any perturbation in the cellular elements or soluble products of these cellular elements, as described above. Several studies, for example, have reported increased numbers of polymorphonuclear cells from samples of BAL fluid during episodes of rejection and infection (156–158).

Although BAL may be sensitive for detecting any pulmonary complication, the more important dilemma has been its inability to distinguish rejection from infection without transbronchial lung biopsy (TBB). A few studies have attempted to identify a marker specific for rejection, even in the presence of infection, by BAL. The Papworth group (156) compared 135 BAL samples in 48 heart-lung recipients with concurrent histologic findings obtained from TBB. Five diagnostic groups were identified: normal (NL), acute rejection (ALR), treated rejection (TR), infection (INF), and chronic rejection (CR). Expression of HLA-DR and IL-2R was amplified in the BAL cells in all diagnostic groups. The highest BAL lymphocyte counts were recovered in the ALR group, primarily from an increase in $CD8^+$ cells. Although the ALR group had a relative BAL lymphocytosis, no distinction could be made from the INF group or any other group because of the large variations in cell numbers. Also, there was no correlation with the percentage of lymphocytes by BAL and the histological grade of rejection. The investigators concluded that BAL offered no further diagnostic utility in the diagnosis of lung rejection in heart-lung recipients.

The Stanford group (158) applied the polymerase chain reaction to evaluate cytokine gene expression in BAL cells and peripheral blood leukocytes in 31 lung allograft recipients in an attempt to find a marker specific for rejection. The transcripts of a number of cytokines were identified in both BAL and peripheral blood samples in this study population. The mRNA transcripts for the cytokines IL-1 through IL-8, TNF-beta, and gamma IFN were identified in BAL cells and peripheral blood lymphocytes (PBL) from these lung recipients. Increased expression of the transcripts for IL-4 were detectable in acute rejection but not during infection. This study concluded that IL-4 transcripts might be useful as a discriminatory rejection marker. Though promising, this finding has not been repeated or validated.

In another study in quest of a specific marker to distinguish acute lung rejection from infection, Wilkes and associates (159) suggested a BAL IgG2/IgG1 ratio $\geqslant 1$ might show promise as a specific marker. Twenty-five bronchoscopies with TBB and BAL were performed on 18 lung allograft recipients; 5 nonsmoking normal volunteers served as controls. The IgG1 and IgG2 levels were measured and the IgG2/IgG1 ratio was calculated in serum and BAL. These results were matched with the morphological findings. The investigators determined that the IgG2/IgG1 $\geqslant 1$ had a specificity of 80%, a sensitivity of 91%, and a positive predictive value of 92%. They also noted no association with CMV culture status in the BAL fluid and the IgG2/IgG1 ratio. These results suggest that, during acute rejection, predominantly Th-1 lymphocytes are activated, which is in opposition to the report by Whitehead et al., who found increased expression of IL-4 gene transcripts, a product of activated Th-2 lymphocytes, during rejection only. This suggests that the dichotomy of Th-1 and Th-2 lymphocytes based on cytokine production may not be absolute or that unknown errors in either Whitehead's or Wilkes's study affected their results. Though half their patients had CMV cultured from their BAL, not one recipient was diagnosed with pneumonitis based on TBB. As they pointed out, they could draw no conclusion regarding the effect of viral or opportunistic infection on the BAL IgG2/IgG1 ratio.

Despite its limited utility in discriminating rejection from infection, BAL has been proven useful for diagnosing opportunistic infections in the transplanted lung and invaluable as a research tool in the understanding of lung allograft immunology. The Pittsburgh group has reported on the alloreactivity of lung allograft-infiltrating lymphocytes employing BAL (147,154,160,161). They analyzed sequential BAL isolates of macrophages and lymphocytes using histocompatibility phenotyping. This analysis determined that the donor macrophages and lymphocytes were replaced rapidly by recipient macrophages and lymphocytes in the first 4 weeks following lung transplantation. This transition was nearly complete 12 weeks after transplantation (162). Most importantly, this study verified that the pulmonary alveolar macrophage originated from the bone marrow. In a separate study, they described the immune response of the lymphocytes obtained from peripheral blood and BAL in heart-lung recipients. Donor-specific alloreactivity in a primed lymphocyte test (PLT) was demonstrated by analyzing the BAL lymphocytes recovered from recipients' allografts during acute rejection (154). The sensitivity of a positive PLT was 91% for rejection; however, a positive PLT was observed in 32% of infection events, including bacterial, CMV, and *P. carinii* pneumonia. The PLT performed on the recipients' PBL was positive in only 45% of acute rejection episodes. Thus, despite the excellent sensitivity of the PLT assay using BAL lymphocytes, this assay was nonspecific. In terms of chronic rejection, defined by a progressive decrease in pulmonary function in conjunction with morphologically proven obliterative bronchiolitis (154), a positive PLT test from the BAL and the PBL was demonstrated in 69 and 60% of chronic rejection episodes, respectively. Also, its specificity was 80% for BAL lymphocytes and 84% for peripheral blood lymphocytes. Thus, the PLT assay may supplement pulmonary function tests and transbronchial lung biopsies in monitoring the allograft for chronic rejection. However, this methodology may not be applicable clinically because of time constraints—it required 3 days of incubation with the recipient's BAL lymphocytes—and the necessity to have stored donor spleen or lymph nodes obtained at the time of organ procurement. In spite of these limitations, this study has been integral to understanding the immunological milieu of the lung allograft.

In summary, BAL has provided the opportunity to sample the panoply of immunological events compartmentalized in the lung allograft. Whether these activities have detectable cellular elements and/or soluble products of these cellular elements in a pattern or patterns specific for the diagnosis of rejection by BAL without transbronchial lung biopsy remains to be determined. Given the potential costs, time, and effort that would be required to validate BAL, the risk of missing a significant rejection event and the long-term impact it might have in an allograft recipient, and given the risk of erroneously treating rejection when there is infection, the TBB is still indicated along with the BAL to evaluate lung allograft recipients for rejection and infection.

B. Chronic Lung Rejection (Obliterative Bronchiolitis)

The development of obstructive airway disease as a result of obliterative bronchiolitis (OB) in the transplanted lung has become one of the foremost threats to the long-term survival of heart-lung and lung transplant recipients (163–165). Currently held to be immunologically mediated and a form of chronic lung rejection, OB is an inflammatory disorder of small airways leading to the obstruction and destruction of pulmonary bronchioles. As a consequence of the inflammatory response in conjunction with probable increases in the activities of fibroblastic growth factors, bronchiolar distortion, narrowing, and plugging with granulation tissue and/or scarring results in the destruction of the bronchioles and the development of severe obstructive airway disease (166,167).

In a more recent characterization, Burke et al. state that chronic rejection of the lung manifests as extensive scarring of the large and small airways. This may be a consequence of repeated or severe acute rejection episodes, or it can represent a separate chronic, insidious, and distinct immunological reaction directed at large and small airways (164).

The initial physiological effect is the development of obstructive airway dynamics of the small airway type, which rapidly progresses to the impairment of the large airway (greater than 2 mm in diameter) as well. Once established, the course is relentlessly downhill without any tendency toward spontaneous remission; it is fatal if left unchecked by early effective therapy.

Although current evidence tends to favor immune mechanisms and chronic rejection as the etiology of OB, other possible pathogenic factors include infection, an interaction between acute rejection and infection (particularly CMV), the transient loss of the bronchial circulation at operation and airway ischemia, the effects of lung denervation resulting in an impaired cough reflex, impaired mucociliary clearance, and impaired local defense mechanisms within the lung. Such factors may contribute to increased infections by pooling of secretions or may predispose the lower respiratory tract to chronic exposure from inhaled or aspirated particles, atmospheric pollutants, or other noxious substances that are normally removed. These, in turn, could all play some role as a continuous source of irritation and inflammation within the airway locally and contribute to the development of OB (163).

Depending upon the clinical series reported, the time of the report, and type of transplant procedure performed, the incidence of OB has been variable and has tended to lessen in recent years. The overall incidence reported for OB has ranged from 10 to 54% in long-term survivors with heart-lung, double-lung, and single-lung transplants (163,165, 168,169). The early experience with OB was derived primarily from patients with HLT. In the initial reports from Stanford, OB developed in 50% of the long-term survivors with HLT who received transplants between 1981 and 1986. The mean onset of disease was 10.4 ± 8.3 (SD) months posttransplant. Other groups at Pittsburgh and Papworth Hospital reported incidences for OB of 54% and 9.6%, respectively, in HLT patients (170,171). The total Stanford experience was again reviewed from 1981 to 1989 by McCarthy et al. (172). The overall incidence of OB for the entire period covered was reduced to 38.6% from the 50% incidence previously reported. In comparing the group of patients transplanted between 1981 and 1986 with those transplanted between 1986 and 1989, the incidence of OB was 63% and 20% for the respective groups. The improvement could be attributed to a number of factors, including the addition of azathioprine to cyclosporine and prednisone as part of the immunosuppressive regimen, improved donor lung preservation technique, increased surveillance of pulmonary function, and bronchoscopic surveillance with serial transbronchial lung biopsies for the early diagnosis and treatment of rejection. Although it would be difficult to assign a specific reason for this reduction in OB, it does seem reasonable to conclude that improvement in overall management can lead to a reduction of this complication. The low reported incidence of OB in the initial Papworth experience may have been due to a similar surveillance-management scheme (173). Recent reassessments at Pittsburgh and Papworth report incidents for OB of 37% and 20% respectively (174,175).

Although the development of OB in lungs transplanted without the heart was once considered to be rare and unusual, this is no longer the case, since OB is being reported in SLT and DLT recipients with increasing frequency. In recent reports, the incidence of OB has ranged from 20 to 58% in SLT recipients (176–178) and from 14 to 80% in DLT recipients (176,177,179). Even though some of these studies involved relatively small numbers of patients, OB should no longer be considered a rare entity in lungs-only transplanted patients. In addition, children are not spared this complication. Pediatric patients develop OB following HLT and LT with an incidence ranging from 25 to 47% (180,181).

The presenting signs and symptoms of OB are nonspecific and are often absent at the time of onset. Currently, OB is often diagnosed clinically much earlier than it was in the past as a result of the close monitoring of pulmonary function and a high index of suspicion in the presence of any respiratory complaint. Onset is frequently insidious, with the detection of obstructive airway dynamics as the only manifestation of disease. When symptoms do appear, the early clinical features are not unique among respiratory disorders. There may be a nonproductive or minimally productive cough, associated with a sense of feeling unwell. The bronchitic symptoms may intensify with the progression of disease, associated frequently but not invariably with recurrent lower respiratory tract infections. The onset of dyspnea is often insidious and usually arises within months of the bronchitic symptoms. Dyspnea is a relatively late manifestation, reflecting extensive airway disease. The clinical course is somewhat similar to that found with chronic obstructive pulmonary disease with the exception that it can be rapidly progressive if unattenuated by effective therapy (163,164).

Although the development of OB can be associated with increases in lower respiratory tract infections, the converse may also be true (164,182). Bacterial and viral pneumonitis or bronchitis in previously well recipients may be followed by the immediate development of OB. Most commonly, CMV infections have been associated with OB, although this relationship still remains unsettled and is a subject of great interest (165,183,184).

On examination, the physical findings in early OB are similarly nonspecific. Although inspiratory squeaks, wheezes, or crackles may be present on auscultation, more often than not the examination is normal in the early stages. In patients with well-advanced disease, the physical findings of chronic airway obstruction are manifest and may include diminished breath sounds, prolonged expiration, rhonchi, crackles, and inspiratory squeaks (163,164).

Late inspiratory high-pitched rhonchi, the inspiratory squeaks referred to above, represent a classic clinical manifestation of OB. When present, these are usually audible in the lung bases bilaterally and may relate to late opening of small airways secondary to accumulation of excess mucus and altered elastic properties (164). Coarse inspiratory crackles and/or rhonchi heard bilaterally in the lung bases may be related to bronchiectasis and fibrosis, which tend to develop in advanced cases of OB associated with recurrent infections.

Hypoxemia and cyanosis as a result of $\dot{V}/\dot{Q}$ mismatch can arise relatively early in the course of severe OB. The hypoxemia is most often associated with hypocapnia secondary to alveolar hyperventilation (i.e., decreased arterial P_{CO_2}). CO_2 retention is usually rare in OB except for end-stage disease, at which time CO_2 retention may be present as part of a terminal event. Because of this characteristic, patients with advanced OB have been referred to as blue puffers, since they may be hypoxic/cyanotic with low arterial P_{CO_2} (163,164).

Since the clinical presentation of early-stage OB may be insidious, nonspecific, and often indistinguishable from the early stages of acute rejection or infection, further investigations are needed for diagnosis. These include chest radiographs, pulmonary function studies with arterial blood gases, and fiberoptic bronchoscopy with TBB and BAL.

The radiographic changes associated with OB are considered to be nonspecific and indistinguishable from other infectious and noninfectious processes affecting the lung parenchyma (185–188).

In the original reports, many of the radiographic findings present with OB probably represented changes associated with far advanced disease. Chest radiographs, tomograms, and computed tomography (CT) scans showed peribronchial and interstitial infiltrates with variable degrees of pleural thickening. The infiltrates tended to have a patchy distribution (186). Many of these findings were probably the results of complicating bacterial bronchitis and bronchiectasis, a frequent finding at autopsy (167). Although they considered many of the changes nonspecific, Skeens and coworkers found the presence of central bronchiectasis in 9 of 11 patients with OB and concluded that it may be a distinctive radiographic finding in this disorder (185).

There are no characteristic changes present on the standard chest radiograph that would permit the early detection of OB. During the initial phases of disease, there may be no significant abnormalities present on the radiograph at all. Early changes may include decreased peripheral vascular markings, slight volume loss, and subsegmental atelectasis (189). With advancing disease, the radiograph may show a variety of parenchymal abnormalities consisting of linear-nodular, nodular, confluent-nodular, or diffuse alveolar opacities (185). Many of these changes probably represent organizing pneumonia or complications as a result of underlying pathology, such as bronchiectasis (165).

On high-resolution or thin-section CT scans, bronchial dilatation and bronchiectasis may be distinctive radiographic findings in OB. Moorish et al. found decreased peripheral vascular markings and peripheral bronchiectasis in patients with OB on high-resolution CT scans (189). In other studies by Halvorsen et al. and Loubeyre et al., it was found that high-resolution or thin-section CT scans may show clear abnormalities consisting of bronchial dilatation, bronchiectasis, air trapping, and patchy areas of consolidation with OB even before any changes are visible in the chest radiograph or routine chest CT (190,191).

In a study utilizing high-resolution CT scans to assess bronchial diameters, Lentz et al. correlated bronchial dilation with pulmonary function measurements in 16 heart-lung transplant patients with OB (192). A close correlation was found between the percentage of bronchi in the lower lobes that were dilated and decreases in FEV_1, FEV_1/FVC, and FEF_{25-75}. No other feature identified on high-resolution CT scans correlated with pulmonary function abnormalities. It was concluded from these studies that dilatation of the lower lobe bronchi is a good indication of OB in this population of patients and that the percentage of dilated bronchi generally increases with increasing pulmonary dysfunction.

Even though the detection of bronchial dilatation by CT scanning techniques appears to be a distinctive feature for identifying OB in the transplanted lung, this finding occurs relatively late in the course of disease and is of less use for early detection.

In the original characterization of OB in heart-lung transplanted patients with far advanced disease, serial measures of pulmonary function revealed severe obstructive airway disease with global reductions of flow to very low levels (163,186). In contrast with classic forms of chronic obstructive pulmonary disease, total lung capacity was often reduced rather than elevated, indicating the coexistence of a restrictive defect. Arterial hypoxemia was always seen, with severe impairment of airway dynamics. As noted earlier, most patients had hypocapnia rather than CO_2 retention. Carbon dioxide retention occurred rarely and only during the terminal phases of the clinical course. Lung carbon monoxide diffusing capacity was moderately reduced, but it did not appear to have a bearing on determining clinical stage or course.

Once the destructive nature of OB was recognized as a threat to long-term survival following transplantation, it became apparent that early detection was imperative. Early detection is possible through the use of serial measurements of pulmonary function and the serial performance of transbronchial lung biopsies. This approach is currently the mainstay of the long-term management in all forms of lung transplantation.

Airway function is monitored with spirometry, which also includes the derivation of flow volume relationships (flow-volume loop) during forced expiratory and inspiratory vital capacity maneuvers. The earliest manifestation of OB is the development of obstructive airway dynamics of the small airway type in particular. The most sensitive measures are decreases in the FEF_{25-75} and FEF_{50}/FVC seen in conjunction with the bowing in of the expiratory flow pattern on the flow-volume loop. The latter is indicative of a disproportionate decrease in flow with respect to lung volume, which, in a normal flow-volume relationship, should be linear with decreasing volume over the last 70% of the FVC maneuver. These early decreases in flow associated with small airway disease are often seen before there are significant reductions in FEV_1 and FEV_1/FVC ratio. Large airway (greater than 2 mm diameter) malfunction develops later with the progression of disease and significant decreases in FEV_1 and FEV_1/FVC ratio are usually present at the time (133,163,193,194).

The early changes in pulmonary function attributed to small airway dysfunction are more readily perceived in HLT and DLT patients. The early decreases in FEF_{25-75} or changes in the shape of the FEF pattern on the flow-volume loop may be more difficult to interpret in SLT patients for detecting OB, particularly in those receiving single lung allografts for emphysema. Although less precise in SLT, significant decreases in FEV_1 or FEF_{25-75}, which quite often fall together with significant airway disease, should raise the possibility of OB. Of note, recent studies have shown decreases in FEF_{25-75} prior to decreases in FEV_1 in SLT patients with OB (178,179).

Both physiological and histological criteria are used for making the diagnosis of OB. An ad hoc working group under the auspices of the International Society for Heart and Lung Transplantation (ISHLT) published a position paper, *A Working Formulation for the Standardization of Nomenclature and for Clinical Staging of Chronic Dysfunction in Lung Allografts*, in which criteria are provided for making the clinical diagnosis of OB (195). The term "bronchiolitis obliterans syndrome" (BOS) was selected to connote graft deterioration secondary to progressive airway disease for which there is no other cause. It is widely presumed but unproved that this is a manifestation of chronic rejection. The term "bronchiolitis obliterans" (we prefer OB) is reserved for histologically proven diagnosis only; BOS does not necessarily require histological confirmation (195).

The ad hoc group also concluded that the FEV_1 was the most reliable and consistent indicator of graft dysfunction provided that other identifiable causes are excluded. Using the FEV_1, four stages of BOS were defined, each with two subcategories to indicate whether or not pathological evidence of OB was present. Based on the severity of functional change for the FEV_1 (percent change from previous best value), the following staging system for BOS was proposed:

Stage 0: No significant abnormality; FEV_1 80% or more of baseline value
Stage 1: Mild OB syndrome: FEV_1 66 to 80% of baseline value
Stage 2: Moderate OB syndrome: FEV_1 51 to 65% of baseline value
Stage 3: Severe OB syndrome: FEV_1 50 or less of baseline value

After analyzing application of the staging system to 120 SLT and DLT recipients and comparing data from SLT recipients whose underlying disease was restrictive disease, obstructive disease, or pulmonary hypertension, the committee felt that the single staging system proposed should be applied to all lung transplant recipients, whether they were HLT, DLT, or SLT recipients. It was further suggested that the staging system be reappraised in approximately 2 years (195).

Although the FEV_1 is perceived as being the most reliable parameter for monitoring the lung allograft for the development of obstructive airway disease, it is usually not the most sensitive for detecting onset. In cases of OB that are moderately severe or worse, the FEF_{25-75} and FEV_1 are comparable and of equal value for detecting obstructive airway disease (194). In the detection of mild or early OB, however, the FEF_{25-75} and FEF_{50}/FVC are more sensitive than the FEV_1 (193,194). In several series reported, decreases in the FEF_{25-75} or FEF_{50}/FVC detected the onset of OB 3 to 15 months sooner than decreases in the FEV_1 in HLT, DLT, and SLT recipients (178,179,193,194).

Lung biopsy is the gold standard for making the diagnosis of OB. Although open lung biopsy provides the best tissue samples for histological examination, the performance of serial open lung biopsies in transplant recipients is impractical. The confirmation of OB by transbronchial lung biopsy is variable, ranging from 17 to 66% in patients with suspected OB by pulmonary function criteria (196,197). These differences in diagnosis may, in part, reflect interinstitutional variation in the number of biopsies obtained, but more than likely they reflect the heterogenous distribution of disease within the lung. Thus, as a result of this variability, OB may become a diagnosis of exclusion based upon pulmonary functional abnormalities.

C. Lung Biopsy

The histopathological examination of lung tissue for acute lung rejection is paramount in the management of patients following lung or heart-lung transplantation because of the nonspecific clinical signs that can mimic rejection. Numerous studies have confirmed the safety and utility of transbronchial biopsies for the diagnosis of acute lung rejection. Pneumothorax is the most common complication associated with transbronchial biopsy and occurs in less than 2% of cases (198). Trulock and associates (199) reported an 8.9% complication rate associated with transbronchial biopsy, which included excessive bleeding, pneumonia, hypoxemia, respiratory decompensation, supraventricular tachycardia, and pleurisy. There were no pneumothoraces or fatalities in this series.

Although controversy exists regarding the need to perform serial surveillance transbronchial biopsies, most transplant centers advocate serial surveillance biopsies for the early detection of acute rejection or infection. Starnes reported that clinically indicated transbronchial biopsies following heart-lung transplantation had an 83% diagnostic rate for infection or rejection and that surveillance transbronchial biopsies had a 15% diagnostic yield for infection or rejection (135). Trulock et al. reported a 69% diagnostic rate for infection and rejection in clinically indicated transbronchial biopsies and a 57% diagnostic rate for surveillance procedures following lung transplantation. In the St. Louis study, the sensitivity of TBB was 72% for acute rejection and 91% for CMV infection (199). The Papworth group previously reported the overall sensitivity and specificity of TBB for the diagnosis of acute lung rejection to be 84 and 100%, respectively (200). The association between the number and severity of acute rejection events in the development of obliterative bronchiolitis argues in favor of surveillance transbronchial biopsies following transplantation (201,202).

Recently, Tazelaar and others showed that five pieces of lung tissue obtained from transbronchial biopsy in mongrel dogs had a sensitivity of 92% for mild rejection (203). This is in accordance with the Lung Rejection Study Group, who recommend a minimum of five transbronchial biopsy specimens to adequately assess for acute lung rejection (204). Transbronchial biopsy has emerged as a safe and reliable means of assessing the condition of the lung allograft and should be considered the gold standard for diagnosing acute lung rejection. It is important to combine bronchoalveolar lavage with transbronchial biopsy for the assessment of opportunistic pulmonary infections.

D. Heart-Lung Allografts

Most principles described individually for the heart allografts and lung allografts can be applied to the combined heart-lung allograft. A few unique circumstances exist, however, that are worthy of mention. Earlier investigations suggested that monitoring the heart for acute rejection events by surveillance right ventricular endomyocardial biopsies would provide a means to monitor lung rejections following heart-lung transplantation (205,206). In both animal models and human subjects, it became apparent that a normal endomyocardial biopsy did not exclude pulmonary rejection (135,207,208). In fact, more lung rejection episodes were occurring in the absence of heart-rejection, so that many programs have now eliminated surveillance biopsies of the heart in HLT.

Most of the complications in heart-lung recipients are primarily pulmonary. Efforts continue to focus on the detection of acute lung rejection in order to prevent chronic complications such as OB. Close surveillance of pulmonary function, including the use of flow-volume loops and arterial blood gases, is essential. The chest radiograph, though insensitive and nonspecific, remains an integral part of the clinical assessment following HLT.

Although most programs have eliminated the surveillance endomyocardial biopsy to detect acute heart rejection in these recipients, they remain at risk for developing graft coronary arteriosclerosis. These patients may present with sudden death, findings consistent with heart failure, myocardial infarction, and/or life-threatening dysrhythmias. Yearly surveillance coronary angiograms in combination with intracoronary ultrasonography should be performed to monitor for graft coronary arteriosclerosis. There are some data to suggest that diltiazem may reduce the incidence of graft atherosclerosis (209). Cardiac transplantation remains the only treatment option for progressive coronary graft disease.

The operative and preservation techniques of heart-lung and lung transplantation have been refined, as has the ability to diagnose lung rejection by transbronchial biopsy. Chronic rejection is now the formidable barrier to the success of heart, heart-lung, and lung transplantation. In the form of graft coronary arteriosclerosis and obliterative bronchiolitis, these long-term sequelae appear to correlate with the number, intensity, and duration of acute rejection events and possibly with infection events, particularly CMV. Most transplant programs have intensified screening procedures in an attempt to modify chronic rejection by the early detection and treatment of acute rejection and infection.

REFERENCES

1. Kennan RJ, Bruzzone P, Paradis IL, et al. Similarity of pulmonary rejection patterns among heart-lung and double-lung transplant recipients. Transplantation 1991; 51:176–180.
2. Egan TM, Kaiser LR, Cooper JD. Lung transplantation. Curr Probl Surg 1989; 26:673–751.
3. Burke MN, McGinn AL, Homans DC, et al. Evidence for functional sympathetic reinnervation of left ventricle and coronary arteries after orthotopic cardiac transplantation in humans. Circulation 1995; 91:72–78.
4. Yeoh TK, Frist WH, Eastburn TE, et al. Clinical significance of mild rejection of the cardiac allograft. Circulation 1992; 86(suppl II):II-267–II-271.
5. Gao SZ, Hunt SA, Wiederhold MA, et al. Characteristics of serial electrocardiograms in heart transplant recipients. Am Heart J 1991; 122:771–774.
6. Scott CD, Dark JH, McComb JM. Arrhythmias after cardiac transplantation. Am J Cardiol 1992; 70:1061–1063.
7. Little RE, Kay N, Epstein AE, et al. Arrhythmias after orthotopic cardiac transplantation. Circulation 1989; 80(suppl III):140–146.
8. Jacquet L, Ziady G, Stein K, et al. Cardiac rhythm disturbances early after orthotopic heart transplantation: prevalence and clinical importance of the observed abnormalities. J Am Coll Cardiol 1990; 16:832–837.
9. Kobashigawa J, Warner-Stevenson L. Noninvasive detection of acute cardiac allograft rejection. In: Kapoor AS, Laks H, Schroeder JS, Yacoub MH, eds. Cardiomyopathies and Heart-Lung Transplantation. New York: McGraw-Hill, 1991:293–303.
10. Keren A, Gillis AM, Freedman RA, et al. Heart transplantation rejection monitored by signal averaged electrocardiography in patients receiving cyclosporine. Circulation 1984; 70(suppl I):123–129.
11. Haberl R, Weber M, Reichenspurner H, et al. Frequency analysis of the surface electrogram for recognition of acute rejection after orthotopic cardiac transplantation in man. Circulation 1987; 76:101–108.
12. Warnecke H, Schuler S, Goetze HJ, et al. Noninvasive monitoring of cardiac allograft rejection by intramyocardial electrogram recordings. Circulation 1986; 74(suppl II):72–76.
13. Koike K, Hesslein PS, Dasmahaptra HK, et al. Telemetric detection of cardiac allograft rejection. Circulation 1988; 78(suppl I):106–112.
14. Rosenbloom M, Laschinger JC, Saffitz JE, et al. Noninvasive detection of cardiac allograft rejection by analysis of the unipolar peak-to-peak amplitude of intramyocardial electrograms. Ann Thorac Surg 1989; 47:407–411.
15. Kemkes BM, Schutz A, Englehardt M, et al. Noninvasive methods of rejection diagnosis after heart transplantation. J Heart Transplant 1992; 11:S221–S231.
16. Schutz A, Kemkes BM, Breuer M, et al. Kinetics and dynamics of acute rejection after heterotopic heart transplantation. J Heart Transplant 1992; 11:289–299.
17. Warnecke H, Muller J, Cohnert T, et al. Clinical heart transplantation without routine endomyocardial biopsy. J Heart Lung Transplant 1992; 11:1093–1102.
18. Losman JG, McDonald J, Levine HD. The variation of the electrocardiographic voltage during the day in the normal adult. J Heart Transplant 1981; 1:39–51.
19. Wahlers T, Haverich A, Schafers JH, et al. Changes of the intramyocardial electrogram after orthotopic heart transplantation. J Heart Transplant 1986; 5:450–455.
20. Stevenson LW, Dadourian BJ, Kabashigawa J, et al: Mitral regurgitations after cardiac transplantation. Am J Cardiol 1987; 60:119–122.
21. Valantine HA, Hunt SA, Gibbons R, et al: Increasing pericardial effusion in cardiac transplant recipients. Circulation 1989; 79:603–609.
22. Sagar KB, Hastillo A, Wolfgang TC, et al. Left ventricular mass by M-mode echocardiography in cardiac transplant recipients with acute rejection. Circulation 1981; 64(suppl I):216–220.

23. Dubroff JM, Clark MB, Wang CYH, et al. Changes in left ventricular image associated with the onset of acute rejection after cardiac transplantation. J Heart Transplant 1984; 3:105–109.
24. Paulsen W, Magid N, Sagar K, et al. Left ventricular function of heart allograft during rejection: an echocardiographic assessment. J Heart Transplant 1985; 4:525–529.
25. Dawkins KD, Oldershaw PJ, Billingham ME, et al. Changes in diastolic function as a noninvasive marker of cardiac allograft rejection. J Heart Transplant 1984; 3:286–294.
26. Valantine H, Fowler M, Hatle L, et al. Doppler echocardiographic indices of diastolic function as markers of acute cardiac rejection. Transplant Proc 1987; 19:2556–2559.
27. Valantine H, Fowler M, Hunt S, et al. Changes in doppler echocardiographic indexes of left ventricular functions as potential markers of acute cardiac rejection. Circulation 1987; 76(suppl 5):86–92.
28. Moriguchi J, Stevenson LW, Kobashigawa JA, et al. Decrease in 2-dimensional echocardiographic ejection fraction during transplant rejection: a study of 400 biopsies. J Am Coll Cardiol 1988; 11:121A.
29. Angermann CH, Schott L, Hart R, et al. Echomonitoring of heart transplant recipients: acute and long-term results and assessment of complications. J Heart Transplant 1986; 5:397.
30. Angermann C, Hart R, Spes C, et al: Computerized quantitative evaluation of the endocardium in serial two dimensional echocardiograms of the left ventricular short axis. IEEF Comp Cardiol 1987; 9:437–440.
31. Starnes VA, Bernstein D, Oyer PE, et al. Heart transplantation in children. J Heart Transplant 1989; 8:20–26.
32. Boucek MM, Mathis CM, Boucek RJ, et al. Prospective evaluation of echocardiography for primary rejection surveillance after infant heart transplantation: comparisons with endomyocardial biopsy. J Heart Lung Transplant 1994; 13:66–73.
33. Kung PC, Goldstein G, Reinherz EL, et al. Monoclonal antibodies defining distinctive human T cell antigens. Science 1979; 206:347–350.
34. Cosimi AB, Colvin RB, Burton RC, et al. Use of monoclonal antibodies to T cell subsets for immunological monitoring and treatment in recipients of renal allografts. N Engl J Med 1981; 305:308–310.
35. English TAH, McGregor C, Wallwork J, et al. Aspects of immunosuppression for cardiac transplantation. J Heart Transplant 1982; 1:280–286.
36. Rabin BS. Immunologic aspects of human cardiac transplantation. J Heart Transplant 1983; 2:188–193.
37. Hammer C, Reichenspurner H, Ertel W, et al. Cytological and immunological monitoring of cyclosporine treated human heart recipients. J Heart Transplant 1984; 3:228–232.
38. Reichenspurner H, Kemkes BM, Osterholzer G, et al. Special control of infection and rejection episodes. Tex Heart Inst J 1986; 13:5–12.
39. Ertel W, Reichenspurner H, Hammer C, et al. Cytoimmunologic monitoring: a method to reduce biopsy frequency after cardiac transplantation. Transplant Proc 1985; 17:204–206.
40. Fieguth HG, Haverich A, Schaefers JH, et al. Cytoimmunologic monitoring for the invasive diagnosis of cardiac rejection. Transplant Proc 1987; 19:2541–2542.
41. Klanke D, Hammer C, Dirschedl P, et al. Sensitivity and specificity of cytoimmunologic monitoring in correlation with endomyocardial biopsies in heart transplant patients. Transplant Proc 1987; 19:3781–3783.
42. Ertel W, Reichenspurner H, Lersch C, et al. Cytoimmunological monitoring in acute rejection and viral, bacterial, or fungal infection following transplantation. J Heart Transplant 1985; 4:390–394.
43. Fieguth HG, Haverich A, Schaefers JH, et al: Cytoimmunologic monitoring in early and late acute cardiac rejection. J Heart Transplant 1988; 7:95–101.
44. Hanson CA, Bolling SF, Stoolman LM, et al. Cytoimmunologic monitoring and heart transplantation. J Heart Transplant 1988; 7:424–429.

45. Wijngaard PLJ, Heyn A, Muelen A, et al. Cytoimmunologic monitoring following heart transplantation. Bibl Cardiol 1988; 43:137–141.
46. Klanke D, Hammer C, Schubel C, et al. Reproducibility and reliability of cytoimmunologic monitoring of heart transplanted patients. Transplant Proc 1989; 21:2512–2513.
47. Jutte NHPM, Daane R, Bend JMG, et al. Cytoimmunologic monitoring to detect rejection after heart transplantation. Transplant Proc 1989; 21:2519–2520.
48. Wijngaard PLJ, Muelen A, Schuurman HJ, et al. Cytoimmunologic monitoring for the diagnosis of acute rejection after heart transplantation. Transplant Proc 1989; 21:2521–2522.
49. Coles M, Rose M, Yacoub M. Appearance of cells bearing interleukin-2 receptor in peripheral blood of cardiac transplant patients and their correlation with rejection episode. Transplant Proc 1987; 19:2546–2547.
50. Molajoni ER, Cinti P, Bachetoni A, et al. Immunological diagnosis of rejection in heart transplant recipients. Bibl Cardiol 1988; 43:142–145.
51. Molajoni ER, Bachetoni A, Cassisi P, et al. Relevance of immunological parameters to detect allograft rejection in heart transplant recipients. Transplant Proc 1989; 21:2534–2536.
52. Mohanakumar T, Hoshinaga K, Wood NL, et al. Enumeration of transferrin receptor expressing lymphocytes as a potential marker for rejection in human cardiac transplant recipients. Transplantation 1986; 42:691–694.
53. Hoshinaga K, Mohanakumar K, Pascoe EA, et al. Expression of transferrin receptors on lymphocytes: its correlation with T helper/T suppressor cytoxic ratio and rejection in heart transplant recipients. J Heart Transplant 1988; 7:198–204.
54. Roodman ST, Miller LW, Tsai CC. Role of interleukin 2 receptors in immunologic monitoring following cardiac transplantation. Transplantation 1988; 45:1050–1056.
55. DeMaria R, Zuccelli QC, Masini S, et al. Nonspecific increase of interleukin 2 receptor serum levels during immune events in heart transplantation. Transplant Proc 1989; 21:440–441.
56. Fieguth HG, Haverich A, Hadam M, et al. Correlation of interleukin 2 receptor positive circulating lymphocytes and acute cardiac rejection. Transplant Proc 1989; 21:2517–2518.
57. Rubin LA, Kurman CC, Fritz ME, et al. Soluble interleukin-2 receptors are released from activated human lymphoid cells in vitro. J Immunol 1985; 135:3172–3177.
58. Lawrence EC, Holland VA, Young JB, et al. Dynamic changes in soluble interleukin-2 receptor levels following lung or heart-lung transplantation. Am Rev Respir Dis 1989; 140: 789–796.
59. Lawrence EC. Diagnosis and management of lung allograft rejection. In: Grossman RF, Maurer JR, eds. Pulmonary Considerations in Transplantation. Clinics in Chest Medicine. Vol. II. No. 2. Philadelphia: Saunders, 1990:269–278.
60. Carrier M, Russel DH, Wild JC, et al. Prolactin as a marker of rejection in human heart transplantation. J Heart Transplant 1987; 6:290–292.
61. Cosson C, Myara I, Guillemain R, et al. Serum prolactin as a rejection marker in heart transplantation. Clin Chem 1989; 35:492–493.
62. Goldman MH, Lippman R, Landwehr D, et al. Beta 2 microglobulin and the diagnosis of cardiac transplant rejection. Transplantation 1983; 36:209–211.
63. Margreiter R, Fuchs D, Hausen A, et al. Neopterine as a new biochemical marker for diagnosis of allograft rejection. Transplantation 1983; 36:650–653.
64. Havel M, Laczkovics A, Teufelsbauer H, et al. Neopterine as a new marker to detect acute rejection after heart transplantation. J Heart Transplant 1989; 8:167–170.
65. Huber C, Fuchs D, Hauser A, et al. Pterdines as a new marker to detect human T cells activated by allogenic or modified self major histocompatibility complex determinants. J Immunol 1983; 130:1047–1050.
66. Womble JR, Larson DF, Copeland JG, et al. Urinary polyamine levels are markers of altered T lymphocyte proliferation/loss and rejection in heart transplant recipients. Transplant Proc 1984; 16:1573–1575.

67. Foegh ML, Khirabadi BS, Shapiro R, et al. Monitoring of rat heart allograft rejection by urinary thromboxane. Transplant Proc 1984; 16:1606–1608.
68. Khirabadi BS, Foegh ML, Ramwell PW. Urine immunoreactive thromboxane B_2 in rat cardiac allograft rejection. Transplantation 1985; 39:6–8.
69. Lund G, Letourneau JG, Day DL, et al. MRI in organ transplantation. Radiol Clin North Am 1987; 25:281–288.
70. Kurland RJ, Kelley S, Wert J, et al. Magnetic resonance imaging to detect heart transplant rejection: sensitivity and specificity. Transplant Proc 1989; 21:2537–2543.
71. Aherne T, Tscholakoff D, Finkbeiner W, et al. Magnetic resonance imaging of cardiac transplants: the evolution of rejection of cardiac allografts with and without immunosuppression. Circulation 1986; 74:145–156.
72. Wisenberg G, Pflugfelder PW, Kostuk WJ, et al. Diagnostic applicability of magnetic resonance imaging in assessing human cardiac allograft rejection. Am J Cardiol 1987; 60: 130–136.
73. Revel D, Chapeon C, Malhieu D, et al. Magnetic resonance imaging of human orthotopic heart transplantation: correlation with endomyocardial biopsy. J Heart Transplant 1989; 8:139–146.
74. Smart FW, Young JB, Weilbaecher D, et al. Magnetic resonance imaging for assessment of tissue rejection after heterotopic heart transplantation. J Heart Lung Transplant 1993; 12: 403–410.
75. Kemkes BM, Schutz A, Engelhardt M, et al. Noninvasive methods of rejection diagnosis after heart transplantation. J Heart Transplant 1992; 11:S221–S231.
76. Mosseaux E, Farge D, Guillemain R, et al. Magnetic resonance imaging of human transplanted hearts with gadolinium-DOTA myocardial enhancement: potential for the detection of rejection. J Am Coll Cardiol 1991; 17:326A.
77. Hall TS, Baumgartner WA, Borkon AM, et al. Diagnosis of acute cardiac rejection with antimyosin monoclonal antibody, phosphorus nuclear magnetic resonance imaging, two-dimensional echocardiography and endocardial biopsy. J Heart Transplant 1986; 5:419–424.
78. Iturralde MP. Radionuclide imaging procedures in the evaluation of heart transplant recipients. In: Kapoor AS, Laks H, Schroeder JS, Yacoub MH, eds. Cardiomyopathies and Heart-Lung Transplantation. New York: McGraw-Hill, 1991:305–326.
79. Dietz RR, Patton DD, Copeland JG, et al. Characteristics of the transplanted heart in the radionuclide ventriculogram. J Heart Transplant 1984; 5:113–121.
80. Novitzky D, Cooper DKC, Boniaszczuk J, et al. Prediction of acute cardiac rejection using radionuclide scanning to detect left ventricular volume changes. Transplant Proc 1985; 17:218–220.
81. Novitzky D, Cooper DKC, Boniaszczuk J. Prediction of acute cardiac rejection by changes in left ventricular volume. J Heart Transplant 1988; 7:453–455.
82. McGiffin DC, Karp RB, Logic JR, et al. Results of radionuclide assessment of cardiac function following transplantation of the heart. Ann Thorac Surg 1984; 37:382–386.
83. Latre JM, Arizon JM, Jimenez-Heffernan A, et al. Noninvasive radioisotopic diagnosis of acute heart rejection. J Heart Lung Transplant 1992; 11:453–457.
84. Bergsland J, Carr EA, Carroll M, et al. Uptake of myocardial imaging agents by rejecting hearts. J Heart Transplant 1985; 4:536–540.
85. McKillop JH, McDougall IR, Goris ML, et al. Failure to diagnose cardiac transplant rejection with T_c-99m-PYP images. Clin Nucl Med 1981; 6:375–377.
86. Meneguetti JC, Camargo EE, Soares J, et al. Gallium-67 imaging in human heart transplantation: correlation with endomyocardial biopsy. J Heart Transplant 1987; 6:171–176.
87. Khaw BA, Fallon JT, Beller GA, et al. Specificity of localization of myosin-specific antibody fragments in experimental myocardial infarction. Circulation 1979; 60:1527–1531.
88. Addonizo LI, Michler RE, Marbol C, et al. Imaging of cardiac allograft rejection in dogs using indium-111 monoclonal antimyosin Fab. J Am Coll Cardiol 1987; 9:555–564.

89. Ueda K, Takeda K, LaFrance ND, et al. Is In-111 antimyosin antibody a useful diagnostic marker for evaluation of early cardiac allograft rejection? Transplant Proc 1988; 20: 778–781.
90. Ballester-Rodes, Carrio-Gasset I, Abdal-Berinin L, et al. Patterns of evolution of myocyte damage after human heart transplantation detected by indium-111 monoclonal antimyosin. Am J Cardiol 1988; 62:623–627.
91. Frist W, Yasuda T, Segall G, et al. Noninvasive detection of human cardiac transplant rejection with indium-111 antimyosin (Fab) imaging. Circulation 1987; 76(suppl V):V81–V85.
92. Baughman KL. Monitoring of allograft rejection. In: Baumgartner WA, Reitz BA, Achuff SC, eds. Heart and Heart-Lung Transplantation. Philadelphia: WB Saunders, 1990:157–164.
93. Caves PK, Stinson EB, Billingham ME, et al. Serial transvenous biopsy of the transplanted human heart. Lancet 1974; 2:821–826.
94. Sakakibara S, Konno S. Endomyocardial biopsy. Jpn Heart J 1962; 3:537–543.
95. Imakita M, Tazelaar HD, Billingham ME. Heart allograft rejection under varying immunosuppressive protocols as evaluated by endomyocardial biopsy. J Heart Transplant 1986; 5: 279–285.
96. Kapoor AS. Endomyocardial biopsy. In: Kapoor AS, Laks H, Schroeder JS, Yacoub MH, eds. Cardiomyopathies and Heart-Lung Transplantation. New York: McGraw-Hill, 1991:327–333.
97. Baughman KL. History and current techniques of endomyocardial biopsy. In: Baumgartner WA, Reitz BA, Achuff SC, eds. Heart and Heart-Lung Transplantation. Philadelphia: Saunders, 1990:165–182.
98. Thompson JC. Production of severe atheroma in a transplanted human heart. Lancet 1969; 2:1088–1092.
99. Bieber CP, Stinson EB, Shumway NE, et al. Cardiac transplantation in man: VII. Cardiac allograft pathology. Circulation 1970; 41:753–772.
100. Uretsky BF, Murali S, Reddy PS, et al. Development of coronary artery disease in cardiac transplant recipients receiving immunosuppressive therapy with cyclosporine and prednisone. Circulation 1987; 76:827–834.
101. Bourge R, Naftel D, Costanzo Nordin M, et al. Pre transplantation risk factors for death after cardiac transplantation: A multi-institutional study. J Heart Lung Transplant 1993; 12: 549–562.
102. Hunt SA. Cardiac transplantation: Complications and management. In: Kapoor AS, Laks H, Schroeder JS, Yacoub MH, eds. Cardiomyopathies and Heart-Lung Transplantation. New York: McGraw-Hill, 1991:233–240.
103. Billingham ME. Histopathology of graft coronary disease. J Heart Lung Transplant 1992; 3:538–544.
104. Hardin NJ, Minick R, Murphy GE. Experimental induction of atheroarterio-sclerosis by the synergy of allergic injury to arteries and lipid-rich diet. Am J Pathol 1973; 73:301–321.
105. Minick CR, Stemerman MB, Insull W. Role of endothelium and hypercholesterolemia in intimal thickening and lipid accumulation. Am J Pathol 1979; 95:131–151.
106. Ross R. The pathogenesis of atherosclerosis—an update. N Engl J Med 1986; 314:488–500.
107. Cramer DV, Qian S, Harnaha J, et al. Cardiac transplantation in the rat: the effect of histocompatibility differences on graft arteriosclerosis. Transplantation 1989; 47:414–419.
108. Pennock JL, Oyer PE, Reitz BA, et al. Cardiac transplantation in perspective for the future: survival, complication, rehabilitation and cost. J Thorac Cardiovasc Surg 1982; 83:168–177.
109. Hess ML, Hastillo A, Mohanakumar T, et al. Accelerated atherosclerosis in cardiac transplantation: role of cytotoxic B-cell antibodies and hyperlipidemia. Circulation 1983; 68(suppl II):94–101.
110. Gao SZ, Schroeder JS, Alderman EL, et al. Clinical and laboratory correlates of accelerated coronary artery disease in the cardiac transplant patient. Circulation 1987; 76(suppl V): V56–V61.

111. Gratten M, Moreno-Cabral C, Starnes V, et al. Cytomegalovirus infection is associated with cardiac graft rejection and atherosclerosis. JAMA 1989; 261:3561–3566.
112. McDonald K, Rector T, Braunlin E, et al. Association of coronary artery disease in transplant recipients with cytomegalovirus infection. Am J Cardiol 1989; 64:354–362.
113. Lopez C, Simmons R, Mauer S, et al. Association of renal allograft rejection with virus infections. Am J Med 1984; 56:280–289.
114. Tourkantonis A, Lazardis A. Interaction between cytomegalovirus infection and renal transplant rejection. Kidney Int. 1983; 23:546–549.
115. O'Grady JG, Sutherland S, Harvey F, et al. Cytomegalovirus infection and donor/recipient HLA antigens: interdependent co-factors in pathogenesis of vanishing bile duct syndrome after liver transplantation. Lancet 1988; 2:302–305.
116. Grundy JE, Ayles HM, McKeating JA, et al. Enhancement of class I HLA antigens expression by cytomegalovirus: role in amplification of virus infection. J Med Virol 1988; 25:483–495.
117. vonWillebrand E, Petterson E, Ahonen J, et al. Class II antigen expression and human kidney allograft rejection. Transplantation 1986; 42:364–367.
118. Bieber CP, Hunt SA, Schwinn DA, et al. Complications in long term survivors of cardiac transplantation. Transplant Proc 1981; 13:207–211.
119. Gao SZ, Alderman EL, Schroeder JS, et al. Accelerated coronary vascular disease in the heart transplant patient: coronary arteriographic findings. J Am Coll Cardiol 1988; 12:234–340.
120. Chenzbraun A, Pinto FJ, Alderman EL, et al. Distribution and morphologic features of coronary artery disease in cardiac allografts: an intracoronary ultrasound study. J Am Soc Echocard 1995; 8:1–8.
121. Eich DM, Quigg RJ, Heroux A, et al. Diagnosis and management of graft atherosclerosis (chronic rejection). In: Cooper DKC, Novitzky eds. The Transplantation and Replacement of Thoracic Organs. Dordrecht: Kluwer, 1990:169–175.
122. McKillop JH, Goris ML. Thallium 201 myocardial imaging in patients with previous cardiac transplantation. Clin Radiol 1981; 32:447–449.
123. Hosenspud JD, Novick RJ, Breen TJ, et al. The registry of the international society for heart and lung transplantation: eleventh official report—1994. J Heart Lung Transplant 1994; 13:561–570.
124. Patterson GA, Todd TR, Cooper JD, et al. Airway complications following double-lung transplantation. J Thorac Cardiovasc Surg 1990; 99:14–21.
125. Kawaguchi A, Gandjbakhch I, Pavie A, et al. Heart and unilateral lung transplantation in patients with end-stage cardiopulmonary disease and previous thoracic operations. J Thorac Cardiovasc Surg 1989; 98:343–349.
126. Starnes VA, Barr ML, Cohen RG. Lobar transplantation: indications, technique and outcome. J Thorac Cardiovasc Surg 1994; 108:403–410.
127. Paradis IL, Duncan SR, Dauber JH, et al. Distinguishing between infection, rejection and adult respiratory distress syndrome after human lung transplantation. J Heart Lung Transplant 1992; 11:S232–S236.
128. Millet B, Higenbottam TW, Flower CDR, et al. The radiographic appearances of infection and acute rejection of the lung after heart-lung transplantation. Am Rev Repair Dis 1989; 140: 62–67.
129. Bergin CJ, Castellino RA, Blank N, et al. Acute lung rejection after heart-lung transplantation: correlation of findings on chest radiographs with lung biopsy results. AJR 1990; 155:23–27.
130. Keenan RJ, Bruzzone P, Paradis IL, et al. Similarity of pulmonary rejection patterns among heart-lung and double-lung transplant recipients. Transplantation 1991; 51:176–180.
131. Theodore J, Jamieson SW, Burke CM, et al. Physiologic aspects of human heart-lung transplantation: pulmonary function status of the post-transplanted lung. Chest 1984; 86:349–357.
132. Burke CM, Theodore J, Baldwin JC, et al. Twenty-eight cases of human heart-lung transplantation. Lancet 1986; 1:517–519.

133. Theodore J, Marshall S, Kramer M, et al. The "natural" history of the transplanted lungs: rates of pulmonary functional change in long-term survivors of heart-lung transplantation. Transplant Proc 1991; 23:1165–1166.
134. Otulana BA, Higenbottam T, Scott J, et al. Lung function associated with histologically diagnosed acute lung rejection and pulmonary infection in heart-lung transplant patients. Am Rev Respir Dis 1990; 142:329–332.
135. Starnes VA, Theodore J, Oyer PE, et al. Evaluation of heart-lung transplant recipients with prospective serial transbronchial biopsies and pulmonary function studies. J Thorac Cardiovasc Surg 1989; 98:683–690.
136. Hoeper MM, Hamm M, Schafers HJ, et al. Evaluation of lung function during pulmonary rejection and infection in heart-lung transplant patients. Chest 1992; 102:864–870.
137. Williams TJ, Grossman RF, Maurer JR. Long-term functional follow-up of lung transplant recipients. In: Grossman RF, Maurer JR, eds. Pulmonary Considerations in Transplantation: Clinics in Chest Medicine. Vol. II. No. 2. Philadelphia: Saunders, 1990:347–358.
138. Bjotuft O, Johansen B, Boe J, et al. Daily home spirometry facilitates early detection of rejection in single lung transplant recipients with emphysema. Eur Respir J 1993; 6:705–708.
139. Marshall SE, Lewiston NJ, Kramer MR, et al. Prospective analysis of serial pulmonary function studies and transbronchial biopsies in single-lung transplant recipients. Transplant Proc 1991; 23:1217–1219.
140. Becker FS, Martinez FJ, Brunstring LA, et al. Limitations of spirometry in detecting rejection after single-lung transplantation. Am J Respir Crit Care Med 1994; 150:159–166.
141. Kramer MR, Marshall SE, McDougall IR, et al. The distribution of ventilation and perfusion after single-lung transplantation in patients with pulmonary fibrosis and pulmonary hypertension. Transplant Proc 1991; 23:1215–1216.
142. Mal H, Andreassian B, Pamela F, et al. Unilateral lung transplantation in end stage pulmonary emphysema. Am Rev Respir Dis 1989; 140:797–802.
143. Trulock EP, Egan TM, Kouchoukos NT. Single lung transplantation for severe chronic obstructive disease: Washington University Lung Transplant Group. Chest 1989; 96:738–742.
144. Stevens PM, Johnson PC, Bell RL, et al. Regional ventilation and perfusion after lung transplantation in patients with emphysema. N Engl J Med 1970; 282:245–249.
145. Veith FJ, Koerner SK, Siegelman SS, et al. Single lung transplantation in experimental and human emphysema. Ann Surg 1973; 178:463–476.
146. Herman SJ. Radiologic assessment after lung transplantation. In: Grossman RF, Maurer JR, eds. Pulmonary Considerations in Transplantation: Clinics in Chest Medicine, Vol. II. No. 2. Philadelphia: Saunders, 1990:333–346.
147. Paradis I, Rabinowich H, Zeevi A, et al. Life in the allogeneic environment after lung transplantation. Lung 1990; (suppl)168:1172–1181.
148. Pearlman E, Kazura J, Hazlett F, et al. Modulation of murine cytokine responses to mycobacterial antigens by helminth-induced T helper-2 cell responses. J Immunol 1993; 151:3478–3488.
149. Moore K, O'Garra A, Malefyt R, et al. Interleukin 10. Annu Rev Immunol 1993; 11:165–190.
150. Jelinek D, Lipsky P. Inhibitory influence of IL-4 on human B cell responses. J Immunol 1988; 141:164–173.
151. Kitani A, Strober W. Regulation of C-gamma subclass germ-line transcripts in human peripheral blood B cells. J Immunol 1993; 141:164–173.
152. Wilkes D, Weissler J. Allogantigen-induced immunoglobulin production in human lung: differential effects of accessory cell populations on IgG synthesis. Am J Respir Cell Mol Biol 1994; 10:339–346.
153. Trulock E. Management of lung transplant rejection. Chest 1993; 103:1566–1576.
154. Rabinowich H, Zeevi A, Paradis I, et al. Proliferative responses of bronchoalveolar lavage lymphocytes from heart-lung transplant patients. Transplantation 1990; 49:115–121.

155. Maurer J, Gouch E, Chamberlain D, et al. Sequential bronchoalveolar lavage studies from patients undergoing double lung and heart-lung transplant. Transplant Proc 21:2585–2587.
156. Clelland C, Higenbottam T, Stewart S, et al. Bronchoalveolar lavage and transbronchial biopsy during acute rejection and infection in heart-lung transplant patients. Am Rev Respir Dis 1993; 147:1386–1392.
157. Gryzan S, Paradis I, Hardesty R, et al. Bronchoalveolar lavage in heart-lung transplantation. J Heart Transplant 1985; 4:414–416.
158. Whitehead B, Stoehr C, Wu C, et al. Cytokine gene expression in human lung transplant recipients. Transplantation 1993; 56:956–961.
159. Wilkes D, Heidler K, Niemeier M, et al. Increased bronchoalveolar lavage IgG2/IgG1 ratio is a marker for human lung allograft rejection. J Invest Med 1994; 42:652–659.
160. Duquesnoy R, Zeevi A. Immunological monitoring of lung transplant recipients by bronchoalveolar lavage analysis. Transplant Rev 1992; 6:218–229.
161. Zeevi A, Fung J, Paradis I, et al. Lymphocytes of bronchoalveolar lavages from heart-lung transplant recipients. J Heart Transplant 1985; 4:417–421.
162. Paradis I, Marrari M, Zeevi A, et al. HLA phenotype of lung lavage cells following heart-lung transplantation. J Heart Transplant 1985; 4:417–421.
163. Theodore J, Starnes VA, Lewiston NJ: Obliterative bronchiolitis. In: Grossman RF, Maurer JR, eds. Pulmonary Considerations in Transplantation: Clinics in Chest Medicine. Vol II. No 2. Philadelphia: Saunders, 1990:309–321.
164. Burke CM, Yousem SA, Corris PA. Heart-lung transplantation. In: Epler GR, ed. Disease of the Bronchioles. New York: Raven Press, 1994:259–274.
165. Maurer JR. Lung transplantation bronchiolitis obliterans. In: Epler GR, ed. Disease of the Bronchioles. New York: Raven Press, 1994:275–289.
166. Yousem SA, Berry G, Brunt E, et al. A working formulation for the standardization of nomenclature in the diagnosis of heart and lung rejection. J Heart Transplant 1990; 9:593–601.
167. Tazelaar H, Yousem SA. Pathologic findings in heart-lung transplantation: an autopsy study. Hum Pathol 1988; 19:1403–1416.
168. Bolman RM, Shumway SJ, Estrin JA. Lung and heart-lung transplantation: evolution and new applications. Ann Surg 1991; 214:456–470.
169. Anzveto A, Levine SM, Bryan CL, et al. Obliterative bronchiolitis in single lung transplant recipients. Am Rev Respir Dis 1992; 145:A700.
170. Paradis I, Dummer S, Dauber J, et al. Risk factors for the development of chronic rejection of the human lung allograft. Am Rev Respir Dis 1989; 139:A529.
171. Scott J, Higenbottam T, Clelland C, et al. The natural history of chronic lung rejection in heart-lung transplantation. Am Rev Respir Dis 1989; 139:A242.
172. McCarthy P, Starnes V, Theodore J, et al. Improved survival following heart-lung transplant. J Thorac Cardiovasc Surg 1990; 99:54–60.
173. Penketh ARL, Higenbottam TW, Hutter J, et al. Clinical experience in the management of pulmonary opportunistic infection and rejection in recipients of heart-lung transplants. Thorax 1988; 43:762–769.
174. Griffith BP, Hardesty RL, Armitage JM, et al. A decade of lung transplantation. Ann Surg 1993; 218:310–320.
175. Wallwork J. Risk factors for chronic rejection in heart and lungs—why do hearts and lungs rot? Clin Transplant 1994; 8:341–344.
176. deHoyas AL, Patterson GA, Maurer JR, et al: Pulmonary transplantation: early and late results. The Toronto transplant group. J Thorac Cardiovasc Surg 1992; 103:295–306.
177. Wahlers T, Haverich A, Schafers HJ, et al. Chronic rejection following lung transplantation: Incidence, time pattern and consequence. Eur J Cardiothorac Surg 1993; 7:319–324.
178. Nathan SD, Ross DJ, Belman MJ, et al. Bronchiolitis obliterans in single-lung transplant recipients. Chest 1995; 107:967–972.

179. Keller CA, Cagle PT, Brown RW, et al. Bronchiolitis obliterans in recipients of single, double and heart-lung transplantation. Chest 1995; 107:973–980.
180. Armitage JM, Fricker FJ, Kurland G, et al. Pediatric lung transplantation: the years 1985 to 1992 and the clinical trial of FK506. J Thorac Cardiovasc Surg 1993; 105:337–346.
181. Whitehead B, Rees P, Sorensen K, et al. Incidence of obliterative bronchiolitis after heart-lung transplantation in children. J Heart Lung Transplant 1993; 12:903–908.
182. Paradis IL, Williams P. Infection after lung transplantation. Semin Respir Infect 1993; 8: 207–215.
183. Keenan RJ, Lega ME, Dummer JS, et al. Cytomegalovirus serologic status and postoperative infection correlated with risk of developing chronic rejection after pulmonary transplantation. Transplantation 1991; 51:433–438.
184. Duncan SR, Grgurich WF, Iacono AT, et al. A comparison of ganciclovir and acyclovir to prevent cytomegalovirus after lung transplantation. Am J Respir Crit Care Med 1994; 150:146–152.
185. Skeens JL, Fuhrman CR, Yousem SA. Bronchiolitis obliterans in heart-lung transplantation patients: radiologic findings in 11 patients. AJR 1989; 153:253–256.
186. Burke CM, Theodore J, Dawkins KD, et al. Post-transplant obliterative bronchiolitis and other late sequelae in human lung transplantation. Chest 1984; 86:824–829.
187. Gosink BB, Friedman RJ, Liebow AA. Bronchiolitis obliterans: roentgenologic-pathologic correlation. Am J Roentgenol 1973; 117:816–832.
188. Halland SA, Sutton LC, McKenzie FN. Radiologic findings in heart-lung transplantation: a preliminary experience. Can Assoc Radiol J 1989; 40:94–97.
189. Morrish WF, Herman SJ, Weisbrod GL, et al. Bronchiolitis obliterans after lung transplantation: findings at chest radiography and high-resolution CT. Radiology 1991; 179: 487–490.
190. Halvorsen RA Jr, Du Cret RP, Kuni CC, et al. Obliterative bronchiolitis following lung transplantation: diagnostic utility of aerosol ventilation lung scanning and high resolution CT. Clin Nucl Med 1991; 16:256–258.
191. Loubeyre P, Revel D, Delignette A, et al. Bronchiectasis detected with thin-section CT as a prediction of chronic lung allograft rejection. Radiology 1995; 194:213–216.
192. Lentz D, Bergin CJ, Berry GJ, et al. Diagnosis of bronchiolitis obliterans in heart-lung transplantation patients: importance of bronchial dilatation on CT. Am J Roentgenol 1992; 159:436–467.
193. Valentine VG, Robbins RC, Berry GJ, et al. Actuarial survival of heart-lung and bilateral sequential lung transplant recipients with obliterative bronchiolitis. J Heart Lung Transplant. In press, 1995.
194. Patterson GM, Wilson S, Whang JL, et al. Physiologic definitions of obliterative bronchiolitis in heart-lung and double lung transplantation. A comparison of FEF 25-75 and FEV 1. J Heart Lung Transplant. 1995.
195. International Society for Heart and Lung Transplantation, JD Cooper chairman of committee: A working formulation for the standardization of nomenclature and for clinical staging of chronic dysfunction in lung allografts. J Heart Lung Transplant 1993; 12:713–716.
196. Kramer MR, Stoehr C, Whang JL, et al. The diagnosis of obliterative bronchiolitis after heart-lung and lung transplantation. J Heart Lung Transplant 1993; 12:675–681.
197. Yousem SA, Paradis IL, Dauber JH, et al. Efficacy of transbronchial biopsy in the diagnosis of bronchiolitis obliterans in heart-lung transplant recipients. Transplantation 1989; 47:893–895.
198. Turner JS, Willcox PA, Heyhurst MD, et al. Fiberoptic bronchoscopy in the intensive care unit—a prospective study of 147 procedures in 107 patients. Crit Care Med 1994; 22:259–264.
199. Trulock EP, Ettinger NA, Brunt EM, et al. The role of transbronchial lung biopsy in the treatment of lung transplant recipients: an analysis of 200 consecutive procedures. Chest 1992; 102:1049–1052.

200. Higenbottam T, Stewart S, Penketh A, et al. Transbronchial lung biopsy for the diagnosis of rejection in the heart-lung transplant patients. Transplantation 1988; 46:532–539.
201. Trulock EP. Management of lung transplant rejection. Chest 1993; 103:1566–1576.
202. Yousem SA, Dauber JA, Keenan R, et al. Does histologic acute rejection in lung allografts predict the development of bronchiolitis obliterans? Transplantation 1991; 52:306–309.
203. Tazelaar HD, Nilsson FN, Rinaldi M, et al. The sensitivity of transbronchial biopsy for the diagnosis of acute lung rejection. J Thorac Cardiovasc Surg 1993; 105:674–678.
204. Yousem SA, Berry GJ, Brunt EM, et al. A working formulation for the standardization of nomenclature in the diagnosis of heart and lung rejection. Lung Rejection Study Group. J Heart Transplant 1990; 9:593–601.
205. Reitz BA, Burton NA, Jamieson SW, et al. Heart and lung transplantation. J Thorac Cardiovasc Surg 1980; 80:360–372.
206. Reitz BA, Gaudiani VA, Hunt SA, et al. Diagnosis and treatment of allograft rejection in heart-lung transplant recipients. J Thorac Cardiovasc Surg 1983; 85:354–361.
207. Griffith BP, Hardesty RL, Trento A, et al. Asynchronous rejection of heart and lungs following cardiopulmonary transplantation. Ann Thorac Surg 1985; 40:488–493.
208. McGregor CGA, Baldwin JC, Jamieson SW, et al. Isolated pulmonary rejection after combined heart-lung transplantation. J Thorac Cardiovasc Surg 1985; 90:623–630.
209. Schroeder JS, Gao SZ, Alderman EL, et al. Preliminary study of diltiazem in the prevention of coronary artery disease in heart-transplant recipients. N Engl J Med 1993; 328:164–170.

15

Imaging Diagnosis in Heart and Lung Transplantation

Fernando R. Gutierrez and Marilyn J. Siegel
Mallinckrodt Institute of Radiology, Washington University School of Medicine, St. Louis, Missouri

L. Santiago Medina
Children's Hospital and Harvard Medical School, Boston, Massachusetts

I. INTRODUCTION

Lung transplantation has become an important technique for treating selected patients with end-stage lung disease. The first successful lung transplantation was performed in 1983 by the Toronto Lung Transplantation Group in an adult with pulmonary fibrosis (1). Subsequently, the number of successful transplants has increased as well as the number of centers performing transplants. The technique of combined lung and heart transplantation also has evolved, and this application is used for patients with end stage lung and cardiac disease (2,3). Heart transplantation also has undergone dramatic growth, and it is an effective method for treating patients with previously fatal heart disease.

This chapter reviews the imaging findings in patients with lung and heart transplants. The focus in lung transplantation is on plain chest radiography and CT scanning, as they are the most frequently performed imaging tests in lung transplantation. However, the findings on magnetic resonance imaging (MRI) and radionuclide imaging are also discussed. In cardiac transplantation, the role of plain radiographs, MRI, echocardiography, and scintigraphy are reviewed in the evaluation of transplant complications.

II. LUNG TRANSPLANTATION

A. Indications and Techniques

Lung transplants can be performed as an en bloc double-lung technique with tracheal or bilateral bronchial anastomoses (4,5), as bilateral sequential lung transplants with bronchial anastomoses (4,6), or as a single lung transplant (4,7–10). Because ischemia is greater with a tracheal than with bronchial anastomosis, the en bloc technique with tracheal anastomosis is rarely performed. Instead, it has been replaced by the bilateral sequential bronchial

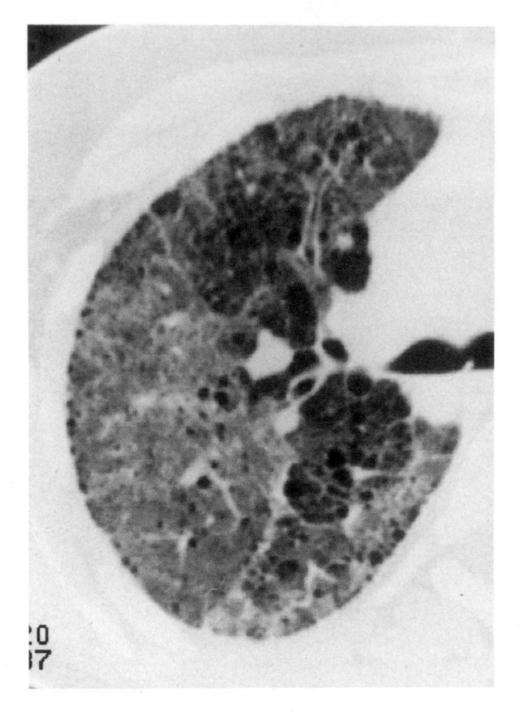

Figure 1 Interstitial fibrosis. Preoperative chest CT reveals honeycombing and diffuse ground-glass opacities.

anastomoses. Moreover, sequential transplant will often avoid the need for cardiopulmonary bypass, which is usually required for en bloc transplantation.

Unilateral lung transplant is selected in patients with interstitial fibrosis (Fig. 1), emphysema from smoking or alpha-1-antitrypsin deficiency, primary or secondary pulmonary hypertension, bronchiolitis obliterans, eosinophilic granuloma, lymphangioleiomyomatosis, and bronchopulmonary dysplasia (7–12). Bilateral lung transplantation is performed in patients with cystic fibrosis (Fig. 2) who have chronically infected lungs and in relatively young patients who are expected to have many years of survival (4,5,6,11).

In some of the earlier lung transplants, an omental flap was wrapped around the tracheal or bronchial anastomosis (11,13). The omentopexy technique is performed by mobilizing omentum from the transverse colon, tunneling it through the chest into the pleural space, and wrapping it around the anastomotic site. Its purpose is to increase anastomotic blood flow, relieve lymphedema, promote healing, and contain a potential dehiscence (13–15). However, because the omental wrap is associated with the additional morbidity of abdominal surgery, it has been replaced by alternative wrapping techniques, such as the use of donor pericardium, internal mammary artery graft and intercostal muscle flap, and more recently the use of a telescoping anastomosis (16,17). In the telescoping technique, the smaller donor bronchus is placed into the larger recipient bronchus with the cartilaginous rings overlapping because this approach provides adequate blood flow to the anastomosis, an omental wrap and associated abdominal surgery can be obviated.

The actuarial survival for all lung transplants is approximately 80% at 30 days and 60% at 1 year (18). Survival also varies with the surgical technique. Survival rates are best for single lung transplantation, followed by the bilateral technique and then the en bloc

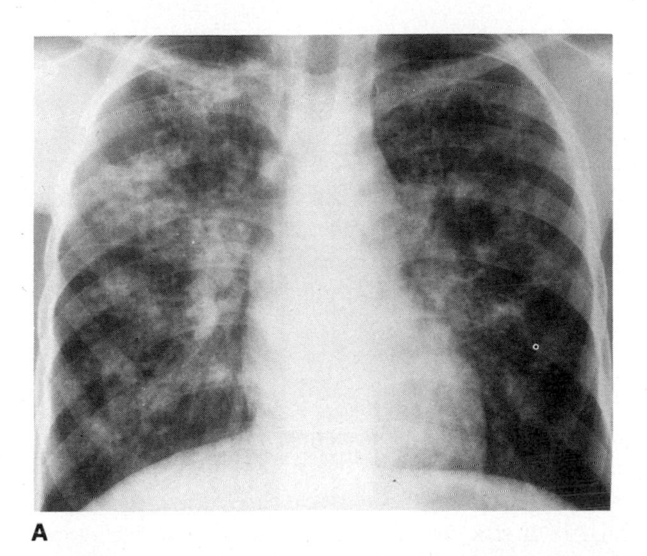

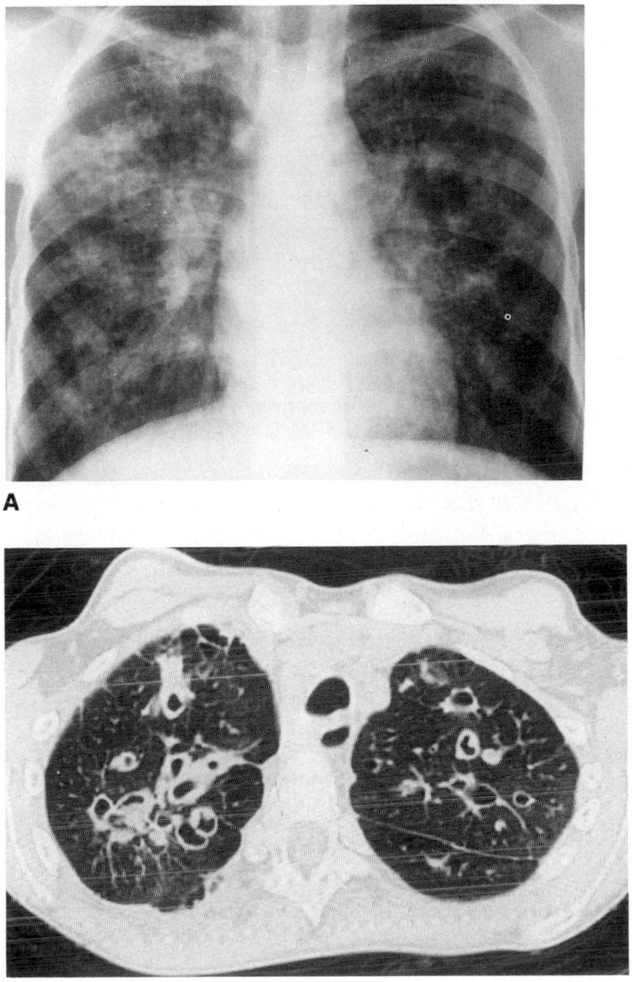

A

B

Figure 2 Cystic fibrosis, pretransplantation chest. (A) Frontal radiograph of a patient with cystic fibrosis reveals bilateral lung hyperexpansion and cystic bronchiectasis. (B) Computed tomography depicts the cystic bronchiectasis with peribronchial thickening.

double technique (18). Principal complications limiting survival include infection, bronchiolitis obliterans, and immunosuppression-induced malignancy.

B. Recipient Selection

Radiographic imaging, especially plain radiographs and computed tomography (CT) are important to detect potential contraindications to transplantation. Extensive pleural and hilar calcifications and pleural adhesions secondary to prior thoracotomy, pleurodesis, or infection can make reimplantation of the donor lung technically difficult and may increase the risk of intraoperative bleeding (9). When chest imaging shows these complications, the least involved side is selected for transplantation.

Chest radiographs and CT scans are also important in identifying occult neoplasms or infection. Patients who undergo lung transplantation because of emphysema secondary to smoking are at increased risk for lung cancer, which can be seen on chest imaging. Imaging may also suggest the presence of active infection, manifested by cavitary nodules, in patients receiving immunosuppression and in those with cystic fibrosis. Such lesions are potential contraindications to transplantation.

In patients undergoing single lung transplantation, differential lung function is important in selecting the lung to transplant. Quantitative ventilation-perfusion scintigraphy is particularly helpful in making this decision. When there is a marked difference in perfusion of the two lungs, the more poorly perfused lung is usually selected for transplantation. In addition, pretransplant scintigraphy offers a baseline to assess future ventilation-perfusion changes after surgery.

C. Donor Organ Selection

Chest radiographs are useful in the selection of a potential donor lung by identifying the presence or absence of parenchymal disease, since a clear chest is the ideal requirement for a lung donor. Nearly all potential donors have sustained a fatal head injury from motor vehicle trauma. As a result, the lung is at risk for pulmonary contusion or laceration. Aspiration is another risk after head injury. Potential donors are by definition brain-dead and hence require intubation and ventilation, which can lead to bacterial colonization of the airway and subsequent parenchymal infection (4,11). Most of these complications are readily identifiable by chest imaging. In addition, chest radiographs can identify prior cardiothoracic surgery, which could potentially contraindicate the use of the donor organ.

D. Imaging Approach: Posttransplant

Radiological imaging is important particularly in the immediate postoperative period and while the patient is in the intensive care unit. Chest radiographs are obtained daily, with additional films obtained as clinically indicated, to identify causes of respiratory compromise, such as pneumothorax and pleural effusion, and to detect pulmonary infiltrates requiring treatment.

If complications develop, CT scanning is performed to evaluate the lung parenchyma, the bronchial anastomosis, and the mediastinum. Most of the relevant information is obtained with axial CT sections. However, spiral CT with multiplanar reconstructions may be useful, especially in complicated cases.

Ventilation-perfusion scintigraphy is also a part of the radiological imaging surveillance and is performed in the immediate postoperative period to document reestablishment of perfusion to the transplanted lung. Additional scans are indicated when respiratory dysfunction develops to determine regional changes in flow or ventilation. Following successful lung transplantation, patients with primary pulmonary hypertension have a significant increase in the percentage of total pulmonary blood flow (flow greater than 90%) to the transplanted lung, compared with patients with chronic obstructive pulmonary disease, alpha-1-antitrypsin deficiency, and idiopathic pulmonary fibrosis (blood flow ranging between 65 and 70%) (11) (Fig. 3).

Magnetic resonance imaging (MRI) is used to assess right ventricular morphology in patients who undergo transplantation for primary pulmonary hypertension. Pretransplant cardiac MRI usually reveals right ventricular hypertrophy, dilatation, and hypokinesis as well as a dilated pulmonary artery and tricuspid regurgitation. After transplantation, decrease or resolution of the right ventricular hypertrophy and hypokinesis can be identified due to the decrease in pulmonary vascular resistance (Fig. 4). Functional and morphological cardiac information can also be obtained with echocardiography and radionuclide ventriculography before and after transplantation.

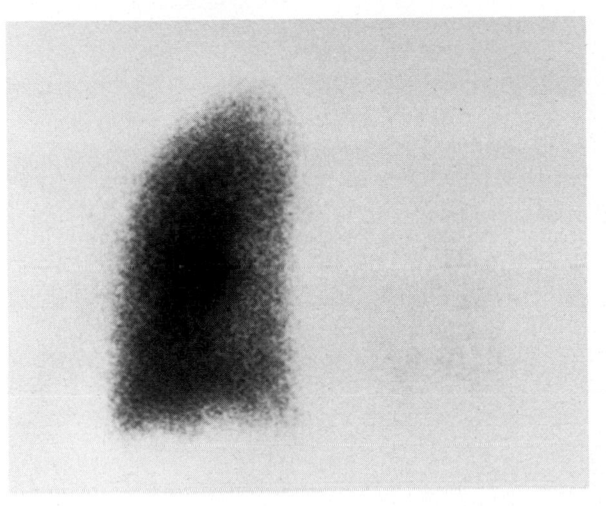

A

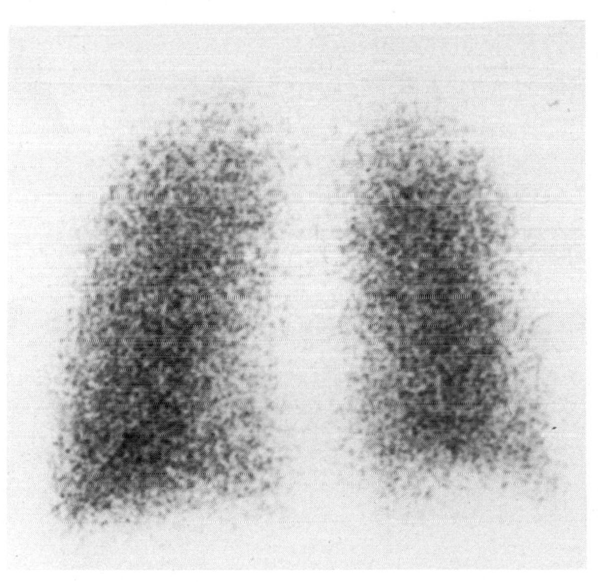

B

Figure 3 Postoperative scintigraphy. (A) Anterior image from a perfusion scintigram in a patient 1 month after a right lung transplant for pulmonary hypertension reveals preferential blood flow in the transplanted lung. (B) Ventilation scintigraphy demonstrates symmetrical ventilation of the transplanted and native lungs.

E. Postoperative Changes

1. Reimplantation Response

The reimplantation response is a frequent reaction to lung transplantation, occurring in virtually all transplanted lungs (4,19,20). It is thought to be a form of noncardiogenic pulmonary edema (21,22) and almost always appears within 48 hr of transplantation. Postulated causes include interruption of lymphatic drainage, ischemia, trauma secondary

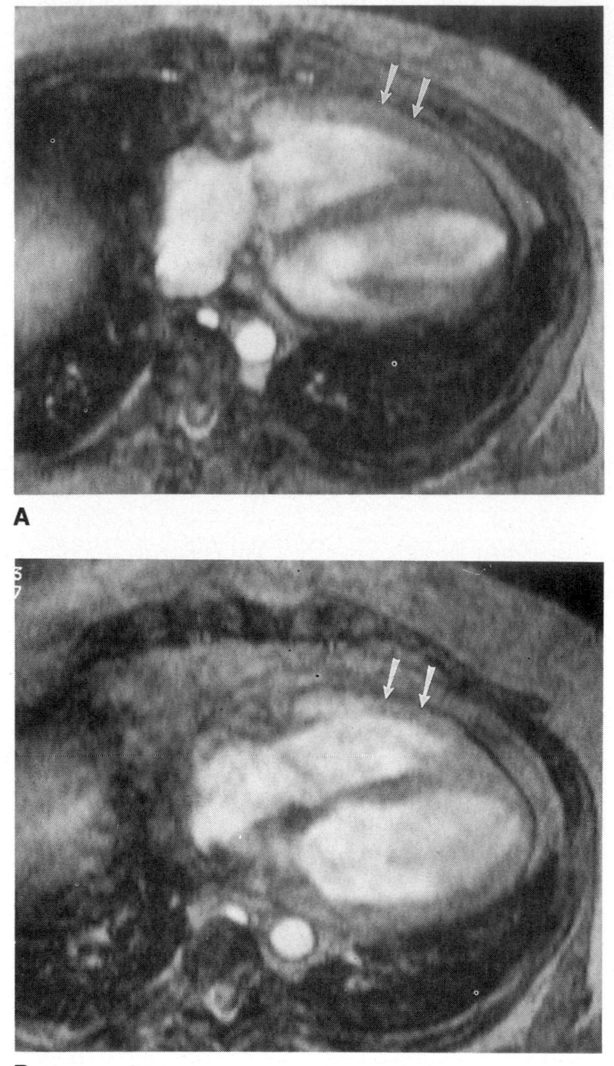

Figure 4 Magnetic resonance imaging. (A) Pretransplant gradient echo image in end diastole demonstrates hypertrophy of the right ventricle (arrows) in a patient with pulmonary hypertension. (B) Comparable follow-up section, 6 months after single-lung transplantation, shows decrease in the right ventricular hypertrophy, reflecting decreased arterial resistance.

to the resection and reimplantation process, and denervation of the transplanted lung (4,19,20,23).

The earliest radiographic finding is perihilar air-space or interstitial infiltrate, which may be present on the immediate postoperative radiograph or may manifest within 2 days of operation (20,24,25). In most patients, the process worsens over time, peaking in severity between the second and fourth postoperative day (20) (Fig. 5). At its severest, it may be confluent, appearing as dense consolidation with air bronchograms. Extension to the lateral

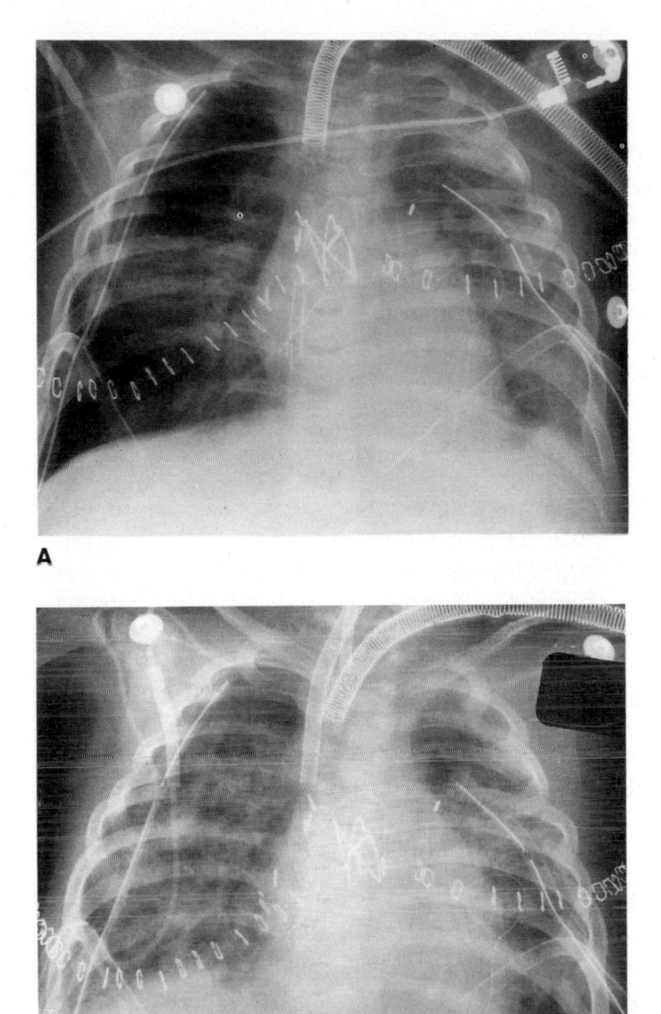

Figure 5 Reimplantation response. (A) Frontal radiograph 1 day after bilateral transplantation reveals mild bilateral perihilar interstitial infiltrates. Also noted are bilateral chest tubes. (B) Follow-up radiography 2 days later demonstrates more diffuse interstitial infiltrates.

chest wall and into the upper and lower lobes can occur, although the extreme peripheral parts of the lungs are almost always spared (19,22). Gradual clearing of the disease begins after the fourth postoperative day, with the time to complete resolution ranging from 11 days to 6 months (20).

The radiographic appearance of the reimplantation response is nonspecific, and fluid overload, infection, rejection, and left ventricular heart failure must be excluded clinically.

As reimplantation edema occurs early in the postoperative course, the development of a pulmonary infiltrate on or after day 5 is more suspicious for infection or rejection (20,25).

2. Acute Rejection

Acute rejection is a major cause of morbidity in patients undergoing lung transplantation (27). It most often occurs within the first 3 postoperative weeks, with a peak incidence during the second week (26,28), but it may occur at any time. Acute rejection occurs at least once in almost all patients, and most recipients usually have two to three episodes within the first 3 postoperative weeks (29). Clinically, patients manifest deterioration of pulmonary function tests and often fever and worsening pulmonary infiltrates on chest radiography (19,29).

Radiographic findings of rejection are variable and include septal lines, pleural effusions, and perihilar or basilar reticular interstitial disease or air-space consolidation (4,19,20,24–26,30,31) (Fig. 6). In heart-lung transplantation, it has been suggested that the combination of new or increasing pleural effusions and septal lines without a concomitant increase in cardiac size, vascular pedicle width, or evidence of vascular redistribution indicates acute lung rejection with a sensitivity of 68% and a specificity of 90% (32). Some authors, however, have suggested that septal lines are insensitive for the diagnosis of acute rejection, occurring in less than 15% of patients (19). Other authors have also described ill-defined perihilar and basilar nodules in acute rejection (31). These nodules sometimes coalesce to form areas of consolidation. In general, the chest radiographic findings are nonspecific and must be differentiated from infection (29–31).

Rejection is usually treated by a bolus injection of corticosteroids (29). Improvement in pulmonary function tests and radiographic infiltrates confirms the diagnosis of acute rejection. Chest radiographs usually return to normal or near normal within the second or third postoperative month, with episodes of acute rejection becoming rare (19). However, if another episode of rejection occurs, the pulmonary infiltrate reappears or progresses (31).

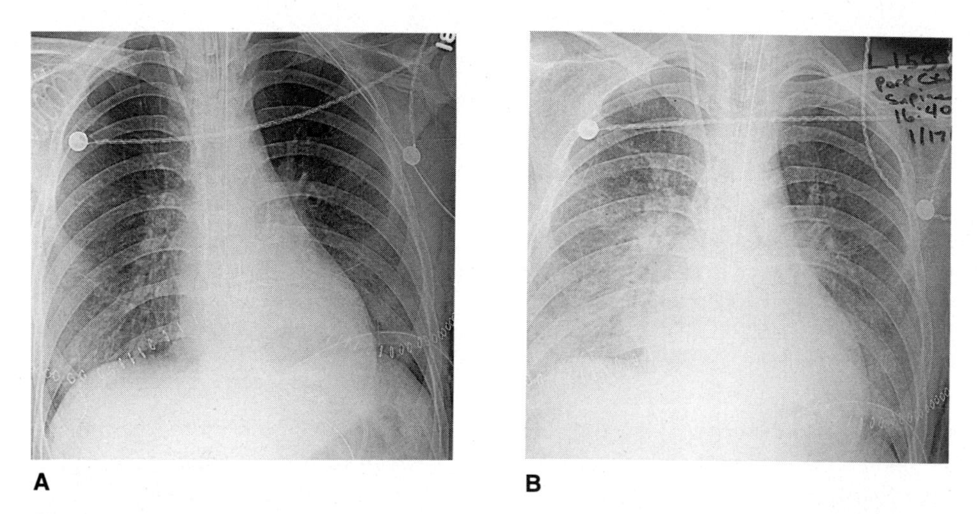

A **B**

Figure 6 Acute lung rejection. (A) Frontal radiograph 1 day after bilateral lung transplantation shows mild bilateral perihilar interstitial infiltrates. (B) Follow-up study 1 day later reveals diffuse infiltrates with basilar predominance. Transbronchial biopsy demonstrated acute rejection.

Radionuclide scans during episodes of acute rejection can be associated with an overall reduction in blood flow to the transplanted lung and a concomitant increase in flow to the native lung in single lung transplantation (29). This appearance is believed to reflect increased pulmonary vascular resistance in the transplanted lung secondary to rejection. However, there is significant overlapping of these findings with other complications, such as infection and bronchiolitis obliterans.

Computed tomography is reported to be a more sensitive method to demonstrate findings of rejection, but as with plain radiographs, the findings on CT are nonspecific (19,33). Findings of rejection on CT include ground-glass opacities, interlobular septal thickening, small nodules (usually less than 1 cm in diameter), decreased vascularity, and air-space consolidation (33,34) (Fig. 7). Currently, CT is not performed routinely to diagnose rejection, but it can be useful to determine the optimal site for transbronchial biopsy.

3. Bronchiolitis Obliterans

Bronchiolitis obliterans is a cause of late morbidity and mortality in lung transplantation (4). It is found in 10 to 50% of long-term survivors of heart-lung transplantation (17,35–38) and to a lesser degree in patients with single or double-lung transplants (38–40). The cause of bronchiolitis obliterans is uncertain, but possible causes include chronic or repeated episodes of subacute rejection, infection, or a combination of infection and rejection leading to small airway injury and subsequent severe obstructive airway disease (38).

Bronchiolitis obliterans usually begins 3 or more months after transplantation. The clinical diagnosis is based on the presence of dyspnea and cough associated with a decrease in the percent of predicted forced expiratory flow between 25% and 75% of vital capacity (4,36,38). Tissue confirmation of the diagnosis can usually be obtained by transbronchial lung biopsy. Occasionally, open lung biopsy is needed for diagnosis. Early detection of this condition is important because early treatment with high doses of steroids may lead to reversal or stabilization of the disease.

The plain chest radiographic findings in chronic rejection are nonspecific and include interstitial opacities, pleural effusions or thickening, decreased vascular markings, patchy air space disease, dilated bronchi, and nodules measuring between 0.5 to 1.5 cm in diameter (19,20,24,30,37–40) (Fig. 8).

The CT findings of bronchiolitis obliterans include bronchial dilatation, diminished peripheral vascularity, ground-glass opacities, and interlobular septal thickening (34, 36,38,40) (Fig. 9). Of these findings, the best predictor of bronchiolitis obliterans is bronchial dilatation relative to the size of adjacent vessels, especially in the lower lobes (36). Upper lobe bronchial dilatation can also occur in bronchiolitis obliterans, but this finding is not as common as lower lobe bronchial dilatation. The bronchi visible on CT are primarily segmental or subsegmental, although in severe bronchiolitis obliterans all bronchial structures can be dilated. The percentage of dilated bronchi closely correlates with the results of pulmonary function tests, including forced expiratory volume in 1 sec, forced vital capacity, and forced expiratory flow between 25 and 75% of vital capacity. The percentage of dilated bronchi generally increases with increasing pulmonary dysfunction (36).

4. Infection

Infection is a common complication in lung transplant patients, with a prevalence as high as 60% (4,19,26,41–44). The causes for the increased susceptibility of the transplanted lung to

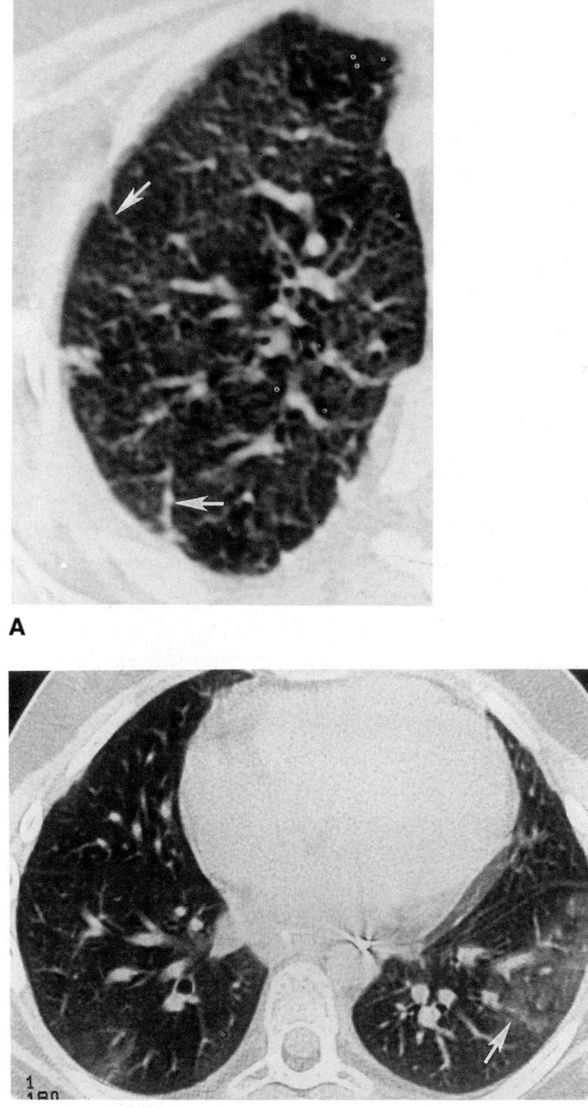

Figure 7 Acute lung rejection. (A) Computed tomography shows interlobular septal thickening (arrows). (B) Computed tomography of another patient depicts ground-glass opacities mainly in the left lower lobe (arrow).

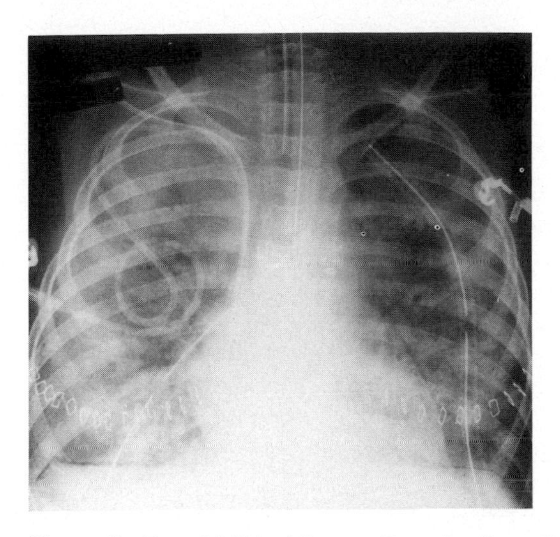

Figure 8 Bronchiolitis obliterans. Frontal radiograph of a patient after bilateral lung transplantation demonstrates bilateral diffuse air-space disease with nearly total consolidation of the right lung.

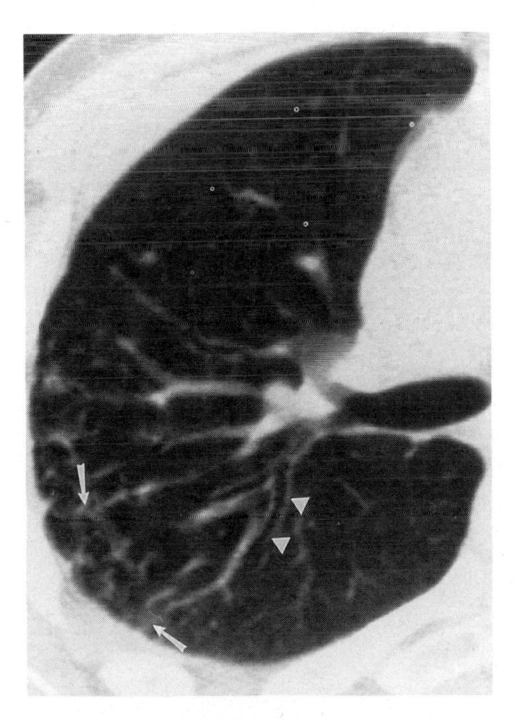

Figure 9 Bronchiolitis obliterans. Computed tomography reveals mild bronchial dilatation (arrowheads) involving the right lower lobe and interlobular septal thickening (arrows). (From Ref. 34.)

infection are multiple and include immunosuppression, denervation (which suppresses the cough reflex), decreased mucociliary clearance, lymphatic interruption, allograft rejection (which depletes the bronchus-associated lymphoid tissue) (45), and possibly direct transmission of infectious organisms, such as cytomegalovirus (41,43).

a. Bacterial Bacterial infections are reported most often in lung transplant patients, with a frequency of 65% (42), but viral and fungal infection can also occur and are more likely to be lethal (42,44). Bacterial infections are most frequent in the first two postoperative weeks, with approximately 75% caused by gram-negative rods, especially *Pseudomonas* and Enterobacteriaceae (42–44). Other less commonly isolated organisms include *Staphylococcus aureus*, *Haemophilus influenzae*, *Streptococcus pneumoniae*, and *Legionella* (42).

On chest radiographs, bacterial infections appear as nodular opacities, focal infiltrates, or lobar consolidation with or without cavitation in the transplanted lung (19,31). Findings on CT include air-space disease, nodules, pulmonary or mediastinal abscess formation, and pleural effusion or thickening (42) (Figs. 10 and 11).

b. Viral. Viral pathogens account for 19 to 23% of infections in lung transplant recipients (43,44). Possible viral pathogens in lung transplant patients include cytomegalovirus (CMV), herpes simplex, Epstein-Barr, and varicella zoster. Of these, CMV is the greatest cause of morbidity and mortality (41–43). Cytomegalovirus infection results when a lung transplant patient who is seronegative or seropositive for CMV receives a lung from a CMV-seropositive donor. The infection in a seronegative recipient who receives a seropositive lung is termed primary, while that in a seropositive recipient receiving a seropositive organ is said to be secondary. The frequency of primary infection among seronegative recipients varies between 50 and 100%, while secondary infection has been reported in 60 to 100% of seropositive recipients (41–43). However, the case fatility rate is highest in CMV-seronegative recipients (46). Viral infections tend to occur between 1 and 6 months postoperatively (41–43).

Chest radiographs in lung transplant patients with viral pathogens, including CMV as well as other viral organisms, demonstrate nonspecific focal or diffuse interstitial or air-

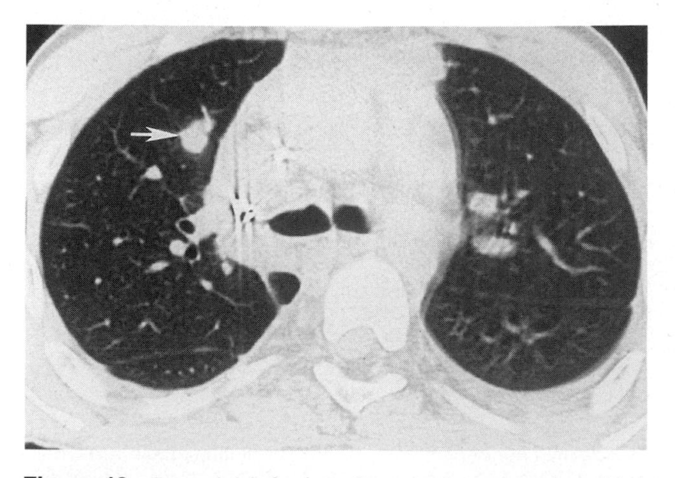

Figure 10 Bacterial infection. Computed tomography with lung window shows a well-defined right upper lobe nodule (arrow). Cultures were positive for *Klebsiella*.

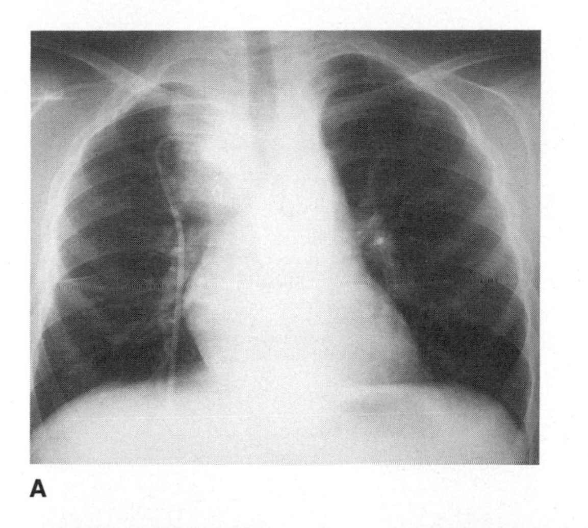

A

B

Figure 11 Mediastinal abscess. (A) Frontal radiograph reveals right greater than left paratracheal widening. (B) Computed tomography shows a low attenuation anterior mediastinal mass (M) with right paratracheal extension (arrow). Aspiration of the anterior mediastinal mass yielded Klebsiella. (From Ref. 26.)

space disease, nodules, and pleural effusions (30–32, 41, 42). On CT, viral disease can produce ground-glass opacities, interlobular septal thickening, and nodules (34) (Fig. 12).

c. Fungal. Fungal infection accounts for approximately 10% of infections and usually occurs in the first 6 months of transplantation, but it can occur later (4,41–44). *Candida albicans* and *Aspergillus* organisms are the most common causes of fungal infection; *Cryptococcus neoformans* is a rare fungal pathogen (4,42–44). As in other infections, fungal infection can manifest as focal nodular opacities or as diffuse infiltrates on plain chest radiographs and CT scans (19) (Fig. 13). Pulmonary cavitary lesions, pleural effusion, airway dehiscence, and adenopathy also can occur.

d. Protozoal. Protozoal organisms, usually *Penumocystis carinii* and rarely *Toxoplasma gondii*, have been identified as causes of infection in 2 to 19% of lung or heart-lung transplants (43,44). Most commonly, the organisms are a late cause of posttransplant morbidity and mortality and are usually detected in the third to sixth postoperative month (41–44). Chest radiographs in protozoal infection show perihilar hazy opacification or air-space consolidation (31,32).

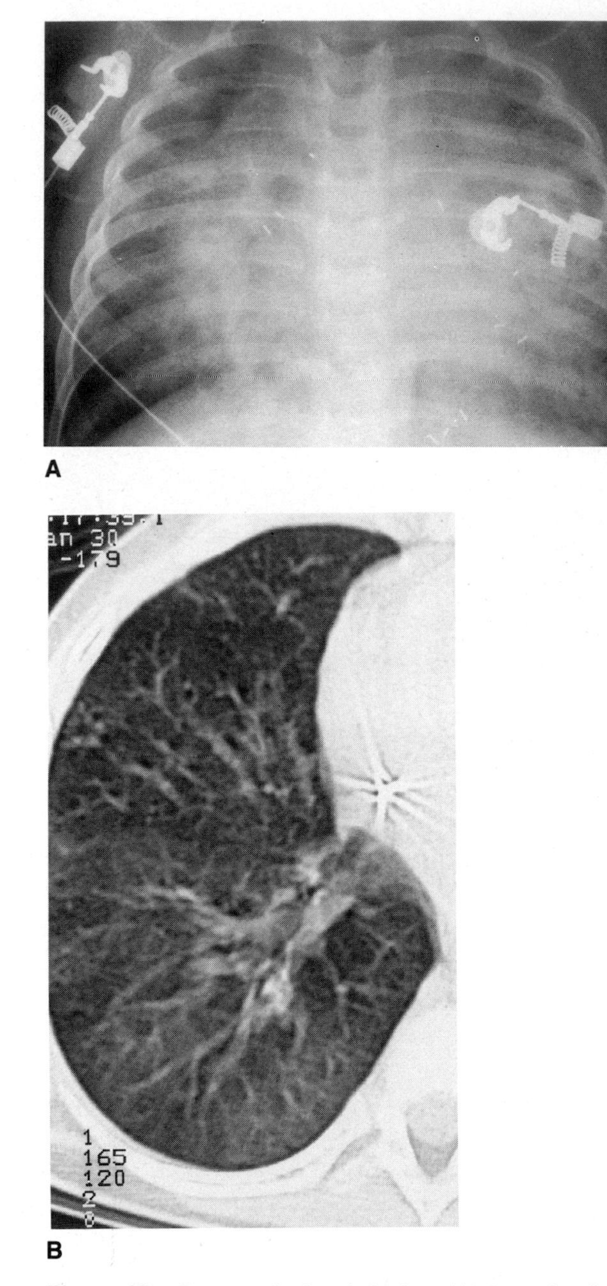

Figure 12 Cytomegalovirus infection. (A) Frontal radiograph reveals diffuse air-space infiltrates which are confluent in the perihilar areas bilaterally. (B) Computed tomography coned down to the right lung in another patient demonstrates diffuse ground-glass opacities posteriorly. Transbronchial biopsy and cultures were consistent with CMV pneumonia.

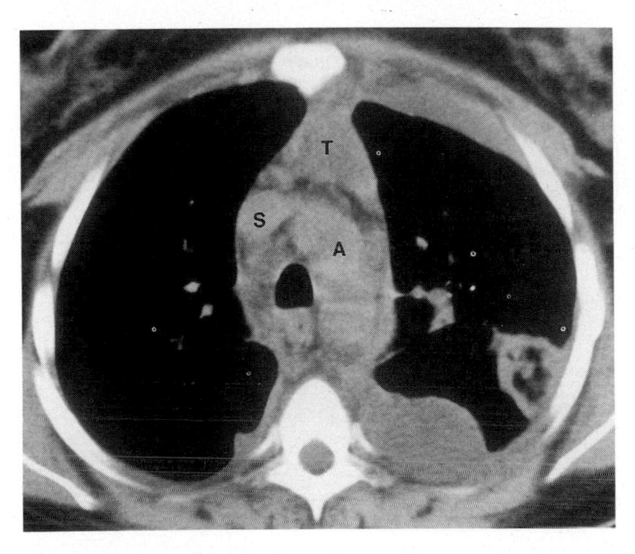

Figure 13 Fungal infection. Computed tomography reveals a cavitary lesion in the left lung. In addition, a loculated left pleural effusion is identified posteriorly. T = thymus; S = superior vena cava; A = aorta.

F. Airway Complications

Bronchial dehiscence and stenosis are the major airway complications after lung transplantation. These complications have been related to airway ischemia at the time of surgery and to the use of perioperative steroids to treat rejection. Steroids appear to have a deleterious effect on healing of the airway anastomosis (19,47). The increased propensity of patients with lung transplantation to develop ischemic changes can be explained by the fact that the systemic or bronchial blood supply is not directly reconnected at surgery. The use of the bronchial omentopexy, pericardial wrapping, bronchial rather than tracheal anastomosis, and, most recently, the telescoping technique for bronchial anastomosis have improved anastomotic blood flow and healing and reduced the frequency of ischemic complications (47). With the use of the telescoping technique, the incidence of airway complications has decreased significantly even with the routine use of perioperative corticosteroid therapy (16,17).

Bronchial dehiscence usually involves only a part of the anastomosis and heals without intervention (19,47). Chest tube placement or direct closure of the bronchial defect has been required in up to 27% of cases (19,47). Stenosis is a late complication of partial or complete dehiscence. Severe strictures may require endobronchial stenting for treatment, while mild to moderate strictures may be treated with laser resection or balloon bronchoplasty (24,48).

CT scanning is useful to complement bronchoscopy in the identification of dehiscence and stenosis, and it is more sensitive than chest radiography in detecting these complications. Following a telescoping anastomosis, minimal irregularity of the bronchus can be noted on CT and is a normal postoperative finding that should not be confused with ulceration or stenosis.

Dehiscence usually is difficult to identify on plain radiography, although chest radiography can occasionally demonstrate extrapulmonary air (Figs. 14 and 15) and lobar or lung collapse, which may accompany dehiscence. Computed tomography can demonstrate an

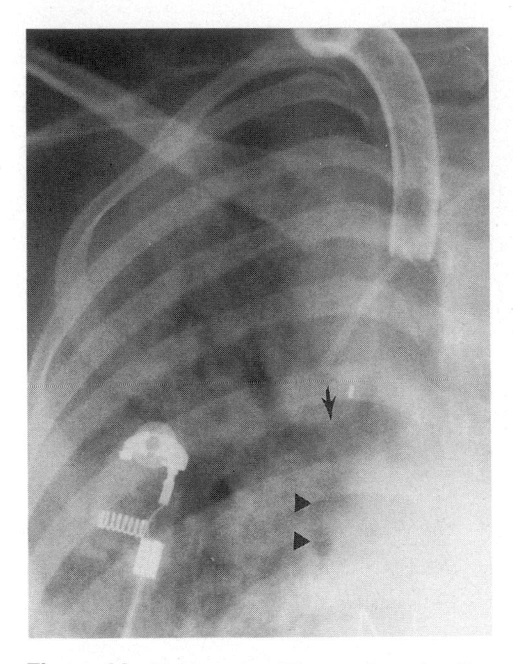

Figure 14 Dehiscence. Closeup frontal radiograph shows a focal area of extraluminal air (arrowheads) in the right hilar area adjacent to the bronchial anastomosis (arrow).

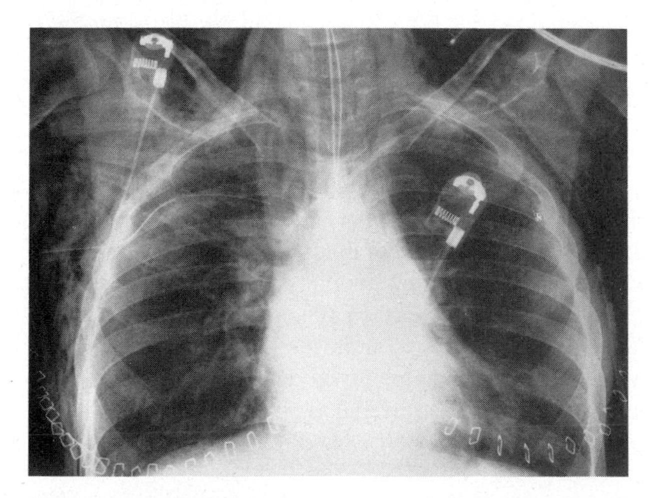

Figure 15 Infected dehiscence. Frontal radiograph reveals mediastinal emphysema as well as extensive subcutaneous emphysema. Bronchoscopy demonstrated dehiscence at the anastomotic site. *Aspergillus* was cultured from airway lavage.

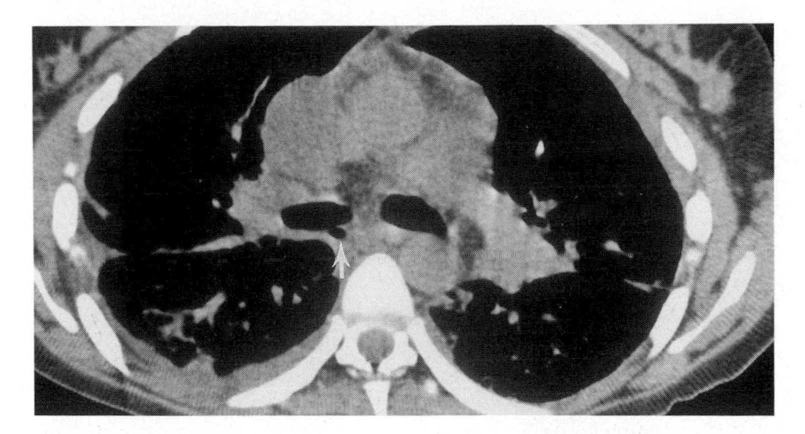

Figure 16 Dehiscence. Computed tomography demonstrates focal area of extraluminal air extending from the right bronchial anastomosis posteriorly (arrow).

extraluminal air collection adjacent to the anastomosis and disruption of the bronchial wall at the anastomotic line (49) (Figs. 16 and 17). In patients who have undergone omentopexy, the extraluminal air may be contained within the omentum. Air also may be noted in the mediastinum or pericardium (Fig. 18). Airway strictures manifest as narrowing of the bronchus and are much better seen by CT than by chest radiography (20) (Fig. 19). Spiral CT with two- and three-dimensional reconstructions may be useful to further delineate the site of dehiscence or stenosis.

Stents used for treatment of bronchial stenosis can be silastic or metallic. Metallic stents are readily identified on plain radiographs. However, silastic stents can be difficult to identify, especially if the radiographs are underpenetrated (Fig. 20). Both stents are virtually always visible on CT, so that their anatomic location can easily be seen. Hence, CT is preferred over plain chest radiographs to document stent migration or displacement (Fig. 21).

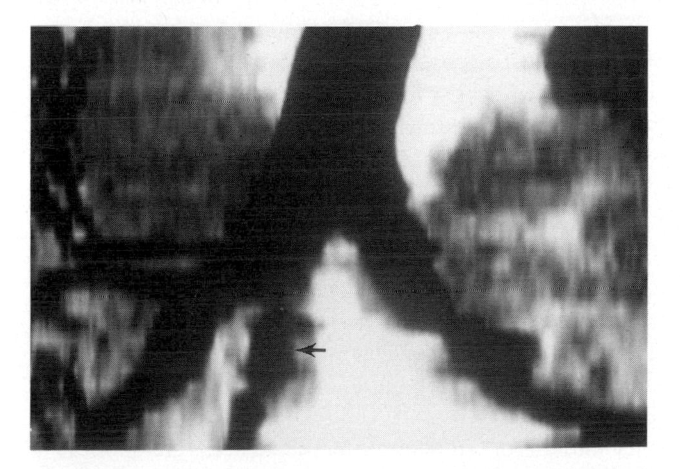

Figure 17 Dehiscence. Coronal three-dimensional CT reconstruction demonstrates a collection of extraluminal air (arrow) extending inferiorly and contiguous with the right bronchial anastomosis. (Reprinted with permission from Ref. 26.)

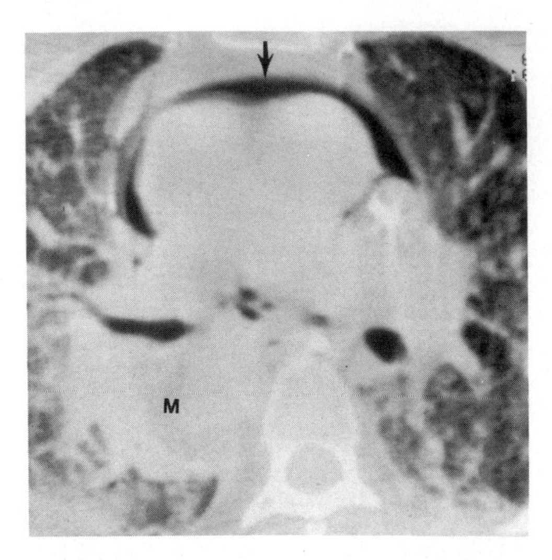

Figure 18 Dehiscence. Computed tomography reveals air in the pericardium (arrow) from a bronchial dehiscence not shown on this image. The soft tissue mass (M) posterior to the right mainstem bronchus is caused by an omental wrap.

On CT, the pitfalls of pseudodehiscence and pseudostenosis must be recognized, so that they are not confused with postsurgical complications. Pseudodehiscence occurs when air insinuates its way between the stent and the airway wall (Fig. 21B). Pseudostenosis occurs when mucous plugs adhere to the airway wall (Fig. 22).

G. Lymphoproliferative Disorders

Lymphoproliferative disorders are believed to be the result of immunosuppression used in transplantation and occur in approximately 2% of organ allograft recipients (50) versus 3.5% of heart and 8% of lung transplant recipients (51). The higher incidence of lymphoproliferative disorders in lung transplantation may relate to the degree of immunosuppression needed to suppress rejection (19). Almost all cases are associated with infection by the Epstein-Barr virus (50) which is believed to have a role in inducing lymphoproliferative disease. The spectrum of lymphoproliferative disease varies from a mild polyclonal proliferation of lymphocytes similar to mononucleosis to an aggressive malignancy similar to non-Hodgkin's lymphoma (19,50). The disease usually occurs within 3 to 4 months of transplantation (51).

The outcome of posttransplant lymphoproliferative disease varies with time of presentation. Early presentation in the first year of transplantation has a lower mortality (approximately 35%), is associated with localized or nodal disease, and responds to a reduction of immunosuppression. Late lymphoproliferative disorders have a high mortality (70 to 80%), often involve disseminated disease at presentation, and do not respond to reduction in immunosuppression (51).

The most common radiological findings of lymphoproliferative disease are multiple or solitary pulmonary nodules and mediastinal and hilar lymphadenopathy (52) (Fig. 23). The pulmonary nodules tend to be well circumscribed soft tissue masses with an average diameter of 2 cm, but, rarely, they can be poorly circumscribed or of low attenuation,

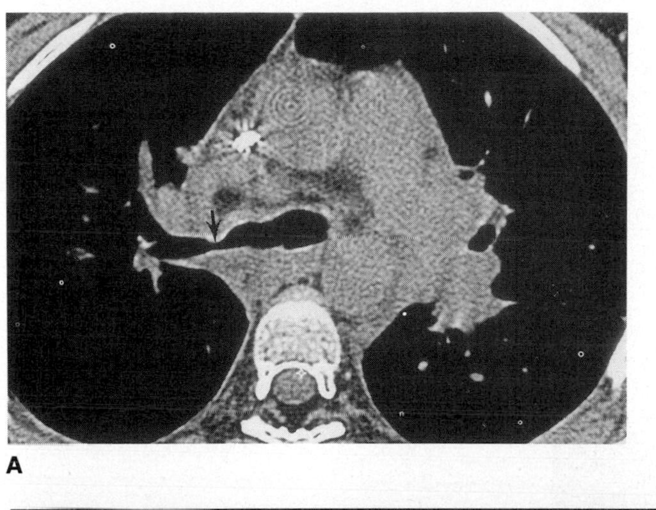
A

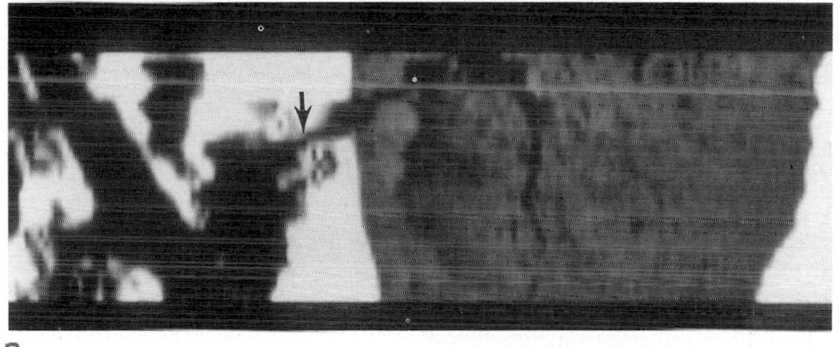
B

Figure 19 Stenosis. (A) Computed tomography reveals a short segment stenosis of the right mainstem bronchus at the anastomosis (arrow). (B) Computed tomography with 3D reconstruction in another patient demonstrates stenosis of the bronchial anastomosis (arrow).

reflecting the presence of necrosis. Mediastinal and hilar lymph nodes also average 2 cm in diameter and have a propensity to involve the paratracheal, anterior mediastinal, and aortopulmonary areas. Less frequent radiographic findings include air-space consolidation (9%), thymic enlargement (6%), pericardial thickening (6%), and pleural effusions (11%) (52). Air-space disease and pleural effusions are nonspecific findings and must be differentiated from pulmonary edema, rejection, and infection. The sensitivity of chest radiography and CT are approximately 40 and 90%, respectively, for identifying intrathoracic tumor in patients with posttransplant lymphoproliferative disorders (52).

H. Postransplant Lung Nodules

Pulmonary nodules in patients undergoing lung transplantation are usually associated with rejection, infection, or lymphoproliferative disorders. Other benign entities that can mimic nodules are healing rib fractures and postbiopsy pseudonodules (19,53). Pseudonodules develop after transbronchial lung biopsy and are believed to be due to hemorrhage. They

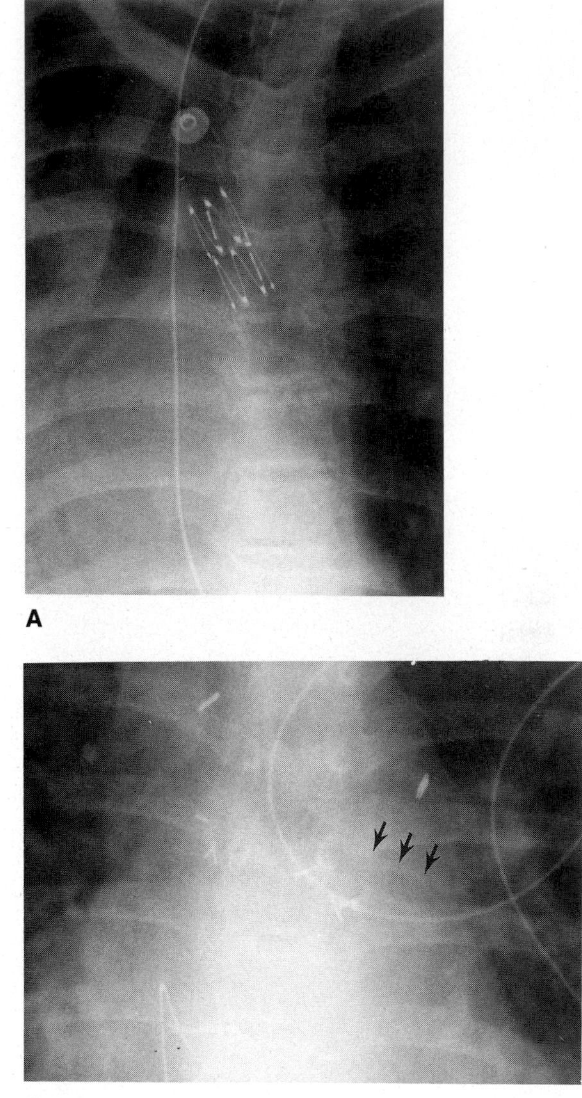

Figure 20 Stents. (A) Frontal radiograph reveals a metallic stent in the left main-stem bronchus. (B) Frontal radiograph of another patient demonstrates a slightly radiopaque silastic stent (arrows) in the left main-stem bronchus. Silastic stents can easily be missed if the film is not well penetrated.

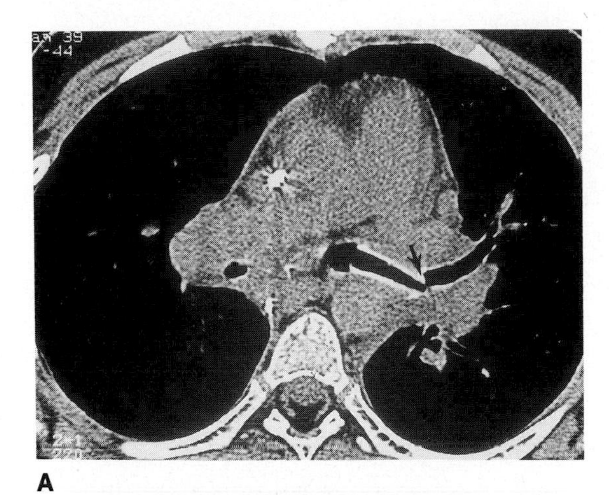

A

B

Figure 21 Stent migration. (A) Computed tomography shows a migration of a silastic stent with associated partial obstruction of the origin of the left upper lobe bronchus (arrow). (B) Follow-up CT shows adequate repositioning of the stent in the left main-stem bronchus. Also noted is a small amount of air (arrowheads) between the stent and the airway wall. This is consistent with a pseudodehiscence and should not be confused with true airway dehiscence.

appear as multiple, ill-defined, rounded opacities in the periphery of the lung on chest radiography (Fig. 24). On CT, they have an appearance similar to that of a laceration, manifesting as small, peripheral, linear parenchymal opacities, some with areas of cavitation (53). The nodules spontaneously resolve over a few days to 2 weeks.

I. Other Postoperative Changes

Pneumothorax, hydropneumothorax, and pneumomediastinum are expected manifestations of resection and reanastomosis of a lung and can be seen on chest radiographs within the

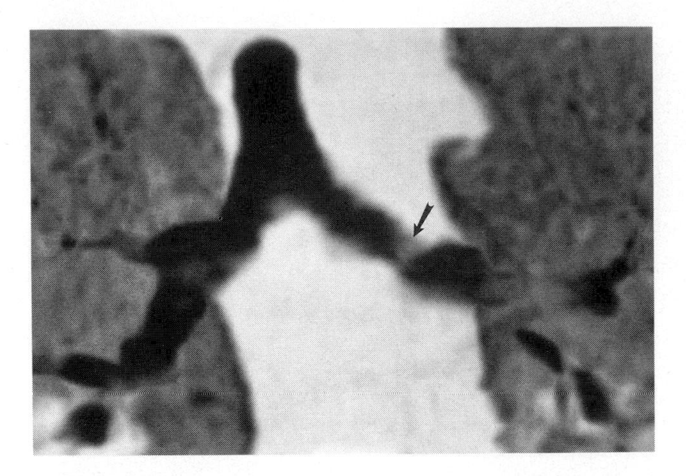

Figure 22 Pseudostenosis. Three-dimensional reconstruction shows apparent narrowing of the left bronchial anastomosis (arrow). At bronchoscopy, a mucous plug was found. The bronchial lumen was widely patent.

first postoperative week. Pneumothorax has been attributed to multiple small tears in the visceral pleura subsequent to the extraction and reimplantation procedure (19). Rarely, pneumopericardium is identified on plain radiographs.

Postoperative CT findings in patients undergoing sternotomy include air and fluid collections in the retrosternal space, poor definition of mediastinal fat planes due to edematous changes, and an increased number of mediastinal lymph nodes. The nodes may be normal in size or enlarged and may represent residual preoperative changes or an acquired postoperative response. Resolution of the retrosternal air and fluid and mediastinal edema is the expected finding on serial CT studies.

Delayed bilateral pneumothoraces have been reported in patients with heart-lung transplants who undergo unilateral biopsy, thoracocentesis, or placement of a central venous catheter (54). The time interval between transplantation and development of bilateral pneumothoraces ranges from 2 weeks to 2 years. The presence of bilateral pneumothoraces is believed to reflect disruption of the anterior mediastinal pleura and the formation of a single pleural cavity in patients who undergo en bloc reimplantation of the heart and lungs (54).

As previously described, some patients may undergo omentopexy or omental wrapping to secure the airway anastomosis and promote healing. The omental wrap can be identified on chest radiography in approximately 50% of patients who undergo omentopexy (13). On the posteroanterior projection, the omental wrap can appear as paraspinal widening, a cardiophrenic angle mass, right paratracheal widening, pseudocardiomegaly, pseudoparenchymal infiltrate, or increased hilar density (Fig. 25). The most frequent findings on the lateral view are increased hilar opacity and pseudoparenchymal infiltrate (13).

On plain chest radiographs, the omental wrap can be a potential interpretative pitfall because it simulates a mass. In problematic cases, the omentum can be easily recognized by CT because of its characteristic attenuation value and course (13). The omentum typically has the same attenuation as fat and often contains linear areas of increased attenuation, representing omental vessels (Fig. 26). Areas of soft tissue attenuation may also be seen in the omentum at its cranial or caudal aspects. The etiology of these soft tissue areas is uncertain, but they are believed to represent areas of edema, hemorrhage, or fibrosis (13). In

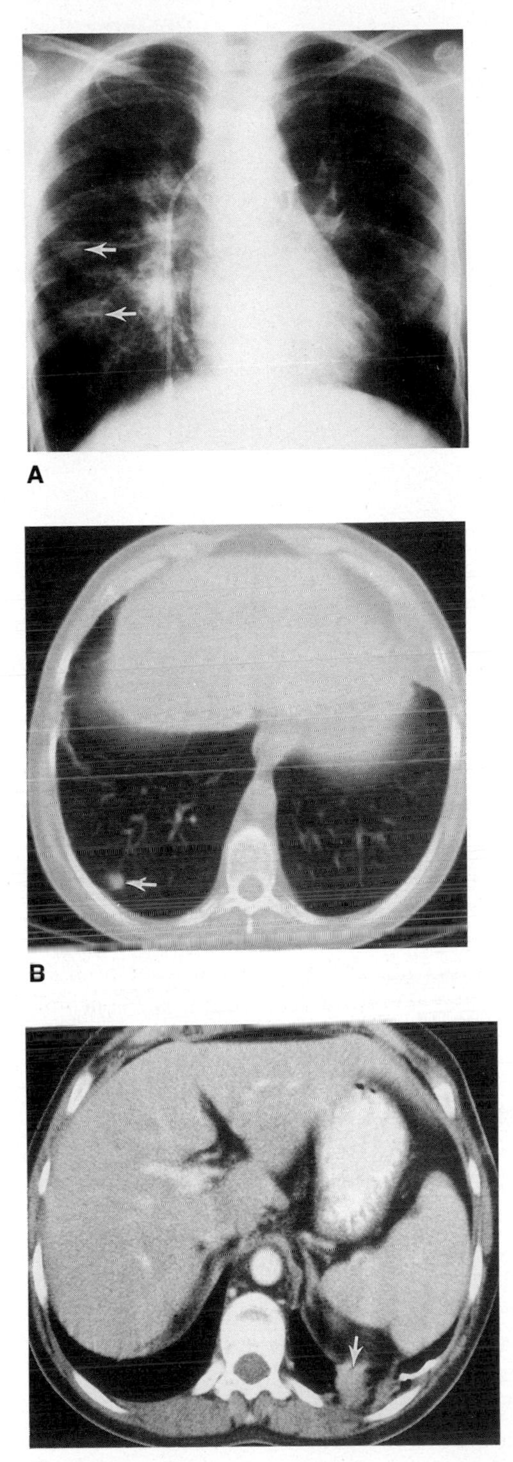

Figure 23 Lymphoproliferative disorder. (A) Frontal radiograph reveals pulmonary nodules (arrows). (B) Computed tomography at a lung window shows a nodule (arrow) in the right lower lobe. (C) Computed tomography with a soft tissue window demonstrates a soft tissue mass in the left costophrenic angle (arrow). (Figure B reprinted with permission from Ref. 26.)

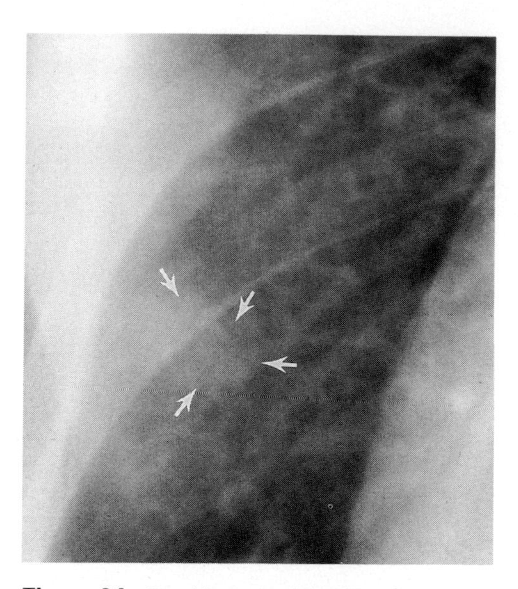

Figure 24 Postbiopsy nodule. Coned-down frontal radiograph of a patient 2 days after lung biopsy reveals an ill-defined focal pulmonary opacity (arrows) consistent with the biopsy site.

patients with bronchial dehiscence, air can be seen in the omental flap adjacent to the bronchial defect.

Pneumoperitoneum may accompany a pneumothorax in patients who undergo omentopexy because, following this procedure, the pleural and peritoneal spaces are in communication (17). In these cases, clinical correlation is important to exclude the possibility of bowel perforation. Another rare complication of transplantation is pseudoaneurysm of the great vessels or heart in patients undergoing repair of congenital heart defects and concomitant lung transplantation (Fig. 27).

III. CARDIAC TRANSPLANTATION

A. Indications

Since the introduction of cyclosporin A for the immunosuppression of patients undergoing cardiac transplantation in 1980 (55), this procedure has gained popularity in the medical community. During 1988, more than 2500 heart transplant operations were performed in more than 170 medical centers around the world (56). Refinements in the administration of immunosuppressive drugs, donor-organ preservation, selection of donor and recipient, and treatment of complications such as infections has allowed significant improvement in the longevity of these patients. The 2-year-survival for heart transplant recipients approaches 90% (57).

Major complications affecting survival include rejection, coronary artery disease, and lymphoproliferative disorders. This section focuses on the imaging diagnosis of these complications.

B. Surgical Techniques

Understanding of the surgical technique and the resulting anatomic alterations is important so that complications can be identified. During the cardiac harvesting procedure, the

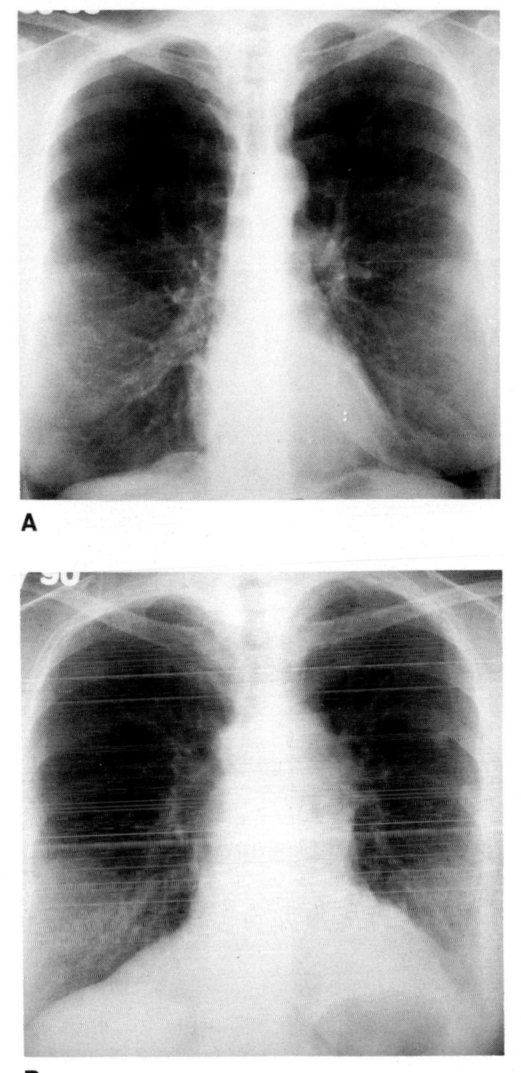

Figure 25 Omental wrap. (A) Frontal chest radiograph before lung transplantation reveals normal width of the mediastinum. (B) Posttransplant radiograph shows prominence of the cardiac silhouette and widening of the superior mediastinum consistent with the omental wrap.

donor's ascending aorta is divided at the level of the mid-ascending portion. The main pulmonary artery is then divided just proximal to its major branches. These two vessels are trimmed and anastomosed to the recipients respective vessels. The most posterior portion of the recipients' left atrium (attached to the native pulmonary veins) remains in place, where it is anastomosed to the new left atrium. The two right atria are anastomosed by means of double-ended sutures.

The donor's superior vena cava is ligated and divided during the harvesting procedure and becomes nonfunctional other than to form part of the newly created right atrium. A small portion of the donor's inferior vena cava accompanies the new heart, since the largest

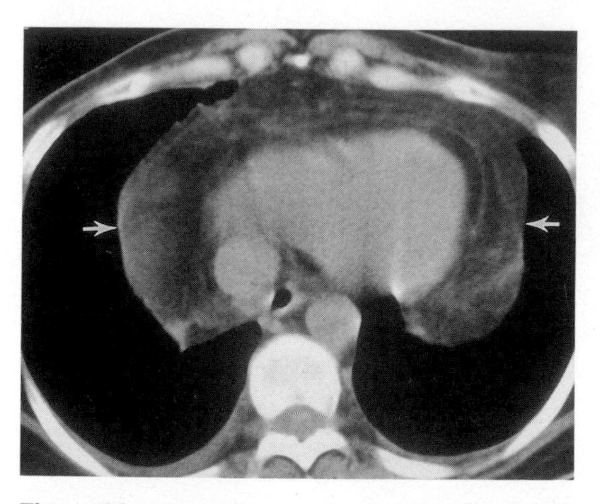

Figure 26 Omental wrap. Computed tomography depicts the greater omentum (arrows) surrounding the heart. Note the soft tissue strands within the fatty tissue consistent with omental vessels.

part of this vessel will accompany the liver, given the fact that multiple organs are harvested from the same donor.

C. Normal Posttransplant Imaging Findings

1. Plain Radiographs

Recognition of normal anatomy is important, so that complications and subsequent appropriate treatment can be instituted (58–60). Common radiographic findings after cardiac

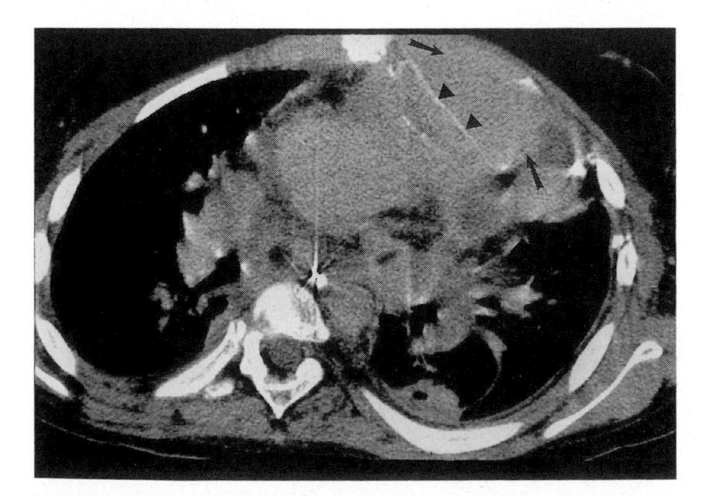

Figure 27 Cardiac pseudoaneurysm. Computed tomography performed in a patient after bilateral lung transplantation and ventricular septal defect repair reveals a soft tissue mass, representing thrombus (arrows), anterolateral to the cardiac suture line (arrowheads). At surgery, dehiscence of the sutures was identified with thrombus barely covering a cardiac pseudoaneurysm.

transplantation include: (a) a step-off at the site of anastomosis between the dilated recipient ascending aorta and the donor's normal-sized aorta—at times, the disparity in size of the two segments of aorta (donor and recipient) can be so striking that it may resemble an aneurysm formation distal to the anastomosis; (b) a double shadow along the lower right heart border, which corresponds to the site where a somewhat dilated recipient right atrium is sutured to a normal donor right atrium (Fig. 28); and (c) convexity in the anterior mediastinum on the lateral view due to positioning of the donor's right atrial appendage (59).

Other postoperative findings include overall increase or decrease in heart size compared to preoperative chest radiographs, and mediastinal widening. A smaller cardiac silhouette may reflect difference in size, shape, and orientation of the new heart. An overall increase in cardiac size usually reflects the presence of pericardial effusion, which is a direct result of placing a smaller heart in a larger pericardial sac. Although the pericardium is left open at the time of surgery, early closure from adhesions or blockage of the drainage tubes can cause fluid to accumulate.

Mediastinal widening is seen in 20% of patients. Mediastinal widening occurs in the immediate postoperative period and clears gradually within 3 weeks. The immediate postoperative mediastinal widening can be attributed to hemorrhage, effusion, edema, or blockage of pericardial fluid drainage.

Other findings are less specific and are related to known thoracic alterations after cardiac surgery. Among these are small pleural effusions, basilar atelectasis, and interstitial edema (60).

After several weeks, the appearance of the chest radiograph gradually returns to normal. Mediastinal widening can reoccur as the result of mediastinal fat deposition in patients receiving corticosteroid therapy.

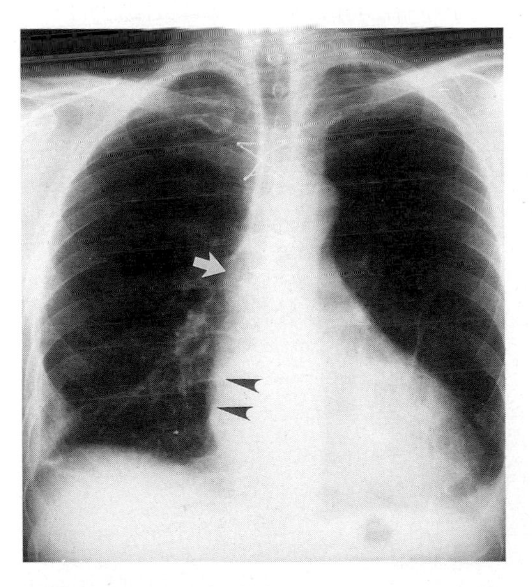

Figure 28 Chest radiography after cardiac transplant. Double atrial shadow (black arrowheads) and aortic dilatation (white arrow) are demonstrated on a frontal radiograph of a patient several months posttransplant.

2. *Computed Tomography*

Computed tomography of the thorax has proven to be a very powerful diagnostic tool in understanding normal and pathological changes in transplanted patients. Again, an understanding of normal postoperative anatomy is necessary so that complications can be identified.

The following CT observations are commonly present (61): (a) small nipplelike protrusion located anterior to the aorta just below the innominate artery, which marks the site of cannula insertion for cardiac bypass (Fig. 29); (b) high-riding main pulmonary artery, which can be at a right angle to the aortic arch—the distance between the main pulmonary artery and the aorta can be increased at times, probably related to the violation of the pericardial membranes at surgery; (c) change in caliber at the point of the surgical anastomosis of either the aorta or main pulmonary artery—a radiopaque Teflon sleeve at the anastomotic site can also be seen (Fig. 30); (d) a small rounded density behind the ascending aorta, sometimes accompanied by a surgical metallic clip, representing the ligated stump of superior vena cava (Fig. 31); (e) separation of the recipient's superior vena cava and the donor's aorta, reflecting an enlarged superior pericardial recess (59); (f) an indentation, termed a left atrial waist, at the site where the pulmonary veins enter the remaining original left atrium posteriorly; (g) an indentation in the anterior as well as the posterior walls of the right atrium, termed a right atrial waist, representing the suture line at this level; (h) inferior vena caval enlargement, reflecting protracted periods of heart failure; (i) fatty infiltration of the superior mediastinum secondary to steroid therapy (this mediastinal fat can sometimes appear infiltrated with soft tissue strands) (62); (j) pericardial effusions, particularly in patients on cyclosporine therapy (63) (Fig. 32); and (k) enlarged mediastinal lymph nodes.

D. Postoperative Complications

1. *Rejection*

Despite the increased survival—due primarily to improvements in immunosuppressive therapy—rejection, whether acute or chronic, remains an important clinical problem. Early

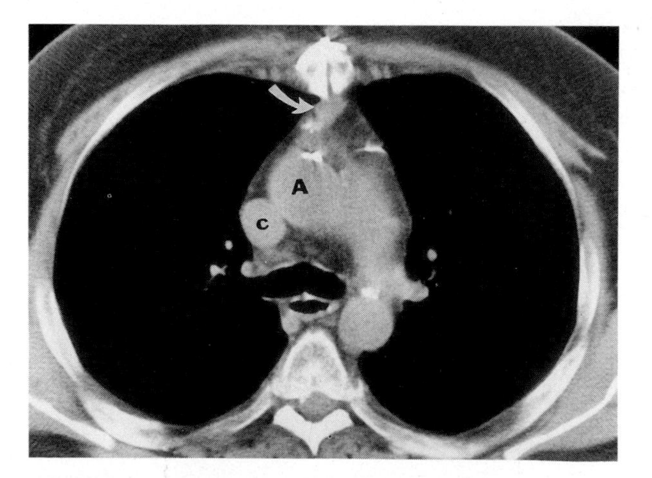

Figure 29 Computed tomography after cardiac transplant. CT demonstrates a nipplelike protrusion (arrow) just anterior to the ascending aorta, most likely representing a sequela from bypass cannulation. A = aorta, C = superior vena cava.

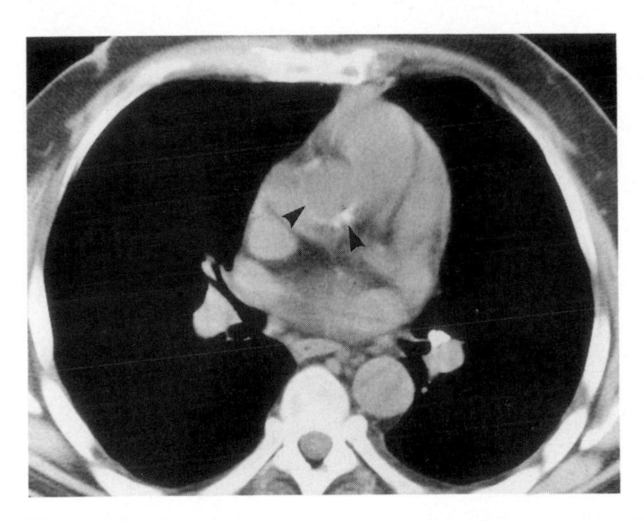

Figure 30 Computed tomography after cardiac transplant. This CT scan demonstrates a radiopaque Teflon sleeve at the aortic anastomosis (arrowheads).

diagnosis of rejection is important because prompt treatment may result in full reversal of the inflammatory changes. Since rejection can often be asymptomatic until the process becomes quite severe, frequent surveillance becomes crucial. Until now, endomyocardial biopsy (EMB) has remained the "gold standard" in the diagnosis of rejection. However, the procedure is invasive and therefore not suitable for frequent monitoring. Among the complications that have been describe following biopsy are arrhythmias, pneumothorax, ventricular perforation, air embolus, and fistula formation (64–66). In addition, since this

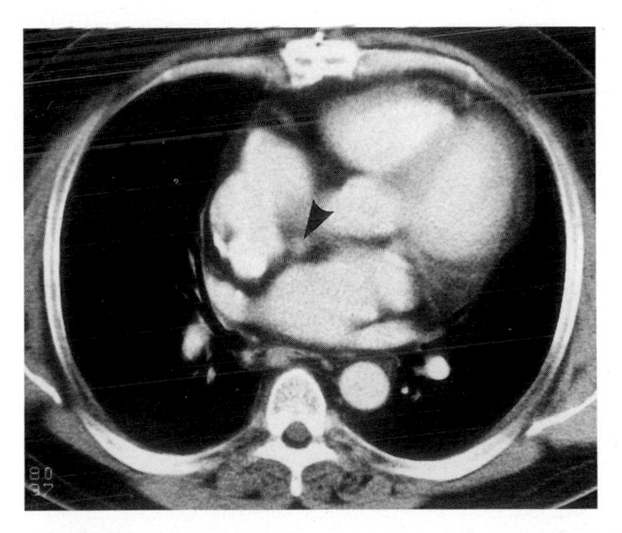

Figure 31 Computed tomography after cardiac transplant. Superior vena cava "stump." Contrast-enhanced CT demonstrates a small rounded density (arrowhead) posterolateral to the aortic root, representing the ligated stump of the superior vena cava.

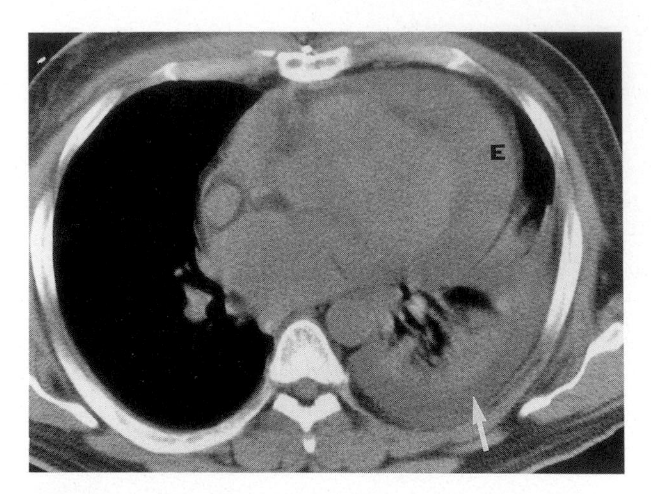

Figure 32 Pericardial effusion. Computed tomography scan several days postoperatively shows development of a pericardial effusion (E). Note also a left pleural effusion (arrow) and adjacent atelectatic lung.

procedure only samples a small focal area of the heart, there is the possibility that rejection can be missed if it has a heterogeneous distribution (67).

a. Chest Radiography. Because it is noninvasive, plain chest radiography has played a role in aiding in the diagnosis of rejection. Plain radiographic changes associated with rejection include cardiomegaly, which may be secondary to a pericardial effusion, pulmonary edema, or congestive heart failure (Fig. 33). These findings are nonspecific, but they can alert the physician that rejection may be present, which can lead to further investigation.

b. MRI. Electrocardiographic-gated MRI also has been used as a noninvasive method in the detection of anatomic changes in rejection. In humans with acute rejection, myocardial thickness has been shown to be increased significantly compared to that of normal volunteers, allograft patients with normal hearts, and allograft patients with resolving rejection (68). Myocardial signal intensity can be normal in patients undergoing immunosuppressive therapy at the time of the procedure, presumably because the therapy decreases edematous changes. However, other authors have reported increased signal intensity on both T_1- and T_2-weighted MRI images (69), agreeing with data from animal studies (70,71). The increased signal has been related to the presence of interstitial edema and infiltration of the myocardium (70,71). The extent of increased signal intensity on T_2-weighted images appears to vary directly with the severity of acute rejection (69). In chronic rejection, MRI is usually normal or nearly normal and hence not helpful in diagnosis (72). In addition to being used in rejection, MRI also can be used to determine the presence and extent of postoperative complications, such as hematoma (Fig. 34).

Contrast-enhanced MRI following administration of gadolinium (Gd) DTPA also can aid in the diagnosis of allograft rejection. Gd-DTPA has been shown to accumulate in areas of tissue inflammation, perhaps due to transudation in areas of increased vascular permeability (73,74). In experimental animals, the extent and distribution of myocardial enhancement corresponds to the severity and distribution of histological rejection (75) (Fig. 35; see also color plate).

At the present time, magnetic resonance spectroscopy does not have a role in evaluation of rejection. Studies evaluating myocardial high-energy phosphate metabolism have been unable to show a direct correlation between metabolic ratios of myocardial phosphocreatine (PCr) to adenosine triphosphate or PCr to inorganic phosphates and the severity of rejection (76).

c. Echocardiography. Echocardiographic techniques have been used to characterize both anatomic and functional changes in cardiac allografts. Anatomic changes in acute rejection include pericardial effusion and increased left ventricular mass. These quantitative changes tend to reflect the histological findings of edema, infiltrates and necrosis (77,78).

Diastolic and systolic function of the allografts is altered with rejection. Altered diastolic function is multifactorial and related to edema, myocardial fibrosis, pericardial effusions and atrial pressure. Functional abnormalities of diastole in rejection include decreased isovolumetric relaxation time (interval between closure of the aortic valve and opening of the mitral valve) and decreased mitral blood flow (79,80). Shortening of the isovolumetric relaxation time is thought to be related to an increase in atrial pressure secondary to edema and inflammation that causes early mitral valve opening (79). This finding has a sensitivity of 87% with a predictive value of 83% for detection of rejection. Alterations in diastolic mitral blood flow and isovolumetric relaxation time are not specific for rejection and can be related to such factors as hypertension and volume loading. For these reasons, alterations in these parameters should be interpreted with caution.

Evaluation of systolic left ventricular function during systole has proven to be an insensitive predictor of cardiac rejection (81), although systolic function, as determined by regional wall motion abnormalities, ejection fraction, and fractional shortening has been used to evaluate response of rejection to therapy (77).

It has been shown that the early stage of acute rejection correlates well with an increase in the ultrasonic integrated backscatter, reflected as increased myocardial echogenicity or gray level (82). It has also been recently demonstrated that the magnitude of the cyclic variation of integrated ultrasonic backscatter in the septum of cardiac allograft recipients with cardiac hypertrophy is different from that of normal subjects. Thus serial echocardiographic studies may hold promise in the detection of acute rejection (83,84) (Fig. 36).

d. Radionuclide Techniques. Radionuclide techniques, using technetium-99m–labeled red blood cells and thallium 201 have been utilized in allograft rejection to evaluate myocardial function and perfusion, respectively. In severe rejection, decreased left ventricular ejection fraction and myocardial blood flow can be identified (85,86). In mild rejection, cardiac imaging is usually normal (Fig. 37).

More recently, leukocytes and platelets, which are known to take an active part in the rejection process, have been labeled with radioisotopes such as indium 111. Experimental work in rats has shown that the radiolabeled platelets accumulate in transplanted allografts with histological findings of rejection (Fig. 38). These changes can be detected as early as 5 days after transplantation before mechanical, functional, and electrocardiographic signs of rejection occur (87–89). Although the results are encouraging for a noninvasive method of diagnosing rejection, similar studies have not yet been performed in a large group of humans.

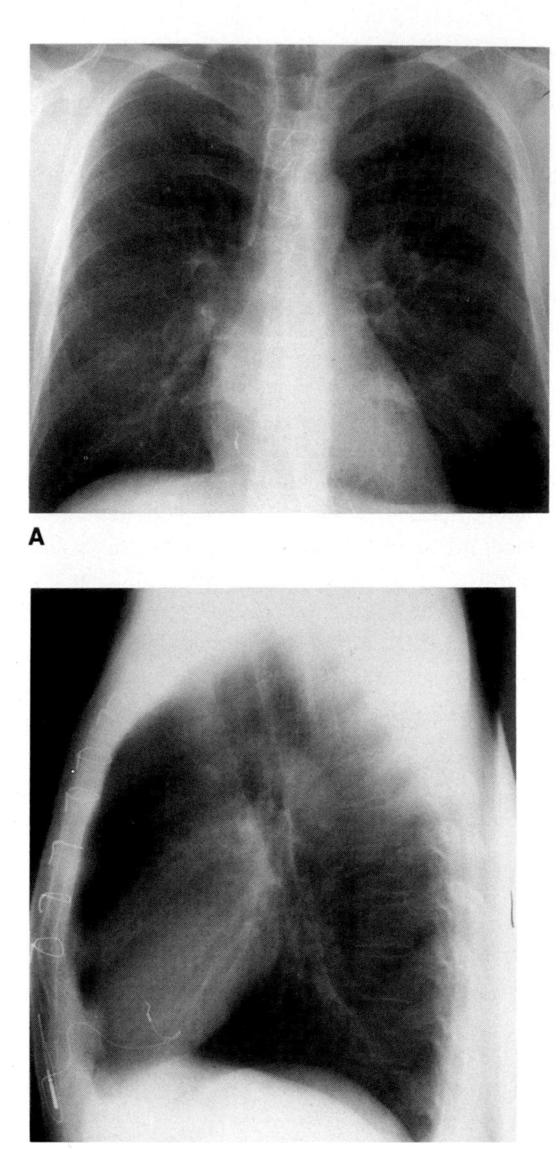

Figure 33 Congestive heart failure resulting from allograft rejection. (A) Frontal and (B) lateral radiographs 2 years posttransplant appear normal. (C) Frontal and (D) lateral radiographs 1 year later, during an episode of severe rejection, show mild cardiac enlargement and interstitial edema, evidence of congestive failure.

E. Imaging Approach—Posttransplant Rejection

In summary, although there is a vast noninvasive imaging armamentarium that has been shown to have some promise and potential clinical application, the fact of the matter is that endomyocardial biopsy still remains the only reliable method to effectively diagnose heart transplant rejection.

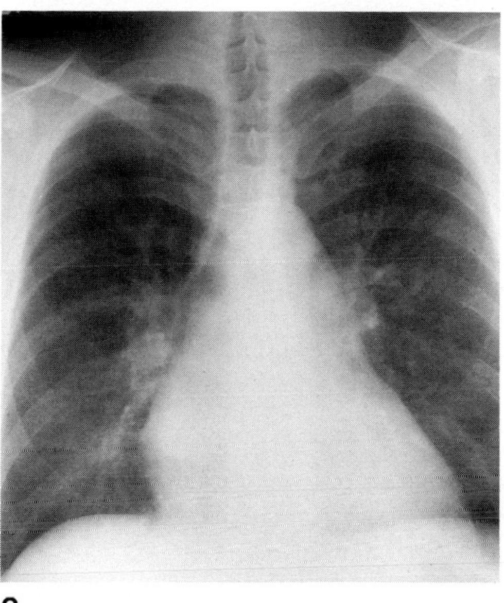

C

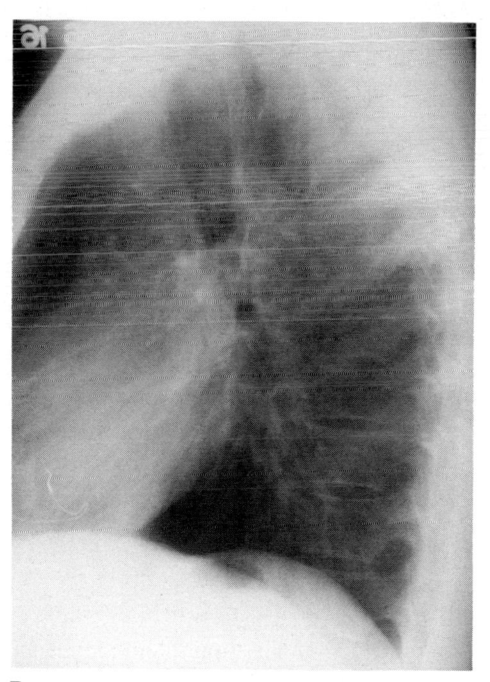

D

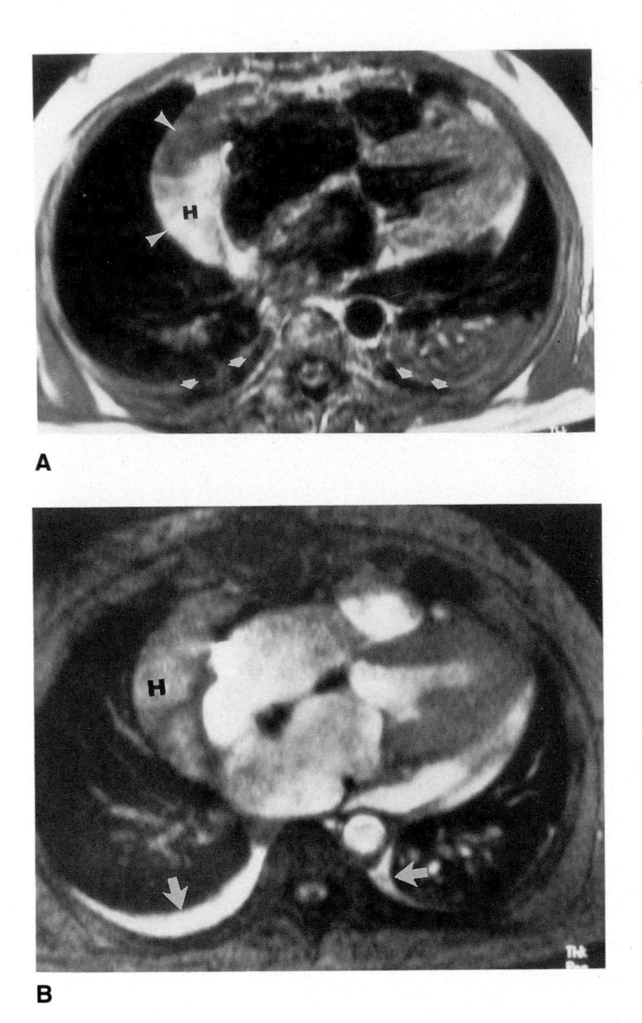

Figure 34 Postoperative hematoma. (A) T_1-weighted spin-echo and (B) gradient echo MRIs several days postoperatively show a pericardial fluid collection, representing hematoma (H). Note different signal intensities (arrowheads) in the pericardial hematoma, reflecting layering of blood (i.e., "hematocrit effect"). Also seen are bilateral pleural effusions (arrows). The pericardial hematoma was subsequently evacuated without complication.

F. Coronary Artery Disease

Although tissue rejection remains an important complication of heart transplant recipients, the development of coronary artery disease in this patient population has been shown to be a limiting factor in their long-term survival. The occurrence of two or more major rejection episodes has been associated with a higher incidence of coronary artery disease. It has been demonstrated that progressive obstructive coronary artery disease can develop over the first 3 years after cardiac transplantation in patients treated with cyclosporine and prednisone immunosuppression (90). The disease affects chiefly the medium and small coronary artery branches. The prognosis is poor because of ischemic complications that occur secondary to these obstructive changes. Coronary arteriography is the usual form of diagnosis. Angio-

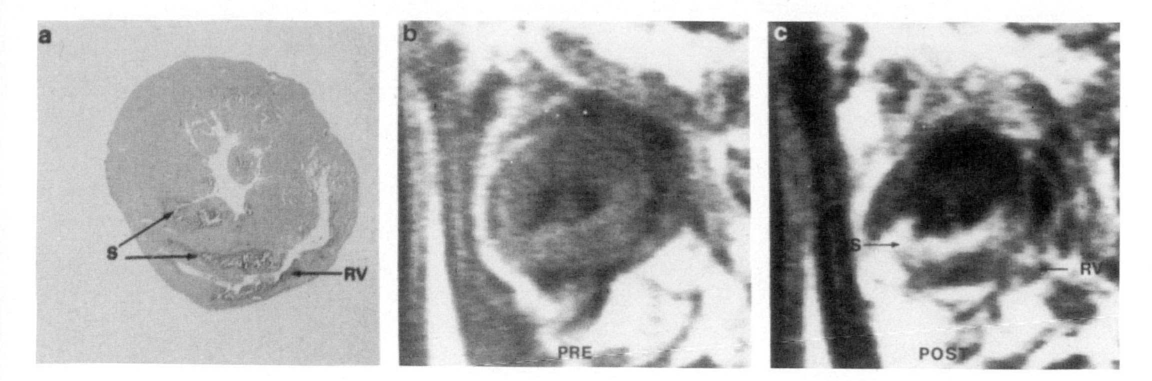

Figure 35 Allograft rejection. (a) Photomicrograph of a histological section in an animal with graft ejection shows areas of inflammatory cell infiltration with associated myocyte necrosis, particularly affecting the interventricular septum (S) and right ventricular (RV) free wall. (b) and (c) Corresponding T_1-weighted images, respectively, before (PRE) and after (POST) Gd-DTPA administration, show zones of intense myocardial enhancement corresponding to the sites of histological rejection. S = interventricular septum; RV = right ventricular free wall. (From Ref. 75.) (For optimal reproduction, see color plate.)

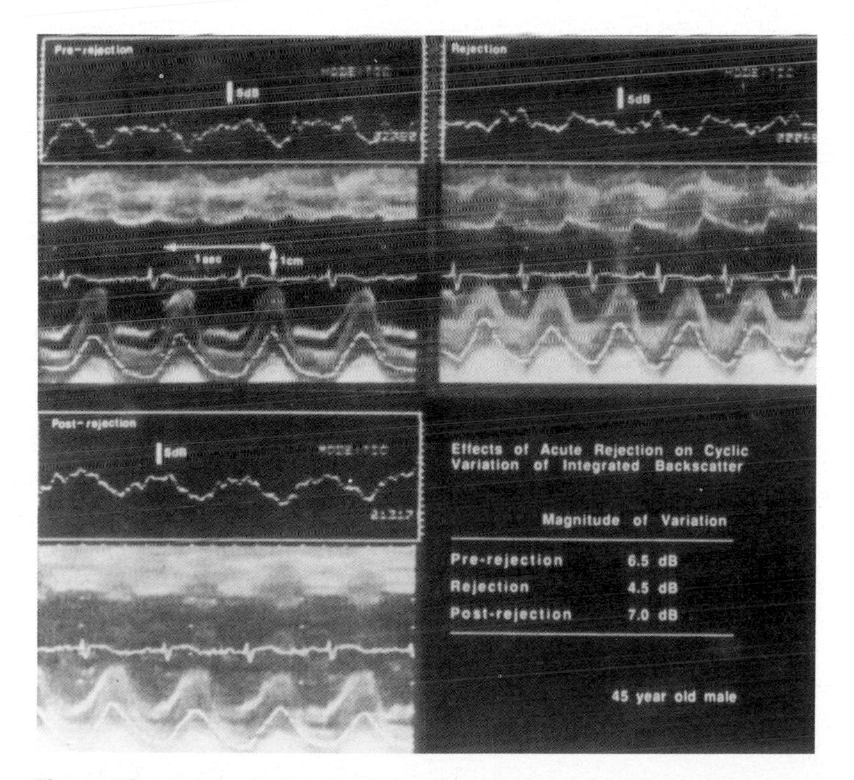

Figure 36 Acute rejection. Representative M-mode images with tracing of area of interest and curve of integrated backscatter (IB) versus time obtained from posterior wall of cardiac allograft at three different time periods: prerejection (upper left panel), during rejection (upper right panel), and postrejection (lower left panel). The magnitude of cyclic variation of IB decreases with rejection and almost fully recovers in the postrejection study. dB, decibels; IB, integrated backscatter; sec, second. (From Ref. 84.)

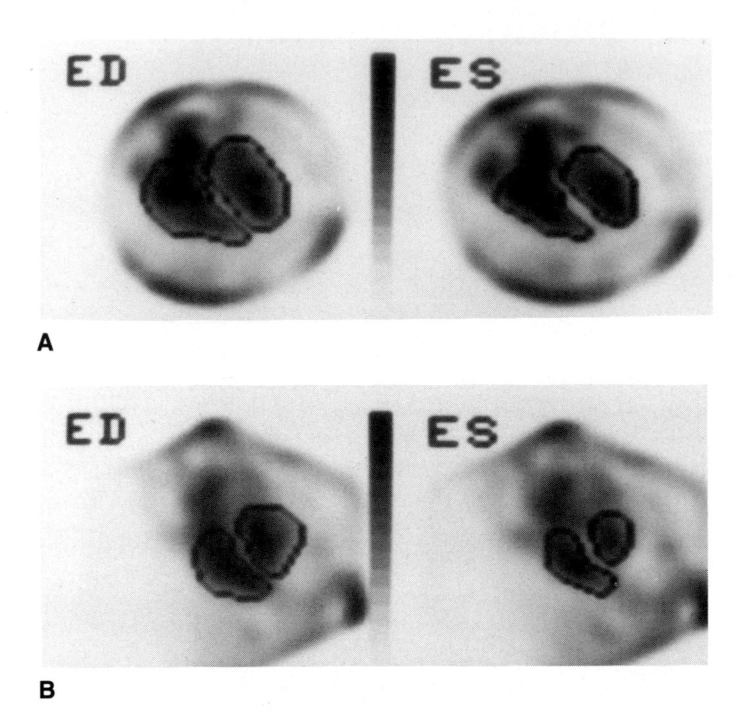

Figure 37 Acute rejection. (A) Tc-99m cardiac blood pool image in a 39-year-old patient with a dilated cardiomyopathy prior to heart transplantation. There is severe biventricular dysfunction and dilatation. (B) A blood pool image two weeks later, and after orthotopic heart transplant, shows normal ventricular function. An endomyocardial biopsy at the time demonstrated mild rejection. (ED = end disatole, ES = end systole.)

graphic findings include irregularity or complete occlusion of distal coronary artery branches (Fig. 39). Intravascular ultrasound also shows promise in defining thickening and vessel walls.

G. Lymphoproliferative Disorders

As previously discussed, lymphoproliferative disorders are believed to be the result of immunosuppression and occur in approximately 3.5% of heart transplants. The most common forms of presentation are multiple or solitary pulmonary nodules (Fig. 40) as well as hilar or mediastinal adenopathy (52). Computed tomography has better sensitivity than plain radiography in detecting these findings.

IV. SUMMARY

Lung and heart transplantation have become important therapeutic alternatives for disease conditions that were untreatable just a few years ago. In addition, the imaging armamentarium available to physicians has become very extensive. An understanding of the most common complications of transplantation and their imaging diagnosis is of crucial importance in the proper management of these patients.

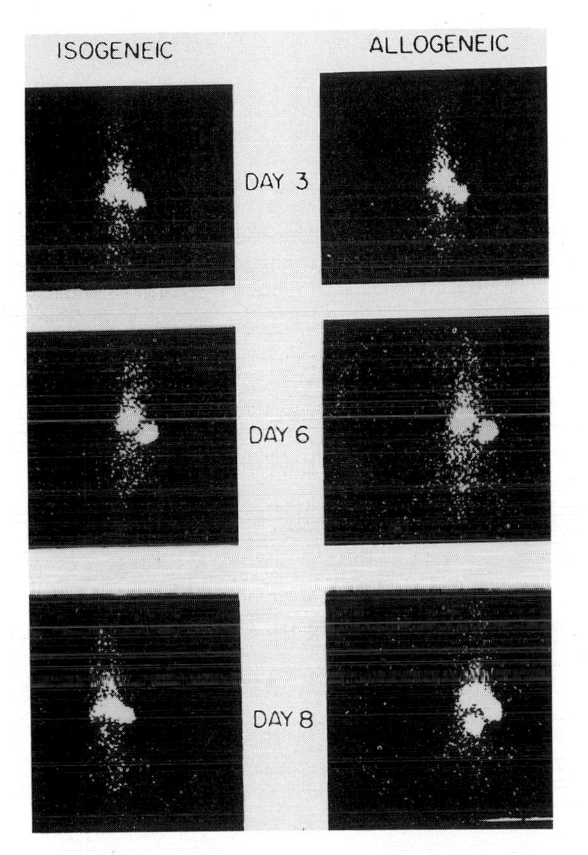

Figure 38 Acute rejection. Comparison scintigraphs, using indium-111-labeled lymphocytes in two rats that had undergone isogeneic and allogeneic cardiac transplants 3 days earlier, show a small amount of cardiac activity in both allografts because of nonspecific surgical inflammation (top panel). Scintigrams at 6 days (middle panel) and 8 days (lower panel) postoperatively show decreasing activity in the isogeneic grafts but increasing activity in the allogeneic transplants. The cardiac activity in the allogeneic transplants represents rejection. (From Ref. 89.)

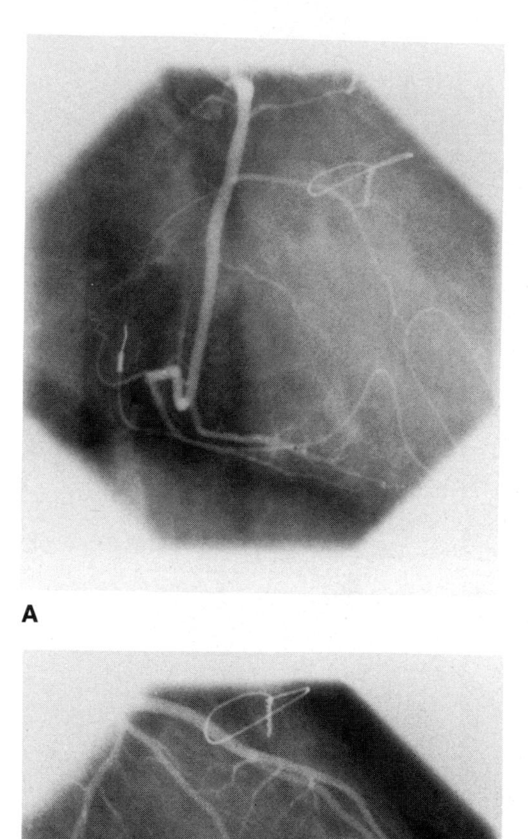

A

B

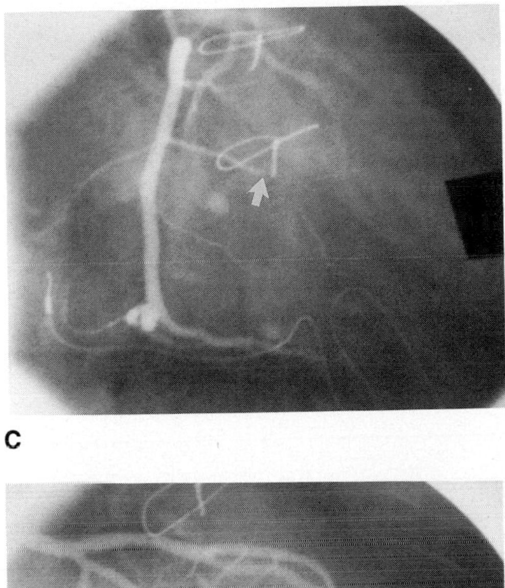

C

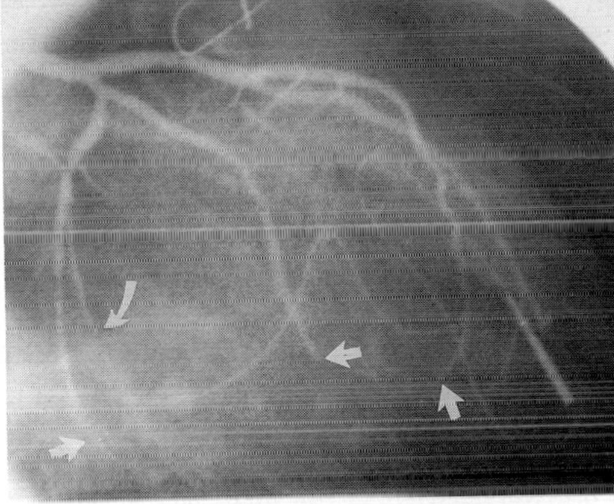

D

Figure 39 Coronary artery disease in a 42-year-old patient 3 years after heart transplantation. (A) Right and (B) left coronary artery angiograms 1 year following cardiac transplant reveal normal coronary artery anatomy bilaterally. (C) and (D) Repeat coronary angiography 2 years later of the right and left coronary arteries, respectively, demonstrates multiple areas of obstruction (arrows).

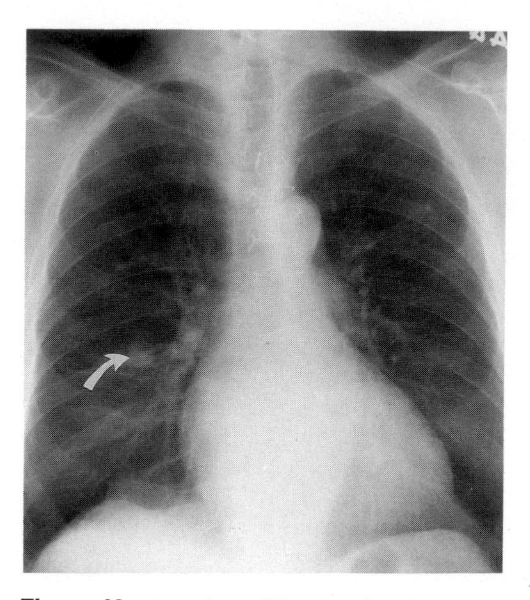

Figure 40 Lymphoproliferative disorder in a 67-year-old patient 2 years after cardiac transplantation. Frontal radiographs shows a single pulmonary nodule (arrow) in the right midlung field.

REFERENCES

1. Toronto Lung Transplant Group. Unilateral lung transplantation for pulmonary fibrosis. N Engl J Med 1986; 314:1140–1145.
2. Kawaguchi A, Gandijbakhch I, Pavie A, et al. Heart and unilateral lung transplantation in patients with end-stage cardiopulmonary disease and previous thoracic operations. J Thorac Cardiovasc Surg 1989; 98:343–349.
3. McCarthy PM, Kirby TJ, White RD, et al. Lung and heart-lung transplantation: The state of the art. Cleve Clin J Med 1992; 59:307–316.
4. Judson MA. Clinical aspects of lung transplantation. Clin Chest Med 1993; 14:335–357.
5. Patterson GA, Cooper JD, Goldman B, et al. Technique of successful clinical double-lung transplantation. Ann Thorac Surg 1988; 45:626–633.
6. Patterson GA. Bilateral lung transplant: Indications and technique. Semin Thorac Cardiovasc Surg 1992; 4:95–100.
7. Egan TM, Cooper JD. Surgical aspects of single lung transplantation. Clin Chest Med 1990; 11:195–204.
8. Trulock EP, Egan TM, Kouchoukos NT, et al. Single lung transplantation for severe chronic obstructive pulmonary disease. Chest 1989; 96:738–742.
9. Trulock EP, Cooper JD, Kaiser LR, et al. The Washington University-Barnes Hospital experience with lung transplantation. JAMA 1991; 266:1943–1946.
10. Waters PF. Single lung transplant: indications and technique. Semin Thorac Cardiovasc Surg 1992; 4:90–94.
11. Kaiser LR, Cooper JD. The current status of lung transplantation. Adv Surg 1992; 25:259–307.
12. Spray TL, Mallory GB, Canter CE, et al. Pediatric lung transplantation for pulmonary hypertension and congenital heart disease. Ann Thorac Surg 1992; 54:216–225.
13. Glazer HS, Anderson DJ, Cooper JD, et al. Omental flap in lung transplants. Radiology 1992; 185:395–400.

14. Morgan E, Lima O, Goldberg M, et al. Improved bronchial healing in canine left lung reimplantation using omental pedicle wrap. J Thorac Cardiovasc Surg 1983; 85:134–139.
15. Pasque MK, Cooper JD, Kaiser LR, et al. Improved technique for bilateral lung transplantation: Rationale and initial clinical experience. Ann Thorac Surg 1990; 49:785–791.
16. Calhoun JH, Grover FL, Gibbons WJ, et al. Single lung transplantation: Alternative indications and technique. J Thorac Cardiovasc Surg 1991; 101:816–825.
17. de Hoyos AL, Patterson GA, Maurer JR, et al. Pulmonary transplantation: Early and late results. J Thorac Cardiovasc Surg 1992; 103:295–306.
18. Knight SR, Dresler C. Results of lung transplantation. Semin Thorac Cardiovasc Surg 1992; 4:107–112.
19. Anderson DJ, Semenkovich JW, Glazer HS, Cooper JD. Radiologic aspects of lung transplantation and complications. In: Fleischner Society, ed. Pulmonary Radiology. Philadelphia: Saunders, 1993:69–80.
20. Herman SJ. Radiologic assessment after lung transplantation. Clin Chest Med 1990; 11:333–346.
21. Prop JM, Ehrie MG, Crapo JD, et al. Reimplantation response in isografted rat lungs: Analysis of causal factors. J Thorac Cardiovasc Surg 1984; 87:702–711.
22. Siegelman SS, Sinha SPB, Veith FJ. Pulmonary reimplantation response. Ann Surg 1971; 177:30–36.
23. Todd TRJ. Early postoperative management following lung transplantation. Clin Chest Med 1990; 11:259–267.
24. Herman SJ, Weisbrod GL, Weisbrod L, et al. Chest radiographic findings after bilateral lung transplantation. AJR 1989; 153:1181–1185.
25. Herman SJ, Rappaport DC, Weisbrod GL, et al. Single lung transplantation: Imaging features. Radiology 1989; 170:89–93.
26. Medina LS, Siegel MJ. CT of complications in pediatric lung transplantation. RadioGraphics 1994; 14:1341–1349.
27. Yousem SA, Berry GJ, Brunt EM, et al. A working formulation for the standardization of nomenclature in the diagnosis of heart and lung rejection: Lung rejection study group. J Heart Transplant 1990; 9:593–601.
28. Lawrence EC. Diagnosis and management of lung allograft rejection. Clinical Chest Med 1990; 11:269–278.
29. Toronto Lung Transplant Group. Experience with single-lung transplantation for pulmonary fibrosis. JAMA 1987; 259:2258–2262.
30. Medina LS, Siegel MJ, Bejarano PA, et al. Pediatric lung transplantation: Radiographic-histopathologic correlation. Radiology 1993; 187:807–810.
31. Millet B, Higenbottam TW, Flower CDR, et al. The radiographic appearances of infection and acute rejection of the lung after heart-lung transplantation. Am Rev Respir Dis 1989; 140: 62–67.
32. Bergin CJ, Castellino RA, Blank N, et al. Acute lung rejection after heart-lung transplantation: Correlation of findings on chest radiographs with lung biopsy results. AJR 1990; 155:23–27.
33. Hruban RH, Ren H, Kuhlman JE, et al. Inflation-fixed lungs: Pathologic-radiologic (CT) correlation of lung transplantation. J Comput Assist Tomogr 1990; 14:329–335.
34. Medina LS, Siegel MJ, Glazer HS, et al. Diagnosis of pulmonary complications associated with lung transplantation in children: Value of CT vs histopathologic studies. AJR 1994; 162:969–974.
35. Burke CM, Theodore J, Dawkins KD, et al. Post-transplant obliterative bronchiolitis and other late lung sequelae in human heart-lung transplantation. Chest 1984; 86:824–829.
36. Lentz D, Bergin CJ, Berry GJ, et al. Diagnosis of bronchiolitis obliterans in heart-lung transplantation patients: Importance of bronchial dilatation on CT. AJR 1992; 159:463–467.
37. Skeens JL, Fuhrman CR, Yousem SA. Bronchiolitis obliterans in heart-lung transplantation patients: Radiologic findings in 11 patients. AJR 1989; 153:253–256.
38. Theodore J, Starnes VA, Lewiston NJ. Obliterative bronchiolitis. Clin Chest Med 1990; 11: 309–321.

39. Williams TJ, Grossman RF, Maurer JR. Long-term functional follow-up of lung transplantation recipients. Clin Chest Med 1990; 11:347–358.
40. Morrish WF, Herman SJ, Weisbrod GL, Chamberlain DW. Bronchiolitis obliterans after lung transplantation: Findings at chest radiography and high-resolution CT. Radiology 1991; 179:487–490.
41. Dauber JH, Pardis IL, Dummer JS. Infectious complications in pulmonary allograft recipients. Clin Chest Med 1990; 11:291–308.
42. DeHoyos A, Maurer JR. Complications following lung transplantation. Semin Thorac Cardiovasc Surg 1992; 4:132–146.
43. Dummer JS, Montero CG, Griffith BP, et al. Infections in heart-lung transplant recipients. Transplantation 1986; 41:725–729.
44. Maurer JR, Tullis E, Grossman RF, et al. Infectious complications following isolated lung transplantation. Chest 1992; 101:1056–1059.
45. Hruban RH, Beschorner WE, Baumgartner WA, et al. Depletion of bronchus-associated lymphoid tissue associated with lung allograft rejection. Am J Pathol 1988; 132:6–11.
46. Smyth RL, Sinclair J, Scott JP, et al. Infection and reactivation with cytomegalovirus strains in lung transplant recipients. Transplantation 1991; 52:480–481.
47. Ramirez J, Patterson GA. Airway complications after lung transplantation. Semin Thorac Cardiovasc Surg 1992; 4:147–153.
48. Kleptko W, Grimm M, Laufer G, et al. One and one-half year experience with unilateral and bilateral lung transplantation. J Cardiac Surg 1992; 7:126–133.
49. Semenkovich JW, Glazer HS, Arcidi J Jr, et al. Bronchial dehiscence in lung transplants: CT evaluation. (abstract) Radiology 1992; 185(p):242.
50. Nalesink MA, Makowka L, Starzl TE. The diagnosis and treatment of posttransplant lymphoproliferative disorders. Curr Probl Surg 1988; 25:365–472.
51. Armitage JM, Kormos RL, Stuart RS, et al. Posttransplant lymphoproliferative disease in thoracic organ transplant patients: Ten years of cyclosporine-based immunosuppression. J Heart Lung Transplant 1991; 877–887.
52. Dodd GD III, Ledesma-Median J, Baron RL, Fuhrman CR. Posttransplant lymphoproliferative disorder: Intrathoracic manifestations. Radiology 1992; 184:65–69.
53. Root JD, Molina PL, Anderson DJ, Sagel SS. Pulmonary nodular opacities after transbronchial biopsy in patients with lung transplants. Radiology 1992; 184:435–436.
54. Paranjpe DV, Wittich GR, Hamid LW, Bergin CJ. Frequency and management of pneumothoraces in heart-lung transplant recipients. Radiology 1991; 190:255–256.
55. Oyer PE, Stinson EB, Jamieson SW, et al. One year experience with cyclosporine A in clinical heart transplantation. Heart Transplant 1980 1:285–293.
56. Heck CF, Shumway SJ, Kaye MP. The Registry of the International Society for Heart Transplantation: sixth official report. J Heart Transplant 1989; 8:271.
57. Bolman RM, Cance C, Spray T, et al. The changing face of cardiac transplantation: The Washington University program, 1985–1987. Ann Thorac Surg 1988; 45:192–197.
58. Singleton EB, Coloquhoun J, Harle TS, et al. Radiological evaluation of cardiac transplantation. AJR 1970; 109:1–11.
59. Silverman JF, Griepp RB, Wexler L. Radiographic changes in cardiac contour following cardiac transplantation. Radiology 1974; 111:302–306.
60. Shirazi KK, Amendola MA, Tisnado J, et al. Cardiovasc Intervent Radiol 1983; 6:1–6.
61. Henry DA, Corcoran HL, Lewis TD, et al. Lower orthotopic cardiac transplantation: Evaluation with CT. Radiology 1989; 170:343–350.
62. Carrol CL, Jeffrey RB, Federle MP, Vernacchia FS. CT evaluation of mediastinal infections. J Comput Assist Tomogr 1987; 11:449–454.
63. Hastillo A, Thompson J, Szentpery S, et al. Cyclosporine-induced pericardial effusions in patients who have undergone heart transplantation. J Heart Transplant 1986; 5:371–373.

64. Przybojewsky JZ. Endomyocardial biopsy: A review of the literature. Cathet Cardiovasc Diagn 1985; 11:287–330.
65. Fowles RE, Mason JW. Role of cardiac biopsy in the diagnosis and management of cardiac disease. Prog Cardiovasc Dis 1984; 27:153–172.
66. Fitchett DH, Forbes C, Guerraty AJ. Repeated endomyocardial biopsy causing coronary arterial-right ventricular fistula after cardiac transplantation. Am J Cardiol 1988; 62:829–831.
67. Haverich A, Scott W, Dawkin KD, et al. Asymmetric pattern of rejection following orthotopic cardiac transplantation in primates. Heart Transplant 1984; 3:280–284.
68. Aherne T, Tscholakoff D, Finkbeiner W, et al. Magnetic resonance imaging of cardiac transplants: The evaluation of rejection of cardiac allografts with and without immunosuppression. Circulation 1986; 74:145–156.
69. Revel D, Chapelon C, Mathieu D, et al. Magnetic resonance imaging of human orthotopic heart transplantation: Correlation with endomyocardial biopsy. J Heart Transplant 1989; 8:139–146.
70. Kemkes BM, Schutz A, Engelhardt M, et al. Noninvasive methods of rejection diagnosis after heart transplantation. J Heart Lung Transplant 1992; 11:221–231.
71. Tscholakoff D, Aherne T, Yee DN, Higgins CB. Cardiac transplantation in dogs: Evaluation with MR. Radiology 1985; 157:697–702.
72. Weisenberg G, Pflugfelder PW, Kostuk WJ, et al. Diagnostic applicability of magnetic resonance imaging in assessing human cardiac allograft rejection. Am J Cardiol 1987; 130–136.
73. Doornbos J, Veerwey H, Essed CE, et al. MR imaging in assessment of cardiac transplant rejection in humans. J Comput Assist Tomogr 1990; 14:77–81.
74. Runge VM, Clanton JA, Price AC, et al. Evaluation of contrast-enhanced MR imaging of a brain-abscess model. AJNR 1985; 6:139–147.
75. Konstam MA, Aronovitz MJ, Runge VM, et al. Magnetic resonance imaging with gadolinium-DTPA for detecting cardiac transplant rejection in rats. Sup Circ 1988; 78:III87–III94.
76. Bottomley PA, Weiss RG, Hardy CJ, Baumgartner WA. Myocardial high-energy phosphate metabolism and allograft rejection in patients with heart transplants. Radiology 1991; 181: 67–75.
77. Hsu DT, Spotnitz HM. Echocardiographic diagnosis of allograft rejection. Prog Cardiovasc Dis 1990; 33:149–160.
78. Valentine HA, Hunt SA, Gibbons R, et al. Increasing pericardial effusion in cardiac transplant recipients. Circulation 1989, 79:603–609.
79. Dawkins KD, Oldershaw PJ, Bilingham ME, et al. Changes in diastolic function as a noninvasive marker of cardiac allograft rejection. Heart Transplant 1984; 3:286–294.
80. Valentine HA, Fowler MB, Hunt SA, et al. Changes in Doppler echocardiographic indexes of left ventricular function as potential markers of acute cardiac rejection. Circulation 1987; 76(suppl 5):86–92.
81. Stinson EB, Caves PK, Griepp RB, et al. Hemodynamic observations in the early period after human heart transplantation. J Thorac Cardiovasc Surg 1975; 69:264–270.
82. Chandrasekaran K, Bansal RC, Greenleaf JF, et al. Early recognition of heart transplant rejection by backscatter analysis from serial 2D echoes in a heterotopic transplant model. J Heart Transplant 1987; 6:1–7.
83. Kemkes BM, Schultz A, Engelhardt M, et al. Noninvasive methods of rejection diagnosis after heart transplantation. J Heart Transplant 1992; 11:S221–S231.
84. Masuyama T, Valentine HA, Gibbons R, et al. Serial measurement of integrated ultrasonic backscatter in human cardiac allografts for the recognition of acute rejection. Circulation 1990; 81:829–838.
85. McGiffin DC, Karp RB, Logic JR, et al. Results of radionuclide assessment of cardiac function following transplantation of the heart. Ann Thorac Surg 1984; 37:382–386.
86. Addonizio LJ. Detection of cardiac allograft rejection using radionuclide techniques. Prog Cardiovasc Dis 1990; 33:73–83.

87. Oluwole S, Wang T, Fawwaz R. Use of indium-111 labeled cells in measurement of cellular dynamics of experimental cardiac allograft rejection. Transplantation 1981; 31:51–55.
88. Wang T, Oluwole S, Fawwaz RA, et al. Cellular basis for accumulation of In-111-labeled leukocytes and platelets in rejecting cardiac allografts: Concise communication. J Nucl Med 1982; 23:993–997.
89. Bergmann SR, Lerch RA, Carlson EM, et al. Detection of cardiac transplant rejection with radiolabeled lymphocytes. Circulation 1992; 65:591–599.
90. Uretsky BF, Murali S, Reddy S, et al. Development of coronary artery disease in cardiac transplant patients receiving immunosuppressive therapy with cyclosporine and prednisone. Circulation 1987; 76:827–834.

16

Clinical Diagnosis of Liver Allograft Rejection

Lorraine C. Racusen
Johns Hopkins University School of Medicine, Baltimore, Maryland

Russell H. Wiesner
Mayo Medical School, Mayo Clinic and Mayo Foundation, Rochester, Minnesota

I. INTRODUCTION

In hepatic allografts, as in allografts of other solid organs, acute and chronic rejection are significant causes of compromised allograft function. Approximately two-thirds of patients will have at least one episode of clinical acute rejection. Over the past decade, however, management of acute allograft rejection has improved to the point that 1-year graft survivals average 70 to 80%, and graft dysfunction due to acute rejection is generally reversible. Chronic allograft injury and dysfunction has become a proportionately more significant problem as these allografts survive beyond the early posttransplant period, with 10 to 15% of patients developing chronic rejection, which is generally irreversible. The incidence of rejection in a number of large series of initial liver allografts is summarized in Table 1 (1–20).

In this chapter, the patterns of graft rejection following liver transplantation are reviewed. The typical patterns of rejection are schematized in Fig. 1. Below, we discuss the clinical monitoring of the hepatic allograft patient throughout the posttransplant course. Criteria for diagnosis of rejection, differential diagnoses, and therapeutic interventions are emphasized (1–20).

II. HYPERACUTE/ANTIBODY-MEDIATED REJECTION

A. Diagnosis

Hyperacute rejection occurs within hours of transplantation and is due to the presence of preformed cytotoxic antibodies. True hyperacute rejection has been detected rarely following hepatic allografting (21), even in cases with ABO incompatibility and positive crossmatch (22). Hepatic allografts may be relatively protected from acute graft loss in this setting due to their dual blood supply (23). However, occasional patients have been described who received both renal and hepatic allografts from the same donor and whose

Table 1 Incidence of Cellular and Ductopenic Rejection in Adults and Children After Initial Liver Transplantation

Medical Center	First Grafts (No.)	Cellular Rejection No.	Cellular Rejection %	Ductopenic Rejection No.	Ductopenic Rejection %	Reference
Adult patients						
Baylor University, Dallas	104	63	61	8	8	1
Birmingham	189	132	70	19	10	2
University of Minnesota	47	36	77	3	6	3
Cambridge—King's College	101	—	—	17	17	4
University of California at Los Angeles	83	83	100	3	4	5
Groningen	83	76	92	9	11	6
Hannover	81	50	62	9	11	7
Pittsburgh	394	201	51	22	6	8
Sydney	28	18	64	3	11	9
Mayo Clinic	164	107	65	15	9	10
University of Wisconsin	127	—	—	3	2	11
Belgium	100	70	70	7	7	12
University of Nebraska	338	—	—	27	8	13
Total	1839	836	66[a]	145	8	
Pediatric patients						
University of California at Los Angeles	68	58	85	3	4	14
Cambridge—King's College	83	53	64	14	17	15
Belgium	139	83	60	8	6	12
University of Minnesota	52	42	81	5	10	16
University of Cincinnati	21	17	81	2	10	17
University of Chicago	50	—	—	5	10	18
Pacific—San Francisco	55	35	64	4	7	19
University of Nebraska	175	—	—	14	8	13
Total	643	288	69[b]	55	9	

[a]Of 1273 adults patients for whom analysis of cellular rejection was reported.
[b]Of 418 pediatric patients for whom analysis of cellular rejection was reported.
Source: From Ref. 20.

renal allografts underwent hyperacute rejection. In these patients, the transplanted liver became necrotic within hours of implantation, likely also representing a hyperacute rejection process (24). These patients presented with primary nonfunction of the hepatic allograft and a severe coagulopathy; one case was reversible. One had a positive preoperative crossmatch, one did not.

It has been suggested that massive hemorrhagic necrosis (MHN) and fulminant graft failure in hepatic allografts may represent an antibody-mediated rejection, at least in some patients (2, 25–27). Developing in 2 to 5% of patients within 2 to 21 days of transplantation, MHN is rare. Patients typically present with a sudden rise in serum transaminases and a prolonged prothrombin time, followed rapidly by hepatic encephalopathy and coma. Extensive hemorrhagic necrosis of the graft is seen on histologic examination; computed

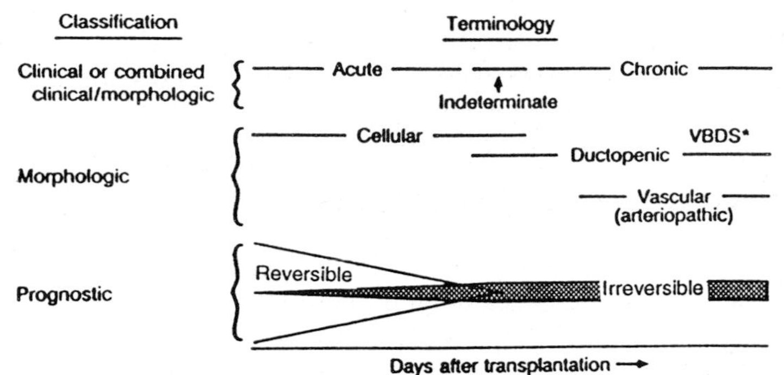

Figure 1 A schematic representation of hepatic allograft rejection depicting relationship of clinical, morphological, and prognostic classifications and occurrence over time. Of course, as noted in the text, acute rejection may occur at any time posttransplant, and ductopenic rejection may be reversible. Note that some cases of rejection never respond to treatment.

tomography (CT) scan has been reported to show large geographic areas of necrosis without specific anatomic distribution (28).

In the immediate posttransplant period, the differential diagnosis of hepatic dysfunction includes harvesting-induced injury and vascular thrombosis. Harvesting-induced injury may result from hypoperfusion in the donor, inadequate perfusion/preservation, and/or prolonged cold or warm ischemia times. The result is extensive ischemic injury to the allograft. Patients present with initial nonfunction, decreased bile flow, and persistent coagulopathy. There is a progressive rise in bilirubin, and serum transaminases are elevated 10- to 20-fold above normal. Hypoglycemia, renal failure, and hepatic encephalopathy often ensue. The incidence of severe preservation injury in a recent large series was 15%, while 69% had minimal and 16% moderate injury; preservation injury did not appear to predispose to development of or enhance the severity of acute rejection (29). The diagnosis is readily established on liver biopsy (see Chap. 8). If the problem is limited to peripheral and subcapsular areas, liver function may recover. Otherwise, retransplantation is necessary; results of retransplantation in this setting have been poor. Vascular thrombosis occurs in a small percentage of adult hepatic allografts (1 to 2%) but is relatively common in pediatric allografts (12%). The typical clinical symptoms include fever, chills, and moderate rise in serum transaminases following initial adequate function. Regional necroses in this setting may be detected by imaging studies. Bile duct necrosis with leakage and even bile peritonitis may occur. Doppler ultrasonography can be used to assess patency of hepatic artery and portal vein, with confirmation by selective angiography.

The mechanisms of MHN are not well defined, but there is some evidence that the process may be immunologically mediated. Extensive MHC antigen expression on hepatocytes and deposition of immunoglobulin on endothelium in these livers, while nonspecific, are consistent with an immunological mechanism. The rapid onset and lack of a cellular infiltrate suggest an antibody-mediated rather than cellular process, though there is no association with preformed cytotoxic antibodies (26) or with matching for HLA or ABO (27). Of note, a similar histologic picture has been described in accelerated humorally mediated liver rejection in an animal model (25).

B. Therapy

Intensive immunosuppression is of little benefit in these patients (2). Urgent retransplantation is the only reported effective therapy (27).

III. CELLULAR REJECTION/ACUTE REJECTION

Cellular rejection is generally defined by the presence of two or more of the following findings on allograft biopsy: portal or periportal hepatitis, destructive or nondestructive nonsuppurative cholangitis, and endothelialitis and phlebitis in branches of portal and hepatic veins (30) (See Chap. 8). While the term "acute rejection" has been used synonymously with "cellular rejection," "acute" connotes onset within the first few weeks following transplantation. Since a cell-mediated rejection process can occur at any time posttransplant, often due to addition of hepatic enzyme-altering drugs to the basic immunosuppressive regimen or poor patient compliance, this term is misleading. In addition, "acute rejection" implies reversibility (2), which is not always the case.

This form of rejection occurs in 50 to 100% of hepatic allograft recipients (see Table 1). Factors predictive of cellular rejection include a double-drug immunosuppressive regimen, young age of recipient, recipient with Rh-positive blood type, and complete HLA-DR donor-recipient mismatch (31). Use of triple-drug immunosuppression has been shown to significantly decrease the incidence of rejection (20). Young age predisposes to rejection in adults (20). In addition, pediatric recipients have an increased incidence of cellular rejection, perhaps related to increased immune reactivity in children (14,15,32).

A. Clinical Diagnosis

Clinically, patients present with fever and malaise. Complaints of abdominal discomfort, anorexia, back pain, or respiratory distress are common. The allograft may be enlarged but is often nontender due to surgical denervation. Biliary drainage becomes pale and watery and output decreases. The earliest change in serum biochemistry is a sharp increase in bilirubin, which is typically followed by increases in alkaline phosphatase and transaminase levels. If the process is severe, prothrombin time may be prolonged.

However, these features are not specific, and other diagnoses must be excluded in these often complicated patients; differential diagnoses in the early posttransplant period include ischemia, perfusion injury, and bile duct abnormalities. Infection in the allograft is another important cause of early allograft dysfunction. Types of infection that may occur include cholangitis and liver abscesses; the latter may develop following ischemic necrosis. Other infections may be due to transfusions, opportunistic organisms, or reinfection of the graft with the agent that produced the original liver disease. Cultures and serologic tests for hepatitis, cytomegalovirus (CMV) and other organisms may be useful in ruling in infection. Infection is discussed in greater detail in Sec. V of this chapter.

Clinical definition of rejection by simple biochemical parameters alone is neither specific nor sensitive as judged by results of protocol liver biopsies (33). No specific pattern of changes in the biochemical parameters appears to correspond to histopathologic findings (34). Assessment of other biochemical, cellular, and molecular markers in serum or bile and the use of appropriate imaging studies may be helpful in establishing the diagnosis of rejection. Biopsy of the allograft is often definitive, as discussed below.

1. Biochemical, Cellular, and Molecular Markers

A variety of other factors have been studied in the search for reliable markers of cellular rejection. These can be broadly divided into biochemical markers and cytokine/effector cell markers. While some appear promising, none of these have been widely tested and none are in widespread use.

Serum levels of acute-phase proteins, including serum amyloid A (SAA) protein and β_2 microglobulin have been proposed as markers of liver allograft rejection (35,36). In a recent study, SAA levels were monitored in 12 consecutive recipients until the 70th posttransplant day. Fourteen rejection episodes were identified in a total of 42 liver biopsies. Two-thirds of rejection episodes were characterized by increases in plasma SAA concentration; 96% of 25 negative biopsies had no associated rise in SAA (36).

Azer et al. have monitored individual serum bile acids as an early marker of rejection (37). They found significantly increased serum concentrations of glycocholate plus glycochenodeoxy cholate and taurocholate/taurochenodeoxycholate ratios in biopsy-confirmed graft dysfunction compared to well-functioning grafts; these changes preceded alterations in conventional biochemical markers and were highly sensitive and specific. Rejections was associated with an early significant increase in the concentration of glycodeoxycholate plus deoxycholate and a decreased cholate/chenodeoycholate ratio compared to "nonrejection graft malfunction." While these results are intriguing, patient numbers were small, and assay of these serum bile acids may not be routinely available.

Gozzo et al. assayed a range of mitochondrial and cytoplasmic enzymes in the plasma of patients to detect and monitor hepatocellular injury and impending rejection (38). They determined activities of mitochondrial aspartate aminotransferase, glutamate dehydrogenase, alanine aminotransferase, aspartate aminotransferase, gamma-glutamyltranspeptidase, and alkaline phosphatase and calculated a "necrosis index" consisting of the percent ratio of mitochondrial over the sum of cytoplasmic and mitochondrial normalized enzyme activities. A ratio higher than 30% was diagnostic of rejection, with sensitivity of 90%, specificity of 80%, and predictive value of 90%.

Soluble class I and class II human leukocyte antigen (HLA) in patient sera have also been monitored. Serum levels of soluble class I HLA (sHLA-I) have been shown to increase sharply in patients with "acute" rejection, beginning 6 days preceding clinically detectable rejection. Moreover, sHLA-I levels declined rapidly in patients following antirejection therapy. Soluble HLA-I levels were positively correlated with transaminase levels and inversely correlated with prothrombin time (39). However, it is not clear whether sHLA-I detection is more useful than these conventional biochemical tests. In contrast, sHLA-II serum concentrations are variable and show no relationship to rejection (40).

Detection of increased eosinophils in blood and/or on graft biopsies may be a useful predictor of hepatic allograft rejection (41,42). One study, including both a retrospective case-control component as well as a prospective study of 20 consecutive graft recipients, concluded that increased blood eosinophilia or abundant eosinophils or their secretion products in liver biopsies are a good indicator of ongoing or recent allograft rejection in the first month posttransplant (42).

Serum and bile interleukin levels have also been evaluated as potential rejection markers. Interleukin-8 (IL-8) and IL-10, derived from monocytes, increase dramatically but transiently after reperfusion of the graft; levels do not correlate with cold ischemia time or rejection episodes (43). Serum interleukin-6 levels rise in cynomologus monkeys following hepatic allografting with no immunosuppressive therapy, before elevations in serum alkaline phosphatase appear (44). There is some evidence that biliary levels of interleukin may be a more accurate reflection of immunologic activity within the allograft than serum levels. Levels of IL-2 receptor and of beta$_2$ microglobulin in bile have also been monitored as rejection markers (45,46). Biliary levels of intercellular adhesion molecule-1 (ICAM-1) have been shown to be elevated specifically in rejection, apparently due to local release/secretion from activated lymphocytes within the liver. ICAM-1 was also elevated in the serum, concomitant with elevated IL-2 receptor; however, these elevations were seen in patients with infective complications as well as in those with rejection (47).

2. Radiology/Imaging

Radiologic methods may aid substantially in the differential diagnosis of acute rejection, and especially in differentiating rejection, infection, vascular thromboses, and biliary tract complications. Duplex ultrasonography is a valuable noninvasive method for evaluating postoperative complications, including patency of vascular anastomoses as well as focal hematomas, infarcts, abscesses, and bilomas in the hapatic parenchyma (48). This technique is considered the optimal approach for screening patients for vascular complications (49,50). T-tube cholangiograms, radionuclide biliary scans, and sonography are useful in detecting bile duct complications.

Detection of a periportal "collar," defined as a large amount of low-attenuation material around the main portal vein or the left or right portal vein, by computed tomography (CT) has been proposed as a reliable predictor of rejection. However, while there is a weak correlation, the sensitivity, specificity, and predictive value of this finding appear to be low (51).

Abnormalities in liver uptake and excretion of radiopharmaceuticals can be detected by hepatobilary scintigraphy in patients with rejection but are also seen in patients without rejection or parenchymal disease (52). Findings useful in predicting graft outcome via this technique include failure to visualize excreted material beyond the biliary anastomosis and persistent or worsening delay in visualization. The scintigraphic finding of delay in excretion is a useful marker for rejection or cholestasis, but does not appear to discriminate between the two (53). A more sophisticated scintigraphic analysis using first-pass and functional time-activity curves to calculate portal perfusion, blood retention, and liver uptake indices enable differentiation of severity of rejection/cholestasis changes but again does not appear to discriminate rejection and cholestasis (54).

Experimental radiologic approaches to rejection diagnosis include use of hepatocyte– and Kuppfer cell–directed magnetic resonance imaging (MRI) contrast agents. Liver enhancement with the former has been found to be delayed and prolonged in allogeneic versus syngeneic grafts (55). Similarly, p-31 nuclear magnetic resonance (NMR) has been used to monitor liver grafts in allogeneic and syngeneic rat models. Using defined parameters, rejecting livers could be detected at a "moderate stage" of rejection (56). These techniques may ultimately be refined further for clinical use.

3. Cytopathology/Histopathology

The "gold standard" for rejection diagnosis remains histopathological assessment. Fine needle aspiration biopsy (FNAB) has been proposed as a relatively noninvasive method for the evaluation of liver allografts. Analysis of inflammatory cells and their level of activation can be used to diagnose rejection; FNAB findings have been shown to correlate with histology with a sensitivity of 69% and specificity of 95% (57). In addition, changes in parenchymal cells can be used to detect cholestasis, preservation damage, hepatotoxic effects, and infections (58,59). Compared to rejection, where activated lymphocytes and blast forms predominate, both hepatitis C virus (HCV) and CMV infection are characterized by infiltration of cells showing less activation and/or rare blast forms (58). In centers with experience with FNAB, this technique can be used for frequent monitoring of the graft in the first weeks posttransplant. However, FNAB is not useful for diagnosis of chronic rejection.

Graft biopsies are routinely used in all transplant centers to evaluate graft dysfunction and to guide antirejection therapy. The criteria for the diagnosis of rejection, described briefly above, are discussed at length in Chap. 8. In general, these diagnostic criteria are reproducible, and there is now consensus agreement on them. However, the transient appearance of portal tract pathological changes consistent with rejection may be seen on protocol biopsies without hepatic dysfunction in approximately 10 to 20% of patients (60).

B. Therapy

Although a detailed discussion of antirejection therapy is outside the scope of this chapter, general aspects of prevention and of induction and maintenance immunosuppressive therapy are discussed briefly here.

1. Prevention

The incidence of significant rejection and graft loss can clearly be reduced by improving HLA compatibility and crossmatching. However, optimal matching is often not possible, since cadaveric hepatic allografting is often an emergent procedure. An optimal approach, which has proved efficacious in renal transplantation and is being increasingly utilized, is the use of living related donors. Grafts from a living donor are generally of superior quality to cadaveric grafts and enable elective transplantation under optimal conditions for the recipient. In some countries where procurement of cadaveric livers is not established, living related donors represent the only source of viable livers for allografting. The most extensive experience with this approach has been in the grafting of segments of liver from an adult donor into a pediatric recipient (61).

As noted above, unlike the situation in other solid-organ allografts, liver grafts from ABO-incompatible donors often do well posttransplant. Indeed, hyperacute rejection is rare in this setting, even in the face of an ABO mismatch. However, ABO incompatibility may have more subtle but significant effects on allograft outcome. Sanchez-Urdazpal et al. compared the incidence of biliary complications in ABO-compatible and incompatible grafts (62). They found that biliary complications developed in 82% of ABO-incompatible grafts versus 6% in ABO matched controls. Cellular rejection was diagnosed in 65%, and 1-year graft survival was 14% in the incompatible group, versus 28% rejection incidence and 78% 1-year survival in controls. Hepatic artery thrombosis occurred in 24% of the incompatible grafts. Donor ABO antigens were expressed on endothelium and on bile duct epithelium up to 150 days posttransplant. These results suggest significant immunologic injury in the incompatible grafts.

A number of studies have found no evidence that HLA-A, B, or DR incompatibility or donor-specific positive crossmatch have an adverse effect on survival of the recipients. However, reductions in graft survival with positive lymphocytotoxic crossmatches have been reported (63). In one large recent study of 800 liver transplant patients, 4-year patient and graft survival were 71% and 67% in recipients with a negative donor-specific T-cell crossmatch and 53% and 50% in those with a positive crossmatch, a statistically significant difference. The majority of T cell–positive crossmatches were in patients with panel-reactive antibody (PRA) > 10%, prompting the authors to recommend crossmatching if logistically feasible in this group of patients. Positive B-cell crossmatch and the presence of PRA had no significant adverse effect (64). In the same study, when effects of HLA mismatching were assessed, patient survival was reduced with increasing antigen mismatches, due to reduced survival following retransplant in those with HLA-DR mismatches in primary transplants requiring intensive immunosuppression. The authors suggest that special immunosuppressive strategies in recipients with HLA incompatibility with the donor might improve these survival rates (64).

Flow cytometry crossmatch (FCXM) testing is an even more sensitive predictor of early graft failures (65). While 11 of the 20 FCXM-positive patients in a recent study had a high PRA, almost half did not. Of the latter, 5 of 9 had graft failure within 1 month, suggesting that low levels of antibody or non-complement-fixing antibody may have a damaging effect.

Another complication associated with prior HLA allosensitization is a doubling of the average need for blood components during surgery. These patients are at risk for poor response to platelet transfusion and may benefit from platelet crossmatching (23).

2. *Induction and Maintenance Immunosuppression*

Immunosuppressive regimens in hepatic allografting have been based largely on regimens developed in renal transplantation. The toxicity of these agents is considered in detail in Chap. 24. The use of a combination of cyclosporine and prednisone in the 1980s substantially enhanced graft and patient survival compared with the earlier regimen of azathioprine plus prednisone (66,67). However, this regimen produced substantial toxic side effects (68,69) (see Chap. 24). A triple-drug regimen consisting of prednisone, azathioprine, and cyclosporine has enabled reduction of doses of cyclosporine and decrease in major side effects of the drug, including hypertension and nephrotoxicity. In several series, a decrease in incidence of both cellular and ductopenic rejection have been reported on this regimen (1,70).

Some investigators have explored the possibility of more individualized immunosuppression with cyclosporin A (CsA). Lemoine et al. studied the relationship between graft cytochrome P-450 3A content and early morbidity posttransplant. Problems related to CsA toxicity were invariably related to low P-450 3A (and consequent reduction in metabolism of CsA). Episodes of early rejection, on the other hand, were related to high P-450 3A levels (71). Dosage adjustment based on levels of this enzyme in the graft could potentially avoid these difficulties. In malabsorbing patients, a new oral form of cyclosporine, Sandimmune-neoral, has shown promising clinical results (72).

Withdrawal of cyclosporine has been attempted in some patients with nephrotoxicity. In one study assessing CsA withdrawl, criteria for inclusion in the protocol included triple immunosuppression, stable graft function for at least 1 year without rejection, and evidence of significant renal dysfunction. Overall, there was no sustained improvement in kidney function, and half of the patients suffered cellular or ductopenic rejection (73).

A "sequential quadruple" regimen has been evaluated in several treatment trials. Typically, induction therapy with OKT3 or antithymocyte globulin is begun posttransplant, followed by triple-drug maintenance therapy instituted 5 to 10 days posttransplant. This regimen delays rejection episodes until the fifth or sixth week posttransplant but does not appear to significantly decrease the overall incidence of rejection compared to triple therapy alone (14,74,75). Untoward effects of the sequential regimen included prolongation of hospitalization due to the late onset of rejection episodes. In addition, the use of OKT3 appears to be associated with a high incidence of infection (76) and an increased risk of Epstein-Barr virus (EBV)-related posttransplant lymphoproliferative disorder (77–79).

A new immunosuppressive regimen undergoing clinical trials is the combination of FK506 and corticosteroid therapy. Initial results suggest antirejection efficacy comparable to cyclosporine, with comparable nephrotoxicity and enhanced neurotoxicity (80). Results of a large multicenter trial comparing FK506 and CsA-based immunosuppressive regimens have recently been published (81). Patient and graft survival at 1 year were very comparable in the two groups, but incidence of acute rejection, steroid-resistant rejection, and refractory rejection were significantly less frequent in the FK506 group. However, FK506-treated patients had a significantly higher incidence of nephro- and neurotoxicity requiring withdrawl from the study. Conversion from CsA to FK506 has proven efficacious in patients with acute or early chronic rejection in spite of apparently optimal CsA therapy (82).

High-dose intravenous corticosteroid therapy is also efficacious for treatment of early acute cellular rejection and appears to be associated with a decrease in the incidence of steroid-resistant rejection and graft failure from rejection (20). OKT3 is widely used to treat rejection episodes resistant to high dose steroids, with good results (83–85). In a recent series, OKT3 produced 1-year patient and graft survivals comparable to patients who had no rejection. Permanent reversal of rejection was achieved in 42 of 71 cases, and there was a temporary response in 12 patients. A second course of OKT3 was attempted in 6; in 4 of these, lymphoproliferative disorder (PTLD) developed (86).

If bolus corticosteroid therapy and antilymphocyte therapy have failed to suppress a rejection episode, FK506 has been advocated as a rescue measure. Results of several uncontrolled trials suggest that this strategy may be useful, at least in some patients (82, 87 90). Up to one half to two-thirds of patients with ductopenic or cellular rejection respond to FK506 "rescue" (91). There is some evidence that success of FK506 rescue therapy may be predicted by the level of serum bilirubin.

Other therapeutic agents and strategies have been used in isolated studies to treat acute cellular rejection episodes. These include mycophenolic acid, which has shown promise in initial studies (92); large-scale studies with this agent are under way. This agent has also been used for maintenance immunosuppression in a small group of patients who could not tolerate CsA/FK506, with some success (93). Evrard et al. have reported successful rescue therapy with a combination of cyclophosphamide and plasmapheresis (94). Other immunosuppressive agents—including rapamycin, brequinar, and 5-deoxyspergualin have shown promise in experimental models and are currently being assessed in human solid-organ transplantation (95).

If all therapeutic initiatives fail to rescue a hepatic allograft, the rejection process will progress to irreversible/chronic rejection. Retransplantation then becomes the only therapeutic option; this is discussed below.

An intriguing aspect of immunosuppressive therapy in hepatic allograft recipients is the possibility of weaning from immunosuppression in long-term grafts. Candidates for weaning are generally 5 to 10 years posttransplant. In a recent series, most of the patients selected for weaning had complications of long-term immunosuppression (96). Of the 59 patients in the study, 27% were weaned completely and the process was progressing in an additional 47%. The attempt failed in 25% without graft loss.

IV. CHRONIC/DUCTOPENIC REJECTION

Ductopenic rejection is less common than the type of rejection described above, occurring in a mean of 5 to 10% of cases. It has been postulated that this low incidence of chronic rejection compared to renal or cardiac allografts may be due to a lower immunogenicity of the liver and/or to its dual blood supply, which protects the organ from effects of obliterative arteriopathy (97). With new immunosuppressive regimens, the incidence is even lower (11,81,98). This process has been referred to by a variety of terms, including "vanishing bile duct syndrome," "chronic rejection," "vascular rejection," and "acute" or "chronic irreversible rejection" (20,99). The severity of this process varies from mild ductopenia with mild cholestasis, which is potentially reversible, to severe bile duct loss with severe cholestasis, often referred to as the vanishing bile duct syndrome and signaling impending irreversible graft failure.

Mechanisms producing this form of rejection are not well understood, though in most cases it is considered to be a form of cell-mediated rejection. Likely mechanisms are depicted in Fig. 2. Indeed, chronic rejection is usually preceded by one or more episodes of acute rejection, which may be severe and/or steroid-resistant. In early stages of ductopenic rejection, there is invasion of biliary epithelium by lymphocytes and degenerative changes in bile duct cells (100). Electron microscopy reveals lymphocytes in contact with degenerating bile duct cells, suggesting direct lymphocytotoxic injury (101). Also, lymphocytes cultured from these patients show cytotoxic activity against donor MHC antigens (102,103). Since class I MHC antigens are constitutively expressed on bile duct epithelium and class II antigens are induced by injury to this epithelium, these, or potentially other, epithelial antigens could serve as targets for cell-mediated immunological attack (104–107). A predominantly $CD8^+$ lymphocytic infiltrate in portal tracts has been associated with an increased risk of chronic rejection (70,108). ICAM-1 is a cell adhesion molecule that is inducible by proinflammatory cytokines. Prolonged and increased expression of ICAM-1 on bile ducts, perivenular hepatocytes, and endothelium that persists despite corticosteroid therapy is associated with chronic rejection (109).

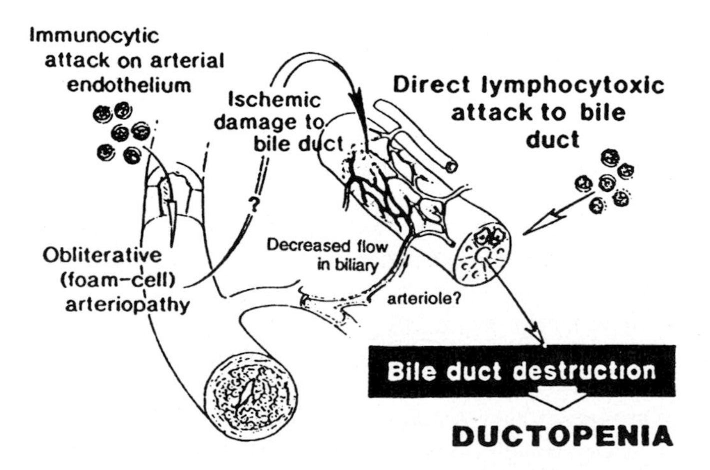

Figure 2 Mechanisms of bile duct destruction leading to ductopenic rejection. Evidence for immunological mechanisms is definitive; the role of ischemia is more speculative.

Foam-cell arteriopathy or foam-cell arteritis is a marker for "chronic rejection," since ductopenia is found in most patients with this finding. This obliterative process could play a pathogenic role in loss of bile ducts, though this has not been proven (110). The association of duct loss and vascular changes is difficult to establish in humans, since the arteriopathic changes occur in medium to large vessels, which are infrequently sampled on liver biopsy. In a dog allograft model, however, ductopenia with severe cholestasis and foam-cell arteriopathy were found together. In the late subtype of ductopenic rejection, it has been suggested that humoral mechanisms may play a role (111,112).

Several clinical factors have been identified in preliminary studies that appear to predict development of this form of rejection in liver allografts. These include primary sclerosing cholangitis as an indication for transplantation, immunosuppression without azathioprine, and a positive lymphocytotoxic crossmatch (10,98,113). Some studies, however, have found no association between positive lymphocytotoxic crossmatch and graft survival. There is also some evidence that HLA-DR mismatch with or without concomitant cytomegalovirus infection may be an additional risk factor (4,114); however, other investigators have found no association between HLA mismatching, CMV infection, and vanishing bile duct syndrome (115). Further investigation of these and other risk factors is needed to resolve these important issues.

A. Diagnosis

1. *Clinical*

The timing of ductopenic rejection posttransplant may vary considerably. The process has been subclassified into early (less than 6 weeks), delayed (6 weeks to 6 months), or late (more than 6 months) ductopenic rejection (2,10). The initial manifestations of early ductopenic rejection are malaise, fever, and an abrupt rise in liver function tests, especially serum aminotransferases. The acute episode generally fails to respond to additional immunosuppressive therapy. As the process progresses, serum aminotransferases decrease and there is a progressive rise in serum bilirubin, alkaline phosphatase, and gamma-glutamyltransferase. Cholestasis persists, and the graft fails as synthetic functions are lost.

Delayed ductopenic rejection, the most common pattern, generally develops after one or several episodes of acute rejection that do not respond to maximal immunosuppressive therapy. Progressive cholestasis develops and graft failure eventually ensues. In rare patients, a late ductopenic rejection is seen. This form often presents insidously, without a history of previous clinically detectable episodes of acute rejection. Progression, marked by developing cholestasis, may be very slow, over a period of months to years, eventually leading to cholestatic graft failure.

Ductopenic rejection is typically progressive and irreversible; however, clinical improvement has been reported in some patients (3,16,116–118). At least some of these patients show marked bile duct proliferation on rebiopsy, suggesting that regeneration of these structures is possible. No clinical, biochemical, or histological findings have been found that can predict which patients will improve and which will relentlessly progress.

2. *Radiology/Imaging*

The hallmark of early ductopenic rejection is cholestasis. Imaging strategies that demonstrate cholestasis are useful but nonspecific, and other causes of cholestasis must be ruled out. Increased echogenicity of periportal areas on ultrasound has been reported and may be useful in differentiating chronic from acute rejection, in which there is decreased parenchymal echogenicity (119), but this observation requires additional testing. Angiography may reveal stenosis of intrahepatic vessels (120) but is not widely used in this setting.

3. *Histopathology*

The diagnosis of ductopenic rejection is defined by allograft biopsy. Histologically, the process is characterized by loss of interlobular and septal bile ducts and is often though not invariably associated with foam-cell arteriopathy (30,99). To diagnose ductopenic rejection, at least a minimum number of bile ducts, usually 20 or more, must be available for evaluation. Foam-cell arteriopathy, if present in the biopsy, is closely correlated with ductopenic rejection. However, ductopenia may be documented without foam-cell arteriopathy; indeed, fewer than 10% of liver biopsy specimens with ductopenic rejection have this finding (120). In some cases, worsening ischemic hepatocellular injury and fibrosis are seen in addition to ductopenia; these cases appear to have a worse prognosis (16). A complete discussion of histologic criteria for this form of rejection can be found in Chap. 8.

In patients with early or delayed subtypes of ductopenic rejection, a progression of changes may be seen on sequential allograft biopsies. In the early phase, biopsies typically show features of nonsuppurative destructive cholangitis. If the process does not respond to immunosuppressive therapy, later biopsies will show persistent cholangitis with ongoing destruction of bile ducts. Finally, bile ducts progressively disappear, there is fibrosis of portal tracts, and inflammatory infiltrates subside. Progressive cholestasis can be documented in the hepatic parenchyma. In the late form, portal inflammatory infiltrates may not be seen, and the dominant findings are ductopenia and degeneration of bile duct epithelium with cholestasis.

B. Treatment

The early phases of ductopenic rejection may respond to immunosuppressive therapy, as outlined above. "Rescue" therapy with FK506 may stabilize patients or produce improved liver function in those with early chronic rejection (87,90). However, in late stages, when inflammatory infiltrates have subsided, additional immunosuppression is generally not helpful (2). With progressive loss of bile ducts and graft failure, retransplantation becomes the only therapeutic option, and is lifesaving in this setting. However, ductopenic rejection develops in a substantial number of these patients in second or subsequent allografts (2,10). The ideal approach to these patients is to prevent this process, perhaps via improved donor-recipient matching or with improved immunosuppressive regimens. As noted above, this complication has become less common with newer immunosuppressive regimens, and additional improvements may be possible as new agents reach clinical trials.

V. DIFFERENTIAL DIAGNOSIS

A variety of processes may cause hepatic allograft dysfunction, requiring differential from a rejection process. Differential diagnoses to be considered with immediate or early allograft dysfunction have been discussed above. Here we discuss additional differential considerations.

A common cause of hepatic dysfunction posttransplant, which must be differentiated from cellular rejection, is CMV hepatitis; diagnosis, treatment, and prevention of CMV infections after liver transplantation has been recently reviewed (122). Ninova et al assessed serum levels of soluble T-cell markers sIL2R, sCD4, and sCD8 as possible differential markers in this setting. They compared small groups of control transplant patients and patients with biopsy-proven cellular rejection or CMV hepatitis, monitoring pretransplant levels and serial measurements posttransplant. Soluble IL2R was elevated in patients with rejection, while both sIL2R and CD8 were elevated in patients with CMV hepatitis, suggesting that these soluble markers could be useful in differentiating late rejection (>20 days) and CMV hepatitis (123). Amplification of CMV DNA in serum by polymerase chain reaction also appears to be a promising approach, with DNA often appearing in the serum before symptomatic infection and clearing with treatment (124,125). Liver biopsy is the definitive diagnostic test, with typical CMV inclusions usually detectable on liver biopsy; in situ hybridization does not improve accuracy of diagnosis compared to routine histopathology (126).

Lymphoproliferative disorder (LPD) induced by EBV almost always occurs in patients receiving OKT3, and is related to cumulative dose, so that presentation is typically 2 to 3 months after transplantation (127). However, LPD may present like rejection in occasional patients (128) and may mimic rejection on liver biopsy. In situ hybridization for EBV and immunostaining for T- and B-cell markers are very useful on biopsy to diagnose this lesion. Hepatitis B and hepatitis C may occur or recur in the allografted liver. In this setting, there is a rise in transaminases, and the clinical picture is generally not typical for rejection. Viral serologies are useful in these patients. Hepatitis can often be diagnosed on liver biopsy.

Chronic rejection requires differentiation from other causes of cholestasis, including biliary obstruction, viral hepatitis, sepsis, and drug toxicity. This differential can be made by histological criteria on liver biopsy. Chronic ductopenic rejection can also produce hilar strictures of the bile duct. These usually develop within the first few months posttransplant and may be caused by hepatic artery occlusion and CMV infection as well as rejection. While percutaneous/transhepatic dilatation of localized strictures is possible, retransplantation may be necessary (129,130).

Late posttransplant, the most difficult dilemma in differential diagnosis comes in patients with liver transplantation for primary biliary cirrhosis. It may be very difficult in this setting to differentiate chronic graft rejection from recurrent disease. Sequential clinical follow-up and biopsies may be helpful in this regard (81,131,132).

VI. SUMMARY

With the refinement of surgical techniques and immunosuppressive therapy, outcomes in liver allografting have markedly improved, and liver transplantation is now the standard therapy for many patients with acute and chronic liver disease (133). The incidence of acute rejection has declined significantly. However, because of implications for graft survival, the diagnosis of acute cellular rejection and its prompt treatment remain very important. There are new molecular and cellular markers that may ultimately prove useful in this regard, and increasingly sophisticated radiologic approaches are also being developed (134). At the present time, however, liver biopsy remains the gold standard for rejection diagnosis, for both acute and chronic rejection. New therapeutic modalities and more refined use of existing agents has led to improved outcome for acute and chronic rejection occurring in allografts. Rejection diagnosis, differential diagnosis, and treatment remain a challenge in this complex patient population.

REFERENCES

1. Klintmalm GBG, Nery JR, Husberg BS, et al. Rejection in liver transplantation. Hepatology 1989; 10:978–985.

2. Adams DH, Neuberger JM. patterns of graft rejection following liver transplantation. J Hepatol 1990; 10:113–119.
3. Snover DC, Freese DK, Sharp HL, et al. Liver allograft rejection: An analysis of the use of biopsy in determining outcome of rejection. Am J Surg Pathol 1987; 11:1–10.
4. O'Grady JG, Alexander GJM, Sutherland S, et al. Cytomegalovirus infection and donor/recipient HLA antigens: Interdependent cofactors in pathogenesis of vanishing bile duct syndrome after liver transplantation. Lancet 1988; 2:302–305.
5. Busuttil RW, Colonna JO II, Hiatt JR, et al. The first 100 liver transplants at UCLA. Ann Surg 1987; 206:387–399.
6. Gouw ASH. Allograft rejection in human liver transplantation: an immunohistologic study (thesis). Groningen, The Netherlands: University of Groningen, 1988.
7. Gubernatis G, Kemnitz J, Tusch G, Pichlmayr R. HLA compatibility and different features of liver allograft rejection. Transplant Int 1988; 1:155–160.
8. Demetris AJ, Markus BH, Esquivel C, et al. Pathologic analysis of liver transplantation for primary biliary cirrhosis. Hepatology 1988; 8:939–947.
9. McDonald JA, Painter DM, Bell R, et al. Human liver allograft rejection: Severity, prognosis, and response to treatment. Transplant Proc 1989; 21:3792–3793.
10. Van Hoek B, Wiesner RH, Krom RAF, et al. Severe ductopenic rejection following liver transplantation: Incidence, time of onset, risk factors, treatment and outcome. Semin Liver Dis 1992; 12:41–50.
11. Pirsch JD, Kalayoglu M, Hafez GR, et al. Evidence that the vanishing bile duct syndrome is vanishing. Transplantation 1990; 49:1015–1018.
12. Otte JB. Recent developments in liver transplantation: Lessons from a 5-year experience. J Hepatol 1991; 12:386–393.
13. Monsour H, Stratta RJ, Markin RS, et al. A case control study of chronic rejection in liver transplant recipients: Results of a multivariate analysis (abstr). Presented at the International Liver Transplantation Society Meeting; 1992; Minneapolis.
14. McDiarmid SV, Millis MJ, Terasaki PI, et al. OKT3 prophylaxis in liver transplantation. Dig Dis Sci 1991; 36:1418–1426.
15. Salt A, Noble-Jamieson G, Barnes ND, et al. Liver transplantation in 100 children: Cambridge and King's College Hospital series. Br Med J 1992; 304:416–421.
16. Freese DK, Snover DC, Sharp HL, et al. Chronic rejection after liver transplantation: A study of clinical, histopathological and immunological features. Hepatology 1991; 13:882–891.
17. Ryckman FC, Schroeder TJ, Pedersen SH, et al. Use of monoclonal antibody immunosuppressive therapy in pediatric renal and liver transplantation. Clin Transplant 1991; 5:186–190.
18. Emond JC, Whitington PF, Thislethwaite JR, et al. Reduced-size orthotopic liver transplantation: Use in the management of children with chronic liver disease. Hepatology 1989; 10: 867–872.
19. Esquivel CO, Nakazato P, Cox K, et al. The impact of liver reductions in pediatric liver transplantation. Arch Surg 1991; 126:1278–1285.
20. Wiesner RH, Ludwig J, Krom RAF, et al. Hepatic allograft rejection: New developments in terminology, diagnosis, prevention, and treatment. Mayo Clin Proc 1993; 68:69–79.
21. Hanto DW, Snover DC, Sibley RK, et al. Hyperacute rejection of a human orthotopic liver allograft in a presensitized recipient. Clin Transplant 1987; 1:304–310.
22. Gordon RP, Fung JJ, Markus B, et al. The antibody crossmatch in liver transplantation. Surgery 1986; 100:705–715.
23. Ramsey G, Sherman LA. Transfusion therapy in solid organ transplantation. Hematol Oncol Clin North Am 1994; 8:1117–1129.
24. Starzl TE, Demetris AJ, Todo S, et al. Evidence for hyperacute rejection of human liver grafts: The case of the canary kidney. Clin Transplant 1989; 3:37–45.
25. Knechtle SH, Kolbeck PC, Tsuchimoto S, et al. Hepatic transplantation into sensitised recipients. Transplantation 1987; 43:8–12.

26. Hubscher SG, Adams DH, Neuberger JM, et al. Massive hemorrhagic necrosis of the liver following transplantation. J Clin Pathol 1989; 42:360–370.
27. McCaughan GW, Huynh JC, Feller R, et al. Fulminant hepatic failure post liver transplantation—clinical syndromes, correlations and outcomes. Transplant Int 1995; 8:20–26.
28. Legmann P, Dousset B, Tudoret L, et al. Hyperacute rejection in liver transplantation: CT findings. J Comput Assist Tomogr 1994; 18:139–142.
29. Katz E, Mor E, Schwartz ME, et al. Preservation injury in clinical liver transplantation—Incidence and effect on rejection and survival. Clin Transplant 1994; 8:492–496.
30. Wiesner RH, Ludwig J, van Hoek B, Krom RAF. Current concepts in cell-mediated hepatic allograft rejection leading to ductopenia and liver failure. Hepatology 1991; 14:721–729.
31. Wiesner RH. Acute cellular rejection following liver transplantation: incidence, risk factors, and outcome in the NIDDK Liver Transplant Database (LTD) study (abstr). Gastroenterology 1992; 102:A910.
32. Ettenger RB, Blifeld C, Prince H, et al. The pediatric nephrologist's dilemma: Growth after renal transplantation and its interaction with age as a possible immunologic variable. J Pediatr 1987; 111:1022–1025.
33. Van Hoek B, Wiesner RH, Ludwig J, Krom RAF. The role of protocol liver biopsies in diagnosis and treatment of early cellular rejection after orthotopic liver transplantation (abstr). Hepatology 1990; 12:866.
34. Henley KS, Lucey MR, Appelman HD, et al. Biochemical and histopathological correlation in liver transplant: The first 180 days. Hepatology 1992; 16:688–693.
35. Malury CPJ, Hockerstedt K, Tepo A-M, et al. Changes in serum amyloid A protein and beta 2-microglobulin in association with liver allograft rejection. Transplantation 1984; 38:551–553.
36. Feussner G, Stech C, Dobmeyer J, et al. Serum amyloid protein (SAA)—A marker for liver allograft rejection in humans. Clin Invest 1994; 72:1007–1011.
37. Azer SA, McCaughan GW, Stacey NH. Daily determinations of individual serum bile acids allows early detection of hepatic allograft dysfunction. Hepatology 1994; 20:1458–1464.
38. Gozzo ML, Avolio A, Forni F, et al. Enzymatic determinations in acute rejection after liver transplantation: Preliminary report on necrosis index. Clin Chim Acta 1993; 214:175–184.
39. Puppo F, Pellicci R, Brenci S, et al. HLA class-1-soluble antigen serum levels in liver transplantation—A predictor marker of acute rejection. Human Immunol 1994; 40:166–170.
40. McDonald JC, Adamashvili I, Hayes JM, et al. Soluble HLA class 1 concentrations. Transplantation 1994; 58:1268–1272.
41. Foster P, Sankary S, Hart M, et al. Blood and graft eosinophilia as predictors of rejection in human liver transplantation. Transplantation 1989; 47:72–74.
42. De Groen PC, Kephart GM, Gleich GJ, Ludwig J. The eosinophil as an effector cell of the immune response during hepatic allograft rejection. Hepatology 1994; 20:654–662.
43. Le Moine O, Marchant A, Durand F, et al. Gelin M, Goldman M, Deviere J. Systemic release of interleukin-10 during orthotopic liver transplantation. Hepatology 1994; 20:889–892.
44. Ohzato H, Monden M, Yoshizaki K, et al. Serum interleukin-6 levels as an indicator of acute rejection after liver transplantation in cynomologus monkeys. Surg Today 1993; 23:521–527.
45. Adams DH, Burnett D, Stockley RA, et al. Biliary beta-2-microglobulin in liver allograft rejection. Hepatology 1988; 8:1565–1570.
46. Adams DH, Wang L, Hubscher SG, Elias E, Neuberger JM. Soluble interleukin-2 receptors in serum and bile of liver transplant recipients. Lancet 1989; 1:469–472.
47. Adams DH, Mainolfi E, Elias E, et al. Detection of circulating intercellular adhesion molecule-1 after liver transplantation—Evidence of local release within the liver during graft rejection. Transplantation 1993; 55:83–87.
48. Morton MJ, James EM, Wiesner RH, Krom RA. Applications of duplex ultrasonography in the liver transplant patient. Mayo Clin Proc 1990; 65:360–372.
49. Taylor KJW, Morse SS, Weltin GG, et al. Liver transplant recipients: Portable duplex US with correlative angiography. Radiology 1986; 159:357–363.

50. Flint EW, Sumkin JH, Zajko AB, Bowen A. Duplex sonography of hepatic artery thrombosis after liver transplantation. AJR 1988; 151:481–483.
51. Stevens SD, Heiken JP, Brunt E, et al. Low-attenuation periportal collar in transplanted liver is not reliable CT evidence of acute allograft rejection. Am J Roentgenol 1991;157:1195–1198.
52. Gelfand MJ, Smith HS, Ryckman FC, et al. Hepatobiliary scintigraphy in pediatric liver transplant recipients. Clin Nucl Med 1992; 17:542–549.
53. Engeler CM, Kuni CC, Nakhleh R, et al. Liver transplant rejection and cholestasis: Comparison of technetium 99m-diisopropyl iminodiacetic acid hepatobiliary imaging with liver biopsy. Eur J Nucl Med 1992; 19:865–870.
54. Brunot B, Petras S, Germain P, et al. Biopsy and quantitative hepatobiliary scintigraphy in the evaluation of liver transplantation. J Nucl Med 1994; 35:1321–1327.
55. Muhler A, Freise CE, Kuwatsuru R, et al. Acute liver rejection: Evaluation with cell-directed MR contrast agents in a rat transplantation model. Radiology 1993; 86:139–146.
56. Bowers JL, Kawano K, Metz KR, et al. P-31 NMR assessment of orthotopic liver rejection in a rat model. Magn Res Med 1994; 32:164–169.
57. Kubota K, Ericzon BG, Reinholt FP. Comparison of fine-needle aspiration biopsy and histology in human liver transplants. Transplantation 1991; 51:1010–1013.
58. Lautenschlager I, Nashan B, Schlitt HJ, et al. Different cellular patterns associated with hepatitis C virus reactivation, cytomegalovirus infection, and acute rejection in liver transplant patients monitored with transplant aspiration cytology. Transplantation 1994; 1339–1345.
59. Schlitt HJ, Nashan B, Ringe B, et al. Differentiation of liver graft dysfunction by transplant aspiration cytology. Transplantation 1991; 51:786–793.
60. Williams JW, Foster PF, Sankary HN. Role of liver allograft biopsy in patient management. Semin Liver Dis 1992; 12:60–72.
61. Broelsch CE, Burdelski M, Rogiers X, et al. Living donor for liver transplantation. Hepatology 1994; 20(suppl):S49–S55.
62. Sanchez-Urdazpal L, Batts KP, Gores GJ, et al. Increased bile duct complications in liver transplantation across the ABO barrier. Ann Surg 1993; 218:152–158.
63. Takaga S, Bronsther O, Iwaki Y, et al. The adverse impact on liver transplantation of using positive cytotoxic crossmatch donors. Transplantation 1992; 53:400–406.
64. Nikaein A, Backman L, Jennings L, et al. HLA compatibility and liver transplant outcome—Improved patient survival by HLA and cross-matching. Transplantation 1994; 58:786–792.
65. Ogura K, Terasaki PI, Koyama H, et al. High one-month liver graft failure rates in flow cytometry crossmatch-positive recipients. Clin Transplant 1994; 8:111–115.
66. Starzl TE, Klintmalm GBG, Porter KA, et al. Liver transplant with use of cyclosporin A and prednisone. N Engl J Med 1981; 305:266–269.
67. Starzl TE, Iwatsuki S, Van Thiel DH, et al. Evolution of liver transplantation. Hepatology 1982; 2:614–636.
68. DeGroen PC, Aksamit AJ, Rakela J, et al. Central nervous system toxicity after liver transplantation: The role of cyclosporine and cholesterol. N Engl J Med 1987; 317:861–866.
69. Myers BD, Ross J, Newton L, et al. Cyclosporine-associated chronic nephropathy. N Engl J Med 1984; 311:699–705.
70. Perkins JD, Rakela J, Sterioff S, et al. Results of treatment in hepatic allograft rejection depend on the immunohistologic pattern of the portal T lymphocytic infiltrate. Transplant Proc 1988; 20:223–225.
71. LeMoine A, Azoulay D, Bries JM, et al. Relationship between graft cytochrome P-450 3A content and early morbidity after liver transplantation. Transplantation 1993; 56:1410–1414.
72. Farber L, Maibucher A, Geissler F, et al. Favourable clinical results of Sandimmune-neoral in malabsorbing liver and heart transplant recipients. Transplant Proc 1994; 26:2988–2993.
73. Sandborn WJ, Hay JE, Porayko MK, et al. Cyclosporine withdrawl for nephrotoxicity in liver transplant recipients does not result in sustained improvement in kidney function and causes cellular and ductopenic rejection. Hepatology 1994; 19:925–932.

74. Cosimi AB, Jenkins RL, Rohrer RJ, et al. A randomized clinical trial of prophylactic OKT3 monoclonal antibody in liver allograft recipients. Arch Surg 1990; 125:781–784.
75. Millis JM, McDiarmid SV, Hiatt JR, et al. Randomized prospective trial of OKT3 for early prophylaxis of rejection after liver transplantation. Transplantation 1989; 47:82–88.
76. Mühlbacher F, Steininger R, Längle F, et al. OKT3 immunoprophylaxis in human liver transplantation. Transplant Proc 1989; 21:2253–2254.
77. Swinner LJ, Costanzo-Nordin MR, Fisher SG, et al. Increased incidence of lymphoproliferative disorder after immunosuppression with the monoclonal antibody OKT3 in cardiac-transplant recipients. N Engl J Med 1990; 323:1723–1728.
78. Canfield CW, Hudnall SD, Colonna JO II, et al. Fulminant Epstein-Barr virus–associated post-transplant lymphoproliferative disorders following OKT3 therapy. Clin Transplant 1992; 6:1–9.
79. Legendre C, Kreis H. Effect of immunosuppression on the incidence of lymphoma formation. Clin Transplant 1992; 6:220–222.
80. Fung J, Abu-Elmagd K, Jain A, et al. A randomized trial of primary liver transplantation under immunosuppression with FK 506 vs cyclosporine. Transplant Proc 1991; 23:2977–2983.
81. Busttil RW, McDiarmid S, Klintmalm GB, et al. A comparison of Tacrolimus (FK 506) and cyclosporine for immunosuppression in liver transplantation. N Engl J Med 1994; 331:1110–1115.
82. Demetris AJ, Fung JJ, Todo S, et al. Conversion of liver allograft recipients from cyclosporine to FK 506 immunosuppressive therapy—A clinicopathologic study of 96 patients. Transplantation 1992; 53:1056–1062.
83. Colonna J, Goldstein L, Brems J, et al. A prospective study on the use of monoclonal anti-T3-cell antibody (OKT3) to treat steroid-resistant liver transplant rejection. Arch Surg 1987; 122:1120.
84. Fung JJ, Demetris AJ, Porter KA, et al. Use of OKT3 with cyclosporin and steroids for reversal of acute kidney and liver allograft rejection. Nephron 1987; 46:19.
85. Samuel D, Gugenheim J, Canon C, et al. Use of OKT3 for late acute rejection in liver transplantation. Transplant Proc 1990; 22:1767–1768.
86. Solomon H, Gonwa TZ, Mor E, et al. OKT3 rescue for steroid-resistant rejection in adult liver transplantation. Transplantation 1993; 55:87–91.
87. Winkler M, Ringe B, Gerstenkorn C, et al. Use of FK 506 for treatment of chronic rejection after liver transplantation. Transplant Proc 1991; 23:2984–2986.
88. Lewis WD, Jenkins RL, Burke PA, et al. FK 506 rescue therapy in liver transplant recipients with drug-resistant rejection. Transplant Proc 1991; 23:2989–2991.
89. D'Alessandro AM, Kalayoglu M, Pirsch JD, et al. FK506 rescue therapy for resistant rejection episodes in liver transplant recipients. Transplant Proc 1991; 23:2987–2988.
90. Shaw BW, Maarkin R, Stratta R, et al. FK506 for rescue treatment of acute and chronic rejection in liver allograft recipients. Transplant Proc 1991; 23:2994–2995.
91. McDiarmid SV, Klintmalm G, Busuttil RW. FK 506 rescue therapy in liver transplantation: Outcome and complications. Transplant Proc 1991; 23:2996–2999.
92. Sollinger HW, Deierhoi MH, Belzer FO, et al. RS-61443—A phase 1 clinical trial and pilot rescue study. Transplantation 1992; 53:428–432.
93. Friese CE, Hebert M, Osorio RW, et al. Maintenance immunosuppression with prednisone and RS-61443 alone following liver transplantation. Transplant Proc 1992.
94. Evrard HM, Miller C, Schwartz M, et al. Resistant hepatic allograft rejection successfully treated with cyclophosphamide and plasmapheresis. Transplantation 1990; 50:702–704.
95. Bumgarder GL, Roberts JP. New immunosuppressive agents. Gastroenterol Clin North Am 1993: 22:421–449.
96. Rames HC, Reyes J, Abuelmayd K, et al. Wearing of immunosuppression in long-term liver transplant recipients. Transplantation 1995; 59:212–217.
97. Lowes JR, Hubscher SG, Neuberger JM. Chronic rejection of the liver allograft. Gastroenterol Clin North Am 1993; 22:401–420.

98. Van Hoek B, Wiesner RH, Ludwig J, et al. Combination immunosuppression with azathioprine reduces the incidence of ductopenic rejection and vanishing bile duct syndrome after liver transplantation. Transplant Proc 1991; 23:1403–1405.
99. Ludwig J. Terminology of hepatic allograft rejection (glossary). Semin Liver Dis 1992; 12:89–92.
100. Vierling JM, Fennel RH Jr. Histopathology of early and late human hepatic allograft rejection: Evidence of progressive destruction of interlobular bile ducts. Hepatology 1985; 5:1076–1082.
101. Fennell RH Jr, Vierling JM. Electron microscopy of rejected human liver allografts. Hepatology 1985; 5:1083–1087.
102. Fung JJ, Zeevi A, Starzl TE, et al. Functional characterization of infiltrating T lymphocytes in human hepatic allografts. Hum Immunol 1986; 16:182–199.
103. Saidman SL, Demetris AJ, Zeevi A, Duquesnoy RJ. Propagation of lymphocytes infiltrating human liver allograft. Transplantation 1990; 49:107–112.
104. Daar AS, Fuggle SV, Fabre JW, et al. The detailed distribution of MHC class II antigens in normal human organs. Transplantation 1984; 38:293–298.
105. Demetris AJ, Lasky S, Van Thiel DH, et al. Induction of DR/IA antigens in human liver allografts: An immunocytochemical and clinicopathologic analysis of twenty failed grafts. Transplantation 1985; 40:504–509.
106. So S, Platt JL, Ascher NL, Snover DC. Increased expression of class I histocompatibility complex antigens on hepatocytes in rejecting human liver allografts. Transplantation 1987; 43:79–85.
107. Steinhoff G, Wonigeit K, Pichlmayr R. Analysis of sequential changes in major histocompatibility complex expression in human liver grafts after transplantation. Transplantation 1988; 45:394–401.
108. McCaughan GW, Davies JS, Waugh JA, et al. A quantitative analysis of T lymphocyte populations in human liver allografts undergoing rejection: The use of monoclonal antibodies and double immunolabelling. Hepatology 1990; 12:1305–1313.
109. Adams DH, Hubscher SG, Burnett D, et al. Immunoglobulins in liver allograft rejection: Evidence for deposition and secretion within the liver. Transplant Proc 1990; 22:1834–1835.
110. Ogura S, Belle S, Starzl TE, Demetris AJ. A histometric analysis of chronically rejected human liver allografts: Insights into the mechanisms of bile duct loss: Direct immunologic and ischemic factors. Hepatology 1989; 9:204–209.
111. Demetris AJ, Markus BH. Immunopathology of liver transplantation. Crit Rev Immunol 1989; 9:67–92.
112. Demetris AJ, Nakamura K, Yagihachi A, et al. A clinicopathological study of human liver allograft recipients harboring performed IgG lymphocytotoxic antibodies. Hepatology 1992; 16:671–681.
113. Batts KP, Moore SB, Perkins JD, et al. Influence of positive lymphocyte crossmatch and HLA mismatching on vanishing bile duct syndrome in human liver allografts. Transplantation 1988; 45:376–379.
114. Donaldson PT, Alexander GJM, O'Grady J, et al. Evidence for an immune response to HLA class I antigens in the vanishing-bile-duct syndrome after liver transplantation. Lancet 1987; 1:945–948.
115. Paya CV, Wiesner RH, Hermans PE, et al. Moore SB, Ludwig J, Smith TF. Lack of association between cytomegalovirus infection, HLA matching and the vanishing bile duct syndrome after liver transplantation. Hepatology 1992; 16:66–70.
116. Hubscher SG, Buckels JAC, Elias E, et al. Reversible vanishing bile duct syndrome after liver transplantation–Report of six cases. Transplant Proc 1991; 23:1415–1416.
117. Snover DC, Freese DK, Sharp HL, et al. Liver allograft rejection: an analysis of the use of biopsy on determining outcome of rejection. Am J Surg Pathol 1987; 11:1–10.
118. Noack KB, Wiesner RH, Batts K, et al. Severe ductopenic rejection with features of vanishing bile duct syndrome: Clinical, biochemical, and histologic evidence for spontaneous resolution. Transplant Proc 1991; 23:1448–1451.

119. Letourneau JG, Day DL, Frick MP, et al. Ultrasound and computed tomographic evaluation in hepatic transplantation. Radiol Clin North Am 1987; 25:323–331.
120. White RM, Zajko AB, Demetris AJ, et al. Liver transplant rejection: Angiographic findings in 35 patients. AJR 1987; 148:1095–1098.
121. Wiesner RH, van Hoek B, Ludwig J, et al. Foam cell arteriopathy in hepatic allografts: incidence, relationship to severe ductopenic rejection, and the sensitivity of needle biopsy for diagnosis (abstr). Hepatology 1992; 16:292A.
122. Wiesner RH, Marin E, Porayko MK, et al. Advances in the diagnosis, treatment, and prevention of cytomegalovirus infections after liver transplantation. Gastroenterol Clin North Am 1993; 22:351–366.
123. Ninova DI, Wiesner RH, Gores GJ, et al. Soluble T lymphocyte markers in the diagnosis of cellular rejection and cytomegalovirus hepatitis in liver transplant recipients. J Hepatol 1994; 21:1080–1085.
124. Patel R, Smith TF, Espy M, et al. Detection of cytomegalovirus DNA in sera of liver transplant recipients. J Clin Microbiol 1994; 32:1431–1434.
125. Drouet E, Colimon R, Michelson S, et al. Monitoring levels of human cytomegalovirus DNA in blood after liver transplantation. J. Clin Microbiol 1995; 33:389–394.
126. Espy MJ, Paya CCV, Holley KE, et al. Diagnosis of cytomegalovirus hepatitis by histopathology and in situ hybidization in liver transplantation. Diagn Microbiol Infect Dis 1991; 14: 293–296.
127. Morgan G, Superina RA. Lymphoproliferative disease after pediatric liver transplantation. J Pediatr Surg 1994; 29:1192–1196.
128. Howard TK, Klintmalm GB, Stone MJ, et al. Lymphoproliferative disorder masquerading as rejection in liver transplant recipients—An early aggressive tumor with atypical presentation. Transplantation 1992; 1145–1147.
129. Ward EM, Kiely MJ, Maus TP, et al. Hilar biliary strictures after liver transplantation: Cholangiography and percutaneous treatment. Radiology 1990; 177:259–263.
130. Zajko AB, Sheng R, Zetti GM, et al. Transhepatic balloon dilation of biliary strictures in liver transplant patients—A 10-year experience. J Vasc Intervent Radiol 1995; 6:79–83.
131. Polson RJ, Portmann B, Neuberger JM, et al. Evidence for disease recurrence after liver transplantation for primary biliary cirrhosis. Gastroenterology 1989; 97:715–725.
132. Lerut JP, Zimmermann A, Gertsch P. Late graft dysfunction after liver transplantation for primary biliary cirrhosis: Disease recurrence versus chronic graft rejection. Am J Gastroenterol 1994; 89:1896–1898.
133. Wood RP, Ozaki CF, Katz SM, et al. Liver transplantation—Last ten years. Surg Clin North Am 1994; 74:1133.
134. Shah AN, Dodson F, Fung J. Role of nuclear medicine in liver transplantation. Semin Liver Dis 1995; 25:36–48.

17

Clinical Diagnosis of Renal Allograft Rejection

M. Roy First
University of Cincinnati Medical Center, Cincinnati, Ohio

I. INTRODUCTION

The introduction in the 1980s of cyclosporine and monoclonal antibodies represented a major therapeutic advance in solid-organ transplantation. The United Network of Organ Sharing (UNOS) has recently released the 1- and 2-year graft and patient survival rates for solid-organ transplants (1). These survival rates are illustrated in Table 1. Currently there are a number of promising new immunosuppressive agents on the horizon, and it appears likely that further advances will be made in our ability to control the immune response (2,3). A dynamic interaction exists between basic immunology and clinical transplantation. Advances in immunobiology have resulted in a better understanding of the immunological events involved in the recognition and response to transplant antigens and led to a better understanding of the action of various immunosuppressive agents. This chapter reviews the clinical approach to the diagnosis and treatment of acute renal allograft rejection.

II. TIMING AND INCIDENCE OF ACUTE REJECTION

Acute renal allograft rejection may occur at any time but is experienced most commonly during the first few months after transplantation. Based upon the analysis of over 40,000 kidney transplants reported to the UNOS Scientific Renal Transplant Registry between October 1987 and August 1992 (4), 24% of recipients of first cadaver grafts experienced one or more rejection episodes during the initial transplant hospitalization, 52% during the first 6 months. At 12 months, only 40% of patients remained rejection-free. Patients who experienced any rejection during the first 6 months had a 72% 1-year graft survival rate, compared with 95% for those who remained rejection-free ($p<0.001$). Recipients of transplants from living donors had a significantly lower incidence of rejection episodes during their initial hospitalization. In these patients, a clear effect of histocompatibility was noted in comparing the incidence of rejection in HLA-identical sibling transplants (8% at discharge, 32% at 1 year) with that in one-haplotype disparate transplants (22% at discharge, 52% at one year; $p<0.01$ at each time point). In other living donors, rejections occurred in 25% at discharge and 56% at 1 year, similar to the figures for cadaver

Table 1 1- and 2-Year Graft and Patient Survival Rates, by Organ, for Transplants Between October 1, 1987, and December 31, 1991

		Graft survival (%)[a]		Patient survival (%)[a]	
Organ	No.	1 Year	2 Year	1 Year	2 Year
Kidney (cadaveric)	30,307	78.9 ± 0.2	72.8 ± 0.3	93.0 ± 0.1	90.0 ± 0.2
Kidney (living)	8,185	91.0 ± 0.3	87.4 ± 0.4	97.1 ± 0.2	95.6 ± 0.2
Liver	9,810	66.7 ± 0.5	62.3 ± 0.5	73.9 ± 0.5	69.4 ± 0.5
Pancreas	1,638	72.7 ± 1.1	65.2 ± 1.3	89.2 ± 0.8	84.1 ± 1.0
Heart	7,032	81.0 ± 0.5	76.2 ± 0.5	81.6 ± 0.4	77.0 ± 0.5
Heart-Lung	197	55.4 ± 3.2	47.7 ± 3.4	55.4 ± 3.2	48.8 ± 3.4
Lung	550	65.8 ± 1.9	53.1 ± 2.6	67.2 ± 1.9	57.7 ± 2.5

[a]Survival rates computed by Kaplan-Meier method (mean ± standard error).

transplants (4). Histocompatibility also influenced the incidence of rejection in first cadaver donor transplants. The incidence of rejection decreased as the recipient age increased; patients under the age of 16 have the highest incidence prior to discharge (28%) and at 1 year (70%), compared with 17% and 47% at the same intervals in patients over 60 years of age. Donor age was also shown to have a significant effect on rejection episodes, with transplants from pediatric and older donors having a higher reported incidence of rejections than those from donors aged 16 to 30 years, especially after hospital discharge. Prior sensitization significantly increased the incidence and severity of rejections that occurred during the transplant hospitalization, and these were more pronounced in retransplanted patients. The incidence of late rejections (>6 months) was significantly higher among black (20%) than among white (13%) or Hispanic (14%) recipients. The majority of acute rejection episodes occur within 60 days of transplantation. In two large series, from the University of Minnesota (5) and Ohio State University (6), approximately two-thirds of acute rejection episodes occurred within this time period.

III. DIAGNOSIS OF ACUTE REJECTION

Acute rejection is the main cause of allograft dysfunction after renal transplantation.

A. Clinical and Biochemical Changes

Acute rejection episodes may be manifest clinically by the development of fever, oliguria, weight gain, edema, hypertension, and the presence of an enlarged, tender graft. However, in cyclosporine-treated recipients, the classic features are frequently absent, and the most common presentation of acute rejection may be an asymptomatic rise in the serum creatinine level. An increase in the serum creatinine level >20% is the cardinal feature of acute rejection in patients on cyclosporine. A variety of tests have been devised in an attempt to increase the diagnostic accuracy of acute rejection. Biochemical changes accompanying the increase in serum creatinine level include an increase in the blood urea nitrogen (BUN), reduced fractional excretion of sodium (7), and increase in urinary protein excretion (8).

B. Evidence of Immune Activation and Nonspecific Graft Injury

Evidence of immune activation may be manifest by increased lymphokine secretion. Measurements of soluble cytokines or their receptors—such as interleukin (IL)-1, IL-2,

IL-2R, IL-6, interferon (IFN)-gamma, and tumor necrosis factor (TNF)-alpha (9–15)—as well as acute-phase proteins (16–18) in the body fluids of renal allograft recipients may give some information on the immunological events. In addition, the appearance of lymphocyturia has been reported to be related to immunological rejection in the graft (19–21).

C. Fine Needle Aspiration Biopsy

Fine needle aspiration biopsy (FNAB) has been used as a noninvasive method for monitoring of renal allograft rejection (22–24). In experienced hands, FNAB has been shown to be a reliable method for diagnosing acute cellular rejection and is most useful during the first postoperative months. It may also help in the differentiation of acute cellular rejection from acute cyclosporine nephrotoxicity. However, it is of limited value in the diagnosis of acute vascular rejection, chronic rejection, chronic cyclosporine nephrotoxicity, and recurrence of original disease (23,24). It must be stressed that FNAB has proven to be an effective adjunct to the diagnosis only in institutions experienced in its use; this has precluded its routine introduction at most transplant centers.

D. Radiological Changes

A number of radiological changes have been described in acute rejection.

1. Duplex Sonography and Doppler Ultrasound

Duplex sonography has been used to detect manifestations of the underlying histopathological process (25). Development of interstitial edema and cellular infiltration may result in an increase in the size of the transplant, which becomes globular in shape. The corticomedullary junction becomes indistinct, while medullary pyramids are larger and more hypoechoic and lose their triangular shape. In more severe cases, the renal cortical echotexture becomes inhomogeneous, with patchy areas of hypoechogenicity, reflecting the underlying cortical edema and areas of increased echogenicity due to infarction and hemorrhage (25,26). Episodes of acute rejection are associated with an increase in the peripheral resistance in graft vasculature due to vasoconstriction, compression of the small vessels by surrounding edema, cellular infiltration, and—in severe cases of vascular rejection—vasculitis and vascular thrombosis. These events may result in a marked increase in the peripheral vascular resistance in the kidney and secondary changes in the Doppler spectral pattern of the transplant vasculature (27). There is a marked increase in the pulsatility of the Doppler waveform with a decrease or absence of forward diastolic flow. Severe cases are associated with dampening of the systolic flow as well as a reversal of flow in diastole. The pulsatility of the waveform results in an increase in the resistive index (RI).

However, limitations exist in renal transplant sonograms. If the rejection episode is mild, the renal transplant may appear normal and the flow pattern may not demonstrate any change. Doppler changes associated with acute rejection are not always specific and may occur in severe cases of acute tubular necrosis, cyclosporine toxicity, or hydronephrosis. Nevertheless, sonography remains a useful diagnostic modality for detecting mechanical problems associated with the allograft, such as peritransplant collections (hematomas, abscesses, urinary leaks, lymphoceles), hydronephrosis, renal vein thrombosis, and renal artery thrombosis.

2. Radionuclide Evaluation

Radionuclides have also been used as an ancillary method for diagnosis of acute allograft rejection (28). These techniques allow assessment of renal perfusion and function and are of greatest benefit when sequential scans are performed (28,29). Acute allograft rejection may be characterized by a marked, sudden decrease in both perfusion and function of the transplanted kidney. Differentiation of acute rejection from acute tubular necrosis and cyclosporine toxicity may be extremely difficult unless repetitive isotope nuclear scans are obtained. The diagnosis of acute rejection superimposed on either acute tubular necrosis or cyclosporine toxicity is also difficult without sequential scans.

3. *Magnetic Resonance Imaging and Spectroscopy*

Magnetic resonance imaging (MRI) and magnetic resonance spectroscopy (MRS) have also been used for evaluating renal allograft dysfunction (30). These techniques are effective in detecting perinephric fluid collections (31). A decrease in the corticomedullary differentiation on MRI has been described in acute rejection. However, MRI has not proven to be sensitive or specific enough in the differentiation of acute rejection from acute tubular necrosis and cyclosporine toxicity. To date, there is little information regarding the value of MRS in human allografts. However, it may be a more sensitive method of differentiating acute rejection from acute tubular necrosis and cyclosporine toxicity.

E. Renal Biopsy

Percutaneous needle biopsy of the allograft remains the most reliable method for the diagnosis of acute rejection and differentiating it from other causes of transplant dysfunction. Percutaneous biopsy of the renal allograft is a safe and effective method for the diagnosis of allograft dysfunction. At the University of Cincinnati Medical Center, sonographically guided biopsies using an automated gun were performed on an outpatient basis in 105 patients (32). Significant hematuria requiring admission occurred in 2% of cases, and adequate tissue for diagnosis was available in 99% of biopsies. Results of the biopsy were available within 6 hr, permitting a decision to be made as to whether acute rejection was present and giving an indication as to the best management for the patient. If findings indicated acute rejection severe enough to require antilymphocyte antibody therapy, patients were then admitted. If the rejection episode was relatively mild and could be treated with steroids, the patient was discharged and treated as an outpatient. If the findings indicated cyclosporine nephrotoxicity, dose adjustments were made and the patient followed as an outpatient. Renal biopsy most accurately confirms the diagnosis of rejection, aids in the differential diagnosis of graft dysfunction, and allows for assessment of the likelihood of response to antirejection therapy. For these reasons, in ideal circumstances allograft biopsy should be done early in all patients with allograft dysfunction (increase in serum creatinine >20% from baseline).

IV. DIFFERENTIAL DIAGNOSIS OF ACUTE ALLOGRAFT DYSFUNCTION

The differential diagnosis of acute allograft dysfunction can be divided into (a) medical and mechanical problems and (b) those occurring earlier (<90 days) and later (>90 days) after transplantation. Acute rejection is the most common cause of graft dysfunction in both the early and late periods. However, the differential diagnosis differs according to the time frame. Acute allograft dysfunction should be thought of in terms of medical and mechanical problems in both time frames. Table 2 illustrates the differential diagnosis of acute allograft dysfunction. The medical and mechanical problems encountered in the early and late periods are outlined according to the probability of occurrence.

The approach to the renal transplant recipient with a rise in serum creatinine level is

Table 2 Differential Diagnosis of Acute Renal Allograft Dysfunction

	Early (0–90 Days)	Late (>90 Days)
Medical	1. Acute rejection	1. Acute rejction
	2. Delayed graft function	2. Cyclosporine nephrotoxicity
	3. Acute cyclosporine nephrotoxicity	3. Chronic rejection
	4. Prerenal/volume contraction	4. Prerenal/volume contraction
	5. Other drug toxicities	5. Other drug toxicities
	6. Infection	6. Infection
	7. Recurrent disease	7. De novo/recurrent disease
Mechanical	1. Lymphocele	1. Renal artery stenosis
	2. Ureteric obstruction	2. Ureteric obstruction
		3. Urine leak
		4. Vascular thrombosis

illustrated in Fig. 1. In the patient who has a rise in the serum creatinine level >20%, a complete physical examination should be the initial approach. Important features include temperature, weight changes, urine output, presence of peripheral edema, blood pressure, and examination of the renal allograft. The state of the extracellular fluid volume (ECFV) must be assessed. If clinical evidence of volume contraction is present, the patient should be given intravenous fluids and then reevaluated. If the ECFV is expanded, diuretics should be administered. In the patient with a normal ECFV, the medications must be checked carefully in order to assess whether the patient is taking medications correctly or taking any medications that may cause renal dysfunction or interfere with cyclosporine metabolism, resulting in either toxic or subtherapeutic levels. Potential cyclosporine drug interactions are indicated in Table 3. If the cyclosporine level is high, the dose should be reduced appropriately and the cyclosporine level and serum creatinine level rechecked. If reducing the dose results in a fall in cyclosporine level to the therapeutic range and a fall in the serum creatinine level, close follow-up is indicated. If the serum creatinine level remains elevated, an ultrasound and possibly a renal scan should be performed. In the patient who has renal dysfunction and a normal or low cyclosporine level, an ultrasound should be the initial approach. If the ultrasound reveals evidence of a mechanical problem (lymphocele, ureteric obstruction, urinary leak), appropriate surgical treatment should be instituted. If no mechanical problem is present and the ultrasound and/or renal scan are suggestive of acute rejection, one might treat the episode by either empirical steroid therapy or proceed directly to allograft biopsy. If empirical steroid therapy results in a good response (serum creatinine level returns to baseline), then maintenance immunosuppression should be increased and the patient followed closely. If there is no response to empirical steroid therapy, an allograft biopsy should be performed without delay and appropriate therapy instituted according to the biopsy findings. However, empirical therapy for suspected rejection might result in overimmunosuppression. Therefore, it is strongly recommended that early allograft biopsy be performed to diagnose the cause of renal dysfunction in patients in whom mechanical factors have been excluded.

V. HISTOLOGICAL CLASSIFICATION OF ACUTE REJECTION

The Banff classification of renal allograft pathology has three distinct diagnostic categories of acute rejection, based on histological severity (33). This classification is reviewed briefly

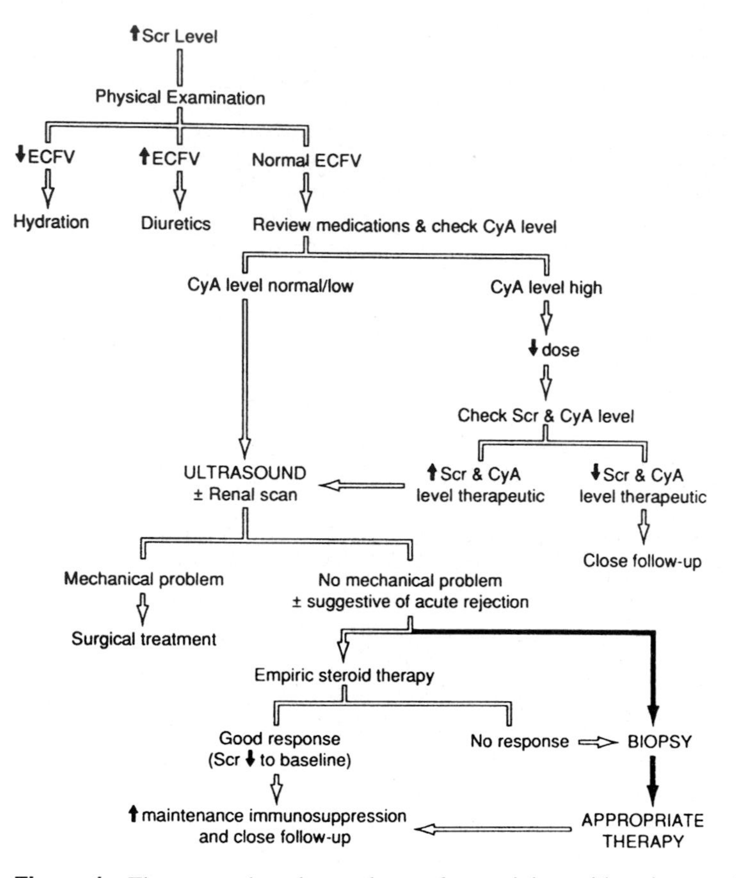

Figure 1 The approach to the renal transplant recipient with an increase in serum creatinine level. Bold lines indicate the suggested approach to be taken in the ideal circumstances.

here, and discussed at length in Chap. 9. The Banff schema is based more on the severity of tubulitis and arteritis than the severity of the interstitial infiltrate.

Acute rejection is classified into grades I (mild), II (moderate), and III (severe). There is also a category referred to as "borderline changes," which is indicated by mild lymphocytic invasion of tubules (tubulitis). In grade I rejection, there is widespread interstitial infiltrate with moderate tubulitis. In grade II rejection, there is widespread interstitial infiltrate with severe invasion of tubules and/or mild or moderate intimal arteritis. In grade III acute rejection, there is a widespread interstitial infiltrate with severe tubulitis and/or severe intimal arteritis and/or transmural arteritis, fibrinoid change, and medial smooth muscle cell necrosis, often with patchy infarction and interstitial hemorrhage.

The introduction of the Banff classification has resulted in a standardized schema for transplant pathology and classification of renal rejection severity. It is hoped that this standardized classification system will be adopted universally and promote international uniformity in the reporting of renal allograft pathology. This may facilitate the performance of multicenter trials of new therapies in renal transplantation and ultimately lead to improvement in the care of renal transplant recipients. The classification has already been adopted for international multicenter trials of many new immunosuppressive agents.

Table 3 Cyclosporin A Drug Interactions

Decreased concentration	Increased concentration	Synergistic nephrotoxicity
Carbamazepine	Ciprofloxacin	Acyclovir
Isoniazid	Erythromycin	Aminoglycosides
Phenobarbital	Fluconazole	Amphotericin B
Phenytoin	Itraconazole	Furosemide
Rifampicin (rifampin)	Ketoconazole	Ganciclovir
	Metoclopramide	H_2 antagonists
	Methylprednisolone	Melphalan
	Nicardipine	Trimethoprim-sulfamethoxazole
	Verapamil	Nonsteroidal anti-inflammatory drugs
		Vancomycin

However, concerns have been expressed about the treatment recommendations made by the Banff group. This is so with regard to the recommendation that borderline changes should not be treated; many clinicians and pathologists believe that the presence of tubulitis in the renal biopsy specimen is indicative of invasion of the allograft by activated lymphocytes and that such changes always warrant treatment. At the other end of the spectrum, the Banff group recommendation—that severe rejection should often not be treated because of poor outcome—is open to dispute. These problems aside, this remains a most important contribution that, it is hoped, will lead to standardizing both the classification and treatment of acute renal allograft rejection.

VI. TREATMENT OF ACUTE REJECTION

The principles of management of acute rejection episodes include rapid and accurate diagnosis and prompt administration of antirejection therapy. Ideally, the doses and duration of antirejection therapy should result in reversal of the rejection episode while at the same time not resulting in excessive impairment of host defence mechanisms and consequent opportunistic infections. Currently, corticosteroids and antilymphocyte antibodies represent the main components of antirejection treatment protocols. There is a wide range of different opinions as to the best method of antirejection therapy.

A. Corticosteroids

Increased doses of corticosteroids have been the mainstay of treatment of acute cellular rejection since the early days of transplantation (34). However, the best route and dosage for steroid treatment of renal allograft rejection remains to be determined, and whether steroids should continue to be the agent of the first choice for acute rejection also is a subject of increasing controversy (35). Intravenous methylprednisolone has been employed as the treatment of first choice by many transplant units. Doses of methylprednisolone have varied between 250 mg and 1 g daily for 3 to 4 days. When low-dose and high-dose intravenous methylprednisolone therapies were compared in double-blind randomized studies, there were no significant differences in rejection reversal or graft function (36,37), although in one study patients receiving high doses tended to have greater reductions in serum creatinine levels, while patients receiving low doses tended to have fewer infections

(36). These studies suggest that the corticosteroid doses in clinical use in the mid-1970s may have been excessive (35). Following the administration of intravenous methylprednisolone, it is common to increase the dose of oral prednisone therapy and then to taper this fairly rapidly. Oral doses of prednisone or prednisolone ranging from 150 to 600 mg/day and tapered over 1 to 3 weeks have also been shown to be effective in reversing acute renal allograft rejection (35). Rejection reversal rates of 56 to 72% have been reported with oral steroids, compared to 60 to 76% with intravenous methylprednisolone (38–40). However, oral steroids were associated with a higher frequency of gastrointestinal bleeding, aseptic necrosis of bone, diabetes, hypertension, fluid retention, and infection (38,39); this higher frequency of adverse effects appears to be related more closely to the duration of therapy than to the total dose administered (37).

B. Polyclonal Anti-T-Cell Antibodies

Polyclonal anti-T-cell antibodies have been shown to successfully reverse more than 90% of acute rejection episodes (41). In a controlled trials, antilymphocyte antibody preparations for first-line treatment of acute rejection have resulted in a more rapid reversal of rejection, fewer repeat rejection episodes, and better long-term graft survival than steroids in living related donor and cadaveric recipients in both azathioprine/steroid-treated and cyclosporine-treated recipients (41–45). These agents have also been effective in the treatment of steroid-resistant rejection episodes (46–50). Anti-T-cell antibody is generally administered for 10 to 14 days, with the dose varying according to the preparation being used. Currently, monoclonal antibody therapy with OKT3 has largely supplanted polyclonal antilymphocyte agents for the treatment of acute rejection episodes.

C. OKT3

In the original multicenter study (51), OKT3 was shown to be effective in reversing first acute rejection episodes in 94% of patients compared to 75% of those treated with intravenous methylprednisolone. One-year graft survival was also significantly improved (62 versus 45%). A number of uncontrolled studies have shown OKT3 to be effective in reversing acute rejection episodes when used as first-line therapy or as rescue therapy (52–58). OKT3 is administered as a daily intravenous dose of 5 mg for 10 to 14 days.

VII. A RATIONAL APPROACH TO THE THERAPY OF ACUTE REJECTION

In deciding upon the approach to the treatment of acute rejection, one must always consider the risk/benefit ratio of doing an early renal biopsy, the value and drawbacks of empiric versus definitive therapy, and the overall effect on the patient of intensifying immunosuppression. The benefits of steroid therapy for acute rejection include the ease of administration; steroids can be administered on an outpatient basis, and are an inexpensive treatment modality. On the other hand, potential problems with steroid therapy must be considered. These include the possibility that if the acute rejection episode is not completely reversed, there is an increased probability of chronic rejection, an increased risk of recurrent rejection episodes, as well as a number of well-known and serious steroid-induced side effects. Moreover, if steroids fail, one would have to intensify immunosuppression further by giving antilymphocyte antibody therapy over and above steroid therapy. The major benefits of antilymphocyte antibody therapy in first-line treatment for rejection are that they have been shown to be significantly more effective than steroids in reversing the rejection process. However, this must be balanced against the fact that they are far more expensive, usually require hospitalization, and carry an increased risk of the development of viral and lymphoproliferative diseases. There are a number of unanswered problems regarding the therapy of acute rejection. Issues that need to be addressed include the following: What constitutes steroid resistance or failure? How long and at what doses should steroids or antilymphocyte preparations be given? What is the best approach to initial therapy? Should prophylactic antiviral therapy be given together with antilymphocyte agents in order to prevent viral and lymphoproliferative disease? Clearly, additional studies are warranted to determine the agent of choice for first-line treatment of allograft rejection (35).

A number of studies have clearly demonstrated the importance of early diagnosis and effective therapy of acute rejection episodes. In the UCLA Transplant Registry (59), the effect of an acute rejection episode during the initial hospitalization on graft survival at 1 and 3 years was calculated. In patients with no acute rejection episodes, 1- and 3-year graft survival rates were 86 and 72%, respectively. In those with one rejection episode, respective graft survival rates were 68 and 53%; and in patients with more than one rejection episode, the survival rates fell to 57 and 46%, respectively. This analysis illustrates the adverse effect of one or more acute rejection episodes on short- and medium-term graft survival. The UCLA Transplant Registry (60) has also examined the severity of the initial acute rejection episode, as measured by the degree of rise in the serum creatinine level, on 1-year graft survival rates. In patients with no rejection, the 1-year graft survival rate was 88%. In those who had a mild increase in the serum creatinine (<1.5 mg/dL), 1-year graft survival was 84% (no significant difference from those patients with no acute rejection). In patients with a moderate rise in serum creatinine (1.5 to 3.5 mg/dL), the 1-year graft survival rate fell to 70% ($p<0.005$ compared to patients with no acute rejection), while in patients with a severe rise in serum creatinine (>3.5 mg/dL), graft survival rate at 1 year was down to 44% ($p<0.001$ compared to patients with no acute rejection). This is the only study that relates severity of rejection, as measured by the increase in the serum creatinine level, with graft outcome. The adoption of the Banff (33) classification will allow for an assessment of the effect of histological severity on graft outcome.

A study from the State University of New York Health Science Center (61), evaluated the effect of early acute rejection on the incidence of late rejection and transplant outcome. The incidence of late rejection in patients who had experienced an early rejection was 35%, compared to 17% in those without an early rejection ($p<0.001$). Serum creatinine levels at 1 and 5 years were significantly lower in those patients who had not experienced an acute rejection episode (2.4 versus 1.7 mg/dL, 2.5 versus 1.7 mg/dL, at 1 and 5 years, respectively). Actuarial graft survival (from 100% at 3 months posttransplant) at 1 year was 93% in those patients without an early acute rejection, compared to 85% in those with an acute rejection episode ($p<0.05$). Corresponding 5-year graft survival rates were 75 and 54%, respectively ($p<0.001$). In the study from Ohio State University (6), actuarial 8-year graft survival was 83% in patients with no rejection episodes, 69% in those with one rejection episode, and 45% in those with more than one rejection episode. In the study from the University of Minnesota (5), in both related donor and cadaveric recipients, biopsy-proven chronic rejection and graft loss due to chronic rejection was an infrequent occurrence in patients who had not experienced a preceding acute rejection episode. These rates increased significantly in patients with early (≤60 days) acute rejection, and the increase was even more pronounced in patients with a late (>60 days) acute rejection episode. These studies clearly illustrate the adverse effect of acute rejection episodes on short- and long-term graft survival. Future immunosuppressive therapy must be aimed at eliminating first rejection episodes and preventing the onset of a devastating second rejection episode.

As outlined above, approaches to the treatment of first episodes of acute rejection remain varied. Treatment of rejection should be tailored to the individual patient. One must consider a number of recipient risk factors, including whether this is the first or a subsequent transplant, the level of sensitization prior to transplantation, and severity of the rejection process. At the University of Cincinnati Medical Center, the decision on treatment of acute rejection has been based on histological severity (58). Mild acute cellular rejection is treated with a 3- to 4-day course of 250 mg of intravenous methylprednisolone, while moderate and severe acute cellular rejection and acute vascular rejection are treated with a 10- to 14-day course of OKT3. Using this approach, first-line treatment with OKT3 has resulted in rejection reversal (serum creatinine level returned to baseline) in over 90% of patients, which is clearly superior to the reversal rate with steroid therapy. In patients receiving OKT3, ganciclovir is administered for 21 to 28 days as prophylaxis against the development of CMV infection and EBV-induced lymphoproliferative disease (62).

VIII. CONCLUSION

At the present time, the only approved drugs for the prevention and treatment of acute renal allograft rejection in the United States are steroids, azathioprine, cyclosporine A, OKT3, and antithymocyte globulin. With these drugs, 1-year cadaveric graft survival rates have been around 80%. However, a significant number of grafts are subsequently lost due to the development of chronic rejection. The rapid advances in immunobiology and immunopharmacology over the past 15 years have led to the promise of an exciting future in organ transplantation. The introduction of new immunosuppressive drugs and monoclonal antibodies holds the promise of improving the results even further. However, the shortage of organs remains a major limitation to the widespread application of solid-organ transplantations throughout the world. In order to meet this demand, it will be necessary to establish successful xenotransplantation programs. It is hoped that the introduction of new and more potent immunosuppressive agents and the exciting developments in molecular biology, genetic engineering, and tolerance induction will allow this to become a practical reality in the future.

REFERENCES

1. *Annual Report of the U.S. Scientific Registry of Transplant Recipients and the Organ Procurement and Transplant Network, Executive Summary*. Washington, DC: U.S. Department of Health and Human Services, 1993:22.
2. First MR. Transplantation in the nineties. Transplantation 1992; 53:1–11.
3. First MR. New immunosuppressive drugs. Am J Kidney Dis 1992; 19:3–9.
4. Koyama H, Cecka JM. Rejection episodes. In: Terasaki PI, Cecka JM, eds. Clinical Transplants 1992. Los Angeles: UCLA Tissue Typing Laboratory, 1993:391–403.
5. Basadonna GP, Matas AJ, Gillingham KJ, et al. Early versus late acute renal allograft rejection: Impact on chronic rejection. Transplantation 1993; 55:993–995.
6. Tesi RJ, Henry ML, Elkhammas EA, Ferguson RM. Predictors of long-term primary cadaveric renal transplant survival. Clin Transplant 1993; 7:345–352.
7. Hong CD, Kapoor BS, First MR, et al. Fractional excretion of sodium after renal transplantation. Kidney Int 1979; 16:167–178.

8. Sethi K, First MR, Pesce AJ, et al. Proteinuria following renal transplantation. Nephron 1977; 18:49–59.
9. Woloszczuk W, Troppmair J, Leiter E. Relationship of interferon-gamma and neopterin levels during stimulation with alloantigens in vivo and in vitro. Transplantation 1986; 41:716–719.
10. Maury CPJ, Teppo AM. Serum immunoreactive interleukin 1 in renal transplant recipients. Transplantation 1988; 45:143–147.
11. McKenna RM, Rush DN, Bakkestad-Legare P, Jeffrey JR. Interleukin 2, interferon, and lymphotoxin in renal transplant recipients. Transplantation 1988; 45:76–81.
12. van Oers MHJ, van der Heyden AA, Aaren LA. Interleukin 6 in serum and urine of renal transplant recipients. Clin Exp Immunol 1988; 71:314–319.
13. Colvin RB, Preffer FI, Fuller TC, et al. A critical analysis of serum and urine interleukin-2 receptor assays in renal allograft recipients. Transplantation 1989; 48:800–805.
14. McLaughlin PJ, Aikawa A, Davies HM. Evaluation of sequential plasma and urinary tumor necrosis factor alpha levels in renal allograft recipients. Transplantation 1991; 51:1225–1229.
15. Schroeder TJ, Helling T, McKenna RM, et al. A multicenter study to evaluate a novel assay for quantitation of a soluble interleukin 2 receptor in renal transplant recipients. Transplantation 1992; 53:34–40.
16. Maury CPJ, Teppo AM, Eklund B, Ahonen J. Serum amyloid A protein: A sensitive indicator of renal allograft rejection in humans. Transplantation 1983; 36:501–504.
17. Edwards LC, Helderman JH, Hamm LL, et al. Noninvasive monitoring of renal transplant function by analysis of beta$_2$-microglobulin. Kidney Int 1983; 23:767–770.
18. Cohen DJ, Benvenisty AI, Meyer E, Hardy MA. Serum c-reactive protein concentrations in cyclosporine-treated renal allograft recipients. Transplantation 1988; 45:919–922.
19. Schumann GB, Burleson RL. Importance of urine cytology in renal transplantation. Transplantation 1977; 23:186–188.
20. Fidler JP, Dajani F, First MR, et al. Value of urine cytology in renal transplantation. Transplantation 1978; 26:133–135.
21. Dooper IMM, Bogman MJT, Hoitsma AJ, et al. Immunocytology of urinary sediments as a method of differentiating acute rejection from other causes of declining renal graft function. Transplantation 1991; 52:266–271.
22. von Willebrand E. Fine-needle aspiration cytology of human renal allografts. Clin Immunol Immunopathol 1980; 17:309–322.
23. Hayry P, von Willebrand E. Monitoring of human renal allograft rejection with fine-needle aspiration cytology. Scand J Immunol 1981; 13:87–97.
24. Belitsky P, Campbell J, Gupta R. Serial biopsy controlled evaluation of fine needle aspiration in renal allograft rejection. Lab Invest 1985; 53:580–585.
25. Sheth S. Evaluation of acute renal transplant rejection with duplex sonography. In: Burdick JF, Racusen LC, Solez K, Williams GM, eds. Kidney Transplant Rejection: Diagnosis and Treatment, 2d ed. New York: Marcel Dekker, 1992:459–470.
26. Rigsby CM, Taylor KW, Weltin GG, et al. Renal allografts in acute rejection: Evaluation using duplex sonography. Radiology 1986; 158:375–378.
27. Rifkin MD, Needleman L, Pasto ME, et al. Evaluation of renal transplant rejection by Doppler examination: Value of the resistive index. Am J Radiol 1987; 148:759–762.
28. Camargo EE, Sostre S. Radionuclides in the evaluation of kidney transplant rejection. In: Burdick JF, Racusen LC, Solez K, Williams GM, eds. Kidney transplant rejection: Diagnosis and treatment, 2d ed. New York: Marcel Dekker, 1992:471–485.
29. Dubovsky EV, Russel CD. Radionuclide evaluation of renal transplants. Semin Nuclear Med 1988; 18:181–198.
30. Tempany CMC, Yang A. Magnetic resonance imaging and magnetic resonance spectroscopy. In: Burdick JF, Racusen LC, Solez K, Williams GM, eds. Kidney Transplant Rejection: Diagnosis and Treatment, 2d ed. New York: Marcel Dekker, 1992:487–502.

31. Geisinger MA, Risius B, Jordan ML, et al. Magnetic resonance imaging of renal transplants. Am J Radiol 1984; 143:1229–1234.
32. Mahoney MC, Racadio JM, Merhar GL, First MR. Safety and efficacy of kidney transplant biopsy: Tru-cut needle vs sonographically guided biopsy gun. Am J Roentgenol 1993; 160: 325–326.
33. Solez K, Axelsen RA, Benediktsson H, et al. International standardization of criteria for the histologic diagnosis of renal allograft rejection: The Banff working classification of kidney transplant pathology. Kidney Int 1993; 44:411–422.
34. Goodwin WE, Kaufman JJ, Mims MM, et al. Human renal transplantation: I. Clinical experience with six cases of renal homotransplantation. J Urol 1963; 89:13–24.
35. Hricik DE, Almwayi WY, Strom TB. Trends in the use of glucocorticoids in renal transplantation. Transplantation 1994; 57:979–989.
36. Kauffman HM, Stromstad SA, Sampson D, Stawicki AT. Randomized steroid therapy of human kidney transplant rejection. Transplant Proc 1979; 11:36–38.
37. Park GD, Bartucci M, Smith MC. High- versus low-dose methylprednisolone for acute rejection episodes in renal transplantation. Nephron 1984; 36:80–83.
38. Mussche MM, Ringoir SMG, Lameire NH. High intravenous doses of methylprednisolone for acute cadaveric renal allograft rejection. Nephron 1976; 16:287–291.
39. Gray D, Shepherd H, Daar A, et al. Oral versus intravenous high-dose steroid treatment of renal allograft rejection. Lancet 1978; 1:117–118.
40. Orta-Sibu N, Chantler C, Bewick M, Haycock G. Comparison of high-dose intravenous methylprednisolone with low-dose oral prednisolone in acute renal allograft rejection in children. Br Med J 1982; 285:258–260.
41. Filo RS, Smith EJ, Leapman SB. Therapy of acute cadaveric renal allograft rejection with adjunctive antithymocyte globulin. Transplantation 1980; 30:445–449.
42. Shield CF, Cosimi AB, Tolkoff-Rubin N, et al. Use of antilymphocyte globulin for reversal of acute rejection. Transplantation 1979; 28:461–464.
43. Nowygrod R, Appel G, Hardy MA. Use of ATG for reversal of acute allograft rejection. Transplant Proc 1981; 13:469–472.
44. Hoitsma AJ, Reekers P, Kreftenberg JG, et al. Treatment of acute rejection of cadaveric renal allografts with rabbit antithymocyte globulin. Transplantation 1982; 33:12–16.
45. Broyer M, Niaudet P, Bijaoui M, Gagnadoux MF. Treatment of acute rejection crisis by antilymphocyte globulins: A randomized prospective study in pediatric kidney transplant recipients. Transplant Proc 1987; 19:1886–1888.
46. Hardy MA, Nowygrod R, Erlberg A, Appel G. Use of ATG in treatment of steroid-resistant rejection. Transplantation 1980; 29:162–164.
47. Light JA, Alijani MR, Biggers JA, et al. Antilymphocyte globulin (ALG) reverses irreversible allograft rejection. Transplant Proc 1981; 13:475–481.
48. Griffin PJA, Williams GT, Salaman JR. Antilymphocyte globulin for the treatment of steroid non-responsive acute renal allograft rejection. Clin Nephrol 1984; 21:115–117.
49. Matas AJ, Tellis VA, Quinn T, et al. ALG treatment of steroid-resistant rejection in patients receiving cyclosporine. Transplantation 1986; 41:579–583.
50. Veremis SA, Maddux MS, Pollak R, et al. Alternative antirejection treatment with steroids or antilymphoblast globulin in renal transplant patients receiving cyclosporine. Transplant Proc 1987; 19:1893–1895.
51. Ortho Multicenter Transplant Study Group. A randomized clinical trial of OKT3 monoclonal antibody for acute rejection of cadaveric renal transplants. N Engl J Med 1985; 313:337–342.
52. Deierhoi MH, Barber WH, Curtis JJ, et al. Treatment of acute rejection by monoclonals: A comparison of OKT3 monoclonal antibody and corticosteroids in the treatment of acute renal allograft rejection. Am J Kidney Dis 1988; 11:86–89.
53. Tesi RJ, Elkhammas EA, Henry ML, Ferguson RM. OKT3 for primary therapy of the first rejection episode in kidney transplants. Transplantation 1993; 55:1023–1029.

54. Cosimi AB, Burton RC, Colvin RB, et al. Treatment of acute renal allograft rejection with OKT3 monoclonal antibody. Transplantation 1981; 32:535–539.
55. Thistlewaite JR, Gaber AO, Haag BW, et al. OKT3 treatment of steroid-resistant renal allograft rejection. Transplantation 1987; 43:176–184.
56. Norman DJ, Barry JM, Bennett WM, et al. The use of OKT3 in cadaveric renal transplantation for rejection that is unresponsive to conventional antirejection therapy. Am J Kidney Dis 1988; 11:90–93.
57. Norman DJ, Shield CF. OKT3: First-line therapy or last option? Transplant Proc 1986; 18: 949–953.
58. Schroeder TJ, Weiss MA, Smith RD, et al. The efficacy of OKT3 in acute vascular rejection. Transplantation 1991; 51:312–315.
59. Terasaki PI, Cecka JM, Lim E, et al. Overview. In: Terasaki P, ed. Clinical Transplants 1991. Los Angeles: UCLA Tissue Typing Laboratory, 1992:409–430.
60. Cecka JM, Terasaki PI. Early rejection episodes. In: Terasaki P, ed. Clinical Transplants 1989. Los Angeles: UCLA Tissue Typing Laboratory, 1990:425–434.
61. Sumrani N, Delaney V, Daskalakis P, et al. The detrimental effect of early rejection on long-term renal allograft outcome. Transplant Proc 1992; 24:1750–1752.
62. Anderson P, Schroeder TJ, Hariharan S, First MR. Incidence of post-transplant lymphoproliferative disease in OKT3 treated renal transplant recipients. Clin Transplant 1993; 7: 582–585.

18

Clinical Diagnosis in Intestinal Allograft Rejection

Sami Asfar
University Hospital, London, Ontario, Canada

Richard Wood
Clinical Sciences Centre, University of Sheffield, Sheffield, England

David R. Grant
University of Western Ontario, London, Ontario, Canada

I. INTRODUCTION

Rejection has been the major barrier to all forms of solid-organ allografting. Early experimental work demonstrated that the small intestine is particularly susceptible to immune attack (1,2). Achieving success in intestinal transplantation depends upon maintaining the integrity of the delicate mucosa of the small bowel. Damage from preservation injury and rejection, in addition to preventing adequate absorption of nutrients, can allow bacteria to translocate from the lumen into the portal venous system, resulting in fatal sepsis. The cocktail of azathioprine and steroids, which provided reasonable immunosuppression for renal and liver transplantation, was unable to control rejection of the small bowel. The large lymphoid component of the gut—comprising the mesenteric lymph nodes, Peyer's patches, lamina propria lymphocytes, and intraepithelial lymphocytes—not only provides a major target for immune attack but also renders recipients susceptible to graft-versus-host disease (GVHD). In clinical practice, late and repeated rejection has been the major barrier to clinical success, particularly with isolated small bowel transplantation. Clinical GVHD has occurred after combined transplantation of the liver and small bowel, but it has been uncommon and rarely associated with any serious ill effects.

At the present time, intestinal transplantation is still an experimental procedure. Therefore, this chapter briefly reviews the indications for small bowel transplantation and the clinical management of intestinal recipients before discussing the clinical diagnosis of graft rejection.

II. INDICATIONS FOR INTESTINAL TRANSPLANTATION

Intestinal failure is defined as the inability to maintain nutrition and/or positive intestinal fluid and electrolyte balance without special measures (3). Home total parenteral nutrition (TPN) is required when the short gut syndrome develops following a massive small bowel resection. Total parenteral nutrition can often be discontinued after 1 or 2 years, as absorption improves, because of adaptation in the residual small bowel. However, some patients must remain on long-term TPN, particularly when less than 100 cm of the ileum has been preserved and the ileocecal valve has been removed (4,5). Long-term TPN is lifesaving, but it has many limitations, including (a) loss of venous access because of catheter infections or thrombosis; (b) development of cirrhosis; (c) lifestyle restrictions imposed by the requirement to infuse the nutrient solutions for 6 to 12 hours each day; and (d) high cost.

Approximately half of the patients with end-stage intestinal failure requiring permanent home TPN are potential candidates for transplantation (3). The need for intestinal transplantation has been estimated at 1 to 3 patients per million population per year (6). So far, success rates have been relatively poor and intestinal transplantation can be recommended only for patients who cannot be maintained on TPN or have developed serious complications related to this treatment. Children are particularly at risk of developing problems with line infections and thrombosis of the vena cava. In addition, infants started on TPN within the first year of life have a significant incidence of hepatic damage due to the inability of the immature liver to handle the TPN solutions. By the time these children reach the age of 4 or 5 years, a significant number will develop irreversible hepatic failure and therefore become candidates for combined liver and small bowel transplantation.

More than half of the transplant operations carried out so far have been performed in infants and children. The indications have included gastroschisis, jejunoileal atresia, malrotation and midgut volvulus, microvillous inclusion disease, neonatal enterocolitis, visceral myopathy, and visceral neuropathy. The indications for transplantation in adults have included massive small bowel resections due to Crohn's disease; strangulated hernias, trauma, or infarction; desmoid tumors; radiation injury; and pseudoobstruction. Malignancy and systemic sepsis are absolute contraindications to transplantation. Frail patients older than 60 years and patients with marginal cardiopulmonary function are poor candidates because of their inability to withstand perioperative complications.

III. SURGICAL TECHNIQUES

A. Procurement of the Intestinal Graft

Intestinal grafts can be procured from most cadaveric donors considered suitable for multiorgan retrieval. It is also possible to procure segmental grafts from a living related donor (7,8). Donors should have the same ABO blood groups as the recipient; ABO-incompatible grafts should be avoided because of the risk of severe hemolysis (9). HLA matching is desirable (but rarely feasible), since it may reduce the risk of rejection (8). Recipients who are seronegative for cytomegalovirus (CMV) should, whenever possible, receive grafts from seronegative donors in order to reduce the risk of refractory CMV disease. In patients with small peritoneal cavities due to prior removal of intrabdominal organs, it is preferable to use donors weighing 20 to 30% less than the recipient.

Broad-spectrum antibiotics are administered intravenously along with oral nystatin, neomycin, and trimethoprim-sulfamethoxazole or erythromycin to decontaminate the donor's gastrointestinal tract prior to organ removal. Mechanical bowel preparations are not used because the fluid-filled bowel can be difficult to manipulate at the time of transplantation. Some centers have advocated treating the donor with antilymphocyte agents in an attempt to deplete lymphocytes from the small bowel and thereby reduce the risk of rejection and GVHD, but this practice has recently fallen out of favor (10,11).

The graft is perfused with 1L of University of Wisconsin (UW) solution through an aortic cannula. The small bowel distal to the duodenojejunal junction as well as the ileocecal valve and portions of the colon are removed after stapling both ends. The mesenteric artery is removed with an aortic cuff along with the superior mesenteric vein and as much of the portal vein as the teams removing the pancreas and liver will allow. The graft is placed in a container of cold UW solution and can be kept on ice for between 6 to 10 hr (11).

B. Recipient Surgery

The superior mesenteric artery with the aortic patch is anastomosed to the infrarenal aorta or the native superior mesenteric artery at the base of the transverse mesocolon. The superior mesenteric vein can be joined to the recipient's portal vein with an end-to-side anastomosis, to the stump of the superior mesenteric vein by an end-to-end anastomosis, or, less commonly, to the anterior surface of the vena cava by an end-to-side anastomosis. Bowel continuity is restored with an anastomosis of the proximal end of the intestinal graft to the upper jejunum or to the recipient's duodenojejunal junction. The distal end of the graft is either exteriorized as a colostomy or ileostomy or it is joined to the rest of the recipient's bowel, in which case a defunctioning ostomy is performed. The ileostomy (or colostomy) is used to observe the viability of the graft and to provide access for endoscopic biopsies to diagnose rejection.

IV. PREVENTION AND TREATMENT OF REJECTION

Rejection has been the primary cause of graft loss following clinical small bowel transplantation. Standard immunosuppressants, including cyclosporine, were unsuccessful in preventing rejection and graft loss (12–15). Two recent developments have facilitated small bowel transplantation in humans. First, a protocol was developed that permitted combined transplantation of the small bowel and liver using cyclosporine (16). Second, isolated intestinal grafting became possible using the potent immune suppressive agent FK506.

The concept of combined liver/small bowel transplantation was stimulated by Sir Roy Calne's experiments in the pig showing that simultaneous liver grafting protected other organ grafts from rejection (17). At University Hospital, there has only been one episode of intestinal graft rejection in seven patients who have undergone combined simultaneous liver and intestinal transplants. Combined transplantation is particularly useful for the treatment of patients with end-stage small bowel failure who have developed liver failure as a complication of long-term TPN. Following the first report of this technique (16), more than 45 combined liver/small bowel transplants have been performed at eight centers with 50 to 70% 1-year actuarial patient survival rates.

The use of FK506 with prostaglandins by Starzl and colleagues in Pittsburgh permitted isolated small bowel transplantation in humans (10,11,18,19). However, recent data from Pittsburgh suggest that further modifications in immune suppression may be required to safely and reliably transplant the small bowel as an isolated graft. The 2-year actuarial graft survival rate is currently only 43%, while patient survival is 66%. In addition, more than 30% of the pediatric intestinal recipients have developed lymphoproliferative disorders (K. Abdu-Almagd, personal communication).

Immunosuppressive protocols for small bowel transplantation are constantly changing in an effort to identify a regimen that will reliably prevent graft rejection without a high rate of sepsis and lymphoproliferative disorders. At University Hospital, recipients are given 500 mL of blood from the donor as an intraoperative transfusion. OKT3 (5 mg IV) is given for 1 to 2 days to reduce the risk of GVHD. FK506 is always used for isolated transplantation, but some centers still give cyclosporine for combined liver/small bowel grafting. Initially, FK506 is given as a continuous IV infusion at 0.1 to 0.15 mg/kg/day; then, within 24 to 48 hr, the patient is switched to oral FK506 at a dose of 0.3 mg/kg/day in two divided doses. Daily FK506 whole blood levels are measured, using intravenous supplementation and oral dose adjustments to achieve a level of 20 to 30 ng/mL during the first 4 weeks and a level of 10 to 20 ng/mL thereafter. Patients are observed for neurotoxicity, nephrotoxicity, or severe glucose intolerance. If these side effects occur, the dose of FK506 is reduced. Methylprednisolone 500 mg IV is given as an intraoperative bolus, followed by 0.5 mg/kg/day IV, then oral prednisone at 0.3 mg/kg/day, which is gradually tapered to 0.1 mg/kg/day. Prostaglandin E_1 0.6 to 0.8 μg/kg/hr is given by a continuous IV infusion, followed by oral misoprostil 200 μg three times daily for 4 to 6 weeks to provide extra immune suppression and protect against the nephrotoxicity of FK506.

Mild rejection is treated by increasing the FK506 dose and giving methylprednisolone 500 mg IV for 3 days. Severe or persistent rejection is treated with OKT3 5 mg/day IV for 7 to 10 days.

Sepsis, related to intense immune suppression, has been a major cause of graft loss and patient death after transplantation. Consequently, most programs are now using aggressive prophylaxis to reduce the risk of bacterial, viral, or fungal infections. At University Hospital, intestinal recipients are given (a) broad-spectrum antibiotics (e.g., imipenem-cilastatin 50 mg/kg IV every 6 hr, starting preoperatively and continuing for 72 hr); (b) acyclovir (200 mg IV every 8 hr for the first few days, then orally at 400 mg four times a day); and (c) fluconazole (200 mg IV/day for a few days then orally 100 mg/day). Some programs also use oral bowel decontamination to prevent bacterial translocation from the graft and give intravenous gamma globulin to reduce the risk of Epstein-Barr virus infections.

V. DIAGNOSIS OF REJECTION

A. Differential Diagnosis of Graft Dysfunction

The intestine has a number of interrelated functions, including motility, absorption, lipoprotein formation, and provision of a barrier against the external environment. As will be discussed later, the tests that are currently used to measure intestinal graft function are relatively crude in comparison to the tests used to monitor other solid-organ grafts such as the heart, kidney, or liver. Unfortunately, we do not yet have a simple, reliable serological test of intestinal graft function comparable to measuring creatinine levels, for example, which are used to monitor kidney graft function. The differential diagnosis of gastrointestinal dysfunction after transplantation is broad and includes preservation injury, vascular compromise, rejection, infection (particularly CMV and pseudomembranous enteritis), lymphoproliferative disorders, GVHD (in the native gut), and recurrence of the primary disease.

B. Clinical Features of Acute Rejection

The signs and symptoms of small bowel allograft rejection are nonspecific. They include abdominal pain, increased stomal output, fever, vomiting, and leukocytosis. With severe rejection, fever, abdominal distension, increased stomal output and/or marked diarrhea, and metabolic acidosis may occur. Blood cultures become positive when patients develop bacterial translocation due to the loss of mucosal barrier function. In extreme cases, respiratory insufficiency and respiratory distress syndrome may result (11).

Visual inspection of the stoma may help in the diagnosis of rejection. Edema of the stoma is expected for the first 7 to 10 days. Thereafter, changes in the color of the stoma from a rosy pink to a cyanotic or dusky appearance should raise the suspicion of rejection and an immediate endoscopic biopsy should be performed.

C. Clinical Features of Chronic Rejection

The incidence of chronic rejection after small bowel transplantation remains unclear. As long-term survival rates improve, it is expected that more cases of chronic rejection will occur. In the cases reported to date, chronic rejection developed from 2 to 22 months after transplantation (11,20). Symptoms have included nausea, vomiting, refractory diarrhea, progressive weight loss, and malnutrition.

D. Endoscopy and Mucosal Biopsies

A thorough endoscopic examination of the lumen of the transplanted bowel is the primary method of diagnosing rejection. Because rejection starts as a patchy process (12), at least 10 to 20 cm of the bowel should be visualized with biopsies of all abnormal areas. The endoscopic findings of early rejection include mucosal edema, hyperemia, and loss of mucosal pattern. Severe cases may show ulceration, mucosal friability or sloughing, bleeding, and loss of peristalsis. Endoscopy of chronic rejection may reveal deep ulcers, pseudomembranes, loss of mucosal folds, and absence of peristalsis.

The histopathology of acute and chronic rejection is described in Chapter 10. It is important to note that mucosal biopsies and routine histology are subject to sampling error, especially when the specimen is taken near the stoma, because of nonspecific inflammation in this area. The biopsy specimens must be carefully examined to exclude infections, particularly CMV. Severe rejection may be difficult to distinguish from other causes of graft damage, such as vascular thrombosis.

VI. SCREENING FOR INTESTINAL GRAFT REJECTION

The development of noninvasive screening tests for intestinal graft rejection has been driven by a desire to (a) screen the entire graft for rejection and thus avoid the risk of sampling errors inherent with a limited endoscopic examination of the graft and (b) avoid the risk of perforation or bleeding associated with endoscopy and mucosal biopsy. The pros and cons of different screening tests are discussed below. Clinical experience with all of these tests is limited and further data are needed to determine their sensitivity, specificity, and accuracy.

A. Immunohistochemistry

Early allograft rejection is associated with increased expression of MHC class II antigens on enterocytes in the rat model (21). The presence of $CD3^+$ T cells in the crypts of the allograft correlated with early clinical intestinal graft rejection, whereas the presence of CD25 cells did not (22). Stimulated macrophages (Ki-M6 and Ki-M7 positive) were also present in large numbers in the submucosa prior to and during rejection of clinical small bowel transplants (22). In another clinical report, treatment with OKT3 reduced the number of $CD3^+$ cells in the lamina propria within 7 days of starting this antirejection therapy (23).

B. Cytokine Levels

Cytokines released by activated lymphocytes and monocytes play an important role in intestinal allograft rejection. Quan et al. have demonstrated an increased gene expression of MHC class II, ICAM-1, TNF-alpha, and IL-1 beta during small bowel rejection in mice (24). Noguchi et al. documented six episodes of clinical and pathological acute intestinal allograft rejection in which serum IL-6 levels increased with acute rejection and decreased after the rejection was successfully treated (25). IL-2 and TNF-alpha were also elevated at times, but levels did not correlate with rejection.

C. Procoagulant Activity

Procoagulant is a protease which converts fibrinogen to fibrin. It is produced by activated macrophages and endothelial cells. Procoagulant activity increases with surgical stress and stimulation by endotoxin (9). Kim et al. have reported that procoagulant activity in peripheral blood monocytes closely correlated with the histological progression of intestinal allograft rejection in rats. However, sepsis can produce similar results and this test has had limited clinical use (26).

D. Hyaluronan

Hyaluronan is a linear polysaccharide produced by mesenchymal cells in the lamina propria in response to inflammatory mediators. Experimental studies in rats have shown increased hyaluronan levels in the lamina propria and subserosal space and a 10-fold increase in the lumenal contents during intestinal graft rejection (27). Monitoring of hyaluronan levels in luminal perfusates may be useful for the early detection of rejection; a profound increase was noted during an episode of intestinal graft rejection in a 14-month old girl (27).

E. *N*-acetylhexaminidase

The assay for lysosomal acid hydrolase, *N*-acetylhexaminidase is simple and rapid; it was initially developed for the detection of Tay-Sachs disease and Sandholf's disease. Serum levels of *N*-acetylhexaminidase increase with minimal ischemia of the small bowel. Measurement of the activity of this enzyme in serum may prove useful in monitoring for transplant rejection; levels were significantly increased with graft rejection in a rat model (28).

F. Brush-Border Enzymes

Deltz, in Kiel, Germany, was one of the first investigators to report a fall in brush-border enzyme activity with early graft rejection in rat and canine transplant models (29–31).

These data suggest that maltase, monoamine oxidase, or diamine oxidase activity in the mucosa of the small bowel may be more sensitive markers of rejection than routine histology.

G. Gut Absorption

Absorption studies are insensitive for the detection of acute intestinal graft rejection, although they may have a role in the detection of chronic rejection. Animal studies have shown that the mucosa must be severely damaged before there are significant changes in absorption (32,33). Moreover, function is commonly abnormal after transplantation even when there is no histological evidence of rejection. D-xylose absorption tests were performed in 43 long-term recipients from Pittsburgh (11). Only 50% of these patients had normal values 22 months after successful transplants. Fat absorption (measured as fecal fat) also remained abnormal for more than a year after transplantation in some patients (11). Despite these abnormal results, most long-surviving recipients of intestinal transplants maintained normal nutritional status. Clinicians in Pittsburgh use serial measurement of D-xylose absorption to monitor intestinal allograft function, but they note that test results may be unreliable in the presence of impaired renal function or abnormal gastrointestinal motility (34).

H. Gut Barrier Function

Gut barrier function is impaired for 1 to 5 days after transplantation because of preservation damage to the gut mucosa. Thereafter, early intestinal graft rejection can be detected by increased intestinal permeability, which precedes the clinical features of graft rejection (35,36). Serial measurement of intestinal permeability using chromium-labeled ethylenediaminetetraacetic acid (^{51}Cr-EDTA) allowed the early detection of rejection in a patient 60 days after combined small bowel/liver transplantation at University Hospital (16). Currently, we perform weekly permeability studies with ^{51}Cr-EDTA until there are two consecutive normal results. Thereafter, the test is repeated whenever rejection is suspected. Because conditions such as ischemia and gastroenteritis can also affect the gut barrier, endoscopy and biopsies must be performed to provide a specific diagnosis. Other agents that can be used to measure intestinal permeability include technetium-labeled diethylenetriaminepentaacetic acid (DTPA), polyethylene glycol, and mannitol (16,37).

I. Radiological Studies

Radiological studies are generally insensitive for intestinal rejection. Gastrointestinal contrast studies and routine flat plates may detect advanced rejection when it produces edema of the bowel wall, intramural air, or perforation with free intraperitoneal air (38). These findings are not specific for rejection; they can also occur with CMV enteritis or ischemia due to vascular anastomotic complications. In addition to identifying problems in the graft, computed tomography may also detect ascites, abscesses, vascular thromboses, and posttransplant lymphoproliferative disease (39).

J. Radioisotope-Labeled White Blood Cell Scanning

Indium-111 white cell scanning has been used to detect abscesses and active inflammatory bowel disease (40,41). Cambridge reported uptake of this agent throughout the entire graft in a patient with rejection who subsequently responded to antirejection therapy (42). The requirement for 100 mL of blood with this test makes it difficult to use for routine screening.

K. Motility

The small intestinal graft is extrinsically denervated; its motor activity is regulated by signals from the intrinsic neural plexus (43,44). Although enteric neurons are highly sensitive to ischemia, major changes in motility occur only after the entire bowel wall has been damaged. Thus, motility studies have not been useful for the early diagnosis of graft rejection (45).

VII. SUMMARY

The small bowel can be transplanted as an isolated graft or as a multivisceral graft, with or without the liver. Despite refinements in surgical techniques and the use of new immune suppressive agents, intestinal transplantation is still hindered by (a) difficulties in diagnosing and controlling graft rejection and (b) a high rate of sepsis and lymphoproliferative disorders. As yet, there is no simple, sensitive, and specific method to screen for early intestinal graft rejection; the definitive diagnosis relies heavily on clinical symptoms, endoscopy, and the histological examination of mucosal biopsies.

ACKNOWLEDGEMENTS

The authors acknowledge the clinical and research contributions of the other members of the Intestinal Transplant Program—P. Atkinson, D. Bach, J. Duff, B. Garcia, C. Ghent, C. Stiller, W. Wall, and R. Zhong,—and Ms. Cate Abbott for editing the manuscript.

REFERENCES

1. Lillehei RC, Goott B, Miller FA. The physiological response of the small bowel of the dog to ischemia including prolonged in vitro preservation of the bowel with successful replacement and survival. Ann Surg 1959; 150:543–560.
2. Lillehei RC, Idezuki Y, Feemster JA, et al. Transplantation of stomach, intestine, and pancreas: Experimental and clinical observations. Surgery 1967; 62:721–741.
3. Lennard-Jones JE. Indications and need for long-term parenteral nutrition: Implications for intestinal transplantation. Transplant Proc 1990; 22:2427–2429.
4. Rombeau JL, Rolandelli RH. Enteral and parenteral nutrition in patients with enteric fisulas and short bowel syndrome. Surg Clin North Am 1987; 67:551–571.
5. Thompson JS. The current status of surgical therapy for the short bowel syndrome. Contemp Surg 1988; 33:27–32.
6. Ingham Clark CL, Lear PA, Wood S, et al. Potential candidates for small bowel transplantation. Br J Surg 1992; 79:676–679.
7. Deltz E, Mengel W, Hamelmann H. Small bowel transplantation: Report of a clinical case. Progr Pediatr Surg 1990; 25:90–96.
8. Fortner JG, Sichuk G, Litwin SD, Beattie EJ. Immunological responses to an intestinal allograft with HLA identical donor-recipient. Transplantation 1972; 14:531–536.
9. Cohen Z, Silverman RE, Wassef R, et al. Small intestinal transplantation using cyclosporine: Report of a case. Transplantation 1986; 42:613–621.
10. Todo S, Tzakis A, Reyes J, et al. Small intestinal transplantation in humans with or without colon. Transplantation 1993; 57:840–848.

11. Todo S, Tzakis AG, Abu-Elmagd K, et al. Intestinal transplantation in composite visceral grafts or alone. Ann Surg 1992; 216:223–234.
12. Grant D, Sommerauer J, Mimeault R, et al. Treatment with continuous high dose intravenous cyclosporine following intestinal transplantation: A case report. Transplantation 1989; 48:151–152.
13. Revillon Y, Jan D, Goulet O, Ricour C. Small bowel transplantation in seven children: Preservation technique. Transplant Proc 1991; 23:2350–2351.
14. Schroeder P, Goulet O, Lear P. Small bowel transplantation: European experience. Lancet 1990; 336:110–111.
15. Tattersall C, Gebel H, Haklin M, et al. Lymphocyte responsiveness after irradiation in canine and human intestinal allografts. Curr Surg 1989; 46:16–19.
16. Grant D, Wall W, Mimeault R, et al. Successful small-bowel/liver transplantation. Lancet 1990; 335:181–184.
17. Calne RY, Sells RA, Pena JR, et al. Induction of immunological tolerance by porcine liver allografts. Nature 1969; 223:472–476.
18. Todo S, Tzakis A, Reyes J, et al. Intestinal transplantation at the University of Pittsburgh. Transplant Proc 1994; 26:1409–1410.
19. Todo S, Tzakis AG, Abu-Elmagd K, et al. Cadaveric small bowel and small bowel-liver transplantation in humans. Transplantation 1992; 53:369–376.
20. Goulet O, Revillon Y, Jan D, et al. Small-bowel transplantation in children. Transplant Proc 1990; 22:2499–2500.
21. Schmid T, Oberhuber G, Korozsi G, et al. Major histocompatibility complex class II antigen expression on enterocytes during rejection of small-bowel allografts. Transplant Proc 1990; 22:2480.
22. Hansmann ML, Hell K, Gundlach M, et al. Immunohistochemical investigation of biopsies in a successful small-bowel transplantation. Transplant Proc 1990; 2502–2503.
23. Goulet O, Revillon Y, Canioni D, et al. Two and one-half year follow-up date after isolated cadaveric small bowel transplantation in an infant. Transplant Proc 1992; 24:1224–1225.
24. Quan D, Grant DR, Zhong RZ, et al. Semiquantitative analysis of cytokine gene expression during intestinal allograft rejection in the mouse. Surg Forum 1993; 8:619.
25. Noguchi K, Yoshida Y, Kita Y, et al. Serum levels of interleukin-6, tumor necrosis factor-alpha, and interleukin-2 in rejecting human small bowel allografts. Transplant Proc 1992; 24:1152.
26. Kim PO, Levy GA, Craig M, et al. Immune responses during small-intestinal allograft rejection: correlation between procoagulant activity and histopathology. Transplant Proc 1990; 22:2477–2479.
27. Wallander J, Johnsson C, Hallgren R, et al. Intestinal distribution and leakage of hyaluronan in small bowel allografting in the rat. Transplant Proc 1992; 24:1100–1101.
28. Maeda K, Schwartz MZ, Bamberger MH, Daniller A. A possible serum marker for rejection after small intestine transplantation. Am J Surg 1987; 153:68–74.
29. Schroeder P, Schweizer E, Hansmann K, et al. Monitoring in small bowel transplantation using cytochemistry and immunochemistry: A comparison of different techniques. Transplant Proc 1991; 23:675–676.
30. Meijssen MAC, Heineman E, deBruin RWF, et al. Diminished functional capacity and compromised mucosal integrity in acute rejecting DLA-matched and mismatched canine small bowel allografts. Transplant Proc 1992; 24:1116–1117.
31. Zhang S, Zhu Y, Ikoma A, et al. Biochemical monitors of transplant rejection in canine small bowel. Transplant Proc 1994; 26:1548–1549.
32. Cohn WB, Hardy MA, Quint J, State D. Absorptive function in canine jejunal autografts and allografts. Surgery 1969; 65:440–446.
33. Stamford WP, Hardy MA. Fatty acid absorption in jejunal autograft and allograft. Surgery 1974; 75:496–501.
34. Kadry Z, Furukawa H, Abu-Elmagd K, et al. The use of the X-xylose absorption test in the monitoring of intestinal allografts. Transplant Proc 1994; 26:1645.

35. Grant D, Lamont D, Zhong R, et al. ^{51}Cr-EDTA: A marker of early intestinal rejection in the rat. J Surg Res 1989; 46:507–514.
36. Grant D, Hurlbut D, Zhong R, et al. Intestinal permeability and bacterial translocation following small bowel transplantation in the rat. Transplantation 1991; 52:221–224.
37. Takara T, Guttman FM, Lubin A, et al. The use of Tc99mDTPA to assess permeability in allogenic rat small bowel transplantation. (abstr 53). Transplant Proc 1994; 26:1513.
38. Bach DB, Hurlbut DJ, Romano WM, et al. Human orthotopic small intestine transplantation: Radiologic assessment. Radiology 1991; 180:37–41.
39. Bach DB, Levin MF, Vellet AD, et al. CT findings in patients with small bowel transplants. Am J Roentgenol 1992; 159:311–315.
40. Heresbach D, Bretagne J, Raoul J, et al. Indium scanning in assessment of acute Crohn's disease. Dig Dis Sci 1993; 38:1601–1607.
41. Giaffer MH, Tindale WB, Senior S, et al. Quantification of disease activity in Crohn's disease by computer analysis of Tc-99m hexamethyl propylene amine oxime (HMPAO) labelled leucocyte images. Gut 1993; 34:68–74.
42. Calne RY, Pollard SG, Jamieson NV, et al. Intestinal transplant for recurring mesenteric desmoid tumor. Lancet 1993; 342:58–59.
43. Malmfors G, Hakanson R, Okmaian L, Sundler F. Peptidergic nerves persist after jejunal autotransplantation: An experimental study in the piglet. J Pediatr Surg 1980; 15:53–55.
44. Johnson CP, Sarna SK, Cowles VE, et al. Motor activity and transit in the autonomically denervated jejunum. Am J Surg 1994; 167:80–88.
45. Ikoma A, Nakada K, Suzuki T, et al. Gastrointestinal motility at immediate postoperative period after intestinal transplantation with special reference to acute rejection. Transplant Proc 1994; 26:1657–1658.

19

Clinical Diagnosis in Pancreatic Allograft Rejection

Rainer W. G. Gruessner and David E. R. Sutherland
University of Minnesota Medical School, Minneapolis, Minnesota

I. INTRODUCTION

The purpose of pancreatic transplantation is twofold: (a) to establish an insulin-independent, euglycemic state and (b) to favorably influence the course of secondary complications of diabetes. The objective is to improve quality of life—not necessarily to save a life, in contrast to liver and heart transplantation (1,2). Just as kidney transplantation is an alternative to dialysis, pancreatic transplantation is an alternative to insulin treatment. While insulin can keep a patient alive, the quality of life may be low; furthermore, imperfect metabolic control may lead to secondary complications (3).

Pancreatic transplantation is the only treatment of type I diabetes mellitus that normalizes hemoglobin A1C levels (HgA1C) for as long as the graft functions (4). For many pancreas recipients, metabolic control alone significantly improves quality of life (5). Insulin independence and its effect on day-to-day living are profoundly important. Evidence is mounting in the literature that pancreatic transplantation favorably affects the course of many secondary complications of diabetes. Diabetic neuropathy improves or stabilizes for most pancreas recipients (6); the high incidence of sudden death among diabetic patients with autonomic neuropathy is also reduced posttransplant (7). A pancreas transplant can prevent diabetic nephropathy in the native kidneys of nonuremic patients in early stages (8); it can also prevent recurrence of diabetic nephropathy in the newly transplanted kidney of uremic patients (9). Diabetic retinopathy tends to stabilize in pancreas recipients with long-term functioning grafts, although progression of advanced retinopathy does not change in the first 3 years posttransplant (10).

Pancreatic transplants can be done for three different patient categories:

1. Simultaneous pancreas and kidney transplant (SPK) *for uremic patients.* This represents the largest pancreas-recipient population: 80% of the 5807 transplants worldwide between January 1968 and April 1994, as reported to the International Pancreas Transplant Registry (IPTR), were for SPK recipients (11). Thus, pancreas transplantation is most widely applied to uremic diabetic patients, i.e., a population in whom complications have already appeared. At this late stage the assumption that pancreas transplants are primarily done to influence far advanced secondary complications is not correct. Instead, the effect on quality of life is most important. Any positive effect of the simultaneously transplanted pancreas on secondary complications is only a bonus. The addition of a pancreas to a kidney transplant is therefore justified for two reasons: (a) the patients are already obligated to immunosuppression due to the kidney transplant, and it is generally accepted that quality of life is better when immunosuppressed and dialysis-free than when nonimmunosuppressed and dialysis-dependent (12), and (b) quality of life improves even if insulin independence is the only benefit achieved other than reversal of uremia (5,13), with only the minimal surgical risk of transplanting a pancreas as well as a kidney.

2. Pancreas after kidney transplant (PAK) for chronically immunosuppressed recipients. As with SPK patients, secondary complications are usually far advanced in this category. A pancreatic transplant is done to improve quality of life by obviating the diabetic control problem. PAK has the potential to become as common as SPK. Some single centers show that pancreas graft survival is equal for PAK and SPK recipients (14). In regard to kidney graft survival, PAK recipients have an advantage over SPK recipients if the kidney is derived from a living related donor. The long-term outcome with kidney grafts from living related donors continues to be significantly better than with cadaver kidneys, based on kidney registry data (15) and single-center experiences (16). Thus, sequential transplants (i.e., living related kidney first, then a cadaver pancreas 6 to 12 months later) are favored by some centers to optimize kidney graft survival.

3. Pancreatic transplant alone (PTA) for nonuremic, nonkidney transplant recipients. Nonuremic diabetic patients face a different situation. For them, unlike SPK and PAK recipients, posttransplant immunosuppression will be given only for the purpose of correcting diabetes. Thus, the penalty for constant normoglycemia in this group of patients is the need for immunosuppression. The main question, therefore, is whether the improvement in quality of life achieved by being nondiabetic can offset the penalty of being immunosuppressed. It is also not known if the risk of immunosuppression exceeds the risk of developing secondary complications. That is why applying pancreatic transplantation to the entire nonuremic diabetic population for the sake of diabetic control alone awaits the development of tolerance or less toxic immunosuppression. The situation is different for diabetic patients with extreme lability of metabolic control and low quality of life. For them, insulin independence and normoglycemia induced by a successful pancreatic transplant justifies immunosuppression (17)—i.e., the problems of diabetes exceed those of immunosuppression for nonuremic diabetic patients. If this is judged to be the case, a pancreas transplant should be done.

Any discussion of rejection must take into account the three different recipient categories, whose outcomes differ. While 1-year pancreatic graft survival rates, according to the International Pancreas Transplant Registry (IPTR), exceed 70% in SPK recipients, pancreatic graft survival for PTA recipients has not matched these results (Fig. 1). The difference in graft survival can be explained largely by the incidence of rejection. Between October 1, 1987, and April 30, 1994, 2720 SPK, 246 PAK, and 178 PTA cadaver transplants were done in the United States, according to the IPTR (18). With a minimum follow-up time of at least 6 months, the most common causes of graft loss were technical failures for 394 (312 SPK, 50 PAK, 32 PTA), rejection for 274 (156 SPK, 64 PAK, 54 PTA), and other (e.g., primary nonfunction) for 36 recipients (28 SPK, 6 PAK, 2 PTA). Overall, rejection is the second most common cause of pancreatic graft failure. There are, however, differences by recipient category: for SPK recipients, technical failures account for 63% and rejection for 31% of all

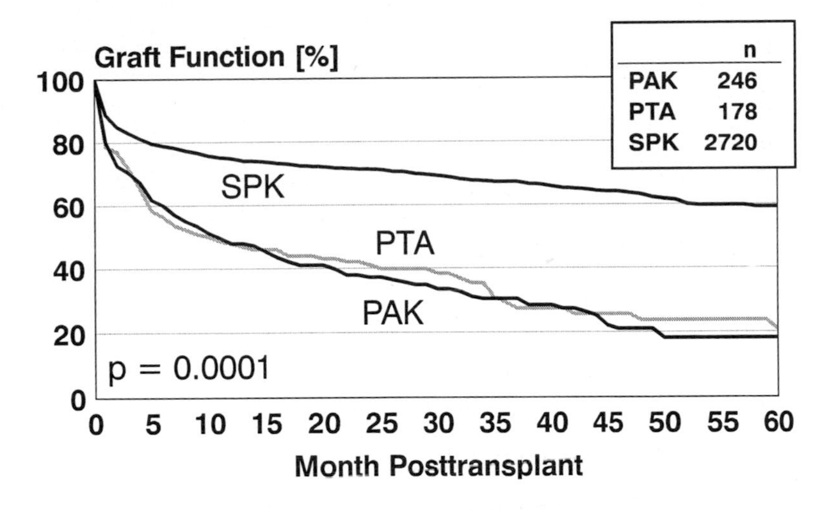

Figure 1 Pancreatic graft survival by recipient category (International Pancreas Transplant Registry, IPTR).

graft losses; for PAK, technical failures for 42% and rejection for 53%: for PTA, technical failures for 36% and rejection for 61%. Thus, for solitary pancreas recipients (PAK, PTA), rejection is the most common cause of graft failure; for SPK recipients, technical failures are more common.

If only technically successful pancreatic transplants are considered, rejection is by far the most common cause of graft loss for all recipient categories. Interestingly, chronic rejection was reported to be responsible for 52% and acute rejection for 47% of all rejection-related graft losses in immunosuppressed patients reported to the IPTR (the remaining 1% are due to patients discontinuing their medication). Thus, acute and chronic rejection—in almost equal numbers—cause pancreatic graft failures.

For technically successful pancreatic transplants (all three recipient categories), 1- and 5-year graft loss rates from rejection were 10 and 13% (11). The IPTR data showed significant differences by category: 1- and 5-year rates for graft loss from rejection for SPK recipients were 6 and 13%; for PAK recipients, 29 and 59%; and for PTA recipients, 32 and 68% (Fig. 2). We noted no difference in the proportions of graft losses from acute or chronic rejection between the three categories.

In contrast to graft survival, patient survival rates were not significantly different between the three pancreas recipient categories (Fig. 3).

Another important aspect of pancreas rejection studies is the analysis of rejection patterns for SPK recipients, since they undergo dual-organ transplants from the same donor. According to IPTR data on 2720 SPK recipients, the distribution of causes of graft failure was different for the pancreas and the kidney (11). In all, 312 recipients lost pancreas grafts from technical failure, 156 from rejection, and 11 from primary nonfunction; 194 died with a functioning pancreas graft. By comparison, 213 recipients lost kidney grafts from rejection, 56 from technical failure, and 6 from primary nonfunction; 186 died with a functioning kidney graft. Thus, technical failures were the most common cause of graft loss for the pancreas; rejection, for the kidney. Eighty SPK recipients lost both the pancreas and the kidney from rejection; this accounts for 51% of all rejection-related pancreas and 38% of all

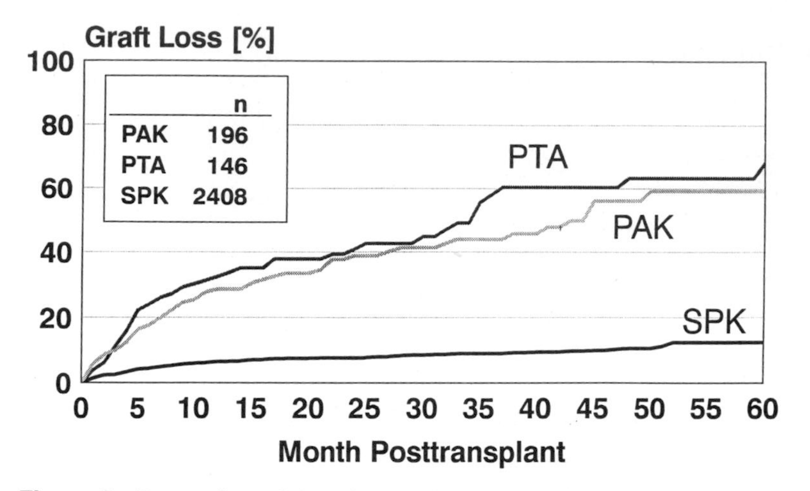

Figure 2 Pancreatic graft loss due to rejection by recipient category (IPTR).

rejection-related kidney graft losses. Thus, 76 SPK recipients lost only the pancreas and 133 only the kidney from rejection. If only one organ of the pair is rejected in an SPK recipient, it is more likely to be the kidney than the pancreas; individual centers have reported a similar phenomenon.

For technically successful SPK transplants only, 1- and 5-year graft loss rates from rejection were 6 and 12% for the pancreas and 5 and 15% for the kidney (Fig. 4); the difference was not statistically significant. Of note, the kidney graft loss rate from rejection was not higher than for diabetic recipients of kidney transplants alone (KTA), per the UCLA kidney registry (19). It is therefore evident that a pancreas does not jeopardize the outcome of a simultaneously transplanted kidney.

Note that the term "rejection" involves two different entities: reversible rejection episodes and graft loss from irreversible rejection. Therefore, the incidence of rejection

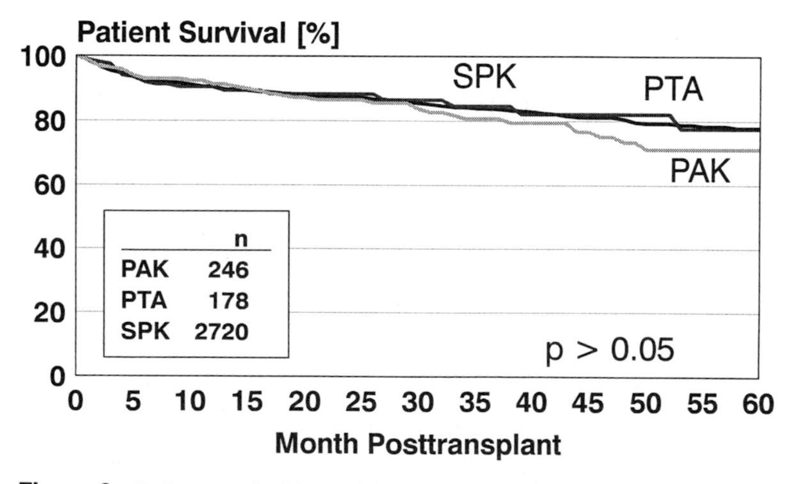

Figure 3 Patient survival by recipient category (IPTR).

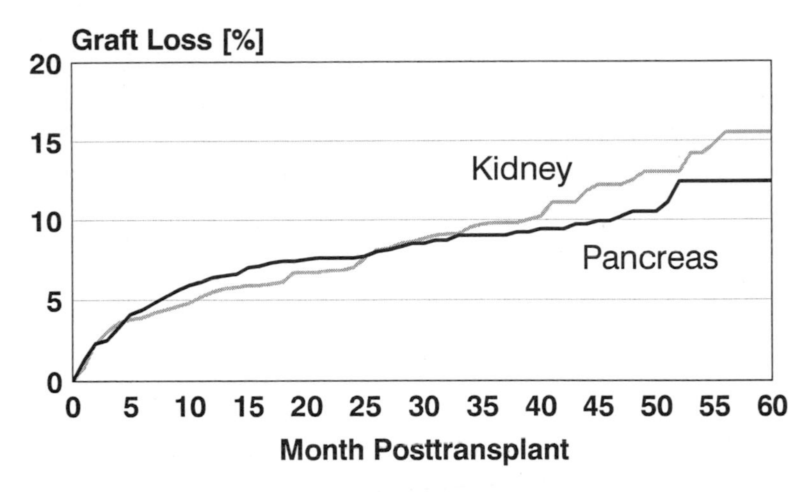

Figure 4 Pancreatic and kidney graft loss due to rejection in 2408 technically successful SPK transplants (IPTR).

episodes and the graft loss rate from rejection must be analyzed separately. In dual-organ transplants (SPK, PAK), rejection episodes and graft loss from rejection can occur in only one organ or in both. The terms "synchronicity" and "dyssynchronicity" describe the potential difference in the timing of rejection episodes or graft loss between two organs from the same donor. Concordance and discordance refer to the rejection grade, which may or may not be identical for both grafts, but both organs are histologically positive for rejection. This standardized nomenclature is needed to avoid differences in interpretation of study results.

II. RESEARCH BACKGROUND

A. Large Animal Studies

1. Studies in Pigs

Of all pancreas rejection models in large animals, the pig model has been studied most extensively. The anatomy of the pig pancreas, as well as its physiological, endocrinological, and immunological function, very much resembles the human pancreas (20–22); the surgical techniques of pancreatic transplantation are the same for pigs and humans (21,23–26). Solitary pancreatic transplants in both pigs and humans are highly immunogenic, and rejection occurs early. With triple immunosuppression—including cyclosporin A (CSA), azathioprine, and prednisone—in dosages similar to the clinical situation, severe interstitial rejection of solitary pancreas transplants in pigs was noted as early as posttransplant day 6 (27); the lack of anti-T-cell therapy in the pig model has resulted in high incidence, early occurrence, and marked severity of rejection.

A major experimental research focus is comparing rejection incidence and severity by recipient category. In a pig study of 36 SPK, 31 PTA, and 36 KTA allotransplants, grafts were biopsied weekly to grade histological severity of interstitial and vascular rejection (27). Pancreatic biopsies were obtained either by open laparotomy or cystoscopically. The latter were done according to the technique described by Marsh et al. (28) in a dog model, but modified by the use of intraoperative ultrasound (which resulted in a higher yield of pancreatic specimens). Pancreatic allograft biopsies at weekly intervals showed a significantly lower incidence of moderate and severe interstitial rejection in SPK (versus PTA) recipients; similarly, vascular rejection was moderate and severe in significantly fewer SPK (versus PTA) pancreatic grafts (27). Immunofluorescent staining with anti-CD2, anti-CD4, anti-CD8, and anti-macrophage antibodies was less intense in pancreatic biopsies of SPK (versus PTA) recipients. Pancreatic graft destruction, as assessed by the number of islet cells staining positive for insulin, was less prominent in SPK (versus PTA) recipients. Pancreatic graft exocrine as well as endocrine function, as assessed by urinary amylase (UA) and plasma glucose levels, was sustained longer for SPK (versus PTA) recipients throughout the observation period. In contrast to the pancreas, kidney allograft biopsies did not show any difference in the incidence of moderate and severe tubulointerstitial rejection for SPK (versus KTA) recipients. The incidence of moderate and severe vascular rejection was significantly lower for SPK (versus KTA) renal allografts at 1 week but not in subsequent weekly biopsies. Kidney allograft functional survival, as assessed by serial serum creatinine determinations, was not significantly different for SPK (versus KTA) recipients. Thus, the clinical and histological progression of pancreatic graft rejection appears less severe for SPK (versus PTA) recipients, suggesting that the kidney downregulates or dilutes the immune attack against the pancreas. Kidney allograft survival is not affected by the addition of a pancreas from the same donor; SPK (versus KTA) transplants do not predispose to more kidney graft losses from irreversible rejection (27).

Another interesting focus of pancreas transplant research in pigs is the hierarchy of rejection for SPK recipients. Transplanting three different organs—pancreas, duodenum, and kidney—allows studies of the host's response to individual grafts. Organ-specific alloantigens have been shown to exist; various organs from the same donor may differ in their susceptibility to rejection damage. For SPK recipients, several different combinations of organ involvement—relative to the incidence of rejection—can be studied: pancreas and kidney, pancreas and duodenum, kidney and duodenum.

For clinical purposes, the first combination is the most relevant. In one pig study, concurrent biopsies of the pancreas and kidney, obtained at weekly intervals posttransplant, were compared (29). Synchronicity (i.e., presence or absence of rejection in both organs) was found in 88% of biopsies at 1 week; dyssynchronicity (i.e., presence of rejection in one organ, absence in the other), in 12%. The severity of interstitial rejection in one organ cannot be used to predict the findings in the other: for pancreatic grafts without interstitial rejection, the corresponding kidney grafts showed moderate or severe rejection; for kidney grafts without interstitial rejection, the corresponding pancreatic grafts showed moderate rejection. Concordance of rejection (i.e., same rejection grades for both grafts) was found in only 25% of all concurrent biopsies; disconcordance (i.e., different rejection grades when both grafts were positive for rejection), in 75%. For interstitial rejection, synchronicity and concordance were not identical between the two organs (possibly due to a different expression of MHC antigens on various parenchymal cells or different non-MHC organ-specific antigens). Yet, one would expect identical grades for vascular rejection because the rejection target—the endothelium—is the same in both organs. However, in this pig study, synchronous vascular rejection in both organs was present in only 54% at 1 week and 71% at 2 weeks; dyssynchronous, 46 and 29%. Concordant rejection was noted in only 46% and discordant rejection in 54% of corresponding biopsies. Conceivably, local interstitial amplification factors may cause a different endothelial response in each organ. The rejection episode usually begins in the parenchyma of the pancreas and kidney. In the study, interstitial rejection was always more advanced than vascular rejection in both organs. The different timing in onset of rejection in the two grafts—as well as organ-specific interaction between parenchymal and endothelial cells—may also explain the different vascular rejection grades, despite identical endothelium in both grafts. In two other pig studies—one using triple immunosuppression (26), the other CSA monotherapy (23)—discordant but not dyssynchronous rejection was confirmed for SPK recipients. Neither study showed isolated pancreatic rejection, but serial biopsies were not taken and histological studies were based on autopsies, missing the early posttransplant period.

Clinical evidence of rejection, as assessed by changes in UA, plasma glucose, and serum creatinine levels, demonstrated a difference between pancreas and kidney in regard to onset of rejection. In one pig study, laboratory manifestation of graft loss from rejection caused first an increase in serum creatinine, then a decrease in UA, and finally an increase in plasma glucose levels (29) (Fig. 5). These results provide evidence that for SPK recipients, rejection of the kidney occurs earlier and more frequently than rejection of the exocrine pancreas: rejection of the exocrine pancreas (based on UA) was diagnosed, on average, 4 ± 2 days before rejection of the endocrine pancreas (based on plasma glucose). In the same study, laboratory parameters (UA, plasma glucose, serum creatinine) correlated poorly with histological results. In the early posttransplant period (first 7 days), no correlation was found at all; at 14 days posttransplant, histological results correlated only with the serum creatinine level. Histological changes usually preceded laboratory (i.e., functional) changes (29).

After the pancreas and kidney, the second most clinically relevant comparison in the hierarchy of rejection is between the pancreas and duodenum. Transplanting the whole pancreas usually includes the second portion of the donor duodenum. In contrast to the pancreas, the duodenum can easily be visualized cystoscopically and is readily accessible to biopsy. Some suggest using the duodenum as a marker of rejection in pancreaticoduodenal transplants. Studies in pigs have examined whether duodenal pathology can predict pancreatic pathology and whether duodenal biopsies can be used to monitor the pancreatic

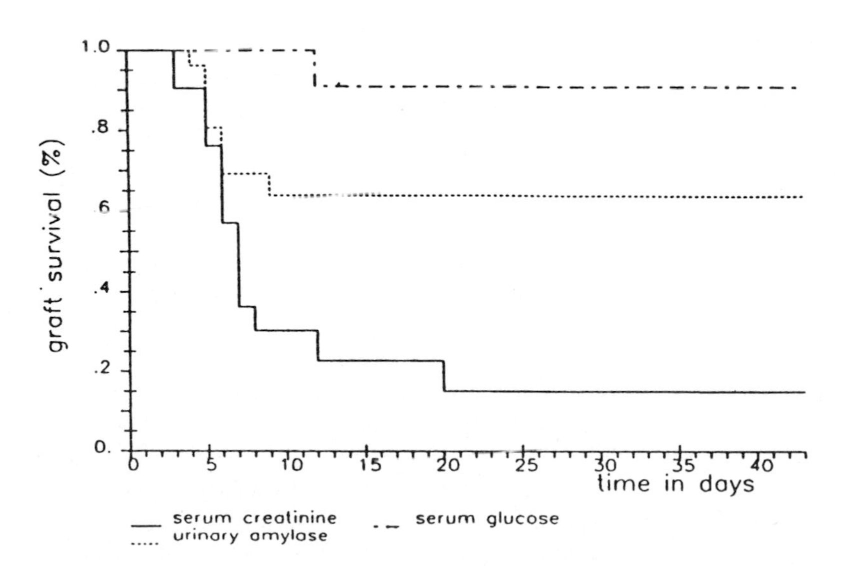

Figure 5 Graft survival after 36 SPK in swine according to serum creatinine, urine amylase, and serum glucose levels.

graft. In one study, concordance of interstitial rejection in both organs was noted in 72% of the biopsies; vascular rejection, in 63% (30). In pigs with discordant rejection, higher rejection grades were found in the pancreas in 78% of interstitial and 58% of vascular rejection; the pancreas seemed to be more prone to rejection than the duodenum.

The results also support the hypothesis that interstitial rejection depends more on tissue-specific factors than vascular rejection. This is not surprising considering the target of rejection. In interstitial rejection, the target cells are acinar and ductal cells in the pancreas and epithelial cells in the duodenum; these cells are developmentally, morphologically, and functionally different. In vascular rejection, the target is the endothelium, whose cells are the same in both organs. Discordance of vascular rejection can be interpreted as a result of differences in local amplification factors, triggered by the parenchyma. From a diagnostic viewpoint, this study indicates that a duodenal biopsy reflects pancreatic pathology more than half the time (30). If the duodenum shows rejection, the likelihood of rejection of the pancreas is high, but if the duodenum is normal, it does not rule out rejection of the pancreas.

The third organ combination, the duodenum and kidney, is also clinically relevant. For SPK recipients, the kidney is generally used as a hallmark of rejection. Since most kidneys transplanted simultaneously with a pancreas are placed intraperitoneally, they are less accessible for biopsy than when placed retroperitoneally, as for KTA recipients. In contrast to both the kidney and pancreas, the duodenum can easily be biopsied by cystoscopy. Sometimes this may be the only way to obtain graft tissue from SPK recipients. Another pig study assessed whether the duodenum can be a marker of kidney rejection (31). Synchronous rejection was noted in 86% of concurrent biopsies. Dyssynchronous rejection was found in 14%; in 10%, the duodenum was free of rejection, while concurrent kidney biopsies showed moderate interstitial rejection; in 4%, rejection was absent in the kidney but present in the duodenum. Concordant rejection was noted in 45%; discordant rejection in 55%. This study suggests that if duodenal biopsies are positive, they are likely to reflect kidney pathology. When negative, they do not rule out kidney graft rejection. In both organs, interstitial rejection preceded vascular rejection; interstitial rejection in the absence of vascular rejection was noted in 50% of duodenal and kidney biopsies, whereas vascular rejection in the absence of interstitial rejection was not observed on any biopsy (31).

Pig autopsy results have also shed light on the hierarchy of rejection by comparing all three organs (32). Rejection was most advanced for the kidney and least advanced for the duodenum: the incidence of moderate or severe interstitial rejection was 77%, kidney; 61%, pancreas; and 46%, duodenum. Concordant rejection was noted in 38% of autopsies, discordant rejection in 62%. Pairwise comparison showed that the incidence of identical rejection grades ranged from 46 to 65% between the possible pairings of the pancreas, duodenum, and kidney. From a diagnostic viewpoint, this indicates that a duodenal biopsy reflects pancreatic pathology no more than two-thirds of the time and reflects kidney pathology less than half the time. One might speculate that the difference in rejection grades between the three allografts does not correlate because the grading schemes do not translate from one allograft to another or that other organ-specific factors pertain; this would, however, explain only a one-way shift in rejection grades. In reality, two-way shifts were noted: the rejection process was more advanced in the duodenum than the pancreas in 22% of biopsies, in the duodenum than the kidney in 7%, and in the pancreas than the kidney in 20% (32). This study is clinically relevant: if only one biopsy were to be done in cases of suspected rejection, the target organ would be the kidney; in a small percentage, isolated pancreatic or duodenal rejection might be missed in those cases without kidney rejection. However, if any two of the three allografts were biopsied at the same time, rejection would not have been missed at all: in none of the cases was rejection absent in more than one allograft.

The impact of simultaneously engrafted lymphoid tissue on pancreatic rejection (simultaneous pancreaticoduodenal and spleen transplants) is different: the spleen presents a greater antigenic load to the host than the simultaneously engrafted kidney. In one pig study, including the spleen was associated with rejection of the pancreas and adversely affected pancreatic graft survival: 63% of pancreas and spleen recipients rejected their graft, on average, 13 days posttransplant; none of the PTA recipients (no simultaneous spleen transplant) rejected their grafts during the 4-week observation period. Interestingly, none of the pancreas and spleen recipients developed signs of graft-versus-host disease (33). Ex vivo irradiation of the donor spleen decreased rejection episodes, compared with simultaneous pancreas and spleen transplants without irradiation. Lymphoid tissue of the donor spleen may sensitize the host and thus induce rejection (34).

2. *Studies in Dogs*

The diagnostic utility of UA monitoring to detect pancreatic allograft rejection was first studied in dogs. Gotoh et al. (35) drained the duct of pancreas grafts to the ureter, as described by Gliedman et al. (36) in humans in the 1970s. This dog study demonstrated that a change in exocrine function, as assessed by UA levels, occurred at least 24 hr before complete breakdown of the pancreatic endocrine function. The change in UA levels occurred earlier than change in serum amylase levels, indicating that UA predicts rejection better.

Prieto et al. (37) drained exocrine secretions of segmental pancreatic transplants into the bladder (ductocystostomy) in totally pancreatectomized dogs. UA levels declined precipitously (<1000 μ/L) before the onset of hyperglycemia: by 1.3 ± 0.2 days in nonimmunosuppressed dogs, by 3.3 ± 1.0 days in dogs on CSA monotherapy, and by 9.4 ± 2.8 days in dogs on triple immunosuppression (CSA, prednisone, azathioprine). In another experiment, dogs received CSA for prophylactic immunosuppression, and antirejection therapy with azathioprine and antilymphocyte globulin was given for 5 days beginning the first day rejection was diagnosed. Rejection was diagnosed when (group A) serum glucose rose to >150 mg/dL or (group B) UA concentrations decreased to <1000 μ/L. Functional graft survival was 9.4 ± 0.8 days in group A and 31.8 ± 6.3 days in group B. These studies clearly show that, for grafts drained into the urinary tract, UA monitoring can diagnose pancreas allograft rejection in its early stage.

In a technically different study, using bladder-drained whole pancreaticoduodenal grafts, Marsh et al. (28) introduced the cystoscopically directed transduodenal pancreatic biopsy technique. A total of 59 biopsy specimens were obtained cystoscopically from 18 dogs; the tissue was adequate for pathological diagnosis in 70% of the specimens. The most frequent complication was bleeding at the biopsy site, all of which stopped within minutes after irrigation began. At autopsy, microscopic hematomas in the pancreatic head were found in three dogs; fistulas, abscesses, or pseudocysts were not noted (28,38).

As an alternative to pancreatic graft biopsies, fine-needle aspiration biopsies (FNAB) were first attempted in a dog model of pancreatic transplantation. Ekberg et al. (39,40) used a 22-gauge needle mounted on a pistol-grip syringe. Although minilaparotomies under general anesthesia were done, no pancreatic fistulas or hemorrhagic complications were encountered after 166 FNAB. Cytocentrifuge FNAB preparations were evaluated by total corrected increment scores (TCI); increases were due to the presence of blast cells and macrophages. In healthy immunosuppressed grafts, TCI remained below 1.6 and was >5.0 when acute rejection or pancreatitis was seen on conventional cytology. Acute rejection and pancreatitis was distinguished by significant differences in increments of monocytes, lymphocytes, and macrophages. The correlation between FNAB and UA was noteworthy: a fall in UA permitted the successful reversal of rejection in 1 of 6 grafts, but 5 of 7 grafts were successfully treated when rejection diagnosis was based on FNAB (40). The authors concluded that earlier diagnosis of rejection is achieved by FNAB than UA measurements, improving the chance to reverse a pancreatic rejection episode. The drawback of this study is the fragility of pancreatic acinar cells, with fragmentation enhanced by cytocentrifugation; this makes the counting of acinar cells difficult, and the cytomorphology is often lost (39,40).

Studies in dogs have also focused on differences in the rejection process between the pancreas and kidney in SPK recipients. In a model of combined kidney and free-draining intraperitoneal pancreatic segmental transplantation, kidney rejection (as assessed by increases in serum creatinine levels) preceded pancreas rejection (as assessed by the onset of hyperglycemia) (41). At the onset of kidney rejection but before hyperglycemia developed, kidney biopsies revealed generalized mononuclear infiltration; pancreatic biopsies showed diffuse interstitial infiltration, but islets appeared to be spared.

In their SPK model, Florack et al. (42) used enteric-drained, segmental pancreatic transplants. Pancreatic graft function was based on plasma glucose levels, kidney graft function on serum creatinine levels. In both nonimmunosuppressed and immunosuppressed (CSA monotherapy, 25 mg/kg/day) dogs, the mean functional survival time of the pancreas was significantly longer than that of the kidney. In comparing graft survival of PTA and KTA recipients without posttransplant immunosuppression, pancreatic grafts showed significantly longer function than kidney grafts. As in the pig model, SPK (versus PTA) pancreatic allografts survived longer, while kidney allograft survival was not different for SPK (versus KTA) recipients. In this model, exocrine secretions were not monitored for rejection (due to the use of enteric drainage) and biopsies at defined intervals were not obtained.

Only a few studies have focused on some of the newer immunosuppressive drugs. Sato et al. (43) studied the impact of FK 506 versus CSA on graft survival after pancreaticoduodenal transplants using enteric drainage to manage exocrine pancreas secretions. Treatment with CSA alone (20 mg/kg/day for 3 weeks, 10 mg/kg/day IM thereafter) resulted in significantly longer pancreas graft survival than with FK 506 (0.1 to 0.3 mg/kg/day IM). FK 506-induced toxicity resulted in loss of appetite and weight. In addition, atrophy of the pancreatic acinar cells was found and ascribed to toxicity of FK 506. In a different study, glucose tolerance tended to be impaired after treatment with FK 506 in dogs. A slight increase of granules in acinar cells suggested possible deterioration of exogenous secretion of the pancreas (44). These FK 506 study findings, however, have not been verified in clinical pancreatic transplantation.

More than anything else, these pig and dog studies have been pivotal to our current understanding of the hierarchy of rejection in dual-organ transplants and in different recipient categories. Crucial steps in the evolution of modern pancreatic transplantation have included UA monitoring to detect rejection at an early stage and the cystoscopic transduodenal pancreatic biopsy technique. These are just a few of the clinically relevant results obtained from research in large animals.

B. Small Animal Studies

According to the above pig and dog studies, pancreas graft survival is better for SPK (versus PTA) recipients. But the impact of pretransplant uremia—present in human SPK but not PTA candidates—has not been experimentally studied in large animals; it is very difficult to keep uremic animals alive. In one of the most elegant small animal pancreatic transplant models, Nakai et al. (45) investigated the impact of preexisting uremia and synchronous kidney transplantation on pancreas allograft survival in rats. In their model, rats were made uremic 2 to 3 weeks pretransplant by a one and four-fifths (1⅘) native nephrectomy. Graft function was monitored by UA concentrations (rejection defined as decline in UA $\leqslant$6000 μ/L or to <100 μ/24 hr), plasma glucose levels (>200 mg/dL), and serum creatinine levels (>3 mg/dL). As in the large animals, the mean functional survival times of both the endocrine and exocrine components of the pancreas were significantly longer for SPK (versus PTA) recipients. Kidney graft survival was not longer in nonuremic SPK (versus nonuremic KTA) recipients. In rats on CSA, graft survival times were longer, but the relative differences between the SPK, PTA, and KTA categories persisted. Preexisting uremia delayed pancreatic rejection for both SPK and PTA nonimmunosuppressed recipients versus their nonuremic counterparts. Kidney graft survival was not significanlty longer for uremic (versus nonuremic) SPK recipients. These data suggest that a synchronous kidney transplant and uremia independently downmodulate the rejection response to a pancreatic graft; the simultaneous pancreatic graft has no detrimental effect on the survival of a kidney graft.

In a study by Vogt et al. (46), not only was a different rat strain used, but also a different immunosuppressive protocol (short-term CSA only) and a different method for managing exocrine secretions (duct ligation). They did not find pancreatic graft survival time longer in SPK (versus PTA) recipients. Of note, they included a group in which a pancreas was transplanted 100 days after a previous kidney allograft from the same donor strain (kidney permanently accepted) and found that the pancreas was rejected within 30 days. In contrast, a subsequent metachronous kidney transplant after a previous kidney transplant from the same donor strain was permanently accepted (>100 days); this was noted without further immunosuppression after removal of the first graft, while unrelated third-party kidney allografts were acutely rejected. These data suggest not only quantitative differences in kidney and pancreatic graft survival, but also differences in the state of immunological unresponsiveness induced by identical CSA immunosuppression. An earlier study by the same group demonstrated that non-MHC antigens coded outside the MHC do induce rejection of the pancreas, but not the kidney (47). Therefore, the stronger immunogenicity of the pancreas (versus the kidney) might be mediated by non-MHC antigens present in the pancreas, but not the kidney.

Earlier pancreatic transplant studies in rats focused on histological patterns of pancreatic rejection. Three distinct patterns of pancreatic graft rejection have been described, depending on the degree of histoincompatibility between donor and recipient (48). MHC incompatibility alone or in combination with non-MHC alloantigens was associated with a morphological pattern of acute rejection. Incompatibility at the RT1.C region resulted in chronic rejection; the two major histological features were (a) embedding of pancreatic ductules and islets in acellular fibrotic material and (b) marked intimal proliferation in major arteries with infiltration of the media. Incompatibility at minor transplant antigens (non-MHC antigens) "prolonged" rejection, characterized by well-preserved proliferated ductules and islets in the process of disintegration. The authors concluded that different patterns of rejection are influenced by the genetic barrier between donor and recipient rats, as well as the strain-specific and individual responder status of the recipient.

Rejection patterns in rats have also been studied with different methods of exocrine drainage: duct ligation, duct obliteration, and duct-open intraperitoneal drainage (49). Early acceleration of graft damage (posttransplant day 6) occurred in the duct-ligated and obliterated allografts, compared with the duct-open group; by day 11, rejection was complete in all three groups. However, compared with pancreatic isografts, the histological diagnosis of rejection can be difficult to define, particularly in the duct-ligated and obliterated groups. In this study, the most useful criterion was localization of cellular infiltrates to the walls of small veins and within islets.

Very few rat studies using pancreas transplant models have investigated some of the newer immunosuppressive drugs. Chen et al. (50,51) studied the synergistic effect of rapamycin and CSA in pancreaticoduodenal transplants. They used rapamycin in two different doses (0.80 and 0.8 mg/kg/day), alone or in combination with CSA; immunosuppressive drugs were delivered continuously by osmotic minipump through a lumbar vein for 14 days. They reported that rapamycin and CSA, used alone, were effective at high doses and significantly prolonged survival of pancreaticoduodenal transplants. At low doses, these agents induced moderate, but still significant, prolongation of graft survival. When both drugs were used in combination, at low doses they already demonstrated a marked in vivo synergism, achieving prolonged survival.

III. CLINICAL DIAGNOSIS OF REJECTION

In most cases of pancreatic allograft rejection, clinical symptoms are subtle or nonexistent. Only 5 to 20% of patients with pancreatic graft rejection present with clinical symptoms (51,53). Graft tenderness is usually the most prominent symptom, but it is difficult to distinguish clinically from pancreatitis. Fever as a clinical symptom of rejection is not common, partly due to CSA maintenance therapy. But if the workup for infection is negative, fever is highly suspicious of rejection. Likewise, paralytic ileus and acute abdomen are rarely seen but can be caused by rejection-induced pancreatitis. Even in the presence of clinical symptoms, the diagnosis of rejection, if a biopsy is not obtained, is usually a composite decision based on clinical and laboratory (e.g., decrease in UA) criteria. Hyperglycemia is considered a late symptom of rejection with a low probability of reversal.

IV. LABORATORY DIAGNOSIS OF REJECTION

A. Urine Markers of Exocrine Rejection

1. Urine Amylase

Bladder drainage is currently the most widely used technique for pancreatic transplantation. Originally advocated to reduce the surgical complication rate, it also allows graft exocrine function to be monitored by measuring pancreatic enzymes secreted directly into the urine (36,54). In clinical and experimental studies, exocrine pancreatic rejection has been shown to precede endocrine rejection (29,37,55); in particular, islets are spared during the early phase of rejection and extensive interstitial rejection can occur with normoglycemia still present (56). Serial urine amylase (UA) measurement has emerged as the standard laboratory test: a decrease in UA activity (relative hypoamylasuria) is the most commonly used biochemical marker of acute rejection in the pancreas alone. By monitoring UA levels, antirejection treatment can begin before hyperglycemia occurs (55). UA measurements are simple and inexpensive, and can be done by any laboratory.

One of the limitations of UA monitoring is that a decrease in activity (hypoamylasuria) does not necessarily mean rejection. It may also be caused by other factors such as preservation injury early post transplant, or pancreatitis, fibrosis, thrombosis, and ductal obstruction (57,58). Prolonged fasting can also cause a decrease in UA activity. Moreover, biochemical factors can influence UA measurement, including extreme acid (pH $\leqslant$ 6) or alkaline (pH $\geqslant$ 9) urine, repeated freezing and thawing of samples, or dilutions with water or saline (57). In one study, incubation of urine samples stored at 37° caused a drop in UA activity as high as 19% in 4 hr and 48% in 9 hr (59). The patient's state of hydration and diuresis can also cause wide fluctuations of UA concentrations; this can be circumvented by measuring UA concentrations per unit of time (units per hour), which tends to correct for dilutional effects, rather than per unit of volume (units per liter). Erroneous interpretation of hypoamylasuria may lead to unnecessary antirejection treatment and may increase the risk of systemic infections. Finally, UA monitoring is a measurement of exocrine or acinar cell function and does not directly reflect the integrity of beta cells (60). Nevertheless, there are no examples of rejection of beta cells without rejection of the exocrine pancreas. Autoimmune recurrence of disease has been described with prevention of exocrine function. Recurrence of disease has not been documented in immunosuppressed recipients of kidney pancreas grafts, only in nonimmunosuppressed recipients of identical twin isografts of minimally immunosuppressed recipients of HLA-identical sibling grafts.

A few studies have correlated hypoamylasuria and pancreaticoduodenal biopsy results. Munn et al. (61) noted 18 episodes of hypoamylasuria (UA decrease $\geqslant$50% from baseline) in 30 SPK and PAK recipients. Histopathological examination of 14 specimens (including 3 kidney graft biopsies) showed rejection in 64% only; fibrosis was noted in 14%, enzymatic necrosis in 7%, cytomegalovirus (CMV) pancreatitis in 7%, and normal pancreatic graft histology in 7%. Nankivell et al. (57) reported a 60% sensitivity when UA activity decreased $\geqslant$50% or was correlated with protocol biopsies. A comprehensive study by Benedetti et al. (52) correlated hypoamylasuria and pancreaticoduodenal biopsy results in three different pancreas recipient categories. They showed that a >25% decrease of UA from baseline on two consecutive measurements correlated with biopsy results in only 55% of specimens. The mean decrease in UA levels did not significantly differ between the positive (67 + 8%) and the negative (57% ± 16%) biopsy group. In assessing the test quality, they found a sensitivity of 100% (stable UA levels meaning no rejection) and a specificity of 30%; the predictive value of a positive test was 53%; of a negative test, 100%. Although previous studies had used >50% decrease in UA to define rejection, a >25% decrease from stable posttransplant baseline levels on 2 consecutive measurements (at least 12 hr apart) turned out to be more helpful in their study: if only >50% decrease were considered to be biochemically consistent with rejection, they would have missed 22% of their patient rejection episodes (28% of all histologically moderate and 18% of all severe rejection episodes). Thus, stable UA levels from a posttransplant baseline reliably rule out rejection, and acute pancreas graft rejection is associated with a decline in UA. However, the test is a nonspecific indicator of rejection. Rather than relying on UA levels, PTA and PAK recipients with hypoamylasuria, as well as SPK recipients with isolated hypoamylasuria (but normal serum creatinine levels), should undergo biopsies whenever possible to avoid unnecessary antirejection treatment. If biopsies cannot be done, from a graft salvage point of view, it is better to treat recipients than to not treat them, since the probability of moderate or severe rejection is $\geqslant$50%.

2. Urine Lipase

Serial urine lipase measurements have not gained widespread application, so there are few data to analyze. No theoretical advantages for measurement of lipase over amylase have been advanced, and it is likely that the same variability and problems with specificity would exist, but until formal testing is done the value of urine lipase measurements is only speculative.

3. Urine Prostaglandin

We know of no reports on clinical prostaglandin measurements after pancreas transplantation. However, in different rat models, urine prostaglandin (PGE2) has been studied as an early marker of pancreatic graft rejection. In a high-responder rat model (ACI to Lewis), with hyperglycemia occurring on day 8 ± 0.5, and in a low-responder model (Fisher to Lewis), with hyperglycemia occurring on day 13 ± 0.5, UA was useful in diagnosing rejection before the onset of hyperglycemia. Elevations of urinary PGE2 were noted in both the minor and major barrier models; these elevations not only correlated with but also preceded changes in UA levels by 2 to 3 days. Elevations of PGE2 occurred 4 to 7 days before loss of endocrine function. PGE2 was also elevated on posttransplant day 1, before stabilizing to baseline levels; this can be interpreted as the response of acinar tissue to preservation and procurement injury. Rats with pancreatitis or infections were not included in this study and biopsies were not done (62).

B. Urine Markers of Endocrine Rejection

1. Urinary C peptides

Urinary C-peptide excretion has been studied as a marker of endocrine pancreatic rejection. C peptide is a proinsulin fragment secreted by beta cells in equimolecular form with insulin; its basal and poststimulated determination in plasma or urine is a reliable method of assessing function of endocrine pancreas for diabetic patients with renal failure (63). When urinary C-peptide excretion was analyzed for 8 SPK and 11 nondiabetic KTA recipients, levels were 10 times lower for the SPK (versus KTA) group (64). In contrast, plasma C-peptide levels and kidney function were similar in both groups. Contamination of urine with pancreatic secretions might be responsible for the decreased urinary C-peptide levels for SPK recipients. Furthermore, recipients with urinary diversion through a nephrostomy catheter had higher urinary C-peptide levels than those with urine and exocrine pancreatic secretions collected directly from the bladder. At the time of pancreatic graft rejection (based on UA decrease and echographic-duplex studies), urinary C-peptide levels increased up to the levels reached for recipients with nephrostomy catheters and pure urine collections (64). The study suggests that the C-peptide molecule is altered by pancreatic exocrine secretions; this is not surprising, considering the proteolytic activity of pancreatic enzymes, such as trypsin, that can cleave proinsulin and insulin molecules (65). In addition, urine pH fluctuations caused by exocrine pancreas secretions can lead to C-peptide alterations. It appears that, for these reasons, urinary C-peptide determination is not useful in monitoring pancreatic graft function.

C. Serum Markers of Exocrine Rejection

Dragstedt et al. (66) showed that extensive destruction of exocrine pancreatic tissue must occur before deterioration in endocrine pancreatic function can be detected. Thus, while hyperglycemia is the ultimate objective measure of pancreatic graft failure, it is a late parameter of rejection and usually becomes apparent only after extensive destruction of islets has taken place. The problem of using pancreas-specific serum markers to detect rejection lies in the pathophysiology of the exocrine pancreas: rejection—as well as pancreatitis, infection, or preservation injury—leads to temporary or constant damage of acinar tissue, with subsequent enzyme and cytokine release. Thus, the causes of destruction of pancreas acinar tissue are multiple and, with pancreas-specific serum parameters only, difficult to differentiate.

This is exemplified by monitoring of the *serum amylase*, a marker of pancreatic inflammation from any cause. An increase in serum amylase may occur with rejection and precede a decline in UA, but it is nonspecific (67–69). Posttransplant hyperamylasemia can be caused by all of the above conditions of acinar tissue damage. In addition, serum amylase is also derived in large part from other tissues, mainly the salivary glands.

Over the last 15 years, a variety of other serum markers were introduced to facilitate early diagnosis of rejection. Most have not reached the level of clinical relevance, either because they are not universally available or are not consistently reliable. Major problems in most studies are use of a clinical definition of rejection, lack of biopsies, and failure to distinguish clearly between kidney and pancreas rejection in SPK recipients.

1. *Serum Anodal Trypsinogen*

Serum anodal trypsinogen (SAT) has been the focus of several experimental and clinical studies. Initial work by Borgström et al. (70) in a pig model compared serum levels of immunoreactive anionic and cationic trypsin; rejection was heralded by a significant increase in immunoreactive anodal trypsinogen by at least 4 or more days before hyperglycemia or histological evidence of rejection in about 80% of the cases. A decrease in immunoreactive cationic trypsin was less sensitive for rejection. In a clinical study of 15 SPK recipients followed between 18 and 134 days posttransplant, a significant increase in anodal trypsinogen levels was noted during a total of 21 rejection episodes (71). However, biopsies were not done. Rejection was diagnosed clinically, but no criteria were defined; rejection was considered real if the patient received a course of antirejection medication (71). Thus, the validity of the study remains in doubt. Two other studies have used SAT to diagnose rejection, but pancreatic graft core biopsies were not obtained in either (68,72). SAT levels are frequently elevated in the early posttransplant period, which may reflect preservation or procurement injury (pancreatitis) rather than rejection; this underscores the need to correlate SAT with pancreatic core biopsy findings. Since the kidneys are the major route for degradation of trypsin, SAT levels may be influenced by renal dysfunction (70–72). Studies of nonuremic PTA recipients with normal renal function have not been done, but determining the impact of renal function would be helpful. SAT can also be elevated due to pancreatitis, trauma, and outlet obstruction. In a small study by Perkal et al., SAT levels and kidney biopsies were obtained in 11 patients (9 SPK, 2 PAK) with a presumptive diagnosis of rejection (73). Biopsies correlated exactly with SAT behavior in all cases of rejection; the conclusion was that an increase in SAT is a reliable marker of pancreas exocrine rejection, but it was not shown to be better than monitoring creatinine in the small subgroup of SPK recipients.

Unlike UA, SAT does not depend on the type of management of exocrine pancreatic secretions. SAT can be used to monitor bladder-drained or enteric-drained grafts, but has not been tested in duct-injected pancreas transplants. Douzdjian et al. (72) compared UA, SAT, and serum amylase in 11 first-time acute rejection episodes in bladder-drained SPK recipients; all rejection episodes were biopsy-proven (core kidney 9, fine-needle kidney 2, fine-needle pancreas 5). They found that serum amylase, although less specific, was as sensitive as SAT, but did not correlate with successful treatment. Both serum amylase and serum creatinine levels positively correlated with SAT at a time when UA changes were not yet apparent. These authors would treat SPK recipients with an elevated SAT level even in the absence of a rise in the serum creatinine, but a large-scale study to calculate specificity and sensitivity was not done. The usefulness of SAT in diagnosing pancreatic graft rejection must be determined in PTA recipients and the frequency with which an increase in SAT and serum amylase precedes a decrease in UA needs to be calculated and correlated with biopsy proven rejection or absence of rejection.

2. *Plasma Pancreatic Secretory Trypsin Inhibitors*

Plasma pancreatic secretory trypsin inhibitor (PSTI) is a pancreatic exocrine protein (6.2-kDa polypeptide consisting of 56 amino acids) that has been used as a marker of acute pancreatitis (74,75). In patients with acinar cell damage, cellular PSTI is released into the pancreatic juice to prevent trypsinogen activation in the pancreatic duct and then released into the blood (76). PSTI elevations after pancreatic transplantation were first reported in a dog model (77). Levels were elevated on posttransplant day 1 (due to preservation injury) and on day 6 due to rejection; the second elevation preceded the onset of hyperglycemia by 3 days. In a clinical study of 17 SPK and 7 KTA recipients, PSTI levels were analyzed during rejection episodes (78). During the rejection course, PSTI levels in SPK recipients increased significantly 1 day before the initial day of rejection diagnosed clinically, and then decreased after rejection treatment. For KTA recipients, PSTI elevation was less dramatic and did not precede the rise in serum creatinine. Pancreas biopsies at the time of rejection were not obtained for SPK recipients. Although the major route for clearance of PSTI is the kidney, PSTI elevations preceded serum creatinine rise; thus, PSTI elevations in the early process appear not to be due to renal dysfunction (78). As with SAT, PSTI needs to be studied in PTA recipients to investigate the true significance of renal dysfunction. The major drawback of PSTI is that, as an acute phase reactant protein, its specificity with respect to pancreatic disease is not sufficient, while its sensitivity is too high (79).

Like SAT, PSTI does not depend on the type of exocrine drainage. It can be used in bladder-drained and enteric-drained transplants, but it has not been tested in duct-injected, pancreatic transplant recipients. Duct injection, with its destruction of exocrine tissue, might destroy the usefulness of all exocrine markers.

3. *Pancreas-Specific Protein*

Elevations of the plasma pancreas-specific protein (PASP) have been reported in recipients with acute pancreatitis and during pancreas graft rejection episodes (80). PASP is also a protein, but it is distinct from PSTI. PASP has a molecular weight of 44.5 kDa and is glutamic acid- and leucine-rich; in contrast, PSTI has a molecular weight of 6.2 kDa and is aspartic acid–rich (81). Fernstad et al. (82) analyzed plasma levels for PASP in 21 SPK recipients and 8 KTA recipients. Diagnosis of rejection in both groups was based on deteriorating renal function; pancreatic biopsies were not obtained. In episodes of kidney rejection, the levels of PASP, but not always of serum amylase, were elevated on "several" occasions; they decreased after antirejection therapy (82). The authors suspected accompanying pancreatic graft rejection. PASP levels and serum amylase levels were stable in KTA recipients and were not affected by serum creatinine levels, renal rejection, or antirejection therapy. One of the drawbacks of PASP in diagnosing rejection is that it is also a marker of graft pancreatitis, with elevations of similar magnitude as for rejection episodes (this may be true for SAT and PSTI as well, but in the studies cited no measurements were reported in patients with pancreatitis). In the Fernstad study, elevation of PASP was also noted before pancreas graft thrombosis was diagnosed; with chronic graft rejection, PASP rose to high levels long before other indications (80). In a follow-up study, 4 PTA patients were included (82). They experienced a total of 7 rejection episodes based on changes in pancreatic juice cytology. PASP elevation started 1 or 2 days before, or at the time of, the diagnosed rejection. Nyberg et al. (83) retrospectively evaluated the clinical course of 15 SPK and 10 PAK recipients in relation to plasma PASP levels. They found an increase in PASP not only during rejection episodes, but also during other conditions of graft damage such as pancreatitis. Of note, at least four "clinically indisputable" pancreas rejection episodes were missed by PASP analysis. Thus, PASP monitoring shows low sensitivity and it is not specific for rejection because it is elevated in pancreatitis. On the other hand, this may be true for all serum markers. If they are not measured under conditions other than rejection, the authors cannot be certain of the specificity of any test.

4. *Pancreatic Elastase 1*

The usefulness of the pancreas specific protein pancreatic elastase 1 in detecting pancreatic rejection was investigated in 27 SPK and 9 PTA recipients (84). Acute rejection episodes were diagnosed primarily by changes in pancreatic juice cytology. During 24 acute rejection episodes, pancreatic elastase 1 was found not to be a sensitive rejection marker during the early postoperative period, because of its slow decline from the peak level. Like most other markers of exocrine pancreatic damage, it was, however, associated with a variety of other conditions such as pancreatitis. In addition, a considerable increase in pancreatic elastase 1 levels was noted in patients with renal dysfunction and without involvement of the pancreatic graft (84,85). It appears that pancreatic elastase 1 is not useful in the laboratory diagnosis of pancreas rejection.

5. *Interleukin-2*

In regard to cytokine measurement, all clinical pancreatic transplant studies have focused on interleukin-2 (IL-2) and the soluble IL-2 receptor (SIL-2R). Secreted by activated T cells, IL-2 is crucial for clonal expansion of T cells and is involved in the T-B cell interaction. IL-2 was studied in the setting of pancreas graft rejection in 8 SPK and 2 PAK recipients (86). A good correlation was noted between the clinical diagnosis of rejection and elevated serum or urinary IL-2 levels; most patients with rejection had elevated IL-2 levels 1 to 3 days before any suggestion of rejection by conventional diagnostic criteria. After successful treatment of rejection episodes, serum and urine IL-2 returned to prerejection baseline levels; whenever postrejection IL-2 levels were higher than prerejection baseline IL-2 levels, recurrent rejection episodes occurred. While acute pancreatitis caused only mild elevation, septic complications unfortunately also raised IL-2 levels comparable to those in patients with rejections.

Perkins et al. (87) analyzed SIL-2R levels of 15 SPK and 3 PAK recipients, including those with acute rejection ($n = 7$), CMV disease ($n = 4$), and both rejection and CMV ($n = 1$). SIL-2R levels were significantly elevated for patients with acute rejection episodes and with CMV disease; for both conditions, levels increased a mean of 7 days before clinical diagnosis of rejection or CMV disease. Interestingly, SIL-2R levels did not increase for patients with acute pancreatitis, wound infection, operative procedures, and CSA nephrotoxicity. In contrast, a study of 22 SPK recipients found an increase of SIL-2R levels not only for those with rejection and viral infections but also for those with pancreatitis (88). The conclusion was that SIL-2R is not rejection-specific. While SIL-2R alone was not useful in diagnosing rejection, the combination of SIL-2R, urinary lipase, and serum creatinine did allow detection of allograft dysfunction, according to this biopsy-proven kidney rejection study (88).

6. *Neopterin*

Neopterin, a marker of T-lymphocyte activation, has been studied in serum, urine, and pancreatic juice samples to assess its usefulness in detecting pancreatic graft rejection. Brattström et al. (89) conducted a study of 10 PTA, 3 PAK, and 3 SPK recipients with a total of 18 rejection episodes. Serum neopterin increased during some of the rejection episodes, but the increase reflected impaired renal function rather than T-lymphocyte activation. In contrast, neopterin in pancreatic juice correlated with rejection. The ratio between pancreatic juice and serum neopterin levels was higher for patients with (versus without) rejection, indicating local production of neopterin by inflammatory cells. Of note, neopterin became detectable in the pancreatic juice before positive cytology. In a different study (90), pancreatic juice neopterin excretion was confirmed to be a specific and sensitive marker for the early detection of acute pancreatic graft rejection in SPK recipients. Diagnosis of rejection was based on clinical symptoms, a decrease in pancreatic juice and amylase, and on juice cytology; the correlation of pancreatic juice and neopterin excretion with rejection was better than that of urinary neopterin. Bacterial contamination and infections were not associated with an increase in pancreatic juice neopterin excretion; patients with pancreatitis, however, were not included in this study.

7. *Phospholipase A_2*

Phospholipase A_2 (PLA_2), a cellular membrane enzyme, has been shown to be a sensitive marker for pancreas acinar cell damage such as acute pancreatitis (91). PLA_2 was studied in 5 SPK recipients, in an attempt to evaluate its diagnostic value in predicting acute pancreas graft rejection. All recipients had biopsy-proven kidney rejection within 1 month posttransplant. PLA_2 levels increased significantly 1 day before the initial day of rejection in two recipients and on the initial day of diagnosed rejection in two recipients. In the fifth recipient, PLA_2 levels did not change. Compared with plasma PLTI, PLA_2 was less sensitive in detecting rejection (79).

8. *Thromboxane and Prostacyclin*

Tissue prostacyclin (PGI_2) and thromboxane (TXA_2) were assessed during acute pancreatic rejection in a rat model (92). Radioimmune assays measured their stable hydrolysis products 6-keto-prostaglandin $F_{1\alpha}$ and thromboxane B_2 (TXB_2). Increased synthesis of these prostanoids was noted during cellular rejection. It was suggested that the change in PGI_2 and TXA_2 may mediate vascular failure by reducing graft perfusion. Vessels supplying the allografted pancreas showed early changes in relative TXB_2 and 6-keto-prostaglandin $F_{1\alpha}$ synthesis, which favors vasospasm and thrombosis. Thus, use of thromboxane inhibitors and prostacyclin analogues may be indicated; they may limit tissue damage resulting from pancreatic graft rejection by restoring a hemeostatic balance, thus reducing the likelihood of vascular thrombosis (92). The clinical value of thromboxane and prostacyclin is still to be determined.

D. Serum Markers of Endocrine Rejection

1. *First-Phase Insulin Release*

To study the disassociation between exocrine and endocrine pancreatic function, Henry et al. (60) evaluated the usefulness of acute first-phase insulin releases after intravenous glucose and glucagon stimulation tests for predicting an impending pancreatic beta-cell failure. The normal first-phase insulin response is a brisk output of preformed insulin in response to a physiological challenge; a blunted response characterizes poor functional reserve and, in the allograft setting, potential graft rejection (93,94). The study involved 3 SPK and 5 PAK recipients diagnosed with presumed pancreatic graft rejection based solely on decreased UA levels. All were normoglycemic and insulin-independent at the time of the study. Despite a remarkable decline in UA levels ($\geq$ 50 to 90%), 5 recipients (group I) had qualitatively and quantitatively normal acute first-phase insulin release; 3 had blunted first-phase insulin release (group II). All of the group I recipients maintained normoglycemia and insulin independence long-term (range, 6 to 44 months) after treatment, while group II recipients suffered pancreatic graft endocrine failure (2 rejections, 1 thrombosis). It was concluded that a decrease in UA alone does not necessarily predict an impending loss from rejection, but they did not have any examples of high UA with decreased endocrine function with proven rejection. Since biopsies were not obtained, they could not really know whether the decrease in UA was from rejection or other causes. The loss or blunting of acute first-phase insulin release to stimulation, however, did appear to be a specific indicator of beta cell damage, presumably indicating a more advanced stage of rejection. In clinical practice, measuring first-phase insulin is fraught with logistical problems (95). It requires drawing C-peptide levels and insulin levels at 1-min intervals for at least 10 min during an intravenous glucose tolerance test; moreover, insulin and C-peptide analyses are not available in every laboratory and are not reproducible or rapidly obtained. Also, there is no evidence that endocrine function tests are more sensitive than UA for rejection. They may be more specific, but relying on endocrine tests rather than UA may mean treating too late to reverse rejections; we do not view them as a substitute for UA in bladder-drained pancreatic grafts, particularly PTA, where serum creatinine cannot be used as a substitute for UA.

2. *Glucose Disappearance Rate*

The glucose disappearance rate (k_G) reflects the first- and second-phase insulin response. In contrast to the first-phase insulin release, a k_G value can be quickly determined from serial blood glucose measurements. Elmer et al. (95) studied glucose disappearance rates of 13 SPK, 4 PTA, and 3 PAK recipients. Pancreatic biopsies for histological confirmation of rejection were obtained for 84% of rejection episodes; the remaining rejection episodes were confirmed by "clear response" to antirejection treatment. A 20% reduction in k_G values had 91% specificity, 84% sensitivity, 75% positive predictive value, 94% negative predictive value, and 89% accuracy. In comparison, sensitivity and negative value were lower for UA (75 and 86%) and SAT (36 and 79%); the specificity was higher for SAT (96%) and the positive predictive value was higher for UA (82%) and SAT (80%). The authors concluded that, in clinical situations, k_G values are particularly useful when other markers provide conflicting data or when monitoring those markers is not possible (95). In such situations, k_G monitoring provides the greatest clinical utility. An additional advantage is its simplicity and economy. A drawback of the study is that patients with pancreatitis and infections were not included, so any calculations of specificity are suspect. Another drawback is the timing of changes. In rejection, a UA decline still precedes a decline in endocrine function, so relying on endocrine function alone may lead to unacceptable delay in antirejection therapy.

E. Summary of Rejection Markers

Despite the wide variety of serum and urinary tests, not a single marker currently can reliably predict pancreatic graft rejection. For SPK recipients, kidney biopsies in conjunction with serial serum creatinine levels have been used to diagnose rejection. For recipients of solitary pancreatic transplants (PTA, PAK), serum creatinine levels cannot be used and laboratory diagnosis by pancreas-specific markers appears to be even more important. In bladder-drained pancreatic transplants, UA remains the most common parameter due to its simplicity and universal availability. Other urinary markers of either exocrine or endocrine graft rejection have not been regularly used in clinical practice. The need for reliable laboratory parameters is most pressing in enteric-drained or duct-injected solitary pancreatic transplant recipients. Some plasma pancreas-specific markers show good promise, particularly SAT; yet clinical usefulness must be correlated with biopsy specimens from PTA recipients. There are no examples of endocrine dysfunction preceding a decline in UA in bladder-drained grafts undergoing rejection, so at best endocrine markers are useful when UA declines. If endocrine function has also declined, the probability of rejection is likely increased, but a study with biopsy correlation has yet to be done. Jointly using several serum and urinary parameters and carefully assessing the patient's clinical course can help detect rejection early and reverse the destructive process when biopsies cannot be obtained. However, pancreatic biopsies remain the gold standard for diagnosing and grading rejection episodes.

V. TISSUE AND CELL DIAGNOSIS OF REJECTION

A. Needle Core Biopsy

For most solid organ transplants (e.g., kidney, liver, heart), histopathological evaluation of graft biopsies became the gold standard of rejection early on. For pancreas transplantation, the development was different for two reasons.

First, isolated pancreatic transplant rejection is rare for SPK recipients, the most common pancreatic transplant category; most rejection episodes involve either the kidney alone or the kidney and pancreas simultaneously (96). This led to the perception that pancreatic graft rejection can be monitored indirectly by relying on serum creatinine changes or kidney graft biopsies. In recipients of solitary pancreatic transplants (PTA, PAK), serum creatinine levels or kidney biopsies cannot be used as markers of rejection; given the inadequacies of laboratory parameters, biopsies are therefore essential for monitoring solitary pancreas transplants. Even for SPK recipients, isolated pancreatic graft rejection can occur and pancreatic graft biopsies may become necessary if a change in exocrine or endocrine laboratory parameters occurs without a change in creatinine.

Second, in the past, pancreatic transplant biopsies were only reluctantly done, due to the potential complications such as pancreatitis, pancreatic fistulas, and bleeding. Before the development of special needles and new imaging techniques—ultrasound, computed tomography (CT), magnetic resonance imaging (MRI)—tissue diagnosis usually required open laparotomy. In one series of 52 open biopsies, 3 (6%) complications were noted: 1

patient bled and 2 patients developed abscesses; in 1 of the latter patients the graft was removed (97). Currently, pancreatic graft biopsies are obtained either percutaneously or cystoscopically and only rarely by open laparotomy. Percutaneous and cystoscopic biopsies should be done under CT or ultrasound guidance.

Percutaneous biopsies of bladder-drained pancreas transplants were first proposed by Allen et al. (98); in their series, percutaneous needle core biopsies were successful in 37 of 40 attempts (93%). A 20-gauge Biopty-cut biopsy needle mounted in an automated biopsy instrument was used. Biopsies were obtained under ultrasound guidance. Transient hyperamylasemia occurred in almost 30% of the patients, with a complete return to baseline in 3 days; one patient developed microscopic hematuria on two occasions; and in one patient, a biopsy of the small bowel was inadvertently taken without subsequent complication. The usefulness of percutaneous "microbiopsies" was confirmed in a study of 10 bladder-drained pancreas recipients (99). Similarly, a 21-gauge needle was used under ultrasound guidance and local anesthesia. Of 14 biopsy specimens, 13 were adequate. Percutaneous biopsies were judged to be more reliable than biochemical markers in diagnosing rejection.

Despite the paucity of major complications and their high success rate, percutaneous biopsy techniques did not initially gain wide acceptance. Not until the cystoscopic transduodenal pancreas biopsy (CTPB) technique was developed by the Mayo Clinic transplant group did pancreatic biopsies increase. In their initial experience, Perkins et al. (100) obtained adequate pancreatic tissue in only 2 of their first 10 biopsy attempts; later, in 21 (91%) of 23 biopsy attempts, adequate pancreatic tissue was obtained. Other groups, using the same modified Menghini needle, were less successful: in a series of 75 cystoscopic biopsies, pancreatic tissue was obtained in only 57% (101). This led to two technical modifications. First, it was suggested that cystoscopic biopsies of pancreatic grafts should be obtained under intraoperative ultrasound guidance, which eventually increased the yield of pancreatic tissue significantly (22,101). Second, modified core-cut needles were developed independently by two groups: Lowell et al. (102) used 18-gauge 40-cm needles, Jones et al. (101) 14- to 18-gauge 50-cm core-cut needles (Fig. 6). As described for the percutaneous technique, the needles are mounted on a regular Biopty gun and introduced into the bladder via a side-viewing, center-channel 26-French nephroscope. Using the modified biopsy needle under intraoperative ultrasound guidance has resulted in a ≥80% yield of pancreatic tissue (101,102).

Another advantage of the cystoscopic biopsy technique is that concurrent duodenal biopsies can be obtained by inserting a gastrointestinal biopsy ("alligator") forceps through the cystoscope. Previous experimental and clinical studies showed that rejection of the duodenum highly correlates with rejection of the pancreas; however, absence of duodenal rejection does not preclude rejection of the pancreas (30,103). For clinical practicality, antirejection treatment in the absence of a pancreas biopsy is justified if the duodenal biopsy shows rejection; if the duodenal biopsy is negative for rejection and the risk:benefit ratio of treating on clinical grounds is high, rebiopsy of the pancreas should be attempted.

Cystoscopic biopsies are associated with a low complication rate: although microhematuria is frequent, postbiopsy macrohematuria is found in less than 10% of patients (52,101,102). In cases of macrohematuria, continuous bladder irrigation using a three-way Foley catheter usually corrects the bleeding. Blood transfusions and surgical reexplorations have not been necessary in the two largest series of cystoscopic biopsies (101,102). In addition, biopsy-related pancreatitis, as defined by an increase in serum amylase levels postbiopsy, is uncommon; even if present, it resolves uneventfully without further therapy.

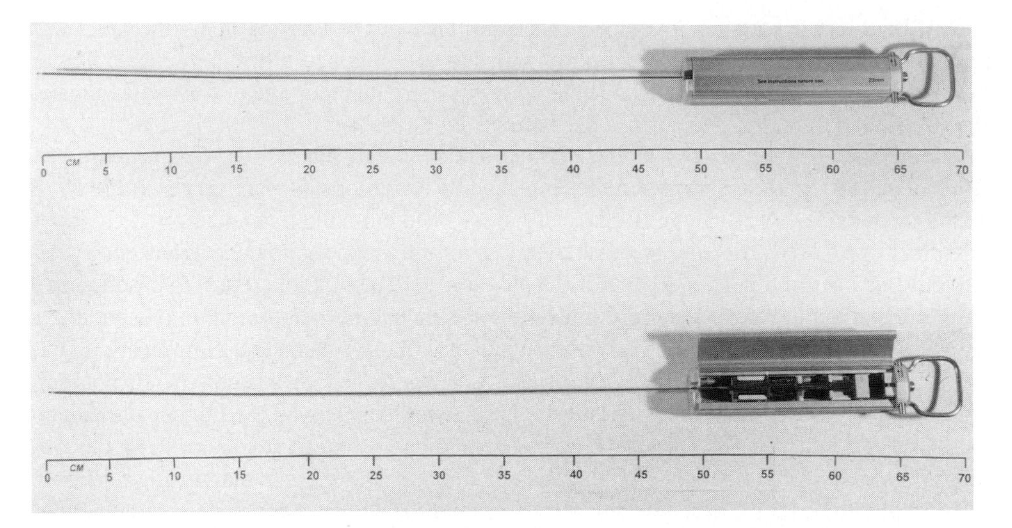

Figure 6 Core-cut biopsy needle mounted on a Biopty gun. The needle is 50 cm in length, 14- to 18-gauge in diameter. The Biopty gun is directed through a side-viewing nephroscope. Biopsies are obtained using intraoperative ultrasound.

A retrospective analysis of open versus cystoscopic biopsies clearly showed that the open procedure is associated with a higher incidence of complications, including graft loss, and is less cost-effective (104).

Cystoscopic and percutaneous biopsies are both relatively easy to do and appear to have a lower complication risk than open biopsies. The choice between cystoscopic and percutaneous biopsies is based on several considerations. Patients undergoing cystoscopic biopsies are usually hospitalized, and general (101) or regional (102) anesthesia is used. In contrast, percutaneous biopsies are equally effective—they also cost less and are done under local anesthesia; the patient may not even require hospitalization. The University of Minnesota transplant group, experienced in all three of these biopsy techniques, favors the following approach: if a biopsy is necessary, the percutaneous approach is attempted first. If pancreatic tissue is obtained and histological assessment is negative for rejection, patients are usually not hospitalized overnight unless complications arise. If tissue cannot be obtained percutaneously under CT or ultrasound guidance (e.g., due to overlying bowel, inadequate tissue sample), then the cystoscopic approach is used for bladder-drained pancreatic recipients. If this fails, and concurrent biopsies of the duodenum are negative despite a clinical suspicion of pancreatic rejection, open biopsy must be considered. Laparotomy may also become necessary for non-bladder-drained pancreas transplant recipients, if percutaneous biopsy attempts fail and if random antirejection treatment is considered riskier than open biopsy.

B. Fine-Needle Aspiration Biopsy

Before needle core biopsies were recognized to be safe and simple, fine-needle aspiration biopsy (FNAB) was considered a useful tool for the early diagnosis of pancreas rejection. In contrast to core-needle biopsy, FNAB is more prone to technical difficulties: the failure rate has been as high as 30% due to either pancreatic fluid or increasing fibrosis (98). False-positive results have also been reported, alluding to another FNAB-specific problem: it largely depends on the expertise of the pathologist (98). Finally, and again in contrast to core-needle biopsies, FNAB results cannot be duplicated and infiltrating cells are not equally sampled. For these reasons, needle-core biopsies are a better way of providing representative samples for histological evaluation.

C. Cytology

The use of pancreatic juice cytology is based on the penetration of inflammatory cells into the pancreatic ducts; these cells appear in the juice as an early sign of rejection. One of the first applications of pancreatic juice cytology was in the setting of temporary external drainage of the pancreatic duct in enteric-drained pancreatic transplants (105). In a study of 6 PTA and 2 PAK recipients, 8 rejection episodes were diagnosed by loss of amylase concentration in the pancreatic juice; in 7 of these cases, cytology revealed increased cellularity with a relative increase in the number of mononuclear cells and the occurrence of lympho- or monoblasts. Among 12 SPK recipients with a total of 30 kidney graft rejection episodes, pancreatic juice cytology was suggestive of pancreatic graft involvement in 3. The appearance of lymphoblasts in the juice preceded the decrease in pancreatic juice amylase activity by 1 to 2 days for all rejection episodes (105). In a study of 1116 cytologic specimens obtained from 35 pancreatic grafts, the sensitivity of pancreatic juice cytology was 87% and the specificity 97% (106). The authors found pancreatic juice cytology helpful in diagnosing other complications such as pancreatitis; bacterial, viral, or fungal infections; and CSA toxicity. According to their definition of acute cellular rejection, two or more of the following criteria had to be detected: (a) increase in cell numbers by ≥30% versus baseline (present in 53% of all rejection episodes in their study); (b) >5% lymphocytes in the differential count (present in 90%); (c) eosinophil granulocytes (present in 60%); and/or (d) necrotic epithelial cells (present in 80%). Changes in pancreatic juice cytology preceded clinical diagnosis by 2 to 5 days (106,107). One of the drawbacks of pancreatic juice cytology is that isolated vascular rejection cannot be detected, theoretically increasing the rate of false-negative results (106,107).

For pancreatic transplant recipients, not only pancreatic juice cytology but also urine cytology has been useful for bladder-drained grafts in diagnosing rejection. In a study by the Nebraska group, 1444 urine cytologic specimens collected from 61 bladder-drained SPK recipients were evaluated; a sensitivity of 75% was reported (108). When the urine cytological score was combined with HLA-DR antigen staining, sensitivity was 93%, specificity 99%, positive predictive value 62%, and negative predictive value 99% (108). HLA-DR antigen staining takes advantage of the association of rejection with induction of MHC class II antigen expression and upregulation on allograft parenchymal cells. In several studies by Radio et al. (108–110), positive cytological signs of immunoactivation preceded exocrine dysfunction by 1 day, and were more sensitive than UA activity, UA concentrations, or serum amylase levels. Limitations of the technique were (a) persistence of HLA-DR antigen staining long after successful antirejection treatment; (b) CMV infections, mimicking positive urine cytology and positive HLA-DR antigen staining and lymphocyturia; and (c) severe pancreatitis (preservation injury) resulting in the shedding of neutrophils and epithelial cells immediately posttransplant (108).

With the availability of percutaneous and cystoscopic pancreatic graft biopsies, the usefulness of urine or pancreatic juice cytology as a substitute for biopsy must be determined by doing both for correlation. If shown to have a good correlation, urine cytology could be an alternative for patients in whom pancreatic biopsies are considered too risky (e.g., those with systemic anticoagulation or graft pancreatitis).

VI. IMAGING TECHNIQUES FOR DIAGNOSIS OF REJECTION

While imaging techniques have been helpful in a variety of pathological conditions after pancreatic transplantation—such as pancreatitis, graft thrombosis, and intraabdominal infection—most techniques have failed to reach the level of clinical relevance in the (early) diagnosis of rejection. There are virtually no correlative studies with biopsies, calling into question most of the conclusions in the published papers.

A. Scintigram

A variety of tracers have been studied in pancreatic transplant recipients: technetium-99 DPTA, technetium-99 sulfur colloid, technetium-99 glucoheptonate, technetium-99 HMPAO, technetium-99 red blood cells, selenium 75 methionine, and indium-111 platelets (111). Clinically, the most frequent tracer is technetium-99 DPTA, due to visualization of the simultaneously transplanted kidney. Computer analysis can generate a quantitative measure of blood flow to the pancreas (technetium index, TI); however, poor visualization of the pancreas has been reported during radionuclide flow studies despite normal allograft function. Therefore, in clinical practice, the results are usually interpreted in conjunction with laboratory data (such as UA) and clinical findings. The Wisconsin group reported a TI prerejection mean of 0.57% (i.e., 0.6% of the total amount of tracer injected into the recipient is sequestered or localized in the pancreas). The TI rejection mean was 0.39%. After rejection therapy, TI >0.3 was associated with a 96% graft survival rate, whereas levels <0.3 resulted in a 73% graft loss rate. It appears that technetium-99 DPTA studies might help predict outcome after rejection treatment (112). Other studies using technetium-99 sulfur colloid or indium-111 platelets have also claimed some usefulness in differentiating rejection from other pathological conditions (113,114). The drawback of all scintigraphic methods, however, is that while they are capable of differentiating grafts with normal versus abnormal function, they are not capable of distinguishing subtle changes, such as early rejection versus mild pancreatitis.

B. Ultrasound, CT, and MRI

Sonographic studies have not been helpful in diagnosing rejection, although patterns of patchy decreased echogenicity have been linked with acute rejection (115). But graft inhomogenicity can also be seen with preservation injury, pancreatitis, or (partial) thrombosis (116,117). Graft enlargement has been noted in association with acute rejection or pancreatitis. Duplex color Doppler flow sonography has been successfully used in one study in the immediate postoperative period for reasons other than rejection: the investigators found that a low splenic vein velocity, associated with absence of pulsatile flow and inadequate glucose control, suggested partial splenic vein thrombosis. For other purposes, such as rejection, duplex color Doppler flow sonography has not been helpful (118). Others have suggested that Doppler sonography of intrapancreatic arterial flow and determination of resistive index values can help diagnose acute rejection. But the intraabdominal location of the pancreas, which causes occasional difficulty with visualization (i.e., overlying gas), and the lack of sensitivity and specificity for resistive indices (as demonstrated for renal and hepatic transplants) have tempered enthusiasm for the use of Doppler sonography in diagnosing rejection (117).

Likewise, CT studies have not been able to reliably diagnose (early) rejection. Graft inhomogenicity can be seen, but is nonspecific (117,119). Irreversible rejection diminishes graft size due to shrinkage and fibrosis (115,119). Computed tomography studies in pancreas recipients are best used to detect major parenchymal abnormalities (e.g., thrombosis, edema, hemorrhage, pseudocyst) and abdominal fluid but not to diagnose rejection (117). No studies correlating the images with biopsies are reported.

A few MRI studies have been conducted in pancreas grafts during rejection. One group noted changes in tissue water content, such as inflammatory edema during rejection and a decrease in congestion after effective treatment (120). However, false-positive results were noted, especially during recovery from acute rejection and in the immediate postoperative period; the false-negative rate was low, suggesting that rejection is unlikely if MRI is negative. In a retrospective study comparing nuclear medicine, ultrasound, and MRI, it appeared that MRI had the highest sensitivity and specificity in detecting rejection (121). MRI, in conjunction with blood flow studies (magnetic resonance angiography, MRA), showed good promise in another study: pancreatic graft and peripancreatic edema was observed in all cases of moderate or severe rejection, but mild rejection could not be detected by MRI/MRA (122). The use of false-positive and false-negative terminology should not be taken as indicative of a definitive study, since the terms were used without correlation with biopsy; instead, correlation was made with the clinical decision to treat. Further studies are needed to investigate whether MRI is more useful in suggesting rejection than CT or ultrasound studies.

In summary, imaging techniques today can help diagnose a variety of pathological conditions after pancreatic transplantation, but unfortunately, are not capable of diagnosing early rejection.

VII. IMMUNOSUPPRESSION

The principles of immunosuppressive therapy for pancreas recipients are basically the same as for recipients of other solid-organ allografts. However, the amount of immunosuppression required appears to be more than for liver, heart, or kidney transplants alone. This is based on a higher incidence of rejection episodes, at least initially.

Combination immunotherapy has been the mainstay of clinical immunosuppression dating back to the first pancreatic transplants in the 1960s (123). Initially, most pancreas recipients were treated with a combination of prednisone and azathioprine; later, a polyclonal antibody was added for induction. Despite these efforts, pancreatic graft survival was poor in the precyclosporine era, with 1-year graft survival rates approaching only 25% (124,125).

The advent of cyclosporine (CSA) had a major impact on the acceptance of pancreas transplantation as an option for selected type I diabetic patients. CSA was used with other agents, most commonly as part of triple therapy with prednisone and azathioprine (123,124). Only a few centers have used CSA alone (126), and CSA monotherapy has not become popular. While triple therapy has become the standard for maintenance, the additional use of anti-T-cell therapy has remained somewhat controversial.

Over the last few years, convincing data have accumulated in support of quadruple immunosuppression for induction. A randomized multicenter Scandinavian study compared triple ($n = 23$) versus quadruple ($n = 20$) induction immunosuppression in SPK recipients. It showed that quadruple induction therapy with polyclonal antibody therapy (ATG) not only postponed the first rejection episode, but also reduced the number of rejection episodes in SPK recipients (127). Others have confirmed the superiority of quadruple over triple immunosuppression for induction. The IPTR analyzed the results with use of anti-T-cell therapy and CSA given either for maintenance only or for both induction and maintenance, and found that the best results were when both were given for induction, but one or the other must be given to prevent inferior results (128).

In a retrospective study at a single center, Sollinger et al. (129) compared the use of monoclonal (OKT3) vs. polyclonal (Minnesota antilymphocyte globulin, MALG) antibody therapy during induction. Pancreatic and kidney graft and patient survival were not significantly different at 1 year posttransplant between groups. For kidney grafts, median serum creatinine levels were equal (1.8 mg/dL) in both groups at discharge. The overall rate of rejection episodes was similar in both groups (93% OKT3, 86% ALG). Likewise, the frequency of rejection during induction (within the first 14 days posttransplant) was no different between groups (40% OKT3, 45% ALG). The only significant difference was the rate of opportunistic infection: it was higher in the OKT3 group. In particular, CMV infections occurred with a significantly higher frequency during the first 6 months posttransplant in the OKT3 group. Based on these data, the authors recommended polyclonal antibody therapy for induction (129).

Others have used the monoclonal antibody OKT3 for induction because of batch homogeneity and predictability, ease of administration (peripheral versus central for ATG or ALG), its selective antilymphocytic effect, and consistent dosing. In addition, outpatient administration of OKT3 is feasible in selected cases and is also more cost-effective. Among the drawbacks are undesirable side effects due to cytokine release. Stratta et al. (130) reported dose-limiting side effects in 21% of 100 pancreas recipients. High-titer anti-OKT3 antibody developed in 6%. While the incidence of acute rejection was 62%, with most rejection episodes occurring in the first 2 months posttransplant, the rate of immunological graft losses was only 5%. The risk of major infection was 41%, with 1 death due to sepsis. The authors cautioned that intraoperatively administering the initial dose of OKT3 is not necessarily protective against cytokine side effects, because diabetic patients are predisposed to pulmonary capillary leak syndrome (130,131).

Another advantage of antibody therapy during induction is that it spares CSA in the immediate posttransplant period, a factor that is most important for SPK recipients. If the transplanted kidney's immediate function is consistent with acute tubular necrosis, the administration of CSA, due to its nephrotoxic side effects, can be delayed; it has been recommended that antibody therapy and CSA overlap for at least 2 to 3 days to achieve therapeutic CSA levels by the time antibody therapy is discontinued.

According to the immunosuppressive protocol used by the University of Minnesota, anti-T-cell therapy is given to SPK recipients for 10 days and to PTA and PAK recipients for 14 days during induction. For PTA and PAK recipients only, CSA is continuously given intravenously immediately posttransplant (daily IV dosage: 3 mg/kg); for SPK recipients, it is usually delayed for 5 days. Thereafter, the dose is tapered to maintain CSA blood levels between 200 and 300 ng/mL for the first 6 months, 150 to 200 ng/mL for the second 6 months, and 100 to 150 ng/mL thereafter. Azathioprine is given at a dose of 2.5 mg/kg/day, and adjusted to maintain a whole white blood count of $\geqslant 3 \times 10^9$ cells per liter. The initial prednisone dose is 2 mg/kg/day, then tapered to 0.5 mg/kg/day by 1 month and 0.2 mg/kg/day by 1 year (123).

The importance of high CSA trough levels during maintenance therapy has been pointed out by several groups (132,133). Dawidson et al. (132), in a study of 20 SPK recipients, noted that rejection episodes occurred only in patients with CSA levels below 300 ng/mL (TDX-specific monoclonal assay). However, 13 biopsies were read as CSA nephrotoxicity, but 9 of the 13 (72%) had CSA levels ⩾400 ng/mL. High CSA levels were achieved by simultaneously administering the calcium antagonist verapamil. While verapamil induced about two times higher blood CSA levels, it also induced markedly improved renal function as well as partial protection from CSA-induced renal dysfunction. It appears that CSA levels between 300 and 400 ng/mL are a practical clinical therapeutic window—eliminating rejection but accepting 20% CSA nephrotoxicity. Cantarovich et al. (133) maintained trough CSA blood levels between 200 and 300 ng/ml (RIA); an episode of CSA-induced nephrotoxicity on renal histology was noted in only 1 of their 50 SPK recipients, requiring CSA tapering and CSA levels of <150 ng/mL. They also noted that the kinetics of CSA blood levels is different for SPK versus nondiabetic KTA recipients: while trough 4- and 6-hr CSA levels were similar in both groups, SPK recipients had significantly lower 2-hr CSA levels; moreover, 25% of SPK recipients had lower 4- and 6-hr CSA levels than the trough levels, versus 9 and 8% of nondiabetic KTA recipients (133). Diabetic enteroneuropathy, present in most of their SPK recipients, could in part explain the difference.

Very few clinical studies have been done using some of the new immunosuppressive agents. FK506 has been used for pancreatic transplantation at some centers to replace CSA, but, so far, no prospective studies have compared the two for either induction or maintenance therapy.

Cantarovich et al. (134), in a prospective randomized trial of 40 SPK recipients, compared the effects of induction with the rat IgG 2a monoclonal antibody 33B3.1 versus rabbit ATG. The rat IgG 2a monoclonal antibody 33B3.1 is directed against the human alpha chain of the Il-2 receptor. Both antibodies were given for 10 days posttransplant at 10 mg/day/patient each. For induction and maintenance, recipients also took azathioprine, low-dose corticosteroids, and CSA. The incidence of rejection episodes during the first 3 months posttransplant was higher but not significantly different in 33B3.1 recipients versus ATG recipients; after the third month, more recipients in the 33B3.1 group experienced rejection episodes and the difference was statistically significant. The onset of rejection episodes was similar in both 33B3.1 and ATG groups. The gravity of the rejection process (as judged by need for rescue therapy) was also similar in the two groups. OKT3 as first-line treatment was highly effective in reversing rejection episodes for either 33B3.1 or ATG recipients, suggesting that previous exposure to anti-IL-2 receptor monoclonal antibody or polyclonal antilymphocyte serum may not interfere with the use of other monoclonal antibodies such as anti-CD3 monoclonal antibody. Immunologic graft losses, although not significantly different, were higher in the 33B3.1 group (2 pancreas, 2 kidney) than in the ATG group (1 kidney), suggesting that 33B3.1 monoclonal antibody was less effective than ATG in preventing rejection. The 3-month and 36-month patient, pancreatic, and kidney actuarial survival rates did not differ between the two groups. The study suggests that 33B3.1 monoclonal antibody is less effective than ATG due to a significantly higher rate of rejection episodes, but long-term graft and patient survival were not significantly different between the 33B3.1 and ATG groups.

At most centers, pancreatic rejection episodes are treated with a 7- to 14-day course of mono- or polyclonal antibody (123,129,135). The Wisconsin group reported on 46 rejection episodes in 21 recipients (13 SPK, 8 PAK) treated with OKT3 (53). Indications for OKT3 use included steroid- or antilymphoblast globulin-resistant rejection. OKT3 was administered for 14 days, concomitant with pulsed corticosteroids. In 62% of recipients, OKT3 rescue therapy was successful, but significant differences by recipient category were noted: for SPK recipients, 92% of rejection episodes were responsive to OKT3; for PAK recipients, only 13%. The mean time to rejection reversal was 8.8 days; graft loss from rejection occurred at a mean of 5.5 days posttransplant. OKT3 therapy was most successful for recipients with early rejection, for SPK recipients with rejection, and for rejection not associated with hyperglycemia. No graft losses were due to infection or patient death after OKT3 treatment. Salvage treatment with OKT3 appears safe and effective in reversing pancreatic rejection (53). The validity of this study, however, was hampered because pancreatic rejection was based on clinical criteria, not on pancreatic biopsies.

The increasing diagnostic usefulness of percutaneous and cystoscopic biopsy techniques may help determine whether pancreatic rejection treatment can be individualized by severity of the rejection episode as graded by a pathologist. It is conceivable that minimal or mild pancreatic rejection may only require steroid boluses or recycling of the steroid taper. Antibody therapy may be necessary only to reverse moderate and severe rejection episodes. These hypotheses must be tested in clinical studies.

Controversy still exists over whether SPK recipients with isolated kidney rejection episodes require anti-T-cell therapy. If the kidney biopsy shows moderate or severe interstitial rejection with or without a vascular component, anti-T-cell therapy is usually recommended; if kidney rejection is graded as mild, treatment with corticosteroids alone can be attempted, but the incidence of ongoing rejection is high (unpublished data, University of Minnesota). Steroid-resistant kidney rejection episodes account for 47 to 96% of all kidney rejection episodes (136,137), a rate that is significantly higher than for steroid-resistant rejection episodes in KTA recipients.

VIII. CLINICAL REJECTION

A. Rejection by Recipient Categories

Most studies comparing graft survival by recipient categories have focused on the kidney rather than the pancreas, due to the greater ease of obtaining kidney biopsies. The most commonly studied recipient categories are SPK and KTA. Very few investigators have compared the incidence of pancreatic rejection for SPK versus PTA recipients; so far, none of these studies is based on pancreatic biopsy results. The PAK group has been included in only one study, in which kidney survival was compared for SPK versus PAK versus KTA recipients and pancreatic survival for SPK versus PAK versus PTA recipients (96).

1. SPK versus KTA

It is widely accepted that the simultaneously transplanted pancreas does not jeopardize the kidney. While this is true for the incidence of graft loss from rejection, some studies have shown a higher rate of reversible kidney rejection episodes for SPK (versus KTA) recipients. This is documented, for example, in a study by the Minnesota group comparing 69 primary cadaver SPK versus 59 primary cadaver KTA recipients (136). The SPK group experienced significantly more episodes of first acute rejections (72%) than the KTA group (39%). There were, however, no differences in regard to the mean number of acute rejection episodes per patient (1.0 ± 0.1 SPK, 1.0 ± 0.2 KTA) and serum creatinine levels at 1 year (1.8 ± 0.1 SPK, 1.9 ± 0.1 KTA). Similarly, the overall actuarial kidney graft survival rates were no different between groups: at 1 year, 80% for SPK and 86% for KTA; at 2 years,

75% for SPK and 86% for KTA recipients. Several other groups have also reported more first acute rejection episodes for SPK (versus KTA) recipients. Sollinger et al. (138) found a rejection rate of 89% for SPK versus 59% for diabetic KTA recipients. The Mayo Clinic group also showed that the mean number of acute kidney rejection episodes per patient was higher for SPK (1.5 ± 1.0) than KTA (0.8 ± 0.6) recipients (137). In addition, SPK recipients experienced rejection episodes throughout the first year, whereas for KTA recipients, rejection episodes occurred only during the first 3 months. Another difference between the two groups was that acute rejection episodes for SPK recipients were relatively refractory to methylprednisolone treatment, particularly if the pancreas was involved: only 2 of 50 combined pancreas and kidney rejection episodes were reversed with methylprednisolone. Isolated kidney rejection episodes were reversed with methylprednisolone in 67% of SPK recipients versus 80% of KTA recipients. As for the two previously discussed studies, there was no difference in regard to kidney graft loss from rejection between the SPK and KTA groups. Schulak et al. (139), in a study of 60 SPK and 28 diabetic KTA recipients, found a 75% incidence of rejection episodes (SPK) versus 54% (KTA). Steroid-resistant rejection episodes were also more common for SPK (47%) than KTA (22%) recipients. Only 1 SPK kidney was lost due to irreversible rejection versus 4 KTA kidneys, all of which developed irreversible rejection.

Differences in induction therapy and the incidence of kidney rejection episodes were studied by Hedman et al. (140). Of 19 SPK recipients, 10 received triple-drug and 9 quadruple-drug induction therapy. Of 15 diabetic KTA recipients, all received triple-drug therapy. There were significant differences between quadruple- versus triple-drug induction therapy for SPK recipients; those receiving triple-drug therapy had more rejection episodes (1.8 ± 1.0 vs. 1.0 ± 0.8), a higher incidence of >1 rejection episode (60% versus 27%), and a higher incidence of ATG treatment for rejection (60% versus 7%). No significant differences were found between triple-drug KTA and quadruple-drug SPK recipients in regard to the number of rejection episodes, the percentage of patients with >1 rejection episode, and the percentage of patients treated with ATG for rejection. Thus, quadruple- but not triple-drug therapy for SPK recipients provides similar results as triple-drug therapy for KTA recipients.

Similarly, Cantarovich et al. (141) observed no significant difference in the incidence of rejection episodes for 67 SPK and 100 nondiabetic KTA recipients; all had received quadruple-drug induction therapy. The 3-month incidence of rejection episodes was 33% for SPK versus 29% for KTA recipients; after the third month, the incidence of rejection was 8% for SPK versus 5% for KTA recipients. Only three patients in each group required rescue therapy. There were no differences between the two groups in regard to the 1-year mean serum creatinine levels and actuarial kidney graft survival rates (91% KTA, 85% SPK).

Two European studies done more than 5 years ago reported a poorer long-term outcome of kidney grafts for SPK (versus KTA) recipients (142,143). The first, a multicenter study orchestrated by Eurotransplant, retrospectively analyzed the early pancreas transplant experience (1979 through 1987) in 16 Eurotransplant centers with 134 SPK and 335 diabetic KTA recipients (137). Kidney graft survival rates at 1 and 3 years were 73 and 52% for SPK versus 78 and 64% for KTA recipients; the difference between both groups failed to reach significance. The less favorable SPK result was explained by poorer HLA matching (142). A single-center study by Hillebrand et al. (143) analyzed the early experience of the Munich group with 53 SPK recipients (1981 through 1986). Kidney graft survival at 4 years was only 26%. The authors stated that long-term survival was better for

KTA recipients, but did not give numbers. As in the multicenter study, the high incidence of mismatches in the SPK group was blamed for the poor results. Both studies, representing early experience with inadequate immunosuppressive protocols, are good examples of the continuing progress achieved in the field of pancreatic transplantation, with constant improvement in outcome over time.

2. SPK versus PTA

Studies of pancreatic rejection comparing SPK versus PTA recipients are scarce. In contrast to SPK, with its higher rate of technical failure during the first year posttransplant, rejection is the major cause of graft loss for PTA recipients during the first year posttransplant. After the first year, very few SPK pancreas grafts are lost from rejection, but rejection remains not only the major but also a frequent cause of PTA graft loss (144). In PTA recipients, only the pancreas can be monitored. The bladder drainage technique has therefore been particularly useful in this group for both laboratory monitoring and cystoscopic biopsies. Results published by the Stockholm, Minnesota, and Munich groups have shown that the incidence of rejection episodes and graft loss from rejection is significantly higher for PTA (versus SPK) recipients. The increasing use of HLA matching to reduce rejection, and the close monitoring of urine amylase to detect early rejection in conjunction with confirmatory biopsy may improve the results for PTA recipients, particularly if early antirejection treatment with anti-T-cell agents is initiated (144–146).

3. SPK versus PTA versus PAK versus KTA

Only one retrospective study has analyzed the incidence of reversible rejection and graft loss from rejection in all four diabetic recipient categories (96). The diagnosis of kidney rejection was based on biopsies; pancreatic rejection, on laboratory and clinical parameters. This study comprised 39 SPK, 31 PTA, 10 PAK, and 48 diabetic KTA recipients. For pancreatic grafts, the cumulative incidence of rejection episodes at 1 year was 61% for SPK, 75% for PAK, and 96% for PTA recipients; for kidney grafts, 71% for SPK and 46% for KTA recipients. When only technically successful cases were analyzed, similar disparities were noted for pancreatic rejection episodes between the SPK and PTA groups and for kidney rejection episodes between the SPK and KTA groups. The incidence of first rejection episodes was higher for recipients of solitary pancreas transplants, as was the number of recipients with multiple rejection episodes. The 1-year pancreas graft loss rate from rejection was 7% for SPK, 17% for PAK, and 42% for PTA recipients: only the difference between SPK and PTA was statistically significant. In contrast to pancreas transplants, no significant difference was found in regard to kidney graft loss from rejection for SPK (11% at 1 year) versus KTA (2%) recipients (96). Based on these data, two conclusions can be drawn. First, a pancreatic graft does not jeopardize the simultaneously transplanted kidney; although the incidence of reversible kidney rejection episodes is higher for SPK (versus KTA) recipients, no differences were found in regard to graft loss from rejection. Second, a simultaneously transplanted kidney downmodulates pancreas graft rejection for SPK (versus PTA) recipients; this justifies the use of a more vigorous immunosuppressive regimen for PTA (versus SPK) recipients in clinical practice.

B. HLA Matching

IPTR data show that HLA matching has an impact on PAK and PTA but not SPK outcome. In an analysis of 2185 registry cases, graft survival rates were compared for 0 to 1 versus 2 to 6 HLA-A, B, and DR antigen mismatches (18). Uni- and multivariate analyses were done for technically successful cases only, thus reflecting the pure impact of HLA matching on graft loss from an immunological cause (rejection).

The univariate analysis showed differences between the three pancreas recipient categories. For SPK recipients, mismatching had no adverse effect: 1-year graft survival rates were 74% in the 0 to 1 and 85% in the 2- to 6-antigen mismatch groups. For PAK recipients, mismatching made a significant difference: 1-year graft survival rates were 85% for 0- to 1- and 58% for the 2- to 6-antigen mismatch groups. For PTA recipients, HLA matching had some effect on outcome: 1-year graft survival rates were 63% for the 0- to 1- and 58% for the 2- to 6-antigen mismatch groups; results with no mismatch were superior to the results with one mismatch. The multivariate analysis showed that HLA matching has a significant effect on both solitary pancreas transplant groups (PTA, PAK).

These data suggest that, in regard to graft loss from rejection, SPK transplants can be done liberally when it comes to HLA matching. For recipients of solitary pancreas transplants (PTA, PAK), however, HLA matching is of great importance: good matching can significantly decrease the incidence of graft loss from rejection. In contrast to some single-center studies (147–149) suggesting that good DR matching decreases the risk of rejection, differences in regard to the antigen loci have not been consistent in registry data (18). However, all outcome results in regard to HLA matching must be considered with caution. While some kidney transplant registries comprise more than 100,000 cases in one recipient category, only a few thousand pancreatic transplants have been done in the three recipient categories. More data must be accumulated to reliably analyze the incidence of graft loss according to HLA loci.

The matching effect in solitary pancreatic transplants is also exemplified by the Minnesota experience with living related pancreas transplants. Of 81 transplants from genetic relatives, 52 were HLA-identical and 48% mismatched for 1 haplotype (150). The incidence of graft loss from rejection was significantly lower in pancreas transplants from living related (30%) versus cadaver (41%) donors. This significant difference was noted despite less immunosuppression for living related pancreas recipients. The incidence of rejection episodes was also significantly lower.

One aspect of pancreatic transplants from living related donors is of special interest: the Minnesota experience with identical twin transplants. In the absence of immunosuppression, the first three twin recipients were susceptible to isletitis and disease recurrence; all three became hyperglycemic 6 to 12 weeks posttransplant. Biopsies showed isletitis and selective beta-cell destruction, and, despite polyclonal antibody therapy, the grafts were not salvageable. The fourth twin received azathioprine prophylactically and was normoglycemic for 3 years. Hyperglycemia then occurred with selective beta-cell destruction, per graft biopsy; the patient initially responded to polyclonal antibody therapy and CSA but resumed insulin 5 years posttransplant. The last three twins received immunosuppression with CSA and azathioprine; all three are normoglycemic 4 to 7.5 years posttransplant (150,151). Although both disease recurrence and rejection can present with hyperglycemia, the latter cause of graft failure does not apply to pancreases from identical twin donors. The diagnosis of disease recurrence is made histologically, as outlined in Chap. 11.

C. Rejection in SPK Recipients

Like all other forms of multiple organ transplants, combined pancreatic and kidney transplants provide an opportunity to study the immunological response of the recipient to different organs from the same donor. The previously discussed large animal studies in pigs and dogs have demonstrated, based on concurrent biopsies, that reversible rejection episodes and graft loss from rejection can occur in each organ independently. In contrast to animal studies, histological proof of this phenomenon in humans is usually not obtained, due to the limited willingness of most centers to obtain concurrent biopsies. In clinical practice, the most accessible allograft is biopsied and indirect measures are used to diagnose rejection in the other graft. The lack of concurrent biopsies—regardless of whether a suspected rejection episode clinically involves only one or more grafts—makes any interpretation of organ-specific involvement in multiple transplants inaccurate and unreliable. In fact, histological inadequacy of most of these clinical studies may lead to over- or underdiagnosis of clinical rejection.

1. Rejection Episodes

Most clinical studies report differences between pancreatic and kidney grafts in regard to timing and severity of rejection episodes. Rejection episodes for SPK recipients can involve both the pancreas and kidney, the kidney alone, or the pancreas alone. Most investigators have found the incidence of isolated pancreatic rejection lower than either combined pancreatic and kidney rejection or isolated kidney rejection. There are, however, study-specific differences as to whether rejection episodes more frequently affect both the pancreas and kidney or the kidney alone.

Several groups have reported that rejection episodes most commonly involve both organs. Margreiter et al. (152), in a study of 26 SPK recipients using three different techniques to manage pancreas exocrine secretions, noted involvement of the pancreas and kidney in 53%, of the kidney alone in 23%, and of the pancreas alone in 23% of all rejection episodes. Dubernard et al. (153) reported on 106 rejection episodes in 72 SPK recipients with enteric drainage: 57% of the rejection episodes involved both the pancreas and kidney, 43% the kidney alone; no biopsies were done of the pancreas, so this is only a study of ramifications. The Wisconsin group, in a series of 52 SPK recipients, found involvement of both the pancreas and kidney in 73% of rejection episodes vs. kidney rejection only in 25% and pancreas rejection only in 2% (68). Again, the incidence of kidney only rejection may be an overestimate in the absence of pancreatic graft biopsies.

An equal number of investigators have reported a higher incidence of isolated kidney rejection episodes. The Minnesota group, in a series of 39 SPK recipients, found that in 47% of all rejection episodes the kidney alone was clinically involved, in 37% the pancreas and the kidney, and in 16% the pancreas alone (96,154). In 44% of all rejection episodes involving the kidney, pancreatic rejection was clinically present or detected; in 69% of all rejection episodes involving the pancreas, kidney rejection was clinically present. Thus, of all pancreatic rejection episodes, the kidney may not have been affected a third of the time, but in the absence of biopsies this is only an estimate. Once treatment is initiated, subclinical rejections may be reversed and not counted as rejections. The overall 1-year cumulative incidence of rejection episodes was 71% for kidney and 61% for pancreatic grafts. The rate of early rejection episodes was high: 49% of the recipients had one, 21% two, and 3% three rejection episodes during the first 4 months. Recipients with two sequential rejection episodes had involvement of the same organ in 54% (with kidney the most common) and different organ combinations in 46% of rejection episodes. Recipients with an early first acute rejection episode (within the first 4 months posttransplant) or with >1 rejection episode had an increased incidence of graft loss from rejection (154).

Tesi et al. (155), in a study of 160 technically successful whole-organ bladder-drained SPK recipients, noted a total of 146 clinical rejection episodes: 55% involved the kidney only, 34% the pancreas and kidney, and 11% the pancreas alone. They also found several other differences between pancreatic and kidney rejection. They not only noted a higher frequency of rejection episodes in the kidney (0.81 per patient) versus the pancreas (0.41 per patient), but also a three times higher frequency of multiple rejection episodes in kidney (20%) versus pancreatic (6%) grafts. The average time to first rejection episodes was 45 days (range, 5 to 190 days) for the kidney and 70 days (range, 15 to 295 days) for the pancreas. Likewise, a total of 71% of first kidney rejection episodes occurred in the first 70 days posttransplant versus only 51% of first pancreatic rejection episodes. In addition, they showed a clear correlation between the number of rejection episodes and graft survival: 4-year graft survival for organs without rejection episodes was 88% for kidney and 97% for pancreatic grafts; for organs with one rejection episode, 97 and 90%; for organs with >1 organ rejection episodes, 56 and 67%. All graft losses in the last group (>1 rejection episodes) were related to acute and chronic rejection (155). These data suggest that the less favorable long-term kidney graft survival was due to the higher frequency of rejection episodes in the kidney versus the pancreas; again, biopsies are lacking.

The Stockholm group (105) was the first to histologically document differences in concomitant biopsies of pancreas and kidney: while the kidney biopsy showed interstitial rejection, the pancreatic biopsy was without histological signs of rejection. So far, only one study, by Barr et al. (156), has investigated organ involvement based on a large series of concurrent biopsies of pancreatic and kidney grafts. They found rejection episodes in both the pancreas and kidney in 42%, isolated kidney rejection in 32%, and isolated pancreatic rejection in 26%. According to their study, the pancreas and kidney reject independently in 58%. This may, however, represent an artificially high percentage, since nearly 50% of the biopsies were obtained on a protocol basis. These data suggest that confirmatory biopsies should be obtained for episodes of clinically suspected pancreatic rejection to avoid overimmunosuppression.

2. *Graft Loss from Rejection*

In his initial series of 14 pancreatic transplants, Lillehei et al. (157) reported on 1 SPK recipient who lost the kidney from acute rejection but kept the pancreas; they suggested that the pancreas might be less antigenic than the kidney when transplanted simultaneously. Most investigators, however, have not found any significant organ-specific prevalence in regard to the incidence of irreversible graft loss from rejection. The Minnesota group reported a cumulative incidence of 1-year graft loss from rejection as 7% for pancreatic and 11% for kidney grafts (96). Likewise, no significant difference was found in a study by Tesi et al. (155) of 160 SPK recipients: 9 (6%) lost the pancreas and 15 (9%) lost the kidney from rejection. Stratta et al. (135), in a study of 82 consecutive SPK recipients, noted 5 kidney graft losses from rejection (2 refractory acute, 3 chronic) and 2 pancreas graft losses from rejection (both chronic); 2 recipients with rejection-related kidney graft loss remained insulin-independent with normal pancreatic graft function.

The Wisconsin group, in a study of 200 consecutive SPK recipients, noted graft loss from rejection in the kidney only in 9 recipients and in the pancreas only in 3 recipients; both the pancreas and kidney were lost from rejection in 14 recipients (158).

The Minnesota group (159), in a study of discordant graft loss for same-donor SPK recipients, found that either the pancreas or kidney from a single donor, in a single recipient, can be discordantly lost from rejection. Based on 158 technically successful SPK transplants, pancreas graft loss from rejection without kidney rejection was noted in 3 recipients, kidney graft loss from rejection without pancreas rejection in 12. Of note was the low incidence of sustained function of the nonrejected graft, which was higher for the pancreas than for the kidney: it appears that the pancreas is more likely to function with the kidney being rejected than vice versa. While a total of 15 recipients lost only one graft from rejection, an additional 5 SPK recipients rejected both grafts and resumed both dialysis and insulin within a month of each other (range, 1 to 23 months posttransplant). Due to the discordant rejection patterns, an "element of chaos" (159) in the immune response or of local immune events cannot be ruled out.

Differences in the rejection response to individual organs from the same donor reflect the influence of factors other than MHC disparities per se, since histocompatibility antigens are absolutely identical for both pancreas and kidney relative to the recipient. Several hypotheses may help explain the different immunologic response of the recipient to various organs from the same donor:

1. The entrapment or consumption hypothesis is based on the suggestion that lymphocytes from peripheral blood are trapped in the kidney due to its greater blood supply and larger amount of endothelium, compared with the pancreas (41,160). More peripheral blood cells become involved in the rejection process in the kidney and then are not available to the pancreas. If this hypothesis were true, only a one-way shift in rejection should occur; this, however, contradicts the above clinical and experimental study results.
2. Another hypothesis is that uremia exerts a nonspecific immunosuppressive effect (161). Posttransplant uremia that occurs with kidney rejection suppresses the immune system and delays pancreatic rejection. This may explain the higher incidence of kidney than pancreatic involvement in rejection episodes. Kidney rejection is diagnosed first, antirejection treatment is initiated, and the pancreas may not experience a rejection episode at all. This explanation, however, is not in line with some research results: when the impact of azotemia on the rejection process was studied in rats, the functional survival time of pancreatic allografts was no different for SPK recipients that were versus were not uremia-free (45). In a clinical study of preemptive versus postdialysis SPK transplants, Stratta et al. showed that the incidence of both acute rejection and chronic rejection, the timing of first rejection episodes, and the incidence of antilymphocyte rescue therapy did not differ between the two groups (162). Uremia per se is therefore not the reason that pancreatic rejection is delayed.
3. According to the dilution hypothesis (41), the immune response is no different for single versus dual-organ transplants. The same number of effector cells are generated, but they have to be distributed to a greater tissue mass; the dilution results in a slower destruction of parenchymal tissue. This hypothesis is not consistent with the clinical observation that adding a pancreas increases the tendency toward rejection episodes of the kidney.
4. It has also been hypothesized that MHC expression is different in the kidney and pancreas; this is based on observations in rats, where it has been postulated that non-MHC antigens have a different distribution in one organ as opposed to another (47). Another explanation is that non-MHC alloantigens in the parenchyma cause intrinsic differences in the expression or distribution of MHC alloantigens and may trigger different responses in each allograft. Alternatively, if organ-specific alloantigens were solely responsible for discordant rejection, the

allele pool should be greater in one of the two organs. Again, this would explain only one-way shifts in rejection, but not two-way shifts.

5. Still another hypothesis is that the increased passenger leukocyte load of antigenic levels associated with dual-organ transplants could increase the tendency for microchimerism, which could have an immunoprotective effect that is different for various organs (135). Although the propensity for rejection appears to be higher for the kidney than the pancreas, predictions cannot be made for individual cases (162).

Most likely there is a complex mix of all of these factors. The target cell of interstitial rejection is different in both organs; they are developmentally, morphologically, and functionally different. In contrast, the target cell of vascular rejection is the endothelium, which is the same in both organs; therefore, identical vascular rejection grades should be expected, but the opposite has been shown in the previously discussed pig studies (22,29,30). Since interstitial rejection is in general more advanced than vascular rejection, local interstitial amplification factors may induce a different endothelial response. Thus, the hypothesis that cell mediated interstitial rejection causes release of local factors, which subsequently lead to an upregulation of class II HLA antigens on endothelial cells, could also explain in part the different immunological response in both organs. No matter what the explanation is, there is obviously a protective effect, since pancreatic rejection is downmodulated by a simultaneous kidney transplant.

D. Rejection of Graft Duodenum

Very few studies have investigated the clinical correlation between pancreatic and duodenal rejection. In one study, 25 cases were reviewed in which both duodenal and pancreatic tissue were obtained by cystoscopic biopsies (103); 18 were positive for rejection. In 12 of these cases, interstitial rejection was diagnosed in both organs; in 6 cases, in 1 organ only (4 duodenum, 2 pancreas). This demonstrates that the duodenum can reject independently of the pancreas. This finding is also supported by a case report of a PTA recipient in whom isolated rejection of the duodenum caused perforation of an enterically drained duodenal segment without evidence of pancreas rejection; a graft duodenectomy with ligation of the pancreatic duct was done, but endocrine function was sustained (163). Barr et al. (156) found the duodenum to be helpful only if positive for rejection; it showed 100% concordance with the pancreas and 80% concordance with the kidney, with no instances of isolated duodenal rejection. Discordant pancreas rejection was present in 47% of negative duodenal biopsies; these data suggest that a negative duodenal biopsy does not rule out pancreas rejection.

E. Impact of Rejection Episodes on Exocrine and Endocrine Function

The Minnesota group studied the influence of rejection episodes on the relationship between exocrine and endocrine function in 381 bladder-drained pancreas transplants (164). Interestingly, there was no consistent relationship between exocrine and endocrine function at 1 year posttransplant. Some recipients with an adequate metabolic regulation had poor exocrine activity of their graft; in contrast, a high UA excretion did not necessarily correlate with good graft endocrine function. While UA monitoring was variable in diagnosing early rejection, it was of no prognostic value in determining long-term endocrine function. Reversible rejection episodes did not necessarily alter long-term exocrine function, since both an increase and decrease in UA values were noted after reversal of rejection. In a very small percentage of patients, exocrine activity can completely disappear, but endocrine function can be preserved. This discordance is explained by the histological finding that islets are rarely infiltrated during rejection episodes, whereas the exocrine tissue and vessels are involved in the process preferentially (165).

Monitoring rejection becomes extremely difficult for recipients of bladder-drained pancreatic transplants who completely lose their exocrine function but remain insulin-free. Barone et al. (166) observed 4 cases (3 SPK, 1 PTA), representing 5% of their series; although loss of UA activity occurred, on average, 5.9 months posttransplant, the recipients remained insulin-free (mean follow-up, 20 months). Interestingly, IV glucose tolerance tests were obtained before and after loss of UA, and no differences were seen, suggesting a normal endocrine function in spite of exocrine functional loss.

In a different study, isolated loss of exocrine function was noted in 29 of 319 (9%) cadaver bladder-drained pancreatic transplants (167). The extinction of exocrine function was commonly due to chronic rejection. Of the 29 recipients who lost exocrine function but remained insulin-free for at least 1 month, 7 were SPK, 12 PTA, and 10 PAK recipients; 13 (45%) were still insulin-independent, and 16 (55%) went back on insulin. Total loss in this study was defined as a residual UA activity <100 units/hr; partial loss was defined as a residual UA activity between 200 and 800 units/hr with a decline of at least 80% of the base level. UA loss was total for 24 (83%) cases and partial for 5 (17%) recipients.

Several risk factors were identified that increased the probability of being insulin-independent. One was the recipient category itself: the probability of being insulin-free at 1 year, despite loss of exocrine function, was 0.69 for SPK versus 0.35 for PTA and PAK recipients. An explanation is that, for SPK recipients, pancreatic rejection episodes can still be detected by monitoring serum creatinine levels, since most SPK rejection episodes involve the kidney (either alone or in combination with a pancreas). Second, the probability of being insulin-independent was higher after partial loss (0.80) than after total loss (0.31) of exocrine function, suggesting that the acinar tissue damage reflects the severity of the process leading to graft failure. Third, the number of previous rejection episodes had an impact: the probability of remaining insulin-independent was higher for recipients with ≤ 2 (0.56) versus >2 rejection episodes (0.21). This supports the hypothesis that the functioning islet mass approaches a critical level; if further rejection episodes occur, inadequate graft function may result. In contrast, the interval between transplantation and loss of UA, as well as the period over which UA levels declined, seemed to have less influence on graft outcome (165). Thus, the definitive loss of pancreatic exocrine function is not inevitably followed by loss of endocrine function; risk factors for subsequent loss of insulin secretions are absence of a kidney from the same donor, total loss of UA, and >2 previous rejection episodes.

F. Transplant Pancreatectomy for Rejection

Pancreatic failure from rejection infrequently requires graft removal. A transplant pancreatectomy usually is indicated if recipients become symptomatic (e.g., fever, graft tenderness, infection). Up to 25% of all irreversibly rejected pancreatic grafts eventually require removal. Troppmann et al. (168), in a study of 77 transplant pancreatectomies, found rejection the second most common cause (19%), surpassed only by vascular graft thrombosis (31%). For those recipients, transplant pancreatectomy results in complete alleviation of symptoms. Most patients with graft failure from rejection, however, have just temporary symptoms or none at all, and do not require transplant pancreatectomy.

IX. SUMMARY AND CONCLUSIONS

The pancreas is rejected similar to other organs with a combination of interstitial and vascular rejection, the first more common and perhaps leading to the other. In SPK transplants, the kidney is more susceptible to endstage rejection than the pancreas. In solitary pancreatic transplants, the rejection rate is higher, perhaps due to loss of ability to monitor a kidney graft as a surrogate marker for rejection in the pancreas. Biochemical markers show exocrine dysfunction before endocrine dysfunction, but no markers are specific or sensitive enough to preclude the need for confirmatory biopsies. Pancreatic rejections are usually steroid-resistant but are reversible with anti-T-cell therapy. Pancreatic transplantation can have a high success rate and deserves wider application.

REFERENCES

1. Sutherland DER. Pancreatic transplantation: An update. Diabetes Rev 1993; 1:152–165.
2. Robertson RP, Abid M, Sutherland DER, Diem P. Glucose homeostasis and insulin secretion in human recipients of pancreas transplantation. Diabetes 1989; 38:97–98.
3. Diabetes Control and Complications Trial Research Group. The effect of intensive treatment of diabetes on the development and progression of long-term complications in insulin-dependent diabetes mellitus. N Engl J Med 1994; 329:977–986.
4. Morel P, Goetz F, Moudry-Munns KC, et al. Long term metabolic control in patients with pancreatic transplants. Ann Intern Med 1991; 115:694–699.
5. Gross CR, Zehrer CL. Health-related quality of life outcomes of pancreas transplant recipients. Clin Transplant 1992; 6:165–171.
6. van der Vliet JA, Navarro X, Kennedy WR, et al. The effect of pancreas transplantation on diabetic polyneuropathy. Transplantation 1988; 45:368–370, 1988.
7. Navarro X, Kennedy WR, Sutherland DER. Autonomic neuropathy and survival in diabetes mellitus: Effects of pancreas transplantation. Diabetologia 1991; 34(suppl 1):S108–S112.
8. Bilous RW, Mauer SM, Sutherland DER, Steffes MW. Glomerular structure and function following successful pancreas transplantation for insulin-dependent diabetes mellitus. Diabetes 1987; 36:43A.
9. Bilous RC, Mauer SM, Sutherland DER, et al. The effects of pancreas transplantation on the glomerular structure of renal allografts in patients with insulin-dependent diabetes. N Engl J Med 1989; 321:80–85.
10. Ramsay RC, Goetz FC, Sutherland DER, et al. Progression of diabetic retinopathy after pancreas transplantation for insulin-dependent diabetes mellitus. N Engl J Med 1988; 318:208–214.
11. Gruessner AC. Results of the International Pancreas Transplant Registry—An update. 1994 (personal communication).
12. Jacobson SH, Fryd DS, Sutherland DER, Kjellstand CM. Treatment of the diabetic patients with end-stage renal failure. Diabetes Metab Rev 1988; 4:191–200.
13. Zehr PS, Milde FK, Hart LK, Corry RJ. Pancreas transplantation assessing secondary complications and life quality. Diabetologia 1991; 34:S138–S140.
14. Sutherland DER, Gruessner RWG, Gillingham K, et al. A single institution's experience with solitary pancreas transplantation: A simultaneous analysis of factors leading to improved outcome. In: Terasaki PI, ed. Clinical Transplants 1991. Los Angeles: UCLA Tissue Typing Laboratory, 1991:141–152.

15. Cecka JM, Terasaki PI. The UNOS scientific renal transplant registry. In: Terasaki PI, Cecka JM, eds. Clinical Transplants 1993. Los Angeles: UCLA Tissue Typing Laboratory, 1993: 1–18.
16. Sutherland DER, Gores P, Farney A, et al. Evolution of kidney, pancreas and islet transplantation for diabetes at the University of Minnesota. Am J Surg 1993; 166:456–491.
17. Sutherland DER. Present status of pancreas transplantation alone in nonuremic diabetic patients. Transplant Proc 1994; 26:379–383.
18. Sutherland DER, Moudry-Munns KC, Gruessner A. Pancreas transplant results in United Network for Organ Sharing (UNOS) United States of America (USA) Registry with a comparison to non-USA data in the international registry. In: Terasaki CI, Cecka JM, eds. Clinical Transplants 1993. Los Angeles: UCLA Tissue Typing Laboratory, 1993:47–69.
19. Hirata M, Terasaki PI. The long-term effect of primary disease on cadaver-donor renal transplant recipients. In: Terasaki CI, Cecka JM, eds. Clinical Transplants 1993. Los Angeles, UCLA Tissue Typing Laboratory, 1993:485–498.
20. Geffrotin C, Popescu CF, Cribiu EP, et al. Assignment of MHC in swine to chromosome 7 by in situ hybridization and serological typing. Ann Genet 1984; 27:213–219.
21. Gruessner RWG, Tzardis PJ, Schechner R, et al. En bloc simultaneous pancreas and kidney allotransplantation in the pig. J Surg Res 1990; 49:366–370.
22. Gruessner RWG, Nakhleh R, Gruessner A, et al. Streptozotocin-induced diabetes mellitus in pigs. Horm Metab Res 1993; 25:199–203.
23. Gänger KH, Mettler D, Böss, et al. Experimental duodeno-pancreatico-renal composite transplantation: A new alternative to avoid vascular thrombosis? Transplant Proc 1987; 19:3960–3964.
24. Calne RY, Sells RA, Marshall VC, et al. Multiple organ grafts in the pig. Br J Surg 1972; 59: 969–977.
25. Gylling SF, Tauber JW, Ward RE, et al. Composite pancreas-kidney transplant in pigs. Curr Surg 1987; 44:408–410.
26. Koyama I, Williams M, Cameron JL, Zuidema GD. Experimental pancreatic allotransplantation in large animals: The role of donor kidney and cyclosporine in modifying rejection. Transplantation 1986; 42:333–336.
27. Gruessner RWG, Nakhleh R, Tzardis P, et al. Rejection in single versus combined pancreas and kidney transplantation in pigs. Transplantation 1993; 56:1053–1062.
28. Marsh CL, Perkins JD, Barr D, et al. Cystoscopically directed biopsy technique in canine pancreaticoduodenal transplantation. Transplant Proc 1989; 21:2816–2817.
29. Gruessner RWG, Nakhleh R, Tzardis P, et al. Differences in rejection grading after simultaneous pancreas and kidney transplantation in pigs. Transplantation 1994; 57:1021–1028.
30. Nahkleh RE, Sutherland DER, Tzardis P, et al. Correlation of rejection of the duodenum with rejection of the pancreas in a pig model of pancreaticoduodenal transplantation. Transplantation 1993; 56:1353–1356.
31. Gruessner RWG, Nakhleh R, Tzardis PH, et al. Correlation between duodenal and kidney rejection: A histologic comparative study in a pig model of pancreaticoduodenal-kidney transplantation. Transplant Proc 1994; 26:541–543.
32. Gruessner RWG, Nakhleh R, Tzardis P, et al. Rejection patterns after simultaneous pancreaticoduodenal-kidney transplants in pigs. Transplantation 1994; 57:756–760.
33. Dafoe DC, Campbell DA, Marks WH, et al. Association of inclusion of the donor spleen in pancreaticoduodenal transplantation with rejection. Transplantation 1985; 40:579–584.
34. Dafoe DC, Rosenberg L, Campbell DA, et al. Clinical pancreaticoduodenal allotransplantation with inclusion of the donor spleen (irradiated and nonirradiated) to prevent thrombosis. Transplant Proc 1988; 20:876–877.
35. Gotoh M, Monden M, Motoki Y, et al. Early detection of rejection in the allografted pancreas. Transplant Proc 1984; 16:781–782.

36. Gliedman ML, Gold M, Whittaker J, et al. Pancreatic duct to ureter anastomosis in pancreatic transplantation. Am J Surg 1973; 125:245–252.
37. Prieto M, Sutherland DER, Fernandez-Cruz L, et al. Urinary amyalse monitoring for early diagnosis of pancreas allograft rejection in dogs. J Surg Res 1986; 40:597–604.
38. Carpenter HA, Barr D, Marsh CL, et al. Sequential histopathologic changes in pancreatico-duodenal allograft rejection in dogs. Transplantation 1989; 48:764–768.
39. Ekberg H, Allen RDM, Greenberg ML, et al. Early diagnosis of rejection of canine pancreas allografts by fine-needle aspiration biopsy. Transplantation 1988; 46:485–489.
40. Ekberg E, Allen RDM, Greenberg ML, et al. Improvement of canine pancreas-allograft survival with diagnosis of rejection by fine-needle aspiration biopsy. Diabetes 1989; 38: 109–110.
41. Severyn W, Olson L, Miller J, et al. Studies on the survival of simultaneous canine renal and segmental pancreatic allografts. Transplantation 1982; 33:606–612.
42. Florack G, Sutherland DER, Sibley RK, et al. Combined kidney and segmental pancreas allotransplantation in dogs. Transplant Proc 1985; 17:374–377.
43. Sato K, Yamagishi K, Nakayama Y, et al. Pancreaticoduodenal allotransplantation with cyclosporine and FK506. Transplant Proc 1989; 21:1074–1075.
44. Takaori K, Inoue K, Nio Y, et al. Basic study on immunologic effects of cyclosporine and FK 506 for application to pancreatic transplantation. Transplant Proc 1992; 24:894–896.
45. Nakai I, Kaufman DB, Field MJ, et al. Differential effects of preexisting uremia and a synchronous kidney graft on pancreas allograft functional survival in rats. Transplantation 1992; 54:17–25.
46. Vogt P, Hiller WFA, Steiniger B, Kelmpnauer J. Differential response of kidney and pancreas rejection to cyclosporine immunosuppression. Transplantation 1992; 53:1269–1272.
47. Hiller W, Klempnauer J, Vogt P, et al. Relevance of non-major histocompatibility complex antigens in pancreas transplantation. Transplant Proc 1987; 19:4274–4275.
48. Steiniger B, Klempnauer J. Distinct histologic patterns of acute, prolonged, and chronic rejection in vascularized rat pancreas allografts. Am J Pathol 1986; 124:253–262.
49. Lindsey NJ, Nolan MS, Slater DN, et al. Rat pancreas allotransplantation: A short term comparison of rejection patterns with different methods of exocrine drainage. J Pathol 1983; 139:259–274.
50. Chen H, Wu J, Xu D, et al. Reversal of ongoing heart, kidney, and pancreas allograft rejection and suppression of accelerated heart allograft rejection in the rat by rapamycin. Transplantation 1993; 56:661–666.
51. Chen H, Wu J, Luo H, Daloze P. Synergistic effect of rapamycin and cyclosporine in pancreaticoduodenal transplantation in the rat. Transplant Proc 1992; 24:892–893.
52. Benedetti E, Najarian JS, Sutherland DER, et al. Correlation between cystoscopic biopsy results and hypoamylasuria in bladder-drained pancreas transplants. Surgery 1995; 118: 864–872.
53. Stratta RJ, Sollinger HW, D'Alessandro AM, et al. OKT3 rescue therapy in pancreas-allograft rejection. Diabetes 1989; 38:74–78.
54. Sollinger HW, D'Alessandro AM, Stratta RJ, et al. Combined kidney-pancreas transplantation with pancreaticocystostomy. Transplant Proc 1989; 21:2837–2838.
55. Prieto M, Sutherland DER, Fernández-Cruz L, et al. Experimental and clinical experience with urine amylase monitoring for early diagnosis of rejection in pancreas transplantation. Transplantation 1987; 43:73–79.
56. Schulak JA, Drevyanko TF. Experimental pancreas allograft rejection: Correlation between histologic and functional rejection and the efficacy of antirejection therapy. Surgery 1985; 98:330–336.
57. Nankivell BJ, Allen RDM, Bell B, et al. Chapman JR: Factors affecting measurement of urinary amylase after bladder-drained pancreas transplantation. Clin Transplant 1991; 5:392–397.

58. Moukarzel M, Benoit G, Charpentier B, et al. Is urinary amylase a reliable index for monitoring whole pancreas endocrine graft function? Transplant Proc 1992; 24:925–926.
59. Lievens MM. Potential pitfalls in the determination of amylase activity in the urine of pancreas-transplanted patients with bladder drainage. Transplantation 1990; 50:526–527.
60. Henry ML, Osei K, O'Dorisio TM, et al. Concomitant reduction in urinary amylase and acute first-phase insulin release predict pancreatic allograft transplant rejection in type I diabetic recipients. Clin Transplant 1991; 5:112–120.
61. Munn SR, Engen DE, Barr D, et al. Differential diagnosis of hypoamylasuria in pancreas allograft recipients with urinary exocrine drainage. Transplantation 1990; 49:359–362.
62. Soon-Shiong P, Zheng TL, Merideth N, Chang YH. Elevation in urinary prostaglandin (PGE2) as an early marker of pancreas allograft rejection. Transplant Proc 1989; 21:2771–2773.
63. Rubenstein HH, Clark JL, Melani F, Steinen DF. Secretion of proinsulin C-peptide by pancreatic β cells and its circulation in blood: Nature 1969; 224:697–699.
64. Esmatjes E, Fernández-Cruz L, Ricart MJ, et al. Urinary C-peptide excretion in pancreas transplantation with urinary drainage. Transplant Proc 1990; 22:1598–1599.
65. Chance RE, Ellis RM, Bromer WW. Porcine proinsulin: Characterization and amino acid sequence. Science 1968; 161:165–167.
66. Dragstedt LR. Some physiologic problems in surgery of the pancreas. Ann Surg 1943; 118: 576–593.
67. Tydén G, Gunnarsson R, Östman J, Groth CG. Laboratory findings during rejection of segmental pancreatic allografts. Transplant Proc 1984; 16:715–717.
68. Ploeg RJ, D'Alessandro AM, Groshek M, et al. Efficacy of human anodal trypsinogen for detection of rejection in clinical pancreas transplantation. Transplant Proc 1994; 26:531–533.
69. Cheng SS, Munn SR. Posttransplant hyperamylasemia is associated with decreased patient and graft survival in pancreas allograft recipients. Transplant Proc 1994; 26:428–429.
70. Borgström A, Marks WH, Dafoe DC, et al. Immunoreactive anionic and cationic trypsins in serum after experimental porcine pancreatic transplantation. Surgery 1986; 100:841–848.
71. Marks WH, Borgström A, Sollinger H, Marks C. Serum immunoreactive anodal trypsinogen and urinary amylase as biochemical markers for rejection of clinical whole-organ pancreas allografts having exocrine drainage into the urinary bladder. Transplantation 1990; 49: 112–115.
72. Douzdjian V, Cooper JL, Abecassis MM, Corry RJ. Markers for pancreatic allograft rejection: Comparison of serum anodal trypsinogen, serum amylase, serum creatinine and urinary amylase. Clin Transplant 1994; 8:79–82.
73. Perkal M, Marks C, Lorber MI, Marks WH. A three-year experience with serum anodal trypsinogen as a biochemical marker for rejection in pancreatic allografts. False positives, tissue biopsy, comparison with other markers, and diagnostic strategies. Transplantation 1992; 53:415–419.
74. Matsuda K, Ogawa M, Shibata T, et al. Postoperative elevation of serum pancreatic secretory trypsin inhibitor. Am J Gastroenterol 1985; 80:694–698.
75. Kitahara T, Takatsuka Y, Fujimoto K, et al. Radioimmunoassay for human pancreatic secretory trypsin inhibitor: Measurement of serum pancreatic secretory trypsin inhibitor in normal subjects and subjects with pancreatic diseases. Clin Chim Acta 1980; 103:135–143.
76. Suzuki Y, Kuroda Y, Kawamura T, et al. Pancreatic secretory trypsin inhibitor as a marker for early detection of rejection in canine pancreas allotransplantation. Transplant Proc 1989; 21:2793–2794.
77. Kuroda Y, Suzuki Y, Kawamura T, et al. Tanaka T, Saitoh Y: Pancreatic secretory trypsin inhibitor as a marker for early detection of rejection in canine pancreas allotransplantation. Transplantation 1988; 46:493–495.
78. Suzuki Y, Kuroda Y, Sollinger HW, et al. Plasma pancreatic secretory trypsin inhibitor as a marker of pancreas graft rejection after combined pancreas-kidney transplantation. Transplantation 1991; 52:504–507.

79. Suzuki Y, Kuroda Y, Sollinger HW, Saitoh Y. Plasma phospholipase A_2 and pancreatic secretory trypsin inhibitor as markers for pancreas graft rejection. Transplant Proc 1994; 26: 538–540.
80. Fernstad R, Skoldefors H, Pousette A, et al. A novel assay for pancreatic cellular damage: III. Use of a pancreas-specific protein as a marker of pancreatic graft dysfunction in humans. Pancreas 1989; 4:44–52.
81. Greene LJ, Pubols MH, Bartelt DC. Human pancreatic secretory trypsin inhibitor. Methods Enzymol 1976; 359:813–825.
82. Fernstad R, Tydén G, Brattström C, et al. Rejection of pancreas grafts—pancreas-specific protein: New serum marker for graft rejection in pancreas-transplant recipients. Diabetes 1989; 38:55–56.
83. Nyberg G, Olausson M, Norden G, et al. Pancreas specific protein (PASP) monitoring in pancreas transplantation. Transplant Proc 1991; 23:1604–1605.
84. Linder R, Sziegoleit A, Brattström C, et al. Pancreatic elastase 1 after pancreatic transplantation. Pancreas 1991; 6:31–36.
85. Linder R, Sziegoleit A, Peters B, et al. Serum pancreatic elastase 1 as a marker of pancreatic graft damage. Transplant Proc 90; 22:1595.
86. Georgi BA, Dempsey RA, Corry RJ. Interleukin-2 assay in serum and urine as a means of monitoring pancreatic allograft rejection. Transplant Proc 1989; 21:2784–2785.
87. Perkins JD, Munn SR, Barr D, et al. Evidence that the soluble interleukin 2 receptor level may determine the optimal time for cystoscopically directed biopsy in pancreaticoduodenal allograft recipients. Transplantation 1990; 49:363–366.
88. Abendroth D, Capalbo M, Illner WD, et al. Critical analysis of rejection markers sIL-2R, urinary amylase, and lipase in whole-organ pancreas transplantation with exocrine bladder drainage. Transplant Proc 1992; 24:786–787.
89. Brattström C, Tydén G, Reinholt FP, et al. Markers for pancreas-graft rejection in humans. Diabetes 1989; 38:57–62.
90. Königsrainer A, Tilg H, Reibnegger G, et al. Pancreatic juice neopterin excretion—A reliable marker of pancreas allograft rejection. Transplant Proc 1992; 24:907–908.
91. Funakoshi A, Yamada Y, Ito T, et al. Misaki A, Kono M: Clinical usefulness of serum phospholipase A_2 determination in patients with pancreatic diseases. Pancreas 1991; 6: 588–594.
92. Johnson BF, Thomas G, Wiley KN, et al. Thromboxane and prostacyclin synthesis in experimental pancreas transplantation: Changes in parenchymal and vascular prostanoids. Transplantation 1993; 56:1447–1453.
93. Henry ML, Davies EA, Elkhammas EA, et al. Pancreatic allograft function as assessed by IMX first-phase insulin assays. Transplant Proc 1994; 26:537.
94. Ganda OP, Srikanta S, Brink SJ, et al. Differential sensitivity to β cell secretagogues in "early," type I diabetes mellitus. Diabetes 1984; 33:516–521.
95. Elmer DS, Hathaway DK, Shokouh-Amiri H, et al. The relationship of glucose disappearance rate (K_G) to acute pancreas allograft rejection. Transplantation 1994; 57:1400–1405.
96. Gruessner RWG, Dunn DL, Tzardis PJ, et al. Simultaneous pancreas and kidney transplants versus single kidney transplants and previous kidney transplants in uremic patients and single pancreas transplants in nonuremic diabetic patients: Comparison of rejection, morbidity and long-term outcome. Transplant Proc 1990; 22:622–623.
97. Sutherland DER, Casanova D, Sibley RK. Monitoring and diagnosis of rejection: Role of pancreas graft biopsies in the diagnosis and treatment of rejection after pancreas transplantation. Transplant Proc 1987; 19:2329–2331.
98. Allen RDM, Wilson TG, Grierson JM, et al. Percutaneous biopsy of bladder-drained pancreas transplants. Transplantation 1991; 51:1213–1216.
99. Martinenghi S, Dell'Antonio G, Secchi A, et al. Percutaneous microbiopsy for the diagnosis of rejection in whole bladder-diverted pancreas transplantation. Transplant Proc 1991; 26:526.

100. Perkins JD, Munn SR, Marsh CL, et al. Safety and efficacy of cystoscopically directed biopsy in pancreas transplantation. Transplant Proc 1990; 22:665–666.
101. Jones JW, Nakhleh RE, Casanova D, et al. Cystoscopic transduodenal pancreas transplant biopsy: A new needle. Transplant Proc 1994; 26:527–528.
102. Lowell JA, Bynon JS, Nelson N, et al. Improved technique for transduodenal pancreas transplant biopsy. Transplantation 1994; 57:752–753.
103. Nakhleh RE, Sutherland DER, Benedetti E, et al. Diagnostic utility and correlation of duodenal and pancreas biopsy tissues in pancreaticoduodenal transplants with emphasis on therapeutic use. Transplant Proc 1995; 27:1327–1328.
104. Casanova D, Gruessner R, Brayman K, et al. Retrospective analysis of the role of pancreatic biopsy (open and transcystoscopic technique) in the management of solitary pancreas transplants. Transplant Proc 1993; 25:1192–1193.
105. Reinholt FP, Tydén G, Bohman SO, et al. Pancreatic juice cytology in the diagnosis of pancreatic graft rejection. Clin Transplant 1988; 2:127–133.
106. Klima G, Margreiter R. Pancreatic juice cytology in the monitoring of pancreas allografts. Transplantation 1989; 48:980–985.
107. Klima G, Margreiter R, Königsrainer A, et al. Pancreatic juice cytology (PJC) for early detection of pancreas allograft rejection. Transplant Proc 1989; 21:2782–2783.
108. Radio SJ, Stratta RJ, Taylor RJ, Linder J. The utility of urine cytology in the diagnosis of allograft rejection after combined pancreas-kidney transplantation. Transplantation 1993; 55: 509–516.
109. Radio SJ, Stratta RJ, Taylor RJ, Linder J. Urine cytology monitoring for rejection after vascularized pancreas transplantation. Transplant Proc 1992; 24:903–906.
110. Radio SJ, Stratta RJ, Linder J, et al. Histologic confirmation of acute rejection detected by urine cytology in pancreas transplant recipients. Transplant Proc 1994; 26:529–530.
111. Kuni CC. Scintigraphy of pancreas transplants. In: Letourneau JG, Day DL, Ascher NL. eds. Radiology of Organ Transplantation. St. Louis: Mosby-Year Book, 1991:249–256.
112. Stratta RJ, Sollinger HW, Perlman SB, et al. Early detection of rejection in pancreas transplantation. Diabetes 1989; 38:63–67.
113. George EA, Salimi Z, Carney K, et al. Radionuclide surveillance of the allografted pancreas. AJR 1988; 150:811–816.
114. Jurewicz WA, Buckels JAC, Dykes JGA, et al. Indium-111 labeled platelets in monitoring pancreatic transplants in humans. Transplant Proc 1984; 16:720–723.
115. Patel B, Markivee CR, Manhanta B, et al. Pancreatic transplantation: Scintigraphy, US and CT. Radiology 1988; 167:685–687.
116. Letourneau JG, Maile CW, Sutherland DER, Feinberg SB. Ultrasound and computed tomography in the evaluation of pancreatic transplantation. Radiol Clin North Am 1987; 25:345–355.
117. Letourneau JG. Sonography, CT, and MRI of pancreas allografts. In: Letourneau JG, Day DL, Ascher NL, eds. Radiology of Organ Transplantation. St. Louis: Mosby-Year Book, 1991: 257–266.
118. Nghiem DD, Ludrosky L, Young JC. Evaluation of pancreatic circulation by duplex color Doppler flow sonography. Transplant Proc 1994; 26:466.
119. Moulton JS, Munda R, Weiss MA, Lubberg DJ. Pancreatic transplants: CT with clinical and pathologic correlation. Radiology 1989; 172:21–26.
120. Yuh WTC, Hunsicker LG, Sato Y, et al. Application of magnetic resonance imaging in pancreas transplant. Diabetes 1989; 38:27–29.
121. Yuh WTC, Wiese JA, Abu-Yousef MM, et al. Pancreatic transplant imaging. Radiology 1988; 167:679–683.
122. Contis JC, O'Connor TP, Holland GA, et al. Noninvasive evaluation of bladder-drained whole pancreaticoduodenal transplants with magnetic resonance angiography. Transplant Proc 1994; 26:464–465.

123. Sutherland DER. Immunosuppression for clinical pancreas transplantation. Clin Transplant 1991; (special issue) 5:549–553.
124. Sutherland DER. Pancreas Transplantation. Curr Opin Immunol 1989; 1:1195–1206.
125. LeFrancois N, Faure JL, Melandri M, et al. Kidney-graft survival in simultaneous kidney-pancreas transplantation. Diabetes 1989; 38:38–39.
126. Ward RG, Gecim E, Bone JM, et al. Cyclosporin monotherapy in pancreaticorenal transplantation. Transplant Proc 1994; 26:548.
127. Brekke IB, Wramner L, Wadstrom J, Ekberg H. Triple vs quadruple induction immunosuppression in pancreas transplantation. XVth World Congress of the Transplantation Society, Kyoto, Japan. Abstract #137:90, 1994.
128. Sutherland DER, Moudry-Munns KC, Gruessner A. Pancreas transplant outcome with or without biological anti-T-cell therapy for induction immunosuppression with use of cyclosporine. Transplant Proc 1994; 26:2752–2755.
129. Sollinger HW, Knechtle SJ, Reed A, et al. Experience with 100 consecutive simultaneous kidney-pancreas transplants with bladder drainage. Ann Surg 1991; 214:703–711.
130. Stratta RJ, Taylor RJ, Lowell JA, et al. OKT3 induction in 100 consecutive pancreas transplants. Transplant Proc 1994; 26:546–547.
131. Beilman DJ, Shield CF, Hughes JD, et al. The effects of intraoperative administration of OKT3 during renal transplantation. Transplantation 1993; 55:490–493.
132. Dawidson I, Lu C, Ar'Rajab A, et al. Cyclosporine levels predict the likelihood of rejection after simultaneous pancreas/kidney transplantation. Transplant Proc 1994; 26:534.
133. Cantarovich D, Dantal J, Hourmant M, et al. Importance of cyclosporine dosage and blood levels in simultaneous pancreas and kidney transplant success. Transplant Proc 1992; 24: 890–891.
134. Catarovich D, LeMauff B, Hourmant M, et al. Prevention of acute rejection episodes with an anti-interleukin 2 receptor monoclonal antibody. Transplantation 1994; 57:198–203.
135. Stratta RJ, Taylor RJ, Bynon JS, et al. Patterns of rejection after combined pancreas-kidney transplantation. Transplant Proc 1994; 26:524–525.
136. Cheung AHS, Sutherland DER, Gillingham KJ, et al. Simultaneous pancreas-kidney transplant versus kidney transplant alone in diabetic patients. Kidney Int 1992; 41:924–929.
137. Rosen CB, Frohnert PP, Velosa JA, et al. Morbidity of pancreas transplantation during cadaveric renal transplantation. Transplantation 1991; 51:123–127.
138. Sollinger HW, Stratta RJ, D'Alessandro AM, et al. Experience with simultaneous pancreas-kidney transplantation. Ann Surg 1988; 208:475–483.
139. Schulak JA, Mayes JT, Hricik DE. Kidney transplantation in diabetic patients undergoing combined kidney-pancreas or kidney-only transplantation. Transplantation 1992; 53: 685–687.
140. Hedman L, Frisk B, Brynger H, et al. Severe kidney graft rejection in combined kidney and pancreas transplantation. Transplant Proc 1987; 19:3911–3912.
141. Cantarovich D, Hourmant M, Dantal J, et al. Is the incidence of kidney rejection episodes higher in combined kidney/pancreas than in single kidney transplant patients? Transplant Proc 1994; 26:535.
142. Zantvoort FA, Persijn GG, vanRood JJ. Renal allograft and patient survival in combined pancreas/kidney transplantation. Transplant Proc 1989; 21:2831–2832.
143. Hillebrand G, Castro LA, Landgraf R, et al. Combined kidney/pancreas transplantation—Poor long-term outcome of renal grafts. Transplant Proc 1987; 19:3909–3910.
144. Gruessner RWG, Dunn DL, Tzardis PJ, et al. Sutherland DER: An immunological comparison of pancreas transplants alone in nonuremic patients versus simultaneous pancreas/kidney transplants in uremic diabetic patients. Transplant Proc 1990; 22:1581.
145. Höhnke C, Illner WD, Abendroth D, et al. 7-year experience in clinical pancreatic transplantation using duct occlusion technique. Transplant Proc 1989; 21:2862–2863.

146. Tydén G, Tibell A, Bolinder J, et al. Pancreatic transplantation with enteric exocrine diversion: Experience with 120 cases. Transplant Proc 1992; 24:771–773.
147. So SKS, Minford EJ, Moudry-Munns KC, et al. DR matching improves cadaveric pancreas transplant results. Transplant Proc 1990; 22:687–688.
148. Mellert J, Hopt UT, Büsing, Hölzer H. Differential immunosuppressive strategies after combined pancreaticoduodenal and isolated kidney transplantation. Transplant Proc 1990; 22: 1584–1585.
149. So SKS, Moudry-Munns KC, Gillingham K, et al. Short-term and long-term effects of HLA matching in cadaveric pancreas transplantation. Transplant Proc 1991; 23:1634–1636.
150. Gruessner RWG, Najarian JS, Gruessner AC, Sutherland DER. Pancreas transplants from living related donors. In: Touraine JL, ed. Organ Shortage: The Solutions. The Netherlands: Kluwer, 1995:77–83.
151. Sutherland DER, Sibley RK, Xu XZ, et al. Twin-to-twin pancreas transplantation: Reversal and reenactment of the pathogenesis of type I diabetes. Trans Assoc Am Physicians 1984; 97: 80–87.
152. Margreiter R, Klima G, Bömüller C, et al. Rejection of kidney and pancreas after pancreas-kidney transplantation. Diabetes 1989; 38:79–81.
153. Dubernard JM, Traeger J, LaRocca E, et al. Experience of the Hopital Edouard Herriot, University of Lyon I, Lyon, France. In: Dubernard JM and Sutherland DER, eds. International Handbook of Pancreas Transplantation 1989. The Netherlands: Kluwer, 1989:389–398.
154. Gruessner RWG, Najarian JS, Gruessner A, Sutherland DER. Comparison of rejection in clinical transplantation of pancreas alone or associated with kidney transplant. In: Touraine JL, Traeger J, Betuel H, et al, eds. Transplantation and Clinical Immunology: Multiple Transplants. Amsterdam, New York, Oxford: Excerpta Medica 1991; 22:47–54.
155. Tesi RJ, Henry ML, Elkhammas EA, et al. The frequency of rejection episodes with combined kidney-pancreas transplant—The impact on graft survival. Transplantation 1994; 58:424–430.
156. Barr D, Bronner MP, Marsh CL, et al. Concordance of histologic rejection in human kidney and pancreas transplantation. Transplantation. In press.
157. Lillehei RC, Ruiz JO, Acquino C, Goetz FC. Transplantation of the pancreas. Acta Endocrinol 1976; 83 (suppl 205):303–320.
158. Sollinger HW, Ploeg RJ, Eckhoff DE, et al. Two hundred consecutive simultaneous pancreas-kidney transplants with bladder drainage. Surgery 1993; 114:736–744.
159. Sutherland DER, Gruessner R, Moudry-Munns K, Gruessner A. Discordant graft loss from rejection of organs from the same donor in simultaneous pancreas-kidney recipients. Transplant Proc 1995; 27:907–908.
160. Kyriakides G, Olson L, Severyn W, et al. Early detection of pancreatic allograft rejection in dogs: Immunologic and physiologic monitoring in simultaneous kidney and pancreas transplantation and response in immunosuppression. World J Surg 1981; 5:430.
161. Lawrence JS. Uremia: Nature's immunosuppressive device. Ann Intern Med 1965; 2:166–168.
162. Stratta RJ, Taylor RJ, Ozaki CF, et al. A comparative analysis of results and morbidity in type I diabetics undergoing preemptive versus postdialysis combined pancreas-kidney transplantation. Transplantation 1993; 55:1097–1103.
163. Gruessner RWG, Manivel C, Dunn DL, Sutherland DER. Pancreaticoduodenal transplantation with enteric drainage following native total pancreatectomy for chronic pancreatitis. Pancreas 1991; 6:479–488.
164. Brayman K, Morel Ph, Chau C, et al. Influence of rejection episodes on the relationship between exocrine and endocrine function in bladder-drained pancreas transplants. Transplant Proc 1992; 24:921–923.
165. Sibley RK, Sutherland DER. Pancreas transplantation: An immunohistologic examination of 100 grafts. Am J Pathol 1987; 128:151–170.

166. Barone GW, Henry ML, Elkhammas EA, et al. Pancreatic exocrine "burnout" following pancreas transplantation. Transplant Proc 1992; 24:831–832.
167. Barrou B, Barrou Z, Gruessner A, et al. Probability of retaining endocrine function (insulin independence) after definitive loss of exocrine function in bladder-drained pancreas transplants. Transplant Proc 1994; 26:473–474.
168. Troppmann C, Gruessner RWG, Dunn DL, et al. Is transplant pancreatectomy after graft failure necessary? Transplant Proc 1994; 36:455.

20

Ultrasound Evaluation of Allograft Rejection

Ulrike M. Hamper and Sheila Sheth
Johns Hopkins University School of Medicine, Baltimore, Maryland

I. ROLE OF COLOR AND DOPPLER SONOGRAPHY IN THE DIAGNOSIS OF RENAL ALLOGRAFT REJECTION

With the large number of renal transplants performed in this country to treat patients with irreversible renal failure, there is a pressing need for noninvasive imaging modalities to diagnose potential complications that may jeopardize graft survival if not recognized and treated promptly. Clinical signs of oliguria, fever, or pain over the graft and laboratory findings indicating worsening renal function are nonspecific, and sonography is often requested to help differentiate between the various causes for graft dysfunction (1,2). Many surgical complications—such as ureteral obstruction and hydronephrosis, thrombosis or stenosis of the major arteries and veins, and peritransplant fluid collections—are readily diagnosed with color and Doppler sonography.

Unfortunately, the role of sonography in the evaluation of parenchymal abnormalities associated with poor graft function—such as acute tubular necrosis, acute rejection, and cyclosporin A nephrotoxicity—is much more controversial and has been the subject of much debate in the recent literature.

A. Technique of Examination

The renal transplant is examined using high-resolution 3.5- and 5-MHz linear, curvilinear, and sector transducers with color and duplex Doppler capabilities. Gray-scale sonography provides morphological information regarding transplant size and echotexture. An oblique approach over the iliac fossa with the transducer oriented parallel and then perpendicular to the graft provides the best overall evaluation of the kidney and allows accurate measurement of the maximum sagittal and anteroposterior diameters.

Color and duplex Doppler modes provide invaluable information concerning the integrity of the main artery and vein supplying the transplant as well as the state of cortical perfusion. Doppler spectral patterns are recorded from the main renal artery and vein and at least two of the peripheral arteries (arcuate, interlobar, or segmental arteries). Analysis of the Doppler waveform allows differentiation between arterial and venous signal as well as assessment of the vascular impedance in the allograft. The two Doppler indices most widely used to measure the pulsatility of arterial waveform in the renal transplant are (3,4):

$$\text{The resistive index (R1): } \frac{\text{Peak systolic velocity} - \text{end diastolic velocity}}{\text{peak systolic velocity}}$$

$$\text{The pulsatility index (P1): } \frac{\text{Peak systolic velocity} - \text{end diastolic velocity}}{\text{mean velocity}}$$

Pathological conditions associated with an increase in the peripheral vascular resistance in the transplant lead to elevation of these indices above normal values.

At our institution, an initial sonogram is obtained routinely within 24 to 48 hr after transplantation. This provides a baseline study for future comparison and greatly facilitates interpretation of subsequent sonograms and detection of subtle pathological changes in the echotexture or flow pattern of the transplanted kidney (1,2).

B. The Normal Renal Transplant

The normal renal allograft is elliptical in shape, with a relatively hypoechoic renal cortex and a strongly echogenic renal sinus (Fig. 1A). Although the appearance of the healthy allograft is similar to that of a normal native kidney (2), fine morphological details are more readily visible because of the superficial location of the transplant and the ability to image with higher-frequency transducers allowing better spatial resolution. Thus, the renal pyramids are easily seen as triangular structures, slightly more hypoechoic than the surrounding cortex (Fig. 1A). The normal arterial flow pattern as demonstrated by Doppler spectral analysis is characteristic of a low-impedance vascular bed: there is continuous forward flow throughout the cardiac cycle, with a rapid systolic upstroke followed by a gradual downslope in diastole (Fig. 1B) (4–7). Measurements of pulsatility or resistive indices allow semiquantitative analysis of renal arterial blood flow (3,4). An RI value of less than 0.7 in the main and peripheral renal arteries indicates normal peripheral resistance in the transplant (3).

C. Morphological Abnormalities Associated with Acute Rejection

The diagnosis of acute rejection, by either morphological or Doppler criteria, is possible if the pathological changes associated with acute rejection are severe enough to translate into recognizable alteration of the sonographic appearance of the transplant. The sonographic abnormalities directly reflect the underlying histopathological process.

In acute interstitial rejection, the interstitium of the kidney is infiltrated with edema and inflammatory cells (8,9). The allograft suddenly increases in size compared to baseline study and becomes more globular in shape (9–12). Since the lymphocyte-mediated immune response is most prominent at the corticomedullary junction, the edematous pyramids become larger, lose their triangular shape, and are more hypoechoic (9,12,13); there is also loss of the normal corticomedullary differentiation (9). The renal sinus echoes hypoechoic and indistinct as adipose tissue is infiltrated by edema and fibrosis (8) (Fig. 2). In severe cases, areas of hemorrhage and infarction are found throughout the renal parenchyma, and the echotexture of the renal cortex becomes inhomogeneous, with scattered patchy areas of decreased echotexture reflecting edema and infarction and areas of hyperechogenicity due to recent hemorrhage (9,13,14). Mild dilatation of the collecting system and thickening of the wall due to submucosal edema can occur (15,16). Peritransplant fluid collection may be

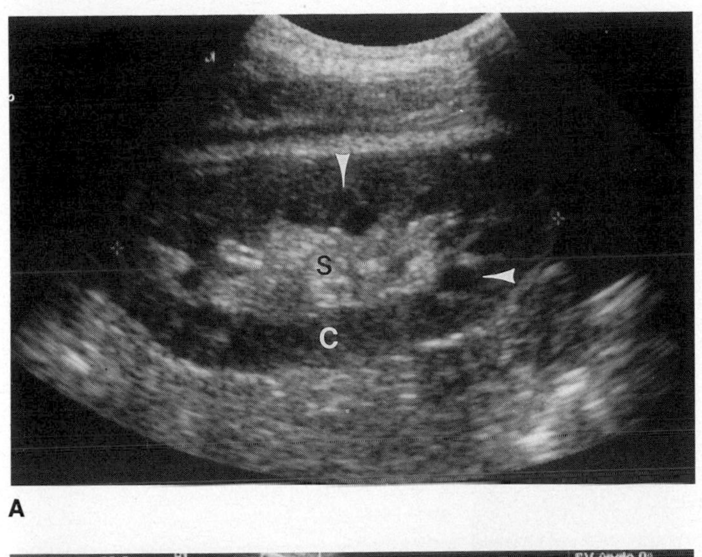

A

B

Figure 1 A: Sagittal sonogram of a normal renal transplant. There is good corticomedullary differentiation and the hypoechoic pyramids are clearly visible (arrowheads). S = renal sinus: C = renal cortex. B: Doppler spectrum obtained in an arcuate artery shows normal flow pattern characteristic of a low-impedance peripheral vascular bed with continuous forward flow in diastole. The resistive index is 0.53.

seen secondary to small areas of cortical disruption along Brodee's line. The overall sensitivity of gray-scale sonography in the diagnosis of acute rejection has been reported to be as low as 52% (17) or as high as 85 to 90% (18,19). The presence of multiple sonographic abnormalities increases the specificity of the diagnosis at the cost of a reduced sensitivity (13,20). However, the combination of a sudden increase in transplant size, enlargement of the pyramids, and inhomogeneity of the renal cortex has been found to be particularly helpful (21). Unfortunately, many cases of acute rejection are not associated with sono-

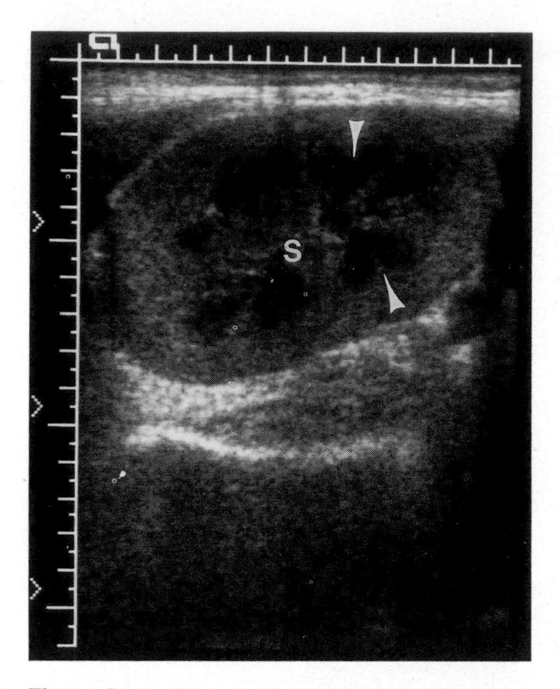

Figure 2 Sagittal sonogram of a transplant with moderate degree of acute rejection. The transplant is enlarged and globular in shape, the pyramids are enlarged (arrowheads), and there is complete loss of the central sinus echoes (S). (From Ref. 70.)

graphically detectable morphological changes in the transplanted kidney, and the absence of sonographic abnormalities does not exclude underlying rejection. In young children, sonography is often inconclusive (12). Whenever there is a strong clinical suspicion of acute rejection, percutaneous biopsy of the allograft is warranted and is usually performed under sonographic guidance, which helps guide the needle toward the area of maximum morphological abnormality.

D. Role of Color and Duplex Color Sonography in the Diagnosis of Acute Rejection

Initial studies evaluating renal transplants with duplex Doppler ultrasound were quite promising and had raised hopes that this modality would be helpful in differentiating acute rejection from other causes of parenchymal dysfunction, such as acute tubular necrosis and cyclosporin A toxicity (2,4,22,23). In the vascular form of acute rejection, the small vessels of the transplant are involved in the pathological process, resulting in vasoconstriction followed by acute necrotizing vasculitis, swelling of the endothelial cells and fibrointimal proliferation with narrowing of the arterial lumen. The resulting increase in vascular impedance is reflected in the Doppler spectral waveform, with loss of the normal diastolic flow and elevation of the resistive and pulsatility indices (Fig. 3B) (3,4,22). Rifkin et al. showed (3) that a resistive index value of 0.80 detected nearly 70% of transplants with acute rejection, and values of RI above 0.9 had a 100% positive predictive value for the diagnosis with, however, a sensitivity of only 13%.

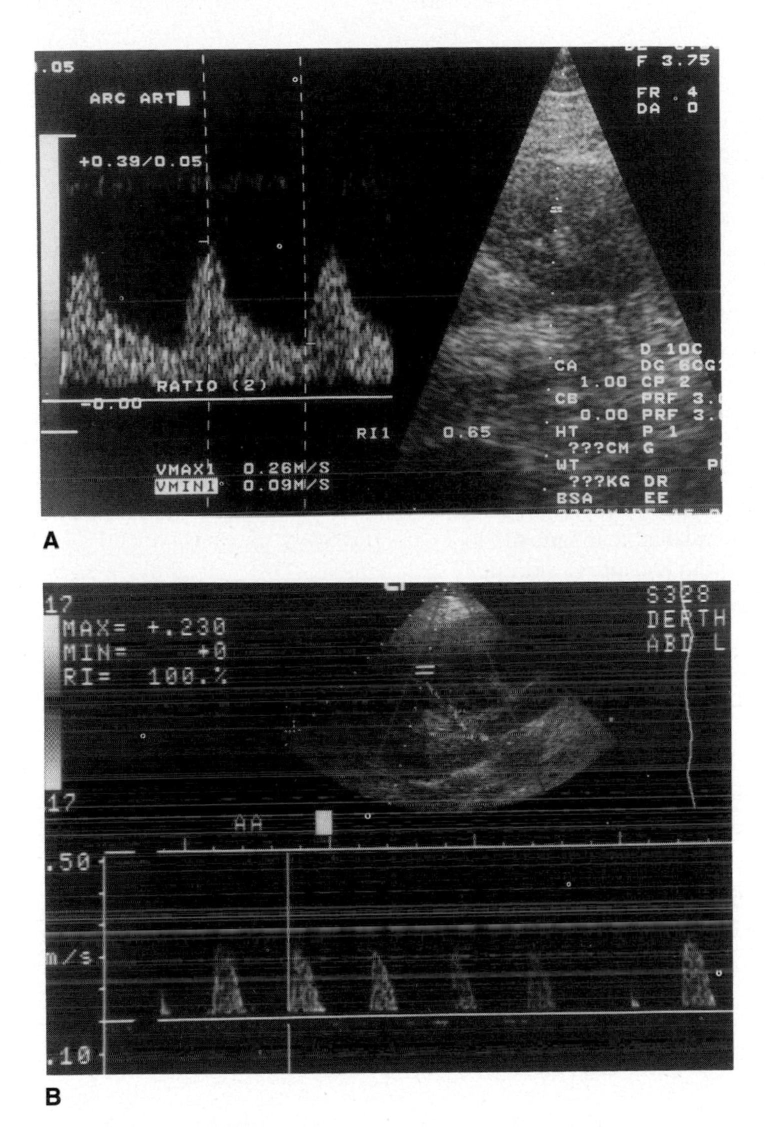

Figure 3 A: Doppler spectrum of the arcuate artery, obtained 4 days after surgery, is normal. The resistive index is 0.65. B: Two days later, the patient experienced a marked decrease in urine output. There has been a dramatic change in the appearance of the Doppler spectrum in the arcuate artery, with complete loss of diastolic flow. The resistive index is 1. Pathological examination revealed there was severe acute rejection with vasculitis.

Initial enthusiasm for measurement of vascular indices in predicting acute rejection has been somewhat dampened as several recent studies have shown that Doppler sonography results do not necessarily obviate the need for biopsy. A significant number of patients with clinically suspected or pathologically proven acute rejection have an RI in the normal (0.7 or less) or indeterminate (<0.8) range (3,24–26). In addition, finding of an abnormal RI is not specific for acute rejection: many other processes affecting the renal transplant—including severe acute tubular necrosis, severe pyelonephritis, acute renal vein thrombosis, obstructive uropathy, and marked compression of the renal parenchyma by a large fluid collection—may affect vascular impedance in the allograft (27,28). However, a highly elevated RI or PI usually indicate poor function of the graft and need for further investigation (29). Even the most severe alteration, reversal of diastolic flow, is not specific for acute rejection but does indicate a poor prognosis (27).

This discrepancy in sensitivity, specificity, and positive and negative predictive value of RI and PI in the diagnosis of acute rejection among various studies can in part be explained by several factors: (a) difference in the prevalence of acute rejection and acute tubular necrosis among the patient population (24) and (b) time elapsed between the initial surgery of the transplant and the time of the Doppler study (29). It is clear that Doppler indices are of little value in the diagnosis of chronic rejection, and as transplants older than 1 year are included in some studies (25,30), the sensitivity and specificity of Doppler ultrasound is altered.

The question that therefore arises is whether we should continue to perform duplex ultrasound evaluation of the transplant kidney. We believe that in fact sonography is, in spite of its limitations, an invaluable diagnostic tool. It is relatively inexpensive and safe, and it can be performed at the bedside in extremely sick patients. The clinical differentiation between parenchymal and surgical complications is often problematic, and sonography will be helpful in recognizing most surgical complications.

Sonography is also essential in providing guidance for percutaneous biopsy of the transplant kidney, and ensuring minimum damage to the organ and maximum safety during the procedure. Finally, while isolated measurements of vascular indices lack specificity and sensitivity for the diagnosis of acute rejection, serial measurements may be more valuable. A rise of RI or PI above baseline may be the first indicator of potentially serious complications requiring rapid diagnosis and intervention (Fig. 3). Doppler parameters often also show improvement after successful therapy of acute rejection (6,31).

In summary, despite its limitations, in the appropriate clinical setting, color Doppler sonography is invaluable in the management of patients with suspected acute rejection of a renal transplant.

II. GRAY-SCALE, DOPPLER, AND COLOR DOPPLER SONOGRAPHY IN THE DIAGNOSIS OF LIVER TRANSPLANT REJECTION

Orthotopic liver transplantation has become an accepted treatment for irreversible end-stage liver disease of various causes in both children and adults. Despite advances in immunosuppressive therapy, allograft rejection remains the major cause of posttransplantation morbidity and mortality, occurring in about 37 to 44% of liver allografts and followed by vascular thrombosis and biliary complications (32,33). Although clinical and laboratory findings as well as imaging studies are of clinical importance in the evaluation of complications that jeopardize graft survival, the diagnosis of rejection usually requires histological confirmation by percutaneous liver biopsy (33,34). Acute rejection is also the leading cause of graft failure, requiring retransplantation (35). The diagnosis of rejection remains difficult because other technical and physiological complications can present in similar fashion, while symptoms and laboratory abnormalities are often nonspecific. The key to treating acute rejection is early detection and timely implementation of powerful immunosuppressive therapy. Duplex sonography has been shown to be useful in detecting hepatic artery thrombosis, biliary obstruction, and postoperative bilomas, hematomas, or seromas

(34,36–42). Measurement of hepatic artery resistive indices has been shown to be unreliable for the diagnosis of rejection (43,44). Measurement of changes in pulsatility of the hepatic veins, however, has shown promise in detecting rejection (45,46).

A. Examination Technique

The hepatic transplant is examined with 3.5- or 5-MHz high-resolution sector or curvilinear transducers with duplex and color Doppler capabilities. With gray-scale sonography, the echotexture of the hepatic transplant as well as intra- or peritransplant fluid collections (hematoma, biloma, seroma) are assessed. The biliary tract is systematically surveyed and postoperative biliary complications—such as biliary obstruction and bile leakage from various causes—are evaluated. Duplex and Doppler examinations of the portal vein, hepatic artery, hepatic veins, and inferior vena cava allow assessment of normal directional arterial and venous vascular supply of the transplant and possible causes of graft failure, such as hepatic artery thrombosis, portal vein and inferior vena cava thrombosis, and anastomotic vascular complications such as aneurysms or pseudoaneurysms of the hepatic artery or portal vein (36,37,42,47,48). Analysis of Doppler waveforms allows measurement of the PI or RI of the hepatic artery as well as evaluation of the hepatic veins.

B. The Normal Liver Transplant

The hepatic parenchyma of a normal transplanted liver shows a uniform and homogeneous echotexture with Doppler ultrasound (49). Characteristic Doppler waveforms are obtained from the hepatic artery, portal vein, hepatic veins, and inferior vena cava. The portal vein shows continuous and relatively low velocity flow with slight decrease in flow during inspiration and mild phasic changes related to the cardiac cycle (Fig. 4A). The hepatic artery demonstrates flow throughout diastole, because of the low vascular impedance of the distal hepatic vascular bed (Fig. 4B). The hepatic veins normally show a triphasic flow pattern with wide moment-to-moment variations of flow with the respiratory and cardiac cycle, reflecting free reflux of blood from the right atrium during systole (Fig. 4C). Flow decreases with expiration and increases with inspiration. Patency as well as normal directional flow (hepatopetal) of especially the hepatic artery and portal vein can easily be seen by duplex or color Doppler ultrasound. Small perihepatic collections (hematomas) or small pleural effusions are infrequently seen in the immediate postoperative period.

C. Morphological Abnormalities Associated with Rejection

Radiographic features reported in rejection have included stretching and attenuation of the intrahepatic bile ducts on cholangiography and diffuse narrowing and stretching of the intrahepatic arterial tree on angiography, all thought to result from swelling of the liver associated with the acute rejection process (44). Letourneau et al. (40) reported that acute rejection was associated with an overall decrease in the echogenicity of the hepatic parenchyma and loss of distinction of the hepatic vein margins, while chronic rejection was characterized by an increase in periportal echogenicity. Kubota et al. (49) reported an increase in echogenicity of the liver parenchyma in their patients. These findings were, however, not a consistent feature in acute rejection. In addition, a normal appearance of the liver parenchyma in a patient with rejection has been described (38). Areas of increased periportal echogenicity have been attributed to transient ischemia or periportal lymphatic

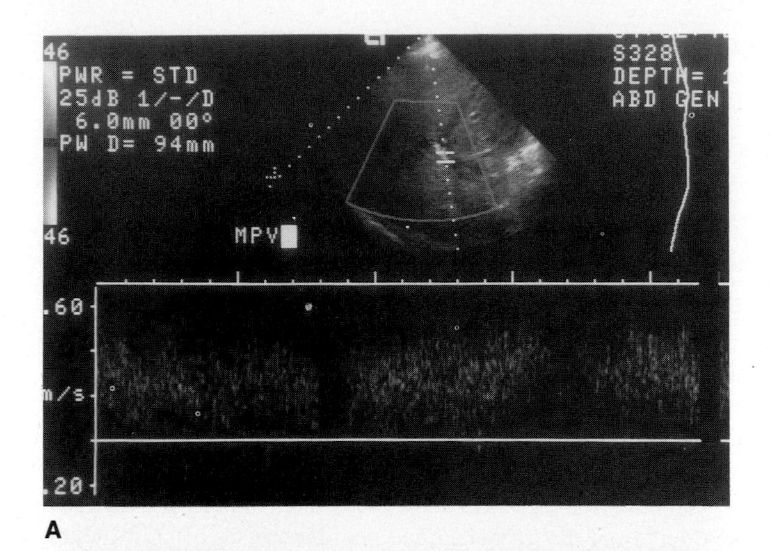
PWR = STD
25dB 1/-/D
6.0mm 00°
PW D= 94mm
S328
MPV
.60
m/s
.20

A

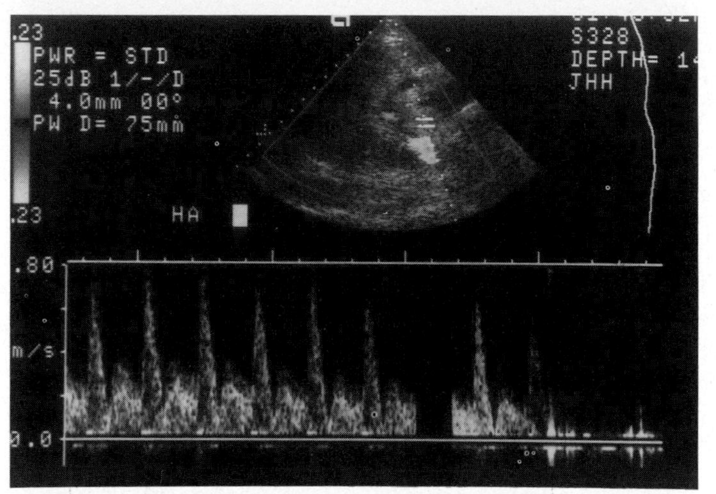
PWR = STD
25dB 1/-/D
4.0mm 00°
PW D= 75mm
S328
JHH
HA
.80
m/s
0.0

B

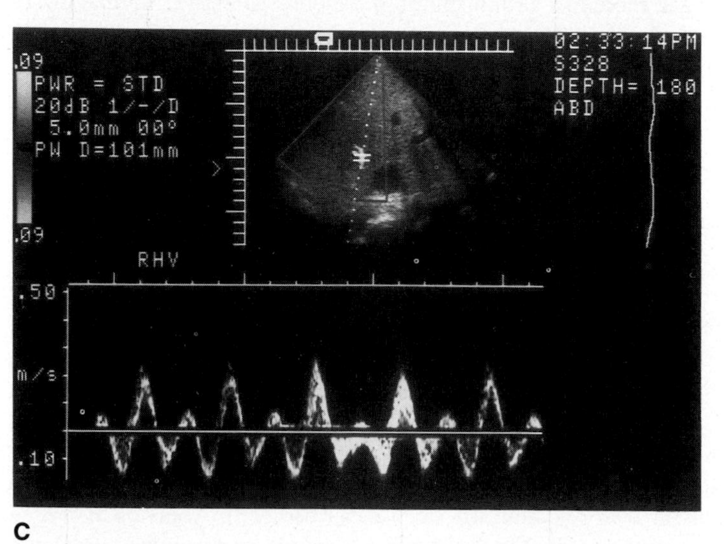
02:33:14PM
S328
DEPTH= 180
ABD
PWR = STD
20dB 1/-/D
5.0mm 00°
PW D=101mm
RHV
.50
m/s
.10

C

engorgement (39). All of the morphological abnormalities described have, however, been nonspecific for the diagnosis of rejection.

D. Role of Duplex and Color Doppler Sonography in the Diagnosis of Acute Rejection

Duplex ultrasonography has been used to measure the RI in the hepatic artery. In contrast to renal allografts, where acute elevation of the RI has been associated with the onset of acute rejection, numerous studies have not shown a similar association in orthotopic liver transplant patients (44,49). Kubota et al. (49) found no statistically significant difference in RI of the hepatic artery in stable grafts, grafts with ischemic damage, acute or chronic rejection, or cytomegalovirus hepatitis. Also, no correlation between the levels of RI and the severity of rejection was found. Coulden et al. (45) reported damping of the normal triphasic waveforms of the hepatic veins in acute rejection, secondary to a distortion of normal hepatic compliance by the inflammatory and edematous response in acute rejection. In their study, an abrupt loss of hepatic vein pulsatility without evidence of cholangitis had a positive predictive value of 78% and a negative predictive value of 100% for rejection. Changes in hepatic vein waveform and hence liver compliance preceded clinical and biochemical evidence of rejection by up to 36 hr (45). Spaeder et al. (46) found a qualitative change (monophasic) in waveforms of at least one hepatic vein (Fig. 5) associated with rejection in the first 14 postoperative days, giving a sensitivity of 73%, specificity of 64% and positive predictive value of 80%. When grouping rejection and cholangitis, which are the leading causes of graft failure, together, the appearance of a monophasic waveform had a sensitivity of 70%, specificity of 86%, positive predictive value of 95%, and negative predictive value of 43%.

In conclusion, duplex and color Doppler ultrasonography is an important diagnostic tool in the assessment of liver transplant patients with graft dysfunction. It reliably provides anatomic information about the graft parenchyma and allows noninvasive assessment of the patency of the vascular system and potential vascular and anastomotic complications. Its role in the evaluation of early rejection, however, is currently limited. Serial Doppler evaluations with particular attention to the damping of the hepatic waveforms in combination with the clinical evaluation may allow earlier diagnosis and treatment of liver rejection and obviate the need for percutaneous biopsy in the diagnosis of acute liver transplant rejection. This, however, is usually possible only after other causes of graft failure and postoperative complications have been excluded.

III. GRAY-SCALE, DOPPLER, AND COLOR DOPPLER SONOGRAPHY IN THE DIAGNOSIS OF PANCREAS TRANSPLANT REJECTION

In recent years, pancreatic transplantation has become an important therapeutic option for patients with type I diabetes, in order to prevent or delay damage to the microcirculation of their critical organs. Complications associated with pancreatic transplantation include

Figure 4 Normal Doppler spectral wave pattern of the hepatic vessels. A: Main portal vein with continuous low-velocity flow and minimal respiratory variation. B: Hepatic artery with pulsatile and forward diastolic flow characteristic of low peripheral vascular resistance. C: Hepatic vein with triphasic flow pattern and variations of flow with the respiratory and cardiac cycle.

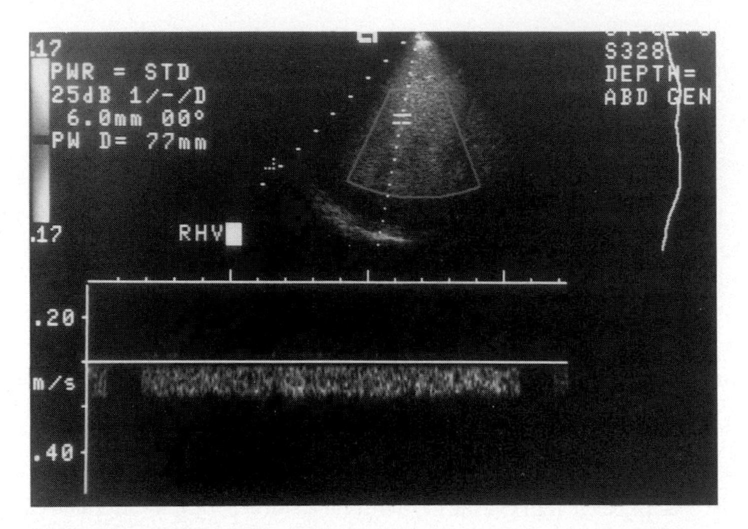

Figure 5 Monophasic waveform of hepatic veins in patient with biopsy-proven rejection. Compare to normal triphasic waveform in Fig. 4C.

vascular thrombosis, rejection, infection, and pancreatitis. The major cause of graft failure after the immediate postoperative phase is rejection (50). The early signs of rejection are, unfortunately, subtle, and graft damage often occurs before rejection is detected and treatment can be instituted (51). Urine chemistry tests and serum glucose, amylase, and lipase levels are the primary noninvasive means of detecting rejection (50–52). Gray scale Doppler and color Doppler ultrasonography (US) allow detection of vascular complications after pancreas transplantation, and are especially useful for detection of graft thrombosis, the presence of intra- or extrapancreatic collections, and assessment of gland size. Its role in the early detection of graft rejection, however, remains uncertain and has been the subject of much controversy in recent years.

A. Examination Technique

The pancreatic transplant is examined with 3.5- or 5-MHz high-resolution sector, linear, or curvilinear array transducers with duplex and color Doppler capabilities. Gray-scale sonography allows morphological evaluation of the transplant echotexture and size as well as peritransplant collections. Duplex and color Doppler exams provide physiological information regarding the vascular supply of the transplant and possible causes of graft failure such as ischemia, hemorrhage, vascular thrombosis, or anastomotic vascular complications (i.e., aneurysms, pseudoaneurysms, or arteriovenous fistulas). The vascular impedance of the pancreatic transplant can be assessed through the analysis of Doppler waveforms and measurement of the PI and RI.

B. The Normal Pancreas Transplant

Transplantation of a whole pancreas or segments of cadaver or living related donor pancreas is performed alone or in combination with a renal transplant. The success rate of pancreatic transplants has improved drastically in recent years due to advancement in surgical techniques and in postoperative care (53,54). The pancreas is transplanted intraperitoneally or extraperitoneally in the iliac fossa. Vascular connections usually include the donor celiac and superior mesenteric arteries on aortic patch grafts anastomosed to the recipient's external iliac artery, with the donor's portal vein draining into the external iliac vein. The exocrine portion of the gland is drained via a segment of donor duodenum anastomosed to the recipient's bladder. Spectral waveform analysis allows demonstration of the circulation in the pancreatic allograft and its vascular anastomoses by duplex Doppler US (55) (Figs. 6A–C). The normal allograft can usually be identified by gray-scale US. Dimensions as well as echotexture of the graft can be assessed. The normal transplant is homogeneous in echotexture and mildly echogenic. Normal allograft anterior-posterior dimensions are usually less than 2 cm (Fig. 7). Occasionally difficulties in visualization are related to large body habitus of the patient or obscuration by adjacent bowel loops. Changes in size and echotexture as well as peritransplant collections are signs of parenchymal disease. Absence of vascular flow is associated with acute vascular thrombosis especially on the venous side and is the second most common cause of graft loss. Increased intraparenchymal resistance with elevated resistive indices (>0.7) have been reported to be associated with graft rejection (56,57).

C. Morphological Abnormalities Associated with Rejection

Changes in size and echotexture of the pancreas, dilatation of the pancreatic duct, and peritransplant fluid collections have been associated with graft failure secondary to rejection (58–60). Diffuse enlargement of the gland with a concomitant decrease in echotexture and indistinct margins can be seen in rejection (Fig. 8A). These findings, however, are not specific for rejection and may be related to pancreatitis and infection (54). Likewise, dilatation of the pancreatic duct and fluid collections can be seen in rejection, infection, or pancreatitis (Fig. 8B). Chronic rejection has been suggested when grafts are small, increased in echotexture, or not possible to visualize (57). A recent report by Wong et al. (61) evaluated gland size, heterogeneity, ductal dilatation, marginal definition, and peripancreatic fluid collections in patients with biopsy-proven rejection and found abnormal morphological appearances to be a nonspecific finding and not diagnostic of transplant rejection. Therefore, since no simple, reliable, noninvasive predictor of early pancreatic transplant rejection has been found to date, percutaneous biopsy is usually required to make this diagnosis. These biopsies can be performed safely and accurately with computed tomographic (CT) or sonographic guidance, avoiding injury to the anastomotic vessels or surrounding organs (61,62), or via a cystoscopic transduodenal approach (63). Ultrasonography is also useful in guiding percutaneous aspirations or drainage of peritransplant fluid collections, including pseudocysts, hematomas, seromas, abscesses, and lymphoceles.

D. Role of Duplex and Color Doppler Sonography in the Diagnosis of Acute Rejection

Doppler US and especially color Doppler studies allow visualization of graft and host vessels in most patients. The most common and critical vascular complication after pancreatic transplantation is graft thrombosis, especially venous thrombosis, occurring in 13 to 20% of cases (64). Conventional and color Doppler studies have been shown to detect graft thrombosis with a reported sensitivity of 80% and specificity of 80% (65–67). In addition, pseudoaneurysms, arteriovenous fistulas, and anastomotic stenoses can be detected (54,57,65). Initial experience with flow velocity indices (RI and PI) in renal transplants had raised hope for the evaluation of acute pancreatic transplant rejection, since the pathological process of vascular rejection is similar in the kidney and pancreas, both

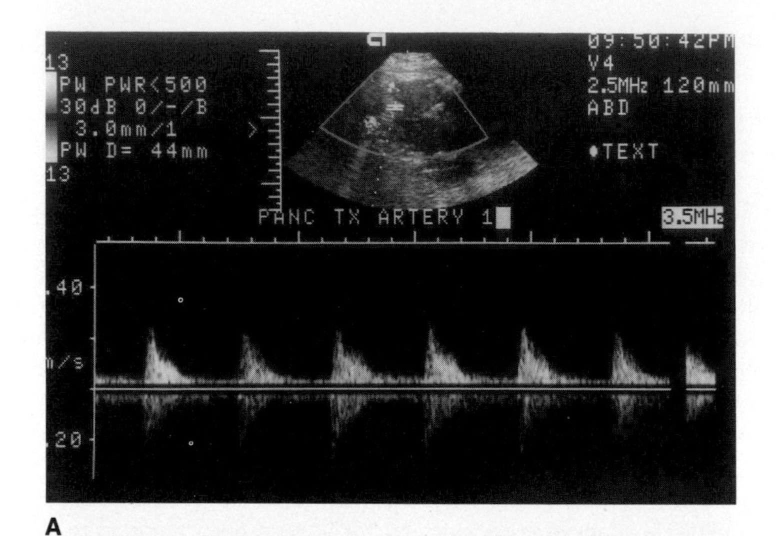

09:50:42PM
V4
2.5MHz 120mm
ABD
•TEXT
13
PW PWR<500
30dB 0/-/B
3.0mm/1
PW D= 44mm
13
PANC TX ARTERY 1
3.5MHz
.40
m/s
.20

A

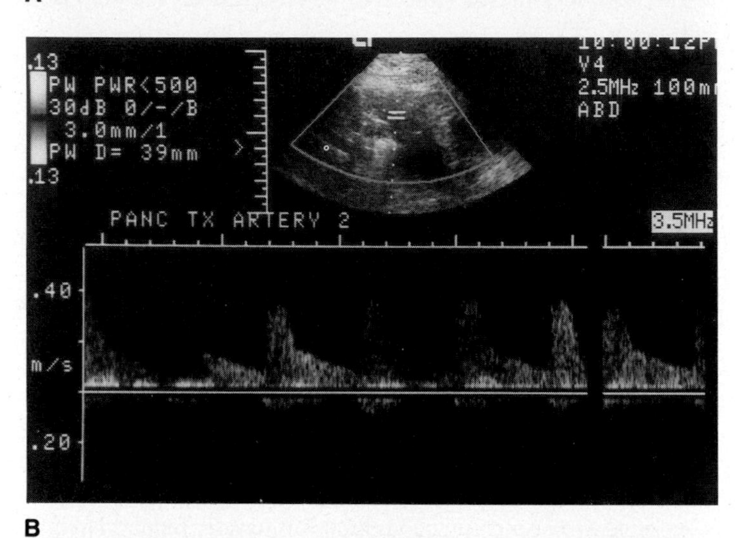

V4
ABD
.13
PW PWR<500
30dB 0/-/B
3.0mm/1
PW D= 39mm
.13
PANC TX ARTERY 2
3.5MHz
.40
m/s
.20

B

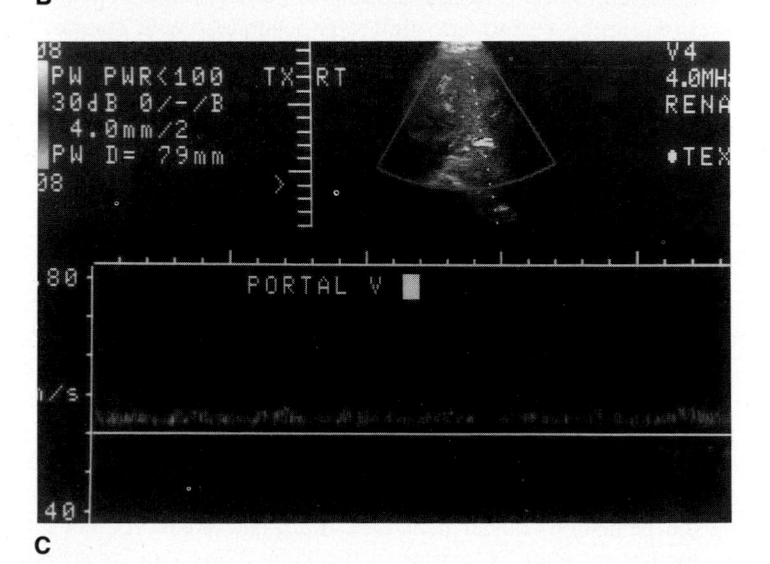

PW PWR<100 TX RT
30dB 0/-/B
4.0mm/2
PW D= 79mm
V4
PORTAL V
.80
.40

C

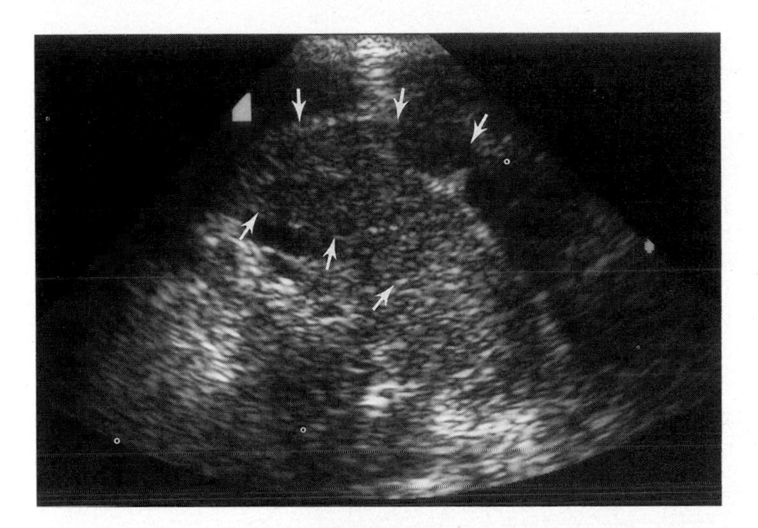

Figure 7 Normal pancreatic allograft (arrows).

leading to increased vascular impedance or resistance to flow and reflected in loss of normal diastolic flow and thus increase in RI and PI.

Patel et al. (58) reported an RI of 0.70 or less in parenchymal vessels of normal transplants and of greater than 0.70 in 87.5% of clinical episodes of rejection. In this study, a positive predictive value of an RI above 0.70 for rejection was 100%, and the negative predictive value of an RI less than 0.70 was 90% in excluding rejection. High RI values were not seen in cyclosporine toxicity, pancreatitis, peripancreatic hemorrhage, or infection. Gilabert et al. (68) showed an increase in RI >0.8 in 18/21 episodes of rejection, with RI normalization (RI <0.63 ± 0.05) after rejection therapy. These initially promising reports, however, could not be corroborated in studies by Kubota et al. (69) and Wong et al. (61). Kubota found acute rejection even when the RI was below 0.7. Wong reported a sensitivity of 23% and specificity of 50% for rejection with an RI >0.7. The discrepancies in these studies may be explained by technical factors (isolated rather than serial RI measurements), availability of different early markers of cellular rejections, and lack of biopsy correlation in most studies. Although the results of the most recent study (61) are discouraging, serial duplex Doppler measurements may be useful, with individual elevations of RI possibly leading to the detection of early rejection. However, more prospective studies are needed before these conclusions can be drawn. Until the usefulness of duplex Doppler US is consistently proven and reproducible results are obtainable, the diagnosis of transplant rejection will require tissue diagnosis, usually by means of US- or CT-guided biopsies.

In conclusion, sonography is an invaluable tool in the evaluation and management of pancreatic transplant patients. Even though parenchymal gray-scale abnormalities are not specific for histopathological diagnoses (rejection versus infection or ischemia), vascular complications such as graft thrombosis, pseudoaneurysms, arteriovenous fistulas, and

---

Figure 6 Doppler spectral pattern of pancreatic transplant vessels. A: Donor superior mesenteric artery with minimal diastolic flow, characteristic of high-resistance flow pattern. B: Donor celiac artery with forward diastolic flow, characteristic of low-resistance flow pattern. C: Donor portal vein anastomosed to recipient external iliac vein with continuous low-velocity flow.

anastomotic stenosis can be diagnosed with duplex and color Doppler US. Likewise, intra- or peripancreatic fluid collections are easily visualized and drained under sonographic guidance. The role of Doppler sonography for the detection of graft rejection, however, is currently limited because of the lack of sensitivity and specificity of isolated RI or PI elevations in rejection. Baseline studies with careful serial follow-up duplex US examination may prove useful in monitoring patients with suspected graft failure due to rejection. Currently, tissue obtained by either percutaneous or US-guided cystoscopic transduodenal pancreas transplant biopsy is required for the diagnosis of acute or chronic rejection.

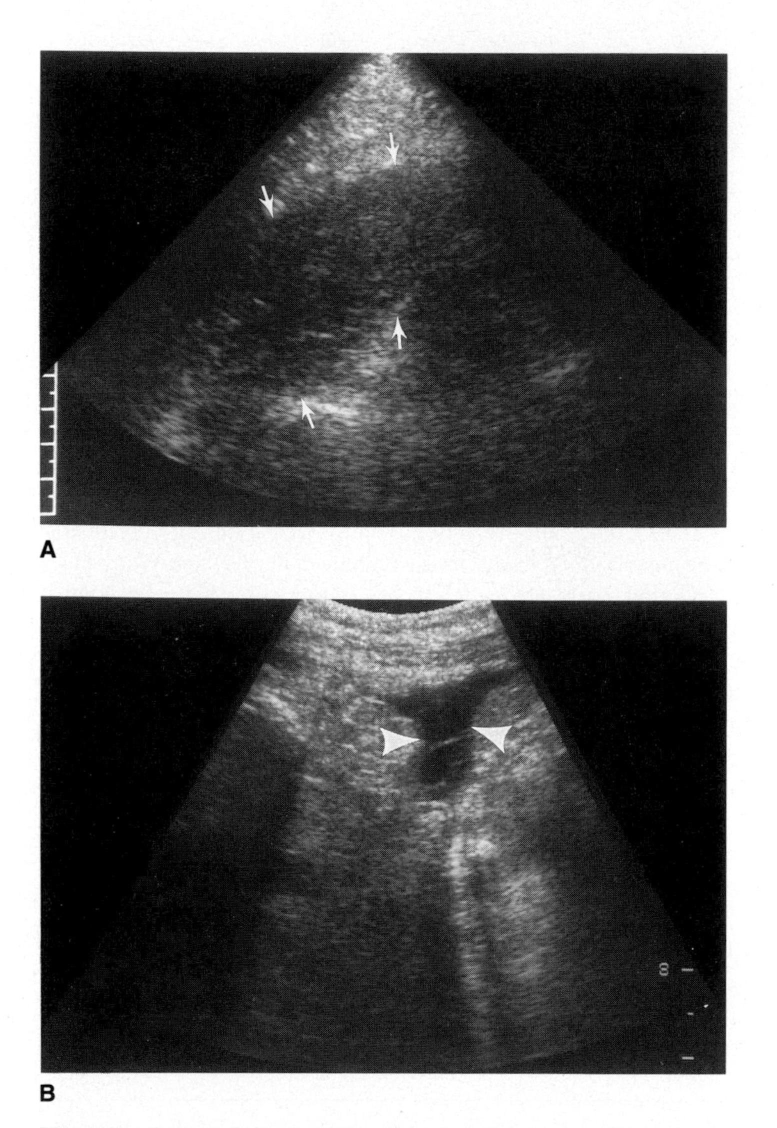

Figure 8 Morphological abnormalities in pancreas transplant rejection. A: Diffuse enlargement of allograft with decreased echotexture and indistinct margins (arrows). B: Complex peripancreatic collection (arrowheads).

REFERENCES

Renal Allograft Rejection

1. Hoddick W, Filly RA, Backman U, et al. Renal allograft rejection: US evaluation. Radiology 1986; 161:469–473.
2. Thomsen HS, Dorph S, Mygind T, et al. The transplanted kidney: Diagnostic and interventional radiology. Acta Radiol Diagn (Stockh) 1985; 26:353–367.
3. Rifkin MD, Needleman L, Pasto ME, et al. Evaluation of renal transplant rejection by duplex Doppler examination: Value of the resistive index. AJR 1987; 148:759–762.
4. Rigsby CM, Burns PN, Weltin GG, et al. Doppler signal quantitation in renal allografts: Comparison in normal and rejecting transplants, with pathologic correlation. Radiology 1987; 162(1, pt 1):39–42.
5. Berland LL, Lawson TL, Adams MB, et al. Evaluation of renal transplants with pulsed Doppler duplex sonography. J Ultrasound Med 1982; 1:215–222.
6. Murphy AM, Robertson RJ, Dubbins PA. Duplex ultrasound in the assessment of renal transplant complications. Clin Radiol 1987; 38:229–234.
7. Rifkin MD, Pasto ME, Goldberg BB. Duplex Doppler examination in renal disease: Evaluation of vascular involvement. Ultrasound Med Biol 1985; 11:341–346.
8. Hricak H, Romanski RN, Eyler WR. The renal sinus during allograft rejection: Sonographic and histopathologic findings. Radiology 1982; 142:693–699.
9. Morley AR. Transplant rejection, in: Williams DI, Chisholm GD, eds. Scientific Foundations of Urology. Chicago: Year Book, 1976:167–171.
10. Hricak H, Cruz C, Eyler WR, et al. Acute post-transplantation renal failure: Differential diagnosis by ultrasound. Radiology 1981; 139:441–449.
11. Hricak H, Toledo-Pereyra LH, Eyler WR, et al. Evaluation of acute post-transplant renal failure by ultrasound. Radiology 1979; 133:443–447.
12. Slovis TL, Babcock DS, Hricak H, et al. Renal transplant rejection: Sonographic evaluation in children. Radiology 1984; 153:659–665.
13. Linkowski GD, Warvariv V, Filly RA, Vincenti F. Sonography in the diagnosis of acute renal allograft rejection and cyclosporine nephrotoxicity. AJR 1987; 148:291–295.
14. Frick MP, Salomonowitz E, Feinberg SB. Sonography of abdominal posttransplant lymphoma. J Clin Ultrasound 1984; 12:383–385.
15. Babcock DS, Slovis TL, Han BK, et al. Renal transplants in children: Long-term follow-up using sonography. Radiology 1985; 156:165–167.
16. Birnholz JC, Merkel FK. Submucosal edema of the collecting system: A new ultrasonic sign of severe, acute renal allograft rejection. A clinical note. Radiology 1985; 154:190.
17. Fried AM, Woodring JH, Loh FK, et al. The medullary pyramid index: An objective assessment of prominence in renal transplant rejection. Radiology 1983; 149:787–791.
18. Frick MP, Feinberg SB, Sibley R, Idstrom ME. Ultrasound in acute renal transplant rejection. Radiology 1981; 138:657–660.
19. Raiss GJ, Bree RL, Schwab RE, et al. Further observations in the ultrasound evaluation of renal allograft rejection. J Ultrasound Med 1986; 5:439–444.
20. Townsend RR, Tomlanovich SJ, Goldstein RB, Filly RA. Combined Doppler and morphologic sonographic evaluation of renal transplant rejection. J Ultrasound Med 1990; 9:199–206.
21. Swobodnik WL, Spohn BE, Wechsler JG, et al. Real-time ultrasound evaluation of renal transplant failure during the early postoperative period. Ultrasound Med Biol 1986; 12:97–105.
22. Rigsby CM, Taylor KJW, Weltin G, et al. Renal allografts in acute rejection: Evaluation using duplex sonography. Radiology 1986; 158:375–378.
23. Buckley AR, Cooperberg PL, Reeve CE, Magil AB. The distinction between acute renal transplant rejection and cyclosporine nephrotoxicity: Value of duplex sonography. AJR 1987; 149:521–525.
24. Perrella RR, Duerinckx AJ, Tessler FN, et al. Evaluation of renal transplant dysfunction by

duplex Doppler sonography: A prospective study and review of the literature. Am J Kidney Dis 1990; 15:544–550.
25. Genkins SM, Sanfilippo FP, Carroll BA. Duplex Doppler sonography of renal transplants: Lack of sensitivity and specificity in establishing pathologic diagnosis. AJR 1989; 152:535–539.
26. Perchik JE, Baumgartner BR, Bernardino ME. Renal transplant rejection: Limited value of duplex Doppler sonography. Invest Radiol 1991; 26:422–426.
27. Warshauer DM, Taylor KJW, Bia MJ, et al. Unusual causes of increased vascular impedance in renal transplants: Duplex Doppler evaluation. Radiology 1988; 169:367–370.
28. Kaveggia LP, Perrella RR, Grant EG, et al. Duplex Doppler sonography in renal allografts: The significance of reversed flow in diastole. AJR 1990; 155:295–298.
29. Taylor KJW, Marks WH. Use of Doppler imaging for evaluation of dysfunction in renal allografts. AJR 1990; 155:536–537.
30. Drake DG, Day DL, Letourneau JG, et al. Doppler evaluation of renal transplants in children: A prospective analysis with histopathologic correlation. AJR 1990; 154:785–787.
31. Rasmussen K, Pedersen E. Doppler ultrasound in the diagnosis of renal allograft rejection and in monitoring the effect of treatment. Scand J Clin Lab Invest 1990; 50:57–61.

Liver Transplant Rejection

32. Legmann P, Dousset B, Tudoret L, et al. Hyperacute rejection in liver transplantation: CT findings. J Comput Assist Tomogr 1994; 18:139–142.
33. Dominguez R, Cuervas-Mons V, Van Thiel DH, et al. Radiographic features of liver allograft rejection. Gastrointest Radiol 1986; 11:326–329.
34. Oliver JH 3d, Federle MP, Campbell WL, Zajko A. Imaging the hepatic transplant. Radiol Clin North Am 1991; 29:1285–1298.
35. Demetris AJ, Lasky S, Van Thiel DH, et al. Pathology of hepatic transplantation: A review of 62 adult allograft recipients immunosuppressed with a cyclosporine/steroid regimen. Am J Pathol 1985; 118:151–161.
36. Koslin DB, Berland LL. Duplex Doppler examination of the liver and portal venous system. J Clin Ultrasound 1987; 5:675–686.
37. Segel MC, Zajko AB, Bowen A, et al. Hepatic artery thrombosis after liver transplantation: Radiologic evaluation. AJR 1986; 146:137–141.
38. Dalen K, Day DL, Ascher NL, et al. Imaging of vascular complications after hepatic transplantation. AJR 1988; 150:1285–1290.
39. Claus D, Clapuyt P. Liver transplantation in children: Role of the radiologist in the preoperative assessment and the postoperative follow-up. Transplant Proc 1987; 19:3344–3357.
40. Letourneau JG, Day DL, Frick MP, et al. Ultrasound and computed tomographic evaluation in hepatic transplantation. Radiol Clin North Am 1987; 25:323–331.
41. Letourneau JG, Day DL, Ascher NL, et al. Abdominal sonography after hepatic transplantation: Results in 36 patients. AJR 1987; 149:299–303.
42. Hall TR, McDiarmid SV, Grant EG, et al. False-negative duplex Doppler studies in children with hepatic artery thrombosis after liver transplantation. AJR 1990; 154:573–575.
43. Taylor KJW, Morse SS, Weltin GG, et al. Liver transplant recipients: Portable duplex US with correlative angiography. Radiology 1986; 159:357–363.
44. Morton MJ, James EM, Wiesner RH, Krom RA. Applications of duplex ultrasonography in the liver transplant patient. Mayo Clin Proc 1990; 65:360–372.
45. Coulden RA, Britton PD, Farman P, et al. Preliminary report: Hepatic vein Doppler in the early diagnosis of acute liver transplant rejection. Lancet 1990; 336:273–275.
46. Spaeder JA, Sheth S, Hamper UM: Hepatic transplant rejection: Duplex evaluation of hepatic vein pulsatility. J Ultrasound Med 1994; 13:S31–S32.
47. Pariente D, Riou JY, Schmit P, et al. Variability of clinical presentation of hepatic artery thrombosis in pediatric liver transplantation: Role of imaging modalities. Pediatr Radiol 1990; 20:253–257.

48. Zajko AB, Campbell WL, Bron KM, et al. Diagnostic and interventional radiology in liver transplantation. Gastroenterol Clin North Am 1988; 17:105–143.
49. Kubota K, Billing H, Ericzon BG, et al. Duplex Doppler ultrasonography for monitoring liver transplants. Acta Radiol 1990; 31:279–283.

Pancreas Transplant Rejection

50. Sutherland DE, Moudry KC. Pancreas transplant registry report. Transplant Proc 1987; 19(4 suppl 4):5–7.
51. Schulak JA, Drevyanko TF. Experimental pancreas allograft rejection: Correlation between histologic and functional rejection and the efficacy of antirejection therapy. Surgery 1985; 98: 330–337.
52. Sollinger HW, Kalayoglu M, Hoffman RM, Belzer FO. Results of segmental and pancreatico-splenic transplantation with pancreaticocystostomy. Transplant Proc 1985; 17:360–362.
53. Perkins JD, Fromme GA, Narr BJ, et al. Pancreas transplantation at Mayo: II. Operative and perioperative management. Mayo Clin Proc 1990; 65:483–495.
54. Day DL, Carpenter BLM, Longley DG. Imaging of the kidney, liver, and pancreas transplant. Ann Chir Gynaecol 1993; 82:121–129.
55. Yang HC, Neumyer MM, Thiele BL, Gifford RRM. Evaluation of pancreatic allograft circulation using color Doppler ultrasonography. Transplant Proc 1990; 22:609–611.
56. Patel B, Markivee CR, Mahanta B, et al. Pancreatic transplantation: Scintigraphy, US, and CT. Radiology 1988; 167:685–687.
57. Yuh WTC, Wiese JA, Abu-Yousef MM, et al. Pancreatic transplant imaging. Radiology 1988; 167:679–683.
58. Patel B, Wolverson MK, Mahanta B. Pancreatic transplant rejection: Assessment with duplex US. Radiology 1989; 173:131–135.
59. Milner LN, Ramos IM, Marks WH, Taylor KJW. Ultrasound imaging of pancreatico-duodenal transplants. J Clin Gastroenterol 1991; 13:570–574.
60. Letourneau JG, Maile CW, Sutherland DER, Feinberg SB. Ultrasound and computed tomography in the evaluation of pancreatic transplantation. Radiol Clin North Am 1987; 25:345–355.
61. Wong JJ, Krebs TL, Klassen D, et al. Evaluation of pancreatic transplant rejection: correlation of ultrasound with biopsy. J Ultrasound Med 1995; 14:S7.
62. Bernardino M, Fernandez M, Neylan J, et al. Pancreatic transplants: CT-guided biopsy. Radiology 1990; 177:709–711.
63. Lowell JA, Bynon JS, Nelson N, et al. Improved technique for transduodenal pancreas transplant biopsy. Transplantation 1994; 57:752–753.
64. Snider JF, Hunter DW, Kuni CC, et al. Pancreatic transplantation: radiologic evaluation of vascular complications. Radiology 1991; 178:749–753.
65. Sutherland DE. Pancreas transplantation. Diabetes Metab Rev 1987; 3:1061–1090.
66. Low RA, Kuni CC, Letourneau JG. Pancreas transplant imaging: An overview. AJR 1990; 155: 13–21.
67. Boiskin I, Sandler MP, Fleischer AC, Nylander WA. Acute venous thrombosis after pancreas transplantation: Diagnosis with duplex Doppler sonography and scintigraphy. AJR 1990; 154: 529–531.
68. Gilabert R, Bru C, Ricart MJ, et al. Pancreatic transplant rejection: Evaluation by duplex-Doppler ultrasound with urinary amylase monitoring correlation. Transplant Proc 1992; 24:11.
69. Kubota K, Billing H, Kelter U, et al. Duplex-Doppler ultrasonography for evaluating pancreatic grafts. Transplant Proc 1990; 22:183.
70. Burdick JF, Racusen LC, Solez K, Williams GM, eds. Kidney Transplant Rejection, 2d ed. New York: Marcel Dekker, 1992; p465.

21

Clinical Diagnosis of Chronic Rejection

Leendert C. Paul and Jeffrey S. Zaltzman
St. Michael's Hospital and University of Toronto, Toronto, Ontario, Canada

I. INTRODUCTION

As the short-term results of organ transplantation have improved (1), concerns regarding the long-term outcome are becoming more important. Chronic rejection is often cited as the single most important cause of graft loss after the first posttransplant year. However, an accurate definition of this condition is still problematic, since neither the clinical signs and symptoms nor most of the histopathological manifestations are specific.

The designation "rejection" in the context of transplantation implies graft destructive allogeneic immune responses of the recipient against incompatible transplantation antigens of the graft. As no test is available to measure such responses accurately, the diagnosis of rejection is usually based on the presence and timing of graft dysfunction alone or in combination with histopathological findings characteristic of rejection that cannot be explained by other causes. The clinical response to antirejection treatments is furthermore frequently used retrospectively as a criterion. Although such an operational definition is often sufficient for the management of patients in the early posttransplant period, it is more difficult to classify late and chronic allograft dysfunction. Interpretational problems arise because the chronicity of the process or processes involved allow enough time for the emergence of tissue repair mechanisms and functional adaptations within the graft that are nonimmunological in nature and do not respond to immunosuppressive drugs.

This chapter reviews the epidemiology, clinical manifestations, and differential diagnosis of chronic allograft loss in various organs with an emphasis on chronic rejection. Attempts to describe the epidemiology are hindered, however, by lack of reliable data; clinical series with long-term follow-up are scarce and reports dealing with specific causes of late graft loss are even rarer; many grafts are not even examined histologically after they have failed, and chronic rejection, when stated as a cause of graft failure, is rarely defined.

II. CHRONIC RENAL TRANSPLANT REJECTION

A. Epidemiology

The fractional renal graft loss due to chronic rejection has been estimated to vary between 4 and 40% in the first 5 years, dependent on the donor source and preservation methods used (2–7). Multivariate analysis have shown that acute rejection episodes substantially increase the likelihood of chronic rejection in the subsequent 5 years; other factors—like retransplantation, infections, low cyclosporin A doses at 1 year, and female gender—are also associated with chronic rejection, but these factors have a low relative risk (6). About 30% of patients who had received a kidney from a living donor and who had experienced one or more acute rejection episodes lost their grafts due to chronic rejection within 5 years; similarly, about 45% of patients with a cadaveric graft who had experienced one or more acute rejection episodes developed chronic rejection, leading to graft failure in 40% of cases (6). The timing of the acute rejection episode(s) seems important, as the prevalence of chronic rejection was 20% in recipients of a living donor kidney who had experienced acute rejection episodes within 60 days versus 43% if the acute rejection episodes occurred after 60 days; similarly, the prevalence of chronic rejection in recipients of a cadaveric graft who had experienced an acute rejection episode within the first 2 months was 36%, versus 63% in patients who had experienced one or more acute rejection episodes later on (6). However, not all studies have found this association (8). Noncompliance with drug therapies is suspected to play an important role in the development of late acute or chronic rejection episodes, but it is difficult to get reliable information on the extent of this problem.

Very little information is available on the prevalence of chronic rejection in transplants that survive for more than 5 years. Data from older studies suggest that 13 to 45% of grafts that have survived for 5 years develop chronic rejection and account for most of the graft failures after exclusion of recipient death (9–11). It is not known whether currently used immunosuppressive drug regimens result in a similar prevalence of late chronic rejections.

B. Clinical Presentations and Differential Diagnosis

The clinical presentation of a patient whose transplant is failing because of chronic rejection is characterized by a progressive decrease in glomerular filtration rate, frequently associated with proteinuria and hypertension (12). It has been postulated that chronic rejection is probably the most common underlying cause of late posttransplant hypertension (13) or the nephrotic syndrome (12), but renal vascular and urological complications as well as other renal parenchymal diseases must be ruled out. Localized renal artery stenosis may be accompanied by an audible bruit over the graft and is confirmed by biplanar arteriography or digital subtraction angiography (14). Late transplant ureteral stenosis is generally due to entrapment of the ureter by scar tissue at the vesicoureteric junction and is usually diagnosed by the hydronephrotic appearance of the graft on ultrasound; the diagnosis is confirmed by percutaneous antegrade pyelography.

The main differential diagnostic challenge is to distinguish chronic rejection from other renal parenchymal lesions, especially chronic cyclosporin A (CsA) nephrotoxicity and recurrent or de novo renal disorders. A renal biopsy is usually necessary, and even this approach may not always be diagnostic. The histopathological manifestations of chronic rejection are characterized by lesions in the vessels, the glomeruli, and the tubulointerstitial compartment (15,16). The vascular changes affect large parts of the arterial and arteriolar tree and consist of concentric narrowing of the lumen due to migration and proliferation of myofibroblasts and fibroblasts from the media into the intima, in conjunction with deposition of extracellular matrix material (Fig. 1). The peritubular capillaries may show characteristic thickening and multilayering of the basement membrane (17). The differential diagnosis of the arterial lesions includes all renal vascular diseases, including arteriosclerotic intimal thickening, thrombotic microangiopathy with involvement of the arteries (as occurs occasionally with CsA immunosuppression), and adaptive intimal fibrosis as seen in chronic renal failure (15).

The glomeruli show a variety of abnormalities, including increased mesangial matrix with partial or complete collapse of the capillary tuft or focal glomerulosclerosis (18). Hamburger et al. were the first to describe a lesion unique to renal transplants and coined the term "rejection glomerulonephritis" (19). This lesion is considered a glomerular manifestation of chronic rejection and has also been called rejection nephropathy (20), transplant glomerular disease (21,22), rejection transplant glomerulopathy (23), transplant glomerulopathy (24), and allograft glomerulopathy (25). It is characterized by widespread reduplication of the glomerular basement membrane, a moderate increase in mesangial matrix, and interposition of matrix and cells (Figs. 2 and 3). Slight or moderate epithelial cell proliferation may be present, typically near adhesions between the capillary tuft and Bowman's capsule. The light microscopic appearance of transplant glomerulopathy may be very similar to that of membranoproliferative glomerulonephritis (26,27), and immunofluorescence and electron microscopic studies are indispensable to exclude the presence of peripheral C3 deposits characteristic of the latter condition (Figs. 3 and 4). The immunofluorescence staining of kidneys with transplant glomerulopathy is usually nondiagnostic or characterized by segmental deposits of IgM and fibrin, sometimes associated with C3. However, some cases have been described with linear deposits of IgG along the glomerular basement membrane (GBM) or the tubular basement membrane (TBM) or with small peripheral granular deposits of IgG or IgA, resembling a membranous pattern (28). The electron microscopy shows widening of the subendothelial space, with interposition of mesangial cells and formation of new lamina densa. Abnormal structures are present in the

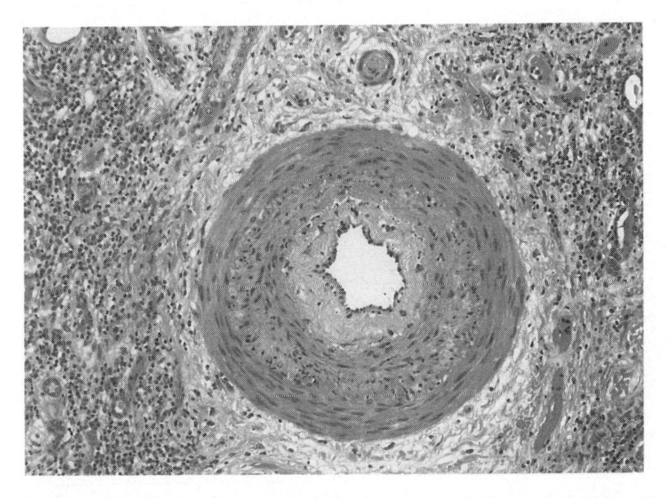

Figure 1 Photomicrograph of a human renal allograft 4 years after transplantation. Marked intimal thickening with proliferation of smooth musclelike cells. (Hematoxylin and eosin stain.) (From Ref. 16.)

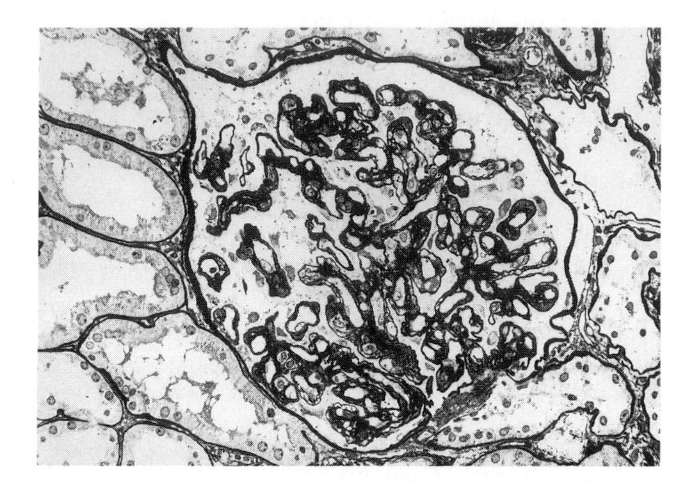

Figure 2 Photomicrograph of a human renal transplant with transplant glomerulopathy. The peripheral capillary walls are markedly thickened, with mesangial interposition.(Periodic acid silver methenamide with toluidine blue counterstain.) (From Ref. 16.)

GBM, between the basement membrane and the endothelium or the epithelium, and in the mesangial matrix (21,22). Immunohistochemistry with antibodies against extracellular matrix proteins has shown peripheral glomerular expansion of collagen 1 alpha (IV) chain, type IV collagen, and fibronectin (28).

Early clinical-pathological studies have found a high incidence of transplant glomerulopathy in chronic rejection (21,22) but more recent studies found the lesion in only 7% of all tissue specimens, representing 23% of the glomerular lesions in renal allografts (29).

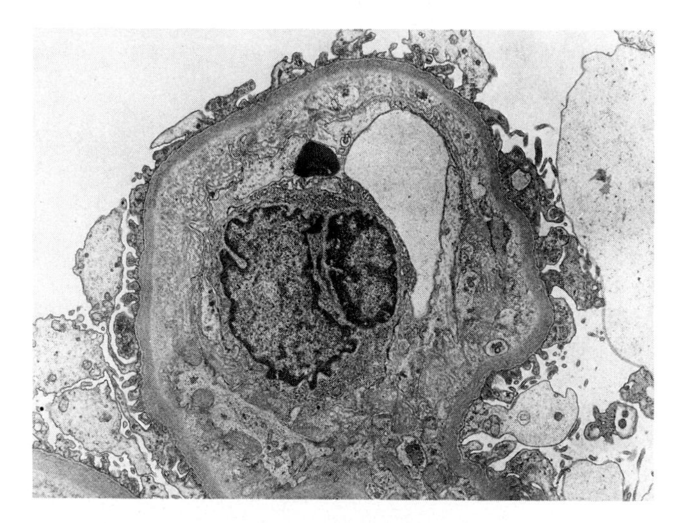

Figure 3 Electron micrograph of a human renal transplant with transplant glomerulopathy. There is a widened subendothelial space containing mesangial cytoplasmic processes and new lamina densa formation. Note the absence of deposits.

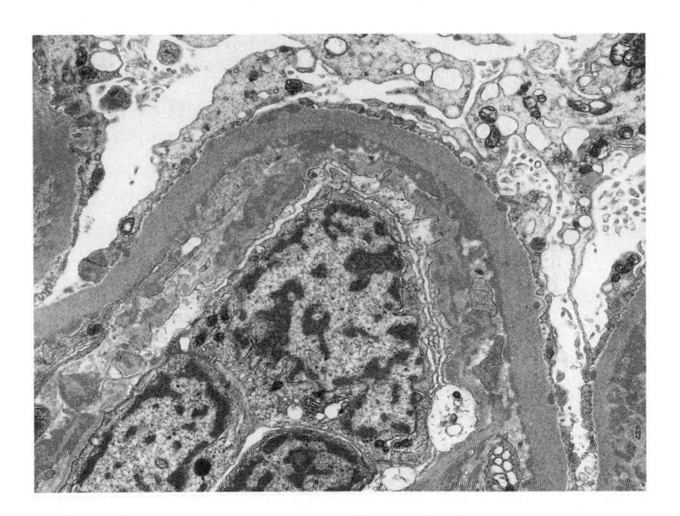

Figure 4 Electron micrograph of a human renal transplant with membranoproliferative glomerulonephritis type I. Portions of the glomerular capillary wall show interposition of mesangial matrix with subendothelial electron-dense deposits.

Transplants with chronic rejection invariably have tubular atrophy, interstitial infiltration, and interstitial fibrosis, and these lesions occasionally dominate the picture. Immunophenotyping of the cellular infiltrate has shown high numbers of plasma cells in the interstitium (30). Since interstitial fibrosis is nonspecific, it cannot be used for the diagnosis of chronic rejection.

Any of the above histological lesions in conjunction with proteinuria and/or declining glomerular filtration rate is considered consistent with chronic rejection after exclusion of other obvious causes of graft dysfunction. However, renal transplant biopsies taken from grafts with normal or slightly increased serum creatinine levels in the first few years after transplantation have shown that up to two-thirds of these grafts have some degree of interstitial fibrosis and tubular atrophy and that more than one-third have some degree of glomerular sclerosis and vascular intimal proliferation. Although the extent of the lesions is usually mild (31,32), it is difficult to use their presence alone as the standard criterion for the diagnosis of chronic rejection. However, the presence of these lesions substantially increases the likelihood of graft dysfunction over the next 2 years (8).

C. Other Parenchymal Renal Diseases

Clinical-pathological studies of transplants with proteinuria of more than 1 g/24 hr for more than 3 months have shown that chronic rejection and transplant glomerulopathy are the leading underlying causes, accounting for 50 to 65% of cases, followed by interstitial fibrosis in 10 to 20% of cases, glomerulonephritis in 10 to 30% of cases, and acute rejection in 10 to 20% of cases (33,34). Chronic CsA nephrotoxicity has been estimated to occur in about 15% of patients (35) and may be difficult to distinguish from chronic rejection. Its clinical manifestation consists of a slowly progressive loss of graft function, usually without proteinuria. Although elevated CsA blood levels may help to distinguish acute nephrotoxicity from chronic rejection, they are usually not excessively high in chronic nephrotoxicity. The histological manifestation of chronic CsA nephrotoxicity is primarily an arteriolar lesion with mucoid endothelial deposits and/or smooth muscle necrosis in conjunction with interstitial fibrosis (15).

Most or all forms of glomerulonephritis may recur or emerge de novo after transplantation (36,37). The recurrence rates vary markedly both among diseases and among different reports for the same disease, presumably because of differences in patient populations, definitions of recurrences, and methods of data acquisition. De novo membranous glomerulopathy, which is the occurrence of membranous nephropathy in recipients whose original renal disease was not membranous nephropathy, has been estimated to occur in 3 to 5% of transplants (38–41) and places this entity second to allograft glomerulopathy as a cause of posttransplant proteinuria, nephrotic syndrome, and renal failure. Recurrence of membranous nephropathy occurs in 10 to 15% of cases (38) and may occur at any time after transplantation. Graft failure occurs more rapidly in de novo than in recurrent disease (42,43).

The most dramatic form of recurrent glomerulonephritis is focal and segmental glomerular sclerosis (FSGS) (44); the reported recurrence rate varied between 5 and 100% in the precyclosporine era, while more recent studies found a recurrence rate of 20 to 50% (45). A recently published single-center study of pediatric patients with FSGS has shown a recurrence rate of 15% (46). In a typical case, massive proteinuria develops within days to months or years without or with persistent or recurrent microscopic hematuria and hypertension. The histopathology is characterized by sclerosis of part of the glomerular tuft in some of the glomeruli; mesangial hypercellularity may be present and electron microscopy shows foot-process fusion of the glomerular epithelial cells. IgM and C3 are commonly found in a granular pattern, but their importance is unclear. A subset of FSGS patients with an increased risk of recurrence has been identified (40,47). This subgroup, diagnosed as having "malignant focal sclerosis," consists of patients typically less than 30 years of age who were severely hypoalbuminemic and hyperlipidemic and who usually progressed from onset of nephrotic syndrome to end-stage renal disease within 30 months (47). The recurrence rate in these patients approaches 50%, and there is an increased likelihood of thrombosis and graft failure. Patients whose original disease was FSGS and who experienced rapid recurrence and accelerated loss of their primary graft have a high likelihood of recurrent FSGS and graft loss in a subsequent graft (45,46,48). High doses of CsA and plasma absorption may control the proteinuria of recurrent disease (46,49).

Recurrent IgA nephropathy is histologically common but is clinically usually benign. The clinical manifestations consist of microscopic hematuria and mild proteinuria; nephrotic syndrome occurs in 10% of cases (36). The histopathology is characterized by mesangial IgA deposits almost always accompanied by C3 and segmental mesangial proliferation. Recurrent disease may be more common in recipients of a kidney from a related donor.

Membranoproliferative glomerulonephritis (MPGN) is difficult to distinguish from transplant glomerulopathy on light microscopic grounds alone. Similarities in the "double contoured" appearance of capillary walls in the two lesions necessitates the use of immunofluorescence and ultrastructural studies (Figs. 3 and 4). Over 150 recurrences of MPGN type I have been reported, representing an overall recurrence rate of 30%, but it leads to graft failure in only 10% of cases. The clinical course is characterized by proteinuria, microscopic hematuria, and—in cases destined for graft failure—progressive loss of function (36). Dense deposit disease or type II MPGN is more virulent, with recurrence rates up to 90%, though it leads to graft failure in less than 10% of cases (50).

Other renal diseases that may recur or emerge de novo include Henoch-Schönlein purpura, anti-GBM nephritis, nephritis of systemic lupus erythematosus, crescentic glomerulonephritis associated with systemic diseases, amyloidosis, and various miscellaneous diseases such as Fabry's disease, cystinosis, and myeloma-induced renal failure. These conditions are rare and have recently been reviewed (51).

Diabetes mellitus is one of the most common causes of end-stage renal disease in adults in the United States and Europe. Both non-insulin-dependent and insulin-dependent diabetes mellitus are major risk factors for allograft loss beyond the first year, largely because of patient death due to cardiovascular complications (52,53). Graft survival in surviving diabetic recipients is similar to that in nondiabetic recipients, although the graft may show features of early diabetic nephropathy within 2 to 3 years (54).

D. Diagnosis of Chronic Rejection

There is currently no test to accurately diagnose chronic renal allograft rejection. Ultrasound and computerized analysis of hippurate and DTPA scans are not sensitive or specific for chronic rejection (55,56). Magnetic resonance imaging may show poor corticomedullary differentiation in the graft, but this is also not specific (57). Graft histology, therefore, remains the gold standard, but several histological features of chronic rejection may be found in routine biopsies from kidneys with no apparent dysfunction (31,33). However, the extent of the histological lesions has a strong predictive value for graft outcome in the subsequent 2 years (8). Therefore, routine graft histology should become an endpoint for studies that evaluate the clinical efficacy of new immunosuppressive drugs. Furthermore, with the emerging interest in intervention studies in established chronic rejection, it will be important to apply a combination of clinical and pathological definitions to assess the efficacy of the intervention on the different functional and tissue expressions of chronic rejection, as proposed recently at the IV Alexis Carrel Conference (58).

III. CHRONIC HEART TRANSPLANT REJECTION

A. Epidemiology

The hallmark of chronic cardiac graft rejection is graft atherosclerosis, a process characterized by diffuse, concentric intimal proliferation in the graft coronary arteries (59). While naturally occurring atherosclerosis consists of focal lesions in the large epicardial vessels, graft atherosclerosis extends along great lengths of both the large and smaller penetrating intramyocardial vessels. It may occur as early as 3 months posttransplantation and may affect individuals of any age. Although graft atherosclerosis is the best-known form of chronic rejection, experimental work in the rat has shown that some forms of chronic rejection are characterized by interstitial fibrosis without vascular involvement (60).

Criteria used for the detection and definition of graft atherosclerosis differ widely in various clinical reports; it is often not clear, for example, whether changes in the small intramyocardial branches have been included in the assessments.

Histopathological assessments of transplants from recipients who had died from various causes furthermore demonstrate that angiography is quite insensitive, as many grafts have vascular changes that were not appreciated on previous angiograms (61–63). With these limitations in mind, it has been estimated that 2 to 14%, 15 to 33%, 26 to 40%, and 42 to 60% of grafts have coronary artery changes after 1, 2, 3, and 5 years respectively (64,65).

Although graft atherosclerosis is the single most important cause of death after the first posttransplant year and accounts for more than 50% of all retransplants (66), it is difficult to evaluate its clinical relevance on these grounds only. Epidemiological data on decreased myocardial function as a result of ischemia or infarction are needed to fully evaluate its clinical bearing.

B. Clinical Presentations and Differential Diagnosis

The clinical manifestations of graft atherosclerosis result from perfusion failure and ischemia. The classic sign of myocardial ischemia, angina pectoris, is usually absent because the transplanted heart is denervated, although some patients report chest discomfort or pain as the presenting symptom (67). Myocardial ischemia and infarction may evoke arrhythmias that are noticed by the patient or recorded during routine or continuous electrocardiographic monitoring. ST-segment changes or development of new Q waves may be observed during routine electrocardiographic follow-up. Mitral regurgitation caused by ischemia or rupture of papillary muscles or by dilatation of the ventricle may be detected by physical examination or by echo-Doppler techniques. Enlargement of the transplanted heart may be noted on chest x-rays when ventricular function decreases; echocardiography or radionuclide angiography demonstrates more specifically dilatation of the ventricles and wall motion abnormalities, before the classic symptoms and signs of heart failure arise. Myocardial perfusion scintigraphy may be helpful to detect ischemia, but transient vasculitis during acute rejection episodes may give a "false-positive" test, while persistent perfusion defects during exercise and rest may be caused by scar tissue after acute rejection episodes. On the other hand, perfusion scintigraphy may not be sensitive enough to detect the sequalae of lesions that are diffusely distributed along the vascular tree (62,68).

Qualitative serial angiographic studies may reveal anatomic changes in the coronary arteries, but—as discussed—this method is relatively insensitive compared with histopathology (69). Serial quantitative angiograms are more suitable to detect gradual changes in luminal diameter (64). A comprehensive description of graft coronary arteriographic findings has been presented (70) and three categories of lesions have been distinguished. Type A lesions are discrete or tubular stenoses in the proximal, middle, or distal segmental branches; type B lesions are diffuse concentric narrowings with onset in the mid-to-distal arteries (type B1: proximal vessel maintaining a normal diameter with abrupt onset of distal concentric narrowing and obliteration; type B2: gradual transition from normal proximal vessel with tapering concentric narrowing, gradually increasing in severity distally); type C lesions are characterized by narrowed irregular vessels with occluded side branches. Heart transplants with atherosclerosis have predominantly type B1, B2, and C lesions in the secondary and tertiary vessels (i.e., major branches of primary epicardial and small side branches of both primary and secondary vessels). Type A lesions are sporadically found in the primary vessels, which is in contrast to nontransplanted hearts with atherosclerosis that show type A lesions only.

Intracoronary ultrasound for the diagnosis of graft atherosclerosis holds great promise but its value must be established. Preliminary data have shown that the majority of patients have, after 1 or more years, ultrasound evidence of intimal thickening that was not apparent by angiography (71). Endomyocardial biopsies may show atherosclerosis, but they often do not contain vessels. Angiography remains, therefore, the cornerstone for the diagnosis of graft atherosclerosis. Although it accounts for most late graft failures, other conditions to be considered in the differential diagnosis include pericardial diseases, interstitial myocardial fibrosis (72,73), recurrent cardiac diseases (73–75), and acute rejection.

IV. CHRONIC LUNG TRANSPLANT REJECTION

A. Epidemiology

During the past decade, both single and double lung transplantation have been used to successfully treat a number of advanced lung diseases, including chronic obstructive disease, pulmonary fibrosis, primary pulmonary hypertension, Eisenmenger's syndrome, cystic fibrosis, and others (76). Improvements in surgical techniques and immunosuppressive regimens have resulted in improved patient survival rates (77,78), but long-term success has been limited by late infectious complications, drug toxicities (79), and chronic rejection (80). Chronic rejection is currently the leading cause of mortality among long-term allograft survivors; it may be more prevalent in patients who have received a combined heart-lung transplant than in patients who received a lung transplant only; as well, recipients of a single lung transplant may be somewhat more protected from chronic rejection than recipients of a double lung transplant (81,82). However, it is conceivable that these differences reflect the larger experience with heart-lung or double lung transplants compared with single lung transplants.

The estimated prevalence of chronic rejection varies between 20 and 40% in patients who survive the first posttransplant year (76). The histopathological hallmark of chronic rejection is obliterative bronchiolitis, a lesion characterized by submucosal fibrosis and chronic inflammation that may ultimately lead to obliteration of the airway lumen. The lesion is, however, not specific, as two forms have been described in lung allografts: an early, cellular, and mostly focal form, chiefly related to infections and aspirations of foreign material, and a late, sclerosing, and acellular type that is attributed to chronic rejection (83) (Fig. 5). Pulmonary atherosclerosis has been found in allograft specimens from patients surviving longer than 3 months (84).

B. Clinical Manifestations and Differential Diagnosis

Chronic lung transplant rejection is characterized by progressive decline in lung function. Different patients have, however, different abilities to return to "normal" lung function because of size mismatches between donor and recipient (85) as well as several recipient factors like chest wall configuration. This makes it difficult to determine the quality of the graft in terms of absolute lung volume. In practice, the best lung volume is measured at 3 months after surgery in the absence of histological evidence of rejection in a transbronchial biopsy. Some patients fail to achieve satisfactory lung volumes because of repeated rejection episodes, while others achieve satisfactory capacity and dynamic volumes but experience a progressive decline in function (86). This functional deterioration seems to correlate with the presence of fibrotic changes in biopsies. Conversely, patients with biopsy evidence of submucosal fibrosis and graft atherosclerosis have lower total lung capacities and dynamic lung volumes than patients with normal biopsies (80). Among patients with histopathological evidence of fibrotic changes, a proportion proceed to develop irreversible airflow obstruction, as shown by a low forced expiratory volume in 1 sec (FEV_1), often in the presence of well-maintained vital capacity. Despite repeated courses of augmented immunosuppression during the period of rapid functional deterioration, these patients

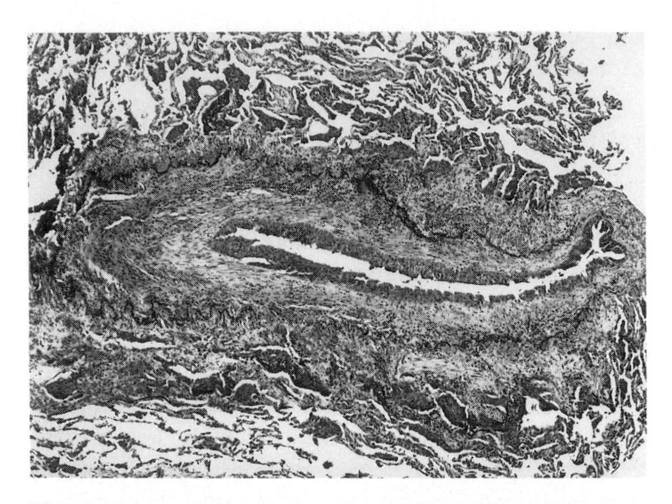

Figure 5 Photomicrograph of a human lung transplant with bronchiolitis obliterans. There is marked submucosal fibrosis with lymphocytic infiltration. (Movat trichrome stain.) (From Ref. 16.)

usually pursue a relentless course until left disabled with much reduced FEV_1 values (87,88).

Chronic rejection of lung transplants is, like that of many other organ transplants, correlated with previous acute rejection episodes (86), but it remains unclear whether it emerges from ongoing immune-mediated tissue damage, chronic rejection-specific immunological reactions, or the repair and scarring in response to damage incurred during acute rejection episodes. In early rejection, perivascular and peribronchiolar mononuclear infiltrates emerge that may be associated with disruption of basement membranes of the airways. In areas with intense rejection, the basement membrane breaks and collagenase-positive histiocytes may be present in the submucosa together with deposition of types III and IV collagen; some of these alterations persist in bronchiolitis obliterans, although the inflammatory infiltrate decreases while the fibrosis increases (Fig. 5) (89,90). Since other forms of lung damage may result in similar changes (91,92), the histopathology is not specific for chronic rejection.

The presenting features of chronic rejection include increasing exertional dyspnea, a dry cough, and wheezing; physical examination reveals tachypnea and basal mid-inspiratory crackles. Immunological and radiographic monitoring have been used, but these techniques have a poor positive predictive value with respect to both diagnosis and follow-up. Measurement of lung function, on the other hand, is the most widely accepted test for both diagnosis and monitoring of progression.

A working formulation for the standardization of nomenclature and clinical staging of chronic lung allograft dysfunction has been derived using spirometric measurements developed by the American Thoracic Society (93,94). The FEV_1 has been recognized as the most reliable and consistent indicator of graft (dys)function, and it has been proposed to use the designation "bronchiolitis obliterans syndrome" to describe graft deterioration secondary to progressive airway disease for which no obvious cause other than allogeneic incompatibility is evident. Histologic confirmation is not required; the description "bronchiolitis obliterans" is, however, reserved for cases in which the diagnosis has been proven histologically (93). The FEV_1 at baseline is used for comparisons with subsequent follow-up studies. Using the average of two FEV_1 measurements, at least 1 month apart, declines in FEV_1 are expressed as a percentage of baseline (93) and the following staging system has been proposed:

0—No significant abnormality: the FEV_1 is 80% or more of baseline value.
1—Mild obliterative bronchiolitis syndrome: the FEV_1 is 66 to 80% of baseline value.
2—Moderate obliterative bronchiolitis syndrome: the FEV_1 is 51 to 65% of baseline value.
3—Severe obliterative bronchiolitis syndrome: the FEV_1 is 50% or less of baseline value.

Within each of the four stages there is an "a" and "b" subcategory based on histological findings; the subcategory "a" designates no pathological evidence of obliterative bronchiolitis, and subcategory "b" designates pathological evidence of obliterative bronchiolitis.

There has been some debate as to how best to obtain tissue for histological diagnosis. An open lung biopsy provides sufficient tissue material, but the inconvenience of the procedure and its associated morbidity makes it a less than ideal approach. Transbronchial biopsies have been used with a reported sensitivity and specificity of 87 and 99% and positive and negative predictive values of 98 and 94%, respectively, when the clinical diagnosis of obliterative bronchiolitis was suspected (95–98). However, not all biopsies were done at the time of clinical evaluation for obliterative bronchiolitis, and biopsies done at the time of clinical diagnosis had a sensitivity of only 59%, although they retained a high degree of specificity (98). Other investigators concluded that transbronchial biopsies are of limited utility in the detection of the early stages of bronchiolitis obliterans because of the focal nature of the process and the size of the tissue samples (99). The complication rate of transbronchial biopsies varies between 9 and 18%, with pneumothorax being the most serious complication, but an infrequent one (95).

Differential diagnostic considerations in the evaluation of deteriorating pulmonary transplant function include acute rejection, congestive heart failure, infections with *Aspergillus* or *Pneumocystis*, viruses like cytomegalovirus and herpes, bacteria, and pulmonary fibrosis not related to chronic rejection. Patients with chronic rejection tend to have had more severe episodes of acute rejection than patients with fibrosis, while the latter group often have more chronic infections. As well, those with chronic rejection had a more significant and ongoing decline in FEV_1 (100).

V. CHRONIC LIVER TRANSPLANT REJECTION

Chronic liver transplant rejection, often referred to as "vanishing bile duct syndrome" or "ductopenic rejection," affects between 3 and 17% of liver transplants in the first few posttransplant years (101). The reported differences in different centers may depend on whether biopsies were done to document the cause of graft dysfunction and the histological criteria used to make the diagnosis.

Ductopenic rejection has been classified based on the time of clinical presentation as either early (<6 weeks), delayed (1 to 6 months) or late (>6 months) (102). Early ductopenic rejection presents as acute cellular rejection with the onset of malaise, fever, and a sharp deterioration in liver function tests, particularly the serum aminotransferase levels, while graft biopsies show cellular rejection. However, increased immunosuppressive medication does not result in functional improvement, and follow-up biopsies show rejection cholangitis with early bile duct degeneration or destruction with mild-to-moderate bile duct loss and inflammatory infiltrates within the portal tracts; large and medium-sized vessels, if present in the biopsy specimen, may show obliterative vasculopathy. As the process progresses, bile ducts continue to disappear and portal tracts become fibrotic while the inflammatory infiltrate subsides; eventually, chronic cholestasis and graft failure ensue. Serum levels of aminotransferase decrease, but the levels of bilirubin, alkaline phosphatase, and gamma glutamyl transferase increase.

Delayed ductopenic rejection (i.e., ductopenic rejection that presents 1 to 6 months after transplantation) is the most common form of chronic rejection. It usually develops after one or more early acute rejection episodes that ultimately fail to respond to increased immunosuppressive medication. The least common form presents insiduously after the initial 6 months, often without a previous episode of acute rejection. The histopathology is characterized by ductopenia with bile duct degeneration but without inflammatory infiltrates. The process usually takes months or years but will eventually lead to severe cholestasis and graft failure (103,104).

While the histopathological definition seems straightforward, the diagnosis may be difficult to make clinically. Multiple or serial graft biopsies may be needed because the diagnosis is subject to a relatively large interobserver variation (105). The rejection is most likely irreversible if 50% or more of the portal tracts lack an interlobular or septal bile duct; however, to ensure that the suggested prognosis of irreversibility is based on adequate tissue samples, it has been proposed that at least 20 portal tracts be examined by an experienced pathologist (100). It is of interest that some cases with severe cholestasis and ductopenia of more than 50% of portal tracts may show recovery of structure and function (106,107).

The differential diagnosis of chronic rejection includes recurrent viral hepatitis, extrahepatic biliary tract obstruction (108,109), and recurrence of primary biliary cirrhosis (110). Ductopenic rejection has a high recurrence rate in subsequent liver grafts (101).

VI. CHRONIC PANCREATIC TRANSPLANT REJECTION

With the recent increase in pancreatic transplant activities, experience with long-term complications and chronic rejection is increasing (111). As in other organ grafts, chronic rejection is emerging as the leading cause of graft loss after the first posttransplant year. It may be more common in patients who have received a solitary pancreatic transplant than in patients who received a simultaneous transplant of kidney and pancreas (112). The reason for this phenomenon has not been elucidated, but it may be because acute renal graft rejection episodes are relatively easily detected and may reflect a simultaneous acute rejection episode in the pancreatic graft (113).

The histopathological lesions of chronic rejection are characterized by subintimal vascular foam cell accumulation, intimal proliferation and fibrosis in conjunction with areas of tissue fibrosis, and chronic inflammation (111). These lesions lead to loss of function and recurrence of the diabetic state. True recurrent diabetes mellitus is characterized by inflammation solely confined to the islets and a selective loss of beta cells. Recurrent disease is, however, rare, since the immunosuppressive drugs taken to prevent rejection are usually sufficient to prevent this (111).

There are no good markers to detect chronically rejecting pancreatic transplants. Thus, unlike acute rejection, which is presumed to be present when there is an acute renal graft rejection episode in recipients of a combined kidney-pancreas transplant, or a decrease in urinary amylase levels in patients with a bladder-drained graft (114), there is no simple biochemical test for the detection of chronic rejection. Hyperglycemia is neither specific nor sensitive for chronic rejection; it is usually a late finding, often indicative of irreversible endocrine dysfunction (115). The diagnosis is ultimately based on biopsy findings; for bladder-drained pancreaticoduodenal grafts, tissue can be obtained via transcystoscopy (116,117), while for intestinally drained and duct-injected grafts, laparoscopy is required to obtain tissue samples, although percutaneous methods have been developed (118). The histological diagnosis is based on the presence of fibrointimal vascular proliferation lesions with intimal foam cell accumulation (111,115).

VII. CHRONIC SMALL BOWEL TRANSPLANT REJECTION

Improvements in surgical techniques and the use of newer immunosuppressive drugs like FK506 have allowed the development of clinical intestinal transplantation. It has been estimated that four or five patients per million population are appropriate candidates for a small bowel transplant alone or in combination with a liver transplant (119). Acute rejection episodes, sepsis, cytomegalovirus infection, and graft-versus-host disease are the major obstacles to successful short-term outcome. The Pittsburgh group reported a survival rate of 19 out of 23 patients followed for a median time of 231 days (range, 67 to 754) (120). A single patient in this group developed chronic rejection. This patient had received an isolated small bowel graft and had experienced multiple acute rejection episodes. Chronic rejection was manifest as intractable diarrhea, abdominal pain, sepsis, weight loss, and intermittent intestinal bleeding. Endoscopy revealed pseudomembranes, ulceration, and thickened mucosal folds, with histological changes consisting of apoptosis of crypt cells and segmental narrowing of the mesenteric artery but with little inflammation (120).

The earliest changes of chronic small bowel graft rejection in a rat model consist of enlargement of Peyer's patches and graft mesenteric lymph nodes, with relative preservation of the mucosa; inflammation of the mesenteric vessels was a consistent early finding, while mucosal inflammation, apoptosis, and cryptitis emerged with time (121). This sequence of events differs from that observed with acute rejection, in which endothelial and crypt damage appears first, followed by progressive destruction of lymphoid tissue and necrosis secondary to inflammation (122,123). The pathophysiology of chronic small bowel rejection thus appears to start with a primary vascular involvement, which may subsequently lead to ischemia and fibrosis. As with other organs, multiple and or poorly controlled acute rejection episodes seem to precede its development. Chronic rejection should be considered in patients who present with diarrhea, fever, weight loss, or intestinal bleeding. Although disaccharide absorption has been used as a diagnostic test, the test is more useful in detecting acute rejection (124). Endoscopy, intestinal biopsy, and mesenteric angiographic findings of segmental vascular narrowing can be used to confirm the diagnosis.

VIII. CONCLUSION

Chronic rejection is currently the main cause of graft failure after the first post-transplant year. Its diagnosis has remained difficult, mainly because the lack of specific tests and the time period over which the lesions develop. Most but not all organs that develop chronic rejection have experienced one or more episodes of acute rejection. The pathophysiological relationship between acute and chronic rejection is, however, not clear. Regardless of the mechanisms involved, it will be of paramount importance to define chronic rejection using a combination of clinical and histopathological criteria, as neither manifestation is specific.

REFERENCES

1. Thorogood J, Van Houwelingen HC, Van Rood JJ, et al. Long-term results of kidney transplantation in Eurotransplant. In: Paul LC, Solez K, eds. Organ Transplantation: Long-Term Results. New York: Marcel Dekker, 1992:33–56.
2. MacDonald AS, Belitsky P, Bitter-Suermann H, et al. Long-term follow-up of cyclosporine-treated renal allograft recipients. Transplant Proc 1988; 20:1239–1242.
3. Foster MC, Rowe PA, Wenham PW, et al. Late results of renal transplantation and the importance of chronic rejection as a cause of late graft loss. Ann R Coll Surg Engl 1989; 71: 41–44.
4. Knight RJ, Kerman RH, Welsh M, et al. Chronic rejection in primary renal allograft recipients under cyclosporine-prednisone immunosuppressive therapy. Transplantation 1991; 51: 355–359.
5. Almond PS, Matas A, Gillingham KJ, et al. Risk factors for chronic rejection in renal allograft recipients. Transplantation 1993; 55:752–757.
6. Basadonna GP, Matas AJ, Gillingham KJ, et al. Early versus late acute renal allograft rejection: Impact on chronic rejection. Transplantation 1993; 55:993–995.
7. Land W, Schneeberger H, Schleibner S, et al. The beneficial effect of human recombinant superoxide dismutase on acute and chronic rejection events in recipients of cadaver renal transplants. Transplantation 1994; 57:211–217.
8. Isoniemi H, Nurminen M, Tikkanen M, et al. Risk factors predicting chronic rejection of renal allografts. Transplantation 1994; 57:68–72.
9. Kirkman RL, Strom TB, Weir MR, Tilney NL. Late mortality and morbidity in recipients of long-term renal allografts. Transplantation 1982; 34:347–351.
10. Parfrey PS, Hutchinson TA, Lowry RL, et al. Causes of late renal transplant failure and role of azathioprine reduction. Transplant Proc 1984; 16:1100–1102.
11. Vanrenterghem Y, Roels L, Lerut T, et al. Long-term prognosis after cadaveric kidney transplantation. Transplant Proc 1987; 19:3762–3764.
12. Cheigh JS, Stenzel KH, Susin M, et al. Kidney transplant nephrotic syndrome. Am J Med 1974; 57:730–740.
13. Luke RG. Hypertension in renal transplant recipients. Kidney Int 1987; 31:1024–1037.
14. Lindsey ES, Garbus SB, Golladay ES, McDonald JC. Hypertension due to renal artery stenosis in transplanted kidneys. Ann Surg 1975; 181:604–610.
15. Mihatsch MJ, Ryffel B, Gudat F. Morphological criteria of chronic rejection: Differential diagnosis, including cyclosporine nephropathy. Transplant Proc 1993; 25:2031–2037.
16. Paul LC, Benediktsson H. Chronic transplant rejection: Magnitude of the problem and pathogenetic mechanisms. Transplant Rev 1993; 7:96–113.
17. Monga G, Mazzucco G, Messina M, et al. Intertubular capillary changes in kidney allografts: A morphologic investigation on 61 renal specimens. Mod Pathol 1992; 5:125–130.
18. Cheigh JS, Mouradian J, Soliman M, et al: Focal segmental glomerulosclerosis in renal transplants. Am J Kidney Dis 1983; 2:449–455.
19. Hamburger J, Crosnier J, Dormont JA. Observations in patients with a well tolerated homotransplanted kidney. Ann NY Acad Sci 1964; 120:558–577.
20. Rossmann P, Jirka J, Malek P, Hejnal J. Glomerulopathies in human renal allografts. Beitr Pathol Bd 1975; 155:18–35.
21. Olsen S, Bohman S-O, Petersen VP. Ultrastructure of the glomerular basement membrane in long term renal allografts with transplant glomerular disease. Lab Invest 1974; 30:176–189.

22. Petersen VP, Olsen TS, Kissmeyer-Nielsen F. Late failure of human renal transplants: An analysis of transplant disease and graft failure among 125 recipients surviving for one to eight years. Medicine 1975; 54:45–71.
23. Busch GJ, Galvanek EG, Reynolds ES. Human renal allografts: Analysis of lesions in long-term survivors. Hum Pathol 1971; 12:253–298.
24. Zollinger HU, Moppert J, Thiel G, Rohr HP. Morphology and pathogenesis of glomerulopathy in cadaver kidney allografts treated with antilymphocyte globulin. Curr Top Pathol 1973; 57: 1–48.
25. Cameron JS, Turner DR. Recurrent glomerulonephritis in allografted kidneys. Clin Nephrol 1977; 7:47–54.
26. Habib R, Antigua C, Hinglais N, et al. Glomerular lesions in the transplanted kidney in children. Am J Kidney Dis 1987; 10:198–207.
27. Manaligod JR, Jao W, Mozes MF, Jonasson O. Glomerular changes in renal allografts. Am J Kidney Dis 1986; 7:29–34.
28. Habib R, Zurowska A, Hinglais N, Gubler M-C, et al. A specific glomerular lesion of the graft: allograft glomerulopathy. Kidney Int 1993; 44(suppl 42):S104–S111.
29. Habib R, Broyer M. Clinical significance of allograft glomerulopathy. Kidney Int 1993; 44(suppl 43):S95–S98.
30. Nadasdy T, Krenacs T, Kalmar KN, et al. Importance of plasma cells in the infiltrate of renal allografts: An immunohistochemical study. Pathol Res Pract 1991; 187:178–183.
31. Isoniemi HM, Krogerus L, Von Willebrand E, et al. Histopathological findings in well-functioning, long-term renal allografts. Kidney Int 1992; 41:155–160.
32. Rush DN, Henry SF, Jeffery JR, et al. Histological findings in early routine biopsies of stable renal allograft recipients. Transplantation 1994; 57:208–210.
33. First MR, Vaidya PN, Maryniak RK, et al. Proteinuria following transplantation: Correlation with histopathology and outcome. Transplantation 1984; 38:607–612.
34. Vathsala A, Verani R, Schoenberg L, et al. Proteinuria in cyclosporin-treated renal transplant recipients. Transplantation 1990; 49:35–41.
35. Lorber MI, Flechner SM, Van Buren CT, et al. Cyclosporine, azathioprine, and prednisone as treatment for cyclosporine-induced nephrotoxicity in renal transplant recipients. Transplant Proc 1985; 17(suppl 1):282–285.
36. Mathew TH. Recurrence of disease following renal transplantation. Am J Kidney Dis 1988; 12:85–96.
37. Morzycka M, Crocker BP Jr, Siegler HF, Tisher CC. Evaluation of recurrent glomerulonephritis in kidney allografts. Am J Med 1982; 72:588–598.
38. Hamburger J, Crosnier J, Noel LH. Recurrent glomerulonephritis after renal transplantation. Annu Rev Med 1978; 29:67–72.
39. Cosyns JP, Pirson Y, Squifflet JP, et al. De novo membranous nephropathy in human renal allografts: Report of nine patients. Kidney Int 1982; 22:177–183.
40. Ramos EL. Recurrent diseases in the renal allograft. J Am Soc Nephrol 1991; 2:109–121.
41. Charpentier B, Levy M. Cooperative study of de novo extramembranous glomerulonephritis in renal allografts in humans: Report of 19 new cases in 1550 renal transplant patients of the transplantation group of the Ile de France. Nephrologie 1982; 3:158–166.
42. Cameron JS. Pathogenesis and treatment of membranous nephropathy. Kidney Int 1979; 15: 88–103.
43. Berger BE, Vincenti F, Biava C, et al. De novo and recurrent membranous nephropathy following kidney transplantation. Transplantation 1983; 35:315–319.
44. Hoyer JR, Vernier RL, Simmons RL, et al. Recurrence of idiopathic nephrotic syndrome after renal transplantation. Lancet 1972; 2:343–348.
45. Artero M, Biava C, Amend W, et al. Recurrent focal glomerulosclerosis: Natural history and response to therapy. Am J Med 1992; 92:375–383.

46. Ingulli E, Tejani A. Incidence, treatment, and outcome of recurrent focal segmental glomerulosclerosis post-transplantation in 42 allografts in children—A single center experience. Transplantation 1991; 51:401–405.
47. Leumann EP, Briner J, Donckerwolcke RA, et al. Recurrence of focal segmental glomerulosclerosis in the transplanted kidney. Nephron 1980; 25:65–71.
48. Stephanian E, Matas AJ, Mauer SM, et al. Recurrence of disease in patients retransplanted for focal segmental glomerulosclerosis. Transplantation 1992; 53:755–757.
49. Dantal J, Bigot E, Bogers W, et al. Effect of plasma adsorption on protein excretion in kidney transplant recipients with recurrent nephrotic syndrome. N Engl J Med 1994; 330:7–14.
50. Turner DR, Cameron JS, Bewick M, et al. Transplantation in mesangial capillary glomerulonephritis with intramembranous dense deposits: Recurrence of disease. Kidney Int 1976; 9: 439–448.
51. Ward HJ, Glassock RJ. Glomerular diseases in renal transplants. In: Paul LC, Solez K, eds. Organ Transplantation: Long-Term Results. New York: Marcel Dekker, 1992:261–281.
52. Fischel RJ, Payne WD, Gillingham KJ, et al. Long-term outlook for renal transplant recipients with one-year function. Transplantation 1991; 51:118–122.
53. Samrani NB, Kelaney V, Ding Z, et al. Diabetes mellitus after renal transplantation in the cyclosporin era: An analysis of risk factors. Transplantation 1992; 51:343–347.
54. Osterby R, Nyberg G, Hedman L, et al. Kidney transplantation in type I (insulin dependent) diabetic patients: Early glomerulopathy. Diabetologia 1991; 34:668–674.
55. Babcock DS, Slovis TL, Han BK, et al. Renal transplants in children: Long-term follow-up using sonography. Radiology 1985; 156:165–167.
56. Schmidlin P, Clorius JH, Lubosch EM, et al. Evaluation of scintigraphic data of renal transplants. Comput Biomed Res 1986; 19:330–339.
57. Te Strake L, Schultze Kool LJ, et al. MR imaging of renal transplants: Its value in the differentiation of acute rejection and cyclosporine A nephrotoxicity. Clin Radiol 1988; 39: 220–228.
58. Paul LC, Häyry P, Foegh M, et al. Diagnostic criteria for chronic rejection/accelerated graft atherosclerosis in heart and kidney transplants: Joint proposal from the Alexis Carrel Conference on chronic rejection and accelerated arteriosclerosis in transplanted organs. Transplant Proc 1993; 25:2022–2023.
59. Billingham ME. Cardiac transplant arteriosclerosis. Transplant Proc 1987; 19:19–25.
60. Cramer DV, Qian QS, Harnaha J, et al. Cardiac transplantation in the rat: I. The effect of histocompatibility differences on graft arteriosclerosis. Transplantation 1989; 47:414–419.
61. Rose EA, Smith CR, Petrossian GA, et al. Humoral immune response after cardiac transplantation: Correlation with fatal rejection and graft atherosclerosis. Surgery 1989; 106:203–208.
62. McKillop JH, Goris ML: Thallium-201 myocardial imaging in patients with previous cardiac transplantation. Clin Radiol 1981; 32:447–449.
63. Chomette G, Auriol M, Cabrol C. Chronic rejection in human heart transplantation. J Heart Transplant 1988; 7:292–297.
64. O'Neil BJ, Pflugfelder PW, Singh NR, et al. Frequency of angiographic detection and quantitative assessment of coronary arterial disease one and three years after cardiac transplantation. Am J Cardiol 1989; 63:1221–1226.
65. Balk AHMM, Weimar WL. Chronic heart graft rejection in the clinical setting. In: Paul LC, Solez K, eds. Organ Transplantation: Long-Term results. New York: Marcel Dekker, 1992: 187–195.
66. Rose AG, Vivier L, Odell JA. Autopsy-determined causes of death following cardiac transplantation: A study of 81 patients and literature review. Arch Pathol Lab Med 1992; 116:1137–1141.
67. Stark RP, McGinn AL, Wilson RF. Chest pain in cardiac transplant recipients—evidence of sensory reinnervation after cardiac transplantation. N Engl J Med 1991; 324:1791–1794.

68. Nitkin RS, Hunt SH, Schroeder JS. Accelerated atherosclerosis in a cardiac transplant patient. J Am Coll Cardiol 1985; 6:243–245.
69. Johnson DE, Gao SZ, Schroeder JS, et al. The spectrum of coronary artery pathologic findings in human cardiac allografts. J Heart Transplant 1989; 8:349–359.
70. Gao SZ, Alderman EL, Schroeder JS, et al. Accelerated coronary vascular disease in the heart transplant patient: Coronary arteriographic findings. J Am Coll Cardiol 1988; 12:334–340.
71. St. Goar FG, Pinto FJ, Alderman EL, et al. Intracoronary ultrasound in cardiac transplant recipients. In vivo evidence of "angiographically silent" intimal thickening. Circulation 1992; 85:979–987.
72. Winters GL. The pathology of heart allograft rejection. Arch Pathol Lab Med 1991; 115: 266–272.
73. Imakita M, Tazelaar HD, Rowan RA, et al. Myocyte hypertrophy in the transplanted heart: A morphometric analysis. Transplantation 1987; 43:839–842.
74. Hosenpud JD. Progression of systemic amyloidosis following cardiac transplantation: Follow-up report of a multicenter survey (abstr). Circulation 1990; 82(suppl III):713.
75. Gries W, Farkas D, Winters GL, Costanzo-Nordin MR. Giant cell myocarditis: First report of disease recurrence in the transplanted heart. J Heart Lung Transplant 1992; 11:370–374.
76. Kriet JM, Kaye MP. The registry of the International Society of Heart and Lung Transplantation: Eighth official report—1991. J Heart Lung Transplant 1991; 10:491–498.
77. Pasque MK, Cooper JD, Kaiser LR, et al. Improved technique for bilateral lung transplantation: Rationale and clinical experience. Ann Thorac Surg 1990; 49:785–791.
78. The Toronto Transplant Group. Experience with single-lung transplantation for pulmonary fibrosis. JAMA 1988; 259:2258–2262.
79. Zaltzman JS, Pei Y, Maurer J, et al. Cyclosporine nephrotoxicity in lung transplant recipients. Transplantation 1992; 54:875–878.
80. Higenbottam T, Clelland C. Heart-lung transplantation and lung transplantation: The challenge of obliterative bronchiolitis. In: Paul LC, Solez K, eds. Organ Transplantation: Long-Term Results. New York: Marcel Dekker, 1992:247–259.
81. Burke CM, Glainville AR, Theodore J, Robin ED. Lung immunogenicity, rejection and obliterative bronchiolitis. Chest 1987; 92:547–549.
82. Kaiser LR, Cooper JD. General thoracic surgery. Am Coll Surg Bull 1989; 74:34–40.
83. Abernathy EC, Hruban RH, Baumgartner WA, et al. The two forms of bronchiolitis obliterans in heart-lung transplant recipients. Hum Pathol 1991; 22:1102–1110.
84. Epler GR, Colby TV. The spectrum of bronchiolitis obliterans. Chest 1983; 83:161–162.
85. Otulana BA, Mist BA, Scott JP, et al. The effect of recipient size on lung physiology after heart-lung transplantation. Transplantation 1989; 48:625–629.
86. Scott JP, Higenbottam TW, Clelland C, et al. The natural history of obliterative bronchiolitis and occlusive vascular disease of patients following heart-lung transplantation. Transplant Proc 1989; 21:2592–2593.
87. Allen MD, Burke CM, McGregor CGA, et al. Steroid-responsive bronchiolitis after human heart-lung transplantation. J Thorac Cardiovasc Surg 1986; 92:449–454.
88. Glanville AR, Baldwin JC, Burke CM, et al. Obliterative bronchiolitis after heart-lung transplantation: Apparent arrest by augmented immunosuppression. Ann Intern Med 1987; 107: 300–311.
89. Yousem SA, Suncan SR, Ohori NP, Sonmez-Alpan E. Architectural remodeling of lung allografts in acute and chronic rejection. Arch Pathol Lab Med 1992; 116:1175–1180.
90. Tazelaar HD, Prop J, Nieuwenhuis P, et al. Airway pathology in the transplanted rat lung. Transplantation 1988; 45:864–869.
91. Keenan RJ, Lega ME, Dummer JS, et al. Cytomegalovirus serologic status and postoperative infection correlated with risk of developing chronic rejection after pulmonary transplantation. Transplantation 1991; 51:433–438.

92. Cerria J, Le Roy LF, Parquin F, et al. Risk factors for obliterative bronchiolitis (OB) after heart-lung (HLT) and double lung transplantation (DLT) (abstr). Am Rev Respir Dis 1992; 145(4; pt 2):A700.
93. International Society for Heart and Lung Transplantation. A working formulation for the standardization of nomenclature and clinical staging of chronic dysfunction in lung allografts. J Heart Lung Transplant 1993; 12:713–716.
94. Gardner RM, Hankinson JL, Clausen JL, et al. Standardization of spirometry—1987 update. Am Rev Respir Dis 1987; 136:1285–1298.
95. Turlock EP, Ehinger NA, Brunt EM, et al. The role of transbronchial biopsy in the treatment of lung transplant recipients. Chest 1992; 102:1049–1054.
96. Higenbottam T, Stewart S, Penketh A, Wallwork J. The diagnosis of lung rejection and opportunistic infection by transbronchial lung biopsy. Transplant Proc 1987; 19:3777–3778.
97. Higenbottam TW, Penketh A, Stewart S, Wallwork J. Transbronchial lung biopsy for the diagnosis of rejection in heart-lung transplant patients. Transplantation 1988; 46:532–539.
98. Yousem SA, Paradis I, Griffith BP. Can transbronchial biopsy aid in the diagnosis of bronchiolitis obliterans in lung transplant recipients? Transplantation 1994; 57:151–153.
99. Kramer MR, Stoehr C, Whang JL, et al. The diagnosis of obliterative bronchiolitis after heart-lung and lung transplantation: Low yield of transbronchial biopsy. J Heart Lung Transplant 1993; 12:675–681.
100. Scott JP, Higenbottam TW, Clelland CA, et al. Natural history of chronic rejection in heart-lung transplant recipients. J Heart Transplant 1990; 9:510–513.
101. Wiesner RH, Ludwig J, Van Hoek B, Krom RAF. Chronic hepatic allograft rejection. A review of ductopenic rejection and the vanishing bile duct syndrome. In: Paul LC, Solez K, eds. Organ Transplantation: Long-Term Results. New York: Marcel Dekker, 1992:197–215.
102. Adams DH, Neuberger JM. Patterns of graft rejection following liver transplantation. J Hepatol 1990; 10:113–119.
103. Ludwig J, Wiesner RH, Batts KP, et al. The acute vanishing bile duct syndrome (acute irreversible rejection) after orthotopic liver transplantation. Hepatology 1987; 7:476–483.
104. Kintmalm GBG, Nery JR, Husberg BW, et al. Rejection in liver transplantation. Hepatology 1989; 10:978–985.
105. Demetris AJ, Belle SH, Hart J, et al. Intraobserver and interobserver variation in the histopathological assessment of liver allograft rejection. Hepatology 1991; 14:751–755.
106. Hubscher SG, Buckels JAC, Elias E, et al. Vanishing bile-duct syndrome following liver transplantation—is it reversible? Transplantation 1991; 51:1004–1010.
107. Roberts JP, Lake JR, Hebert M, et al. Reversal of chronic rejection after treatment with FK506 and RS61443. Transplantation 1993; 56:1021–1023.
108. Rubin R, Munoz SJ. Clinicopathological features of late hepatic dysfunction in orthotopic liver transplants. Hum Pathol 1993; 24:643–651.
109. Rubin R, Munoz SJ, Moritz M. Rejection-independent cholangitis and cirrhosis following orthotopic liver transplantation. Hum Pathol 1993; 24:996–1002.
110. Balan V, Batts KP, Porayko MK, et al. Histological evidence for recurrence of primary biliary cirrhosis after liver transplantation. Hepatology 1993; 18:1392–1398.
111. Sutherland DER, Moudry-Munns K, Gillingham K, Nakhleh R. Long-term outcome of pancreas transplants functioning at one year. In Paul LC, Solez K, eds. Organ Transplantation: Long-Term Results. New York: Marcel Dekker, 1992:217–246.
112. Tydén G, Tibell A, Bolinder J, Östman J, et al. High incidence of late rejections in the preuremic recipients of pancreas transplants either provided alone or in combination with renal transplants. Transplant Proc 1990; 22:1582–1583.
113. Gruessner RWG, Nakhleh R, Tzardis P, et al. Rejection patterns after simultaneous pancreaticoduodenal-kidney transplants in pigs. Transplantation 1994; 57:756–760.
114. Prieto M, Sutherland DER, Fenandez-Cruz L, et al. Experimental and clinical experience with

urinary amylase monitoring for early diagnosis of rejection in pancreas transplantation. Transplantation 1987; 43:73–79.
115. Nakhleh RE, Sutherland DER. Pancreas rejection: Significance of histopathologic findings with implications for classification of rejection. Am J Surg Pathol 1992; 16:1098–1107.
116. Perkins JD, Munn SR, Marsh CL. Safety and efficacy of cystoscopically directed biopsy in pancreas transplantation. Transplant Proc 1990; 22:665–666.
117. Lowell JA, Bynon JS, Nelson N, et al. Improved transduodenal pancreas transplant biopsy. Transplantation 1994; 57:752–753.
118. Allen RDM, Wilson TA, Grierson JM, et al. Percutaneous pancreas transplant fine needle aspiration and needle core biopsies are useful and safe. Transplant Proc 1990; 22:663–664.
119. Talsma SE, Marks WH, Marks C, Brady M. Potential recipients for small-bowel transplants in the United States and the United Kingdom. In: Deltz E. Theide A, Hamelmann H, eds. Small Bowel Transplantation. Berlin: Springer-Verlag, 1986:258.
120. Abu-Elmagd KM, Tzakis A, Todo S, et al. Monitoring and treatment of intestinal allograft rejection in humans. Transplant Proc 1993; 25:1202–1203.
121. Langrehr JM, Banner B, Lee KKW, Schraut WH. Clinical course, morphology, and treatment of chronically rejecting small bowel allografts. Transplantation 1993; 55:242–250.
122. Madara JL, Kirkman RL. Structural and functional evolution of jejunal allograft rejection in rats and the ameliorating effects of cyclosporine therapy. J Clin Invest 1985; 75:502–512.
123. Rosemurgy AS, Schraut WH. Small bowel allografts: Sequence of histologic changes in acute and chronic rejection. Am J Surg 1986; 151:470–475.
124. Teitelbaum DH, Wise WE, Sonnino RE, et al. Monitoring of intestinal transplant rejection. Am J Surg 1989; 157:318–322.

22

Molecular Biology in Diagnosis of Rejection

Dilip S. Kittur and Lloyd E. Ratner
Johns Hopkins University School of Medicine, Baltimore, Maryland

Joyce Nair-Menon
University of South Carolina School of Medicine, Columbia, South Carolina

I. INTRODUCTION

Molecular biology promises to revolutionize transplantation by providing clues for early diagnosis and treatment of rejection. The two fields of molecular biology and transplant immunology started almost simultaneously in the middle of this century and have expanded exponentially. The seminal studies of Medawar and colleagues established the cellular basis of transplant rejection. At about the same time, in the late 1940s and early 1950s, Snell, Gorer, and coworkers identified the major histocompatibility complex (MHC), thus providing a genetic basis for rejection of allografts. These studies provided the foundations for clinical transplantation. Inspired by these studies, groups in Boston and elsewhere quickly demonstrated the feasibility of transplanting organs between monozygotic twins. This pioneering work underlies the modern field of transplant biology.

In this same era, a breakthrough in the understanding of the genetic basis of inheritance launched the nascent field of molecular biology. Discovery of the structure of DNA, RNA, and the genetic code quickly led to recognition of the central tenet of biology: DNA → RNA → protein. Restriction enzymes, which were soon discovered, allowed precise manipulation of DNA. The subsequent tremendous increase in enzymes, including DNA polymerase, and other reagents to manipulate DNA and RNA made genetic engineering a reality. The discovery of reverse transcriptase, which converts RNA to DNA, greatly expanded the potential of molecular biology as both a research tool and a therapeutic modality, greatly facilitating the cloning and propagation of genetic material. The evolution of molecular biology was further accelerated by technological advances such as the polymerase chain reaction (PCR) and the development of highly efficient vectors for cloning and transfer of genes from one organism to another. These advances in molecular biology have had a major impact on all branches of biology and medicine, including transplant biology.

In this chapter we provide an overview of the advances in molecular biology and discuss their impact on the diagnosis of rejection and development of strategies to prevent rejection. The format of this chapter is similar to our previous review (1), in which basic molecular techniques are described along with their applications to transplantation biology. A significant difference between this and the earlier review, however, is the integration into the current chapter of the exponentially increased data accumulated over the last few years. We emphasize the basic molecular approaches and describe the applications in brief; however, references to the applications are provided to direct the reader interested in a particular approach to the most recent work in the field. Detailed procedures for the techniques described can be found in several practical handbooks on molecular biology (e.g., Refs. 2–13).

This chapter is divided into three sections. In the first, we discuss current applications of molecular biology in HLA typing. We then describe molecular approaches to rejection diagnosis using the basic methods of molecular biology, such as analysis of DNA and RNA by Southern and Northern blotting, respectively. Included in this section are gene amplification, gene localization in cells or tissues using the PCR technology and the use of in situ hybridization. In the next section, we describe strategies utilizing genetic techniques to identify, clone, and characterize genes that are important in rejection. Included in this section are discussions of in vitro alteration of genes by site-directed mutagenesis, or recombination with other genes by exon shuffling, and transfection of abnormal genes into appropriate cells so that their expression can then be studied in vitro. The last section describes the in vivo approaches that are currently being used to determine the importance of several genes in allo- and xenorejection. These approaches include in vivo gene transfer to organs as well as the creation of transgenic animals and of animals with genes "knocked out" by homologous recombination.

II. CURRENT CLINICAL APPLICATIONS OF MOLECULAR BIOLOGY IN TRANSPLANTATION

A. HLA Typing

It is generally believed that HLA-matched kidney grafts, especially those matched at six antigens, enjoy better graft survival, although there is some controversy regarding the role of HLA typing in solid-organ transplantation. Moreover, HLA matching is an integral part of allocation of organs for simultaneous kidney and pancreas transplantation in the United States.

Recent molecular analysis of the major histocompatibility complex (MHC) has revealed a rich diversity of genes within this complex. In addition to the well-known HLA-A, B, and DR loci, the class I and class II regions each encode at least 20 more loci (14). Furthermore, there are several other immune-related genes within this complex. The conglomeration of these several immune-related genes in a short stretch of the genome raises the possibility that the MHC is a genetic blueprint of an intracellular immunological organ. The basic components of this organ are the MHC class I (HLA and A and B) and II (HLA DR) proteins, proteosomes (15), and peptide transporters (16). Since genes for all these proteins are encoded within the MHC complex, it is possible that the MHC may have evolved as a complex of genes that efficiently processes (intra- and extracellularly) degraded proteins into peptides, which are transported to the cell surface for presentation to the immune system.

The human leukocyte antigen (HLA) locus contains A-, B-, C-, and D-region genes. A high degree of polymorphism at the A, B, and DR genes had been detected by the use of serological methods. However, DNA analysis has revealed further polymorphism at the nucleotide level. For instance, over 60 alleles have been identified at the DRβ locus (17). Similarly, HLA-A and B are also very polymorphic; over 100 alleles exist at these loci (18).

The molecular techniques for HLA typing have evolved in the last decade. Earliest DNA analysis efforts utilized restriction fragment length polymorphism (RFLP) (19). In RFLP, DNA is cleaved with restriction enzymes, so called because they cut (restrict) DNA at specific sites determined by a specific nucleotide sequence. Therefore, if a gene has a different nucleotide than its polymorphic allele *and* if this nucleotide is at the site of action of a particular restriction enzyme (RE), the RE will cut one allele but not the other. Thus, cutting the DNA with that RE will produce fragments of the genes that are of unequal (different) lengths. Gel electrophoresis is then applied to the restricted DNA fragments to fractionate them by size, and the fragments are then transferred (Southern blotted) to a solid support such as nitrocellulose or nylon. The transferred fragments are then hybridized to a DNA probe, which detects fragments of the gene of interest, enabling detection of the polymorphism.

For bone marrow transplantation, DR typing by DNA typing methods is replacing serological typing. For solid-organ transplantation, DNA typing for DR is not yet commonplace, but it is performed in some institutions for recipient typing. Donor typing is still done primarily by serological methods. However, in the future, automated DNA typing will likely replace serological typing completely.

Polymerase chain reaction technology (discussed below) is becoming the preferred DNA method for HLA typing. Two PCR methods used for tissue typing are SSP and SSOP at lower or higher resolution. There are several other DNA-based typing techniques (20,21), which have not yet found general acceptance. The SSP method (22–24) uses PCR primers that are specific for the common DR allele to amplify the number of molecules of that allele (Fig. 1). Presently, primers for 18 different DR alleles are employed. While the SSP technique is specific, its sensitivity is limited by the number of primers employed in amplification.

The SSOP technique (25) is used when high-resolution typing at the allele level is required, as in bone marrow transplantation. In SSOP PCR primers for a given HLA locus (e.g., DR region) are used to amplify the number of molecules of that locus. This, then, allows DNA hybridization with primers for numerous specific alleles (Fig. 2). The SSOP technique can identify a single nucleotide difference between various alleles. Consequently the 40 to 50 known DR alleles can be unambiguously identified by SSOP.

An important difference between the two techniques is the degree of labor intensity. As stated above, SSP involves PCR amplification of DNA (described below) with DR allele–specific primers. Gel electrophoresis of the products leads to determination of the DR genotype of the individual. The whole procedure can be completed in 3 to 4 hr. On the other hand, SSOP is done on DNA amplified by PCR using generic DNA probes. The amplified DNA is probed with (labeled) allele-specific oligonucleotide probes. Hybridization of an allele-specific probe identifies the DR genotype of the individual. Since hybridization and detection are time-intensive steps the whole procedure can take 2 to 3 days. Nonetheless, when high resolution is required, as in bone marrow transplantation, the SSOP procedure can be performed in large batches.

Current major goals are to develop DNA methods to type class I (HLA A and B) genes (26,27) and to automate the procedure. The complexity of the MHC class I genes is

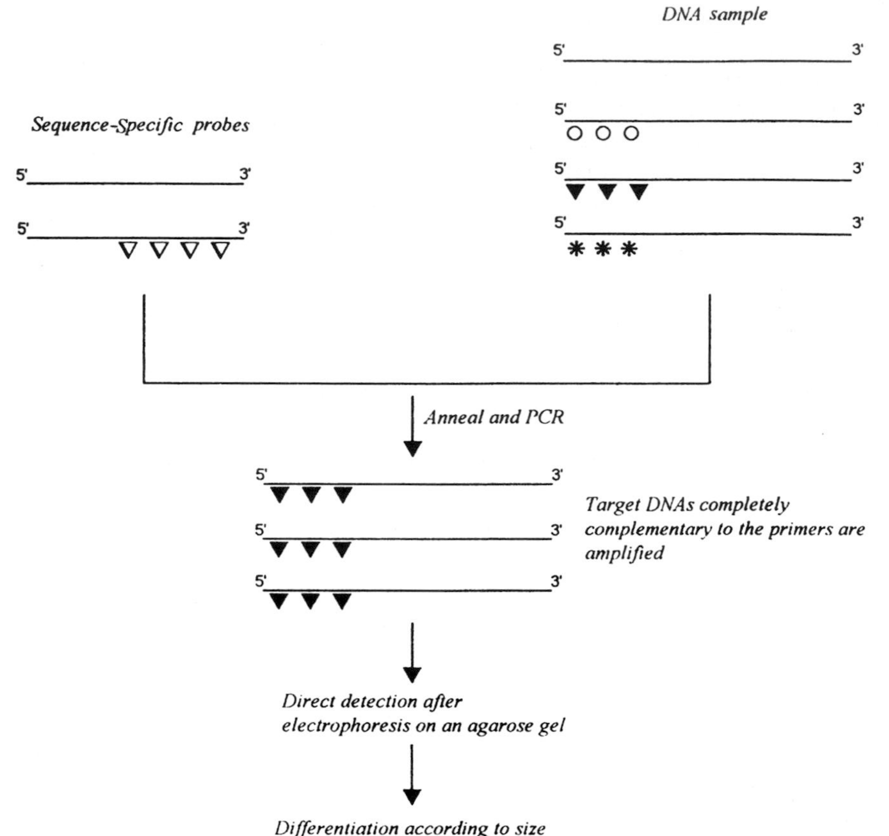

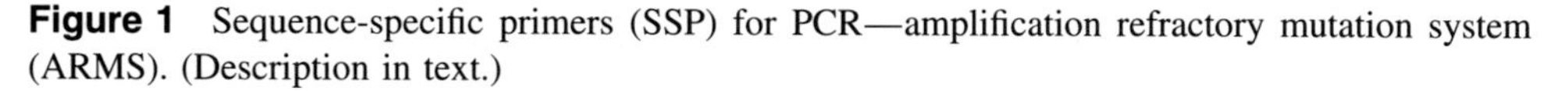

Figure 1 Sequence-specific primers (SSP) for PCR—amplification refractory mutation system (ARMS). (Description in text.)

significantly greater than that of class II. There are more than 100 alleles at the HLA A and B loci (18). Consequently a larger set of primers is necessary to type these two loci. Efforts to generate such primers are under way.

Typing of cadaveric donors (especially pretyping prior to the time of organ harvest) by serological techniques can sometimes be difficult due to the relative paucity of lymphocytes in their peripheral blood. Though DNA typing can overcome this problem, it is not currently used because the methods are not completely standardized. Automation of PCR and detection of PCR products by enzyme-linked immunosorbent assay (ELISA) techniques will lead to standard, commercially available assays. Eventually an unambiguous and quick method of DNA typing will enable molecular typing of cadaveric organ donors and lead to better donor and recipient matching.

In summary, HLA typing using molecular methods is very sensitive and may be of more value in bone marrow transplantation than in organ transplantation. Nonetheless, some data suggest that fine matching leads to better results in solid-organ transplantation (28,29). Currently, organ allocation is largely dependent upon HLA matching. However, many variations in HLA antigens are not picked up by routine serological methods. DNA

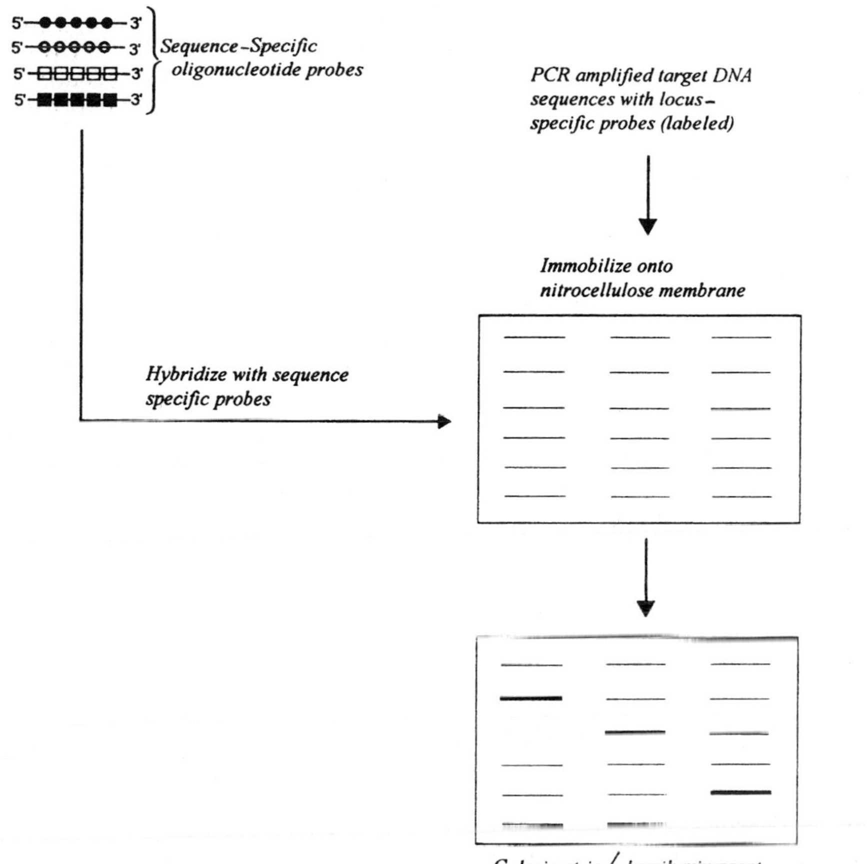

Figure 2 Sequence-specific oligonucleotide probes (SSOP) for allele typing. (Description in text.)

typing provides a more sensitive way of discriminating between the various subtypes and may improve our ability to match organs.

III. MOLECULAR BIOLOGICAL APPLICATIONS TO DETERMINATION OF PATHOGENESIS AND TO EARLY DIAGNOSIS OF REJECTION

A. Introduction

Transplant rejection is a multifactorial process involving multiple interactions between the donor and recipient cells. A current emphasis in molecular biology is to elucidate the role of these interactions and ultimately derive molecular markers of early rejection. The interaction between MHC and T-cell receptor is an important determinant of acute cellular rejection. However, as discussed elsewhere in this book, several other interactions, notably those between costimulatory and adhesion molecules, also play an important role in the rejection process (30,31). Additionally, an array of cytokines and growth factors are active participants in rejection. Since many of these molecules have been discovered in the last decade, their relative importance in the pathogenesis of rejection is not completely delineated. With this in mind, discussion in this section concentrates on the strategies and approaches employed to elucidate the role of different molecules in rejection rather than on the specifics of the individual molecules.

B. Strategies to Determine the Role of Known Genes in Rejection

A common strategy to derive molecular markers for early diagnosis of rejection is to determine whether certain genes/gene products are expressed in allografts and whether this expression correlates with rejection. Generally, the first step in this process has been to elucidate the role of previously cloned genes in allograft rejection by Northern blot analysis or, recently, by PCR. In this correlative approach, genes that are preferentially expressed in rejecting allografts are considered candidate genes. These genes can be grouped into two types: (a) genes coding cell-surface molecules that directly influence the immune system of the recipients and (b) genes resulting in the amplification of the immune response. Examples of the former group are MHC class I and class II genes, adhesion molecules, and costimulatory molecules such as B7 (reviewed in Ref. 31). These gene products are somewhat specific in their action on the immune system of the recipients; that is, the cell-surface molecules on the antigen-presenting cells interact directly with a limited number of cells. Thus, these gene products account for the specificity of the host response against the graft.

The second set of genes amplify the immune response. This category consists of the extracellular secreted molecules such as cytokines, and growth factors which act in an autocrine or paracrine fashion to amplify signals extracellularly. It also consists of the less familiar molecules such as signal transducers (32) and transcription factors (33), which act intracellularly. By acting on multiple genes, these latter molecules amplify the effects of the extracellular immune signals within the cell. For example, the transcription factors c-*fos* and c-*jun* bind to an AP site in the promoter region of several genes and activate the transcription of these genes (34). Genes such as MHC class II and interleukin-2 (IL-2) have identical AP sites in their promoter regions (35,36). Therefore, a stimulus that increases the intracellular levels of c-fos and c-jun can simultaneously increase secretion of IL-2 and transcription of MHC class II genes, thus amplifying the original signal and leading to increased immunogenicity. Although these latter molecules are not as directly implicated in rejection as are cytokines and lymphokines, their ability to amplify the expression of other genes is a potential target for antirejection therapy.

If any of these candidate genes are found to be preferentially expressed in the allografts by Northern blot analysis and/or PCR and if their expression correlates with the onset of rejection, the next confirmatory step usually consists of in situ hybridization of the candidate gene in tissue sections from rejecting allografts. The main drawback of the correlative approach, however, is that its use is restricted to genes or proteins that have been previously characterized.

1. *Northern Blot Analysis*

Understanding of the pathophysiological mechanisms involved in rejection or allograft dysfunction from a molecular standpoint often requires confirmation that gene products are produced. This is commonly done with the highly sensitive molecular biological techniques of Northern and Western blot analysis, which detect posttranscriptional (mRNA) and posttranslational (protein) gene products respectively. These techniques continue to be of great value in transplantation research and are becoming increasingly important in clinical practice.

Knowledge of the genetic sequence of a particular gene of interest enables one to detect whether transcription has occurred and mRNA gene products are present. The principle that RNA molecules will hybridize with DNA molecules of complementary sequence is the underlying rationale for Northern blot analysis. Molecular DNA probes of variable lengths can be constructed with specific sequences identical to those of the gene exons of interest.

Northern blot analysis is useful for detecting abundant mRNA species (Fig. 3). Using standard techniques, total RNA can be isolated from either cells in culture or fresh or snap-frozen tissue specimens. Messenger RNA (mRNA), which represents only a small fraction of total RNA, can be further separated out by virtue of its polyadenylated tail; hybridization

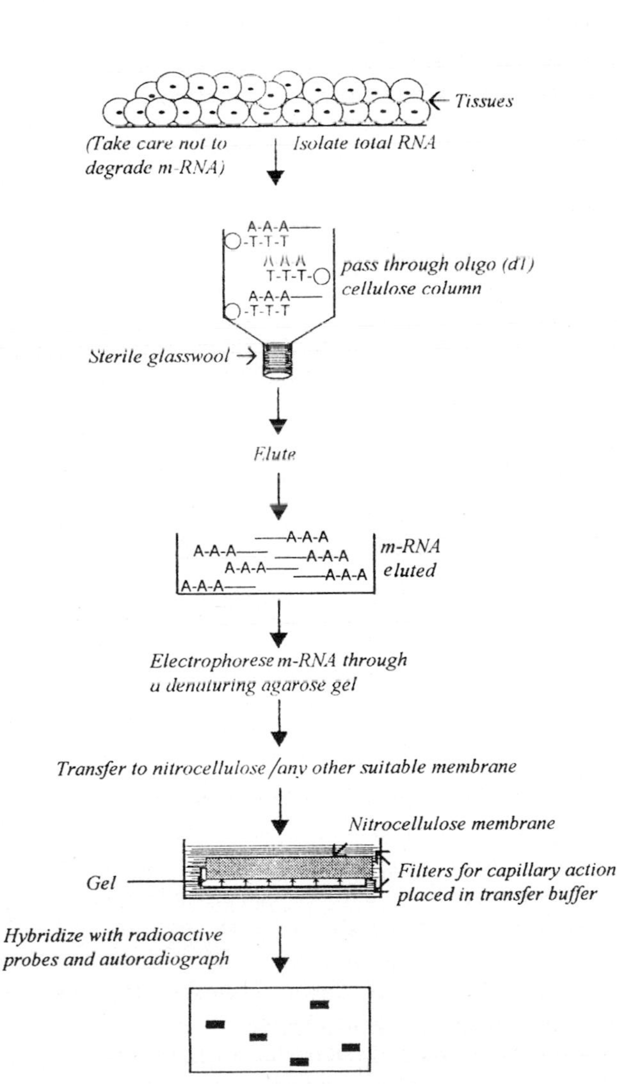

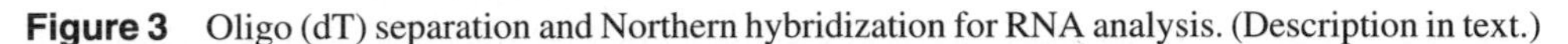

Figure 3 Oligo (dT) separation and Northern hybridization for RNA analysis. (Description in text.)

with oligo-dT bound to a solid-phase support and subsequent elution of the mRNA results in a highly pure mRNA. RNA molecules of differing size are then separated by gel electrophoresis and the RNA can then be transferred to a nitrocellulose or nylon filter and immobilized. Radiolabeled or chemilumenescent DNA probes can then be hybridized to the immobilized RNA. Detection and quantification of the RNA species in question is achieved by autoradiography with radiolabeled probes or by enzymatic activation and visual inspection of chemilumenescent labeled probes.

One of the limitations of Northern blot analysis is that a fairly substantial quantity of the mRNA species of interest is required for detection. This can be problematic when the gene product of interest is present in small numbers. Such is often the case when the molecule of interest is a cytokine. Limited specimen size (e.g., from a clinical allograft biopsy) may also yield insufficient RNA for Northern analysis.

Many of the technical difficulties that were previously associated with the Northern blot procedure have now been obviated. RNA is highly sensitive to degradation by nucleases and, since many tissues have endogenous RNAse, isolation of RNA from tissues frequently yielded degraded RNA. The agar gels used for electrophoresis similarly led to degradation of the RNA. Recently however, several commercial kits have placed isolation and analysis of even minute (submicrogram) quantities of RNA within the reach of most laboratories.

2. *Western Blot Analysis*

Western blot analysis is employed to confirm the presence of a specific protein or to aid in its characterization. Protein preparations from serum, tissue, cells, or cell compartments are separated (usually by molecular weight) by polyacrylamide gel electrophoresis (PAGE). The separated proteins are then transferred electrophoretically from the gel to a nylon or nitrocellulose membrane. Antibody specific for the protein in question is applied to the membrane, and a labeled secondary antibody is then utilized to allow detection. Generally, best results are obtained when a polyclonal primary antibody is used. However, monoclonals have also been utilized successfully. Recently, Western blotting has been employed to identify and characterize the porcine antigens recognized by human xenoreactive natural antibody.

3. *Polymerase Chain Reaction*

The PCR is a molecular biological technique that enables one to analyze small quantities of rare species of nucleic acids. It has numerous applications in transplantation biology. As stated above, it can be used to detect genes or gene products of low frequency. It has been successfully employed to determine cytokine expression (37), TCR V_β repertoire (38–41) and to detect microchimerism (42–44), in which a small number of donor cells are present in the host. Additionally, it has greatly facilitated the process of gene cloning by replacing some tedious conventional molecular biological techniques that often took weeks to perform.

The PCR results in amplification of a highly specific DNA sequence with great fidelity. Utilizing an enzymatic reaction (as described below), the DNA sequence of interest is copied numerous times, yielding an extremely large number of DNA molecules with exactly the same nucleotide sequence as the original. This amplification thus provides sufficient DNA for analysis or for manipulation for gene cloning.

The polymerase chain reaction entails several basic steps that are then repeated many times (Fig. 4). First, the target DNA of interest is denatured by heating, (usually to 95°C), thus separating the two strands. Specific oligonucleotide primers that share a complemen-

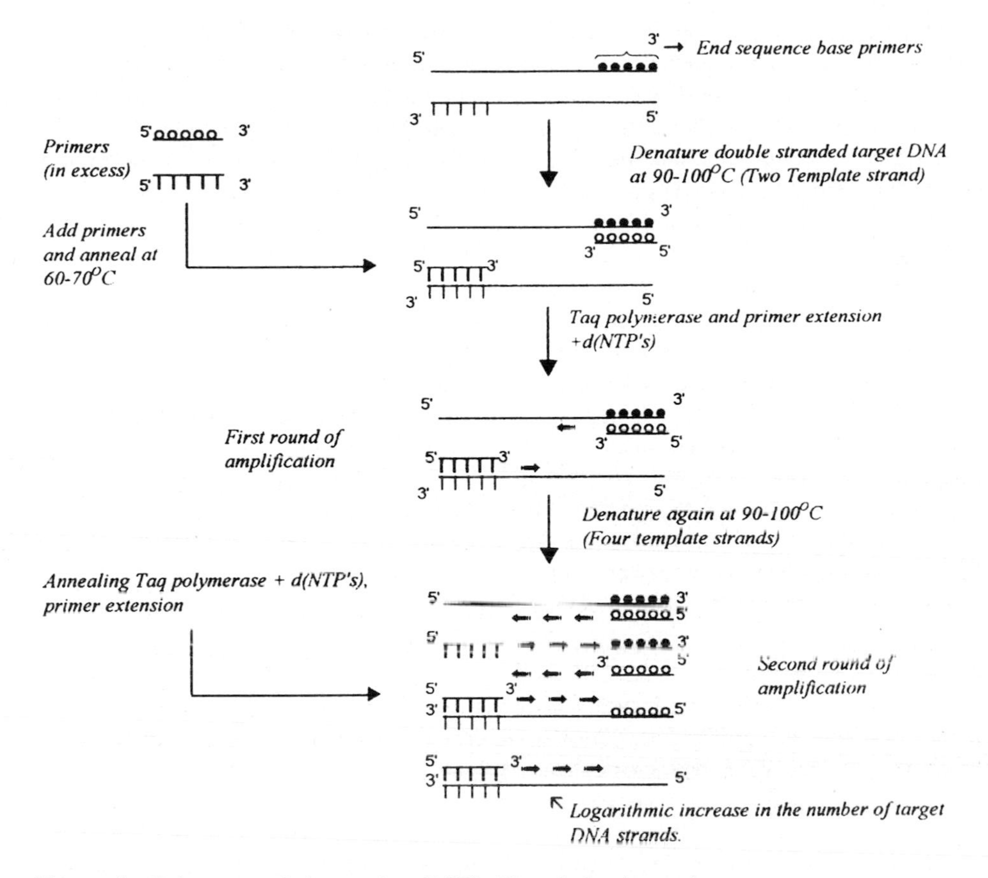

Figure 4 Polymerase chain reaction (PCR). (Description in text.)

tary sequence with the target DNA, commonly 15 to 30 bases long, are allowed to hybridize or anneal with the target DNA by lowering the temperature (55 to 65°C). The primers serve as an initiation site for DNA polymerase, which extends the DNA molecule, using the original target DNA as a template. In the extension phase, temperature is elevated to 72°C. The process is subsequently begun again by separating the newly replicated DNA. The DNA polymerase employed, Taq polymerase, is stable at extremely high temperatures. Consequently, the process can be performed repeatedly with minimal loss of enzymatic activity. The reaction mixture also contains the oligonucleotide primers and deoxytriphosphate nucleotides in vast excess of what is required. Therefore, the limiting factors that determine how much the target DNA is amplified is the number of times that the process is repeated and the efficiency of DNA replication. Using an automated temperature cycler, each cycle takes just minutes. Typically, the reaction is run for 30 to 40 cycles. Hence, the amplification is exponential.

The degree of DNA amplification can be calculated by the following formula:

$$A = A_0(1 + E)^n$$

where A is the final number of DNA molecules produced, A_0 is the initial number of target molecules, E is the efficiency of amplification, and n is the number of cycles performed.

In addition to amplifying DNA, PCR can discriminate between alleles of a gene by detecting small changes in nucleotide sequences (45). If the target gene sequence has allelic variations, the primers hybridize only to that allele, which is perfectly homologous to the sequence of the primers. The perfectly matched allele is therefore amplified, while the mismatched alleles are not. This principle is used to detect chimerism by using primers specific for donor HLA alleles or specific for Y chromosomes (42–44).

The PCR can also be employed when the nucleic acid in hand is RNA. Reverse transcriptase will produce a complementary DNA (cDNA) copy of the RNA of interest. This reaction also requires the use of an oligonucleotide primer as a starting point for the reverse transcriptase. Specific primers designed for oligo (dT) can be utilized to make cDNA copies of all mRNA present. The PCR can then be performed on the cDNA.

This procedure of reverse transcription followed by PCR (RT-PCR) is frequently used in transplantation to determine the expression of genes involved in rejection. For instance semiquantitative RT-PCR can estimate Vβ TCR usage by recipient's T cells that respond to alloantigens (39–41). The effect of exposure to xenoantigens on the recipient's T-cell repertoire can be similarly analyzed by this technique (38). It is important, however, to keep in mind that RT-PCR is at best semiquantitative and that the results of this assay should ideally be validated by another assay.

The PCR technique in general is highly versatile and has several applications of interest in transplantation. cDNA or genomic clones can readily be isolated from libraries by this technique and subcloned directly in specifically designed vectors. Gene sequencing is currently performed on single-stranded DNA synthesized by PCR (45). Segments of cloned genes can be shuffled (exon shuffling) to create chimeric genes. The chimeric genes are used to elucidate the function of the encoded protein, as, for example, the detection of binding sites for adenovirus type II receptors on MHC molecules (46). Alternatively, chimeric genes with desired function can be used to produce novel immunosuppressive agents such as IL-2/diphtheria toxin conjugates (described below).

C. Reverse Genetics to Identify Novel Genes Relevant to Rejection

1. Introduction

Finding novel genes by reverse genetics is a tedious but fruitful approach to understanding the molecular mechanisms of allograft rejection. Novel genes can be cloned relatively easily if one has antibody or other probes to the proteins or genes of interest. One approach is to purify and sequence proteins recognized by antibodies. With the protein sequence information, oligonucleotide probes are synthesized with which genes are cloned from a genomic library. Alternatively, clones in a cDNA library that express fusion proteins can be directly probed by the antibody (if the protein of interest does not need eukaryotic post-translational processing).

In the absence of specific probes for the gene or protein of interest, the more laborious technique of differential hybridization allows cloning of novel genes. The relevance of the genes cloned by differential hybridization to rejection has to be determined by further correlative or transgenic experiments.

2. cDNA Cloning

As mentioned above, novel genes can be readily cloned with specific probes such as antibodies elicited during (or after) rejection. cDNA cloning traditionally involves expressing the genetic message in prokaryote (bacteria) as a fusion protein. The fusion protein can be detected by antibodies specific for the protein of interest. In this manner the gene of interest can be isolated. The first step in cDNA cloning is to isolate messenger RNA from cells that are an abundant source of the protein of interest. The mRNA is converted into cDNA by reverse transcription, using the enzyme reverse transcriptase. The cDNA is then made into a double-stranded DNA, which is then introduced into a vector for further amplification (Fig. 5).

In procaryotic expression cloning, the cDNA cloned in either phage or plasmid vectors is expressed in bacteria to isolate the gene of interest. Lambda phage vectors (λgt 11) are in

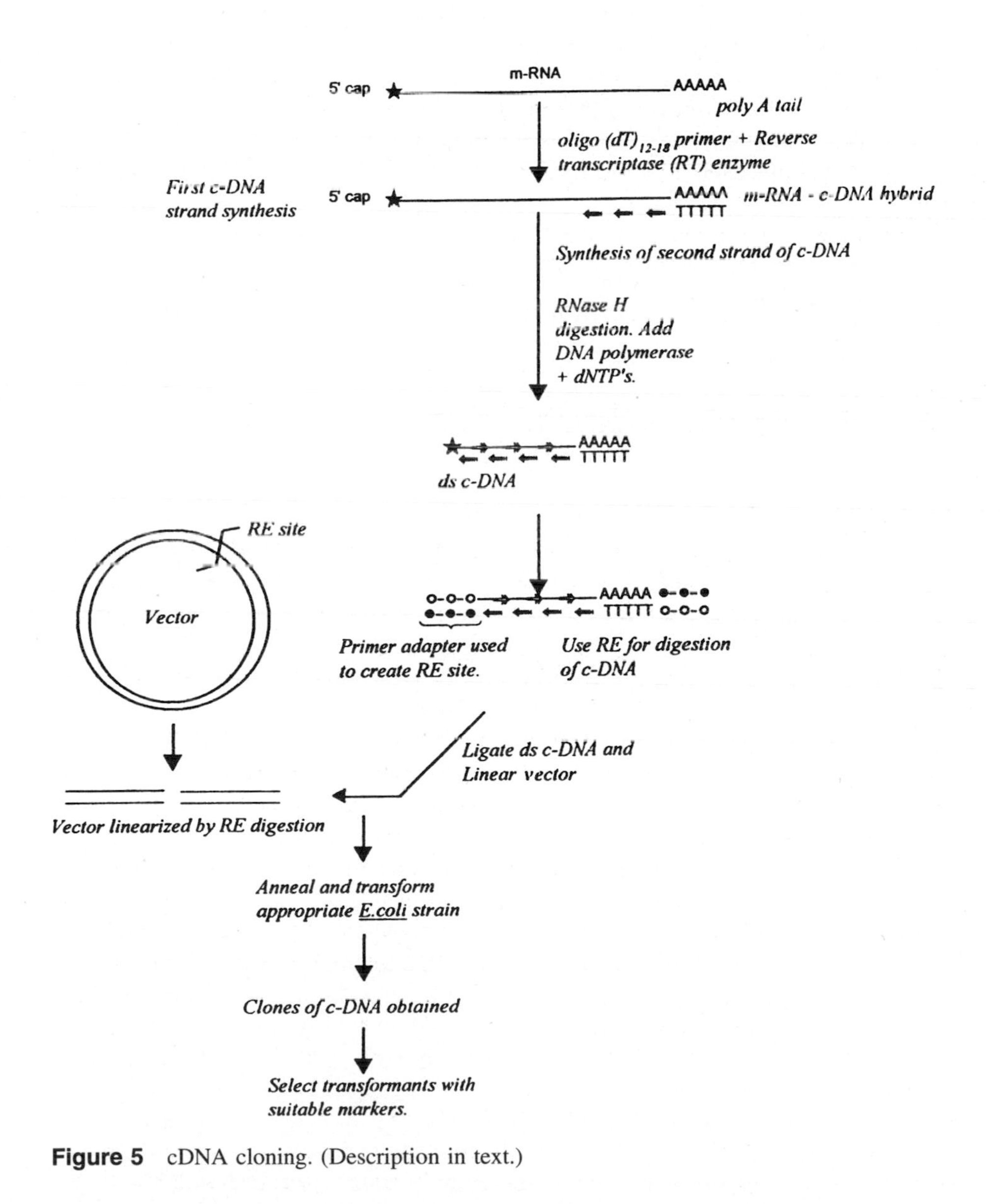

Figure 5 cDNA cloning. (Description in text.)

common use because of the ease in cloning, propagating, and storing the inserted cDNA in phage vectors. The genes in the inserted cDNA are expressed as fusion proteins, since the cDNA is cloned within the LacZ gene of the phage. The expressed proteins are transferred to nitrocellulose filters. Antibodies labeled either with radioactive material or with enzymes (e.g., horseradish peroxidase) are used to detect the clones expressing the desired cDNA. Further rounds of amplification and detection purify the clone to homogeneity.

After having gone through a period of disrepute, plasmid vectors have been resurrected for cDNA cloning by incorporation of some desirable features of the phage vectors. These "phagemid" vectors facilitate cloning in sites that can be cut with several enzymes (multicloning sites). Additionally, the inserted double-stranded cDNA can be amplified as single-stranded phage DNA. The single-stranded DNA is used in several applications such as sequencing, synthesizing high-specific-activity probes, and nuclease protection assays. Synthetic RNA can also be transcribed from the phagemid vectors. Finally, some plasmid vectors are designed to express the inserted genes in certain eukaryotic cells. This last feature is highly desirable in isolating genes that need eukaryotic posttranscriptional processing such as glycosylation, which cannot be accomplished in procaryotic expression cloning.

Several genes such as those in the MHC, antigens involved in antibody-mediated kidney rejection (47,48), and several others of relevance to transplantation have been cloned by cDNA cloning. In general, antibodies continue to be the preferred probes for cloning. Alternatively, *N*-amino-terminal sequencing of immunoprecipitated proteins yields valuable information even prior to actual cloning of the gene. For example, Platt et al. sequenced the *N*-amino terminals of the GP 115/135 complex recognized by naturally occurring human antiporcine xenoantibodies. Interestingly, the three glycoproteins in this complex appear to be homologous with human integrins (49).

3. Subtractive Hybridization

Differential or subtractive hybridization is the procedure of choice when antibody or other probes are not available to isolate genes of interest. In the early 1980s, this procedure was utilized to clone the genes for the T-cell receptor. Since then, several variations of this procedure have been described (see Refs. 2–4).

Subtractive hybridization is performed with two species of mRNA: one that has abundant mRNA of interest and the other that does not have the mRNA of interest but has all other mRNA. One species of mRNA (usually the former) is converted into cDNA and is hybridized with a vast excess (up to 10-fold) of the other mRNA. The resulting mixture contains cDNA/mRNA hybrids and unhybridized cDNA encoding the gene(s) of interest. The cDNA/mRNA hybrids are removed, leaving behind cDNA, which are then cloned into suitable vectors. In practice the hybridization and removal (subtraction) process is repeated three or four times to ensure sufficient enrichment of the cDNAs of interest. Frequently, despite the rounds of substraction, the enriched cDNA contains other genes besides those of interest. The last step, therefore, is to develop additional methods of validating the cDNA clones of interest.

In the past, removal of the unwanted cDNA/mRNA hybrids was accomplished by chromatography on a hydroxyapatite column. Although this method was quite effective, the chromatographic conditions were harsh and led to degraded cDNA. Currently PCR has been used in conjunction with gentler methods of separating the undesired hybrids from the cDNA of interest. Nonetheless, subtractive hybridization remains a tedious, complex procedure to be used by those experienced in the difficulties associated with it.

4. Genomic Cloning

Almost all eukaryotic genes have large introns between expressed exons. Since cDNA cloning isolates only exons, characterization of the entire gene requires cloning the genomic DNA in vectors that can replicate large (> 4 to 5-Kb) pieces of DNA. This genomic cloning is performed in cosmid vectors, or modified plasmid vectors that carry a recombinant segment of DNA (Cos) from phage vectors. The Cos segment allows packaging of the genomic DNA in phage particles. These vectors can carry segments of foreign DNA that are approximately 35 to 45 Kb in length. Similar to cDNA cloning, these vectors are introduced into bacteria and amplified. However, the detection of the DNA fragments of interest is different from that used with cDNA cloning. In genomic cloning, the bacterial colonies are transferred to nitrocellulose and lysed. However, to expose cosmid DNA (containing the cloned fragments) the previously isolated cDNA is used as a probe to select the fragments containing the gene of interest, with adjacent stretches of genomic DNA. The appropriate order of these fragments is determined by restriction mapping, which utilizes multiple restriction enzymes. Unique sites for a particular enzyme in each of the DNA fragments allows precise mapping of the relative position of each fragment. This map allows "walking" along the chromosomal region.

Most recently, the time-consuming steps of cosmid cloning have been shortened by cloning larger fragments of DNA with which one can "jump" along the chromosomal region. Yeast artificial chromosomes (YAC) vectors recently derived from telomeres of yeast chromosomes (50) accommodate DNA fragments up to 1 to 2 megabases, which facilitates mapping and "jumping" along chromosomal regions (Fig. 6). For example, a large part of the 2 million bp region of human MHC extending between HLA-E to HLA-F was recently cloned and mapped with YACs (51). A large genomic region contained within YAC vectors has also been used as a probe to isolate a GTP-binding protein-encoding gene near the HLA-E locus (52) and seven (7) novel genes around the HLA-A locus (53). Finally, although technically very difficult, it is possible to express entire gene complexes by transfecting eukaryotic cells with YAC vectors.

D. Localization of Genetic Markers

1. In situ Hybridization

Confirmation of the mere presence of a gene or gene product in a tissue specimen by Northern blot or PCR is occasionally insufficient information. Using a technique known as in situ hybridization, nucleic acids of specific sequence can be identified and localized within the tissue in question. This technique has been useful in identifying cells of donor origin (54) and in demonstrating the presence of growth factor transcripts in vessel walls. Clinically, it is being employed with increasing frequency. Its most common clinical application relevant to transplantation is in the confirmation of cytomegalovirus, hepatitis B, or C viral genome within a specimen.

IV. MOLECULAR BIOLOGICAL STRATEGIES TO PREVENT REJECTION

A. Introduction

Besides being a powerful approach to early diagnosis of rejection, molecular biology holds promise in promoting allograft tolerance by providing several approaches to prevent

Vector should contain sequences of yeast and a plasmid capable of replicating in E. coli,
e.g.,
- *gene associated with a phenotypic character, with a cloning site like SUP4;*
- *gene for autonomous replication like ARS;*
- *gene providing centromere function like CEN;*
- *a couple of extra genes like TRP1 and URA3 at the ends of the arm carrying all the other genes.*

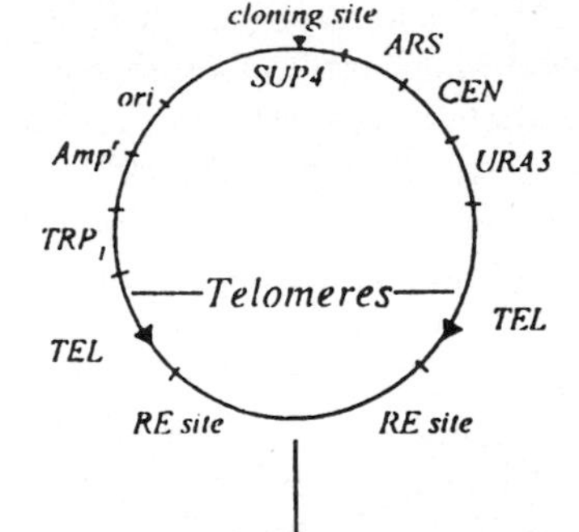

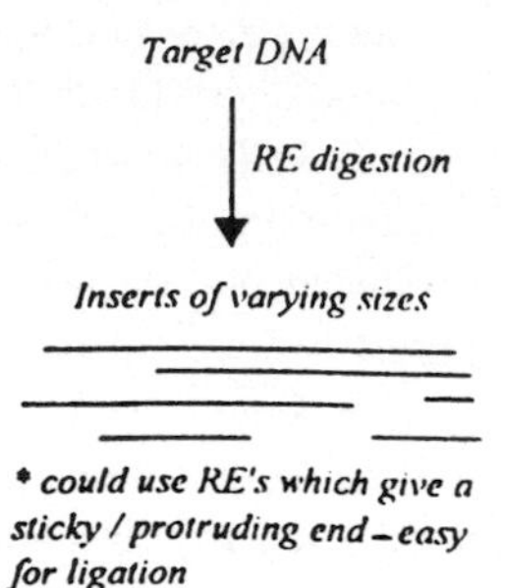

Compatible RE digestion (could also be a double digestion)

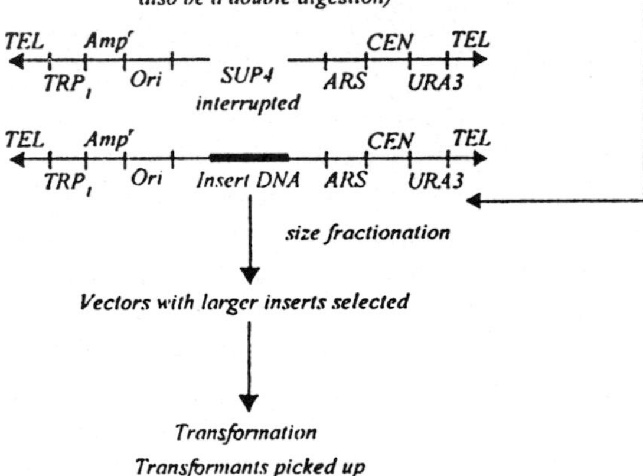

Figure 6 Yeast artificial chromosome (YAC). (Description in text.)

rejection. A common approach is to synthesize immunosuppressive chimeric or fusion proteins with recombinant DNA techniques. Introducing antisense nucleic acid sequences to an immunoregulatory gene is another approach to prevent rejection. An even more exciting approach is to use gene therapy strategies. Clinical trials of several gene therapy approaches are under way in patients with cancer and metabolic disorders. It is anticipated that similar trials will begin shortly in transplantation. A final approach that holds promise in the future is to create genetically engineered animals whose whole organs can be made either to express a gene that will prevent rejection or to "knock out" a gene that causes rejection.

B. Antirejection Agents Made by Molecular Biological Methods

Several antirejection agents have been synthesized in vitro with molecular biological techniques. These can be broadly categorized into protein or nucleic acid (e.g., antisense

RNA) agents. Proteins that are membrane-bound can be transformed into soluble proteins by deleting the exon encoding the transmembrane region from the gene. Examples are soluble MHC molecules and soluble complement receptor type I (sCRI). The latter prolongs xenograft survival significantly when administered to primate recipients of porcine heart xenografts (55,56).

Another interesting strategy is to synthesize chimeric molecules by joining exons of two genes. The utility in producing chimeric molecules is twofold. First, this technique enables molecules that are generally membrane-bound to be secreted. Thus, they can be used as soluble protein reagents. An example is CTLA-4 Ig, which inhibits T-cell costimulation and thus prevents rejection. Second, in chimeric molecules, one molecule possesses two functions. An example is diphtheria toxin/IL-2 conjugate, which kills activated T cells (discussed below).

1. Chimeric Proteins to Induce T-cell Anergy: CTLA-4 Ig

CTLA-4 Ig is a fusion protein made by joining the genes encoding the receptor binding domain of CTLA-4 and the FC part of human IgG2. The CTLA-4 portion acts as a competitive inhibitor by binding to costimulatory molecules that belong to the B7 family on antigen presenting cells (reviewed in Ref. 57). This inhibits the binding of CD28 and CTLA-4 molecules on T cells to the costimulatory molecules on APCs. Inhibiting costimulation with CTLA-4 Ig in vitro leads to anergy of T cells to the antigens presented by the APCs. Administration of CTLA-4 Ig prevents rejection of islet xenografts and heart allografts in rodents (58). Recipients of islet xenografts and of mouse allografts show donor specific unresponsiveness suggestive of in vivo T cell anergy. CTLA-4 molecule is highly conserved in evolution and is the same in humans and rodents. It is anticipated that CTLA-4 Ig will produce similar donor-specific unresponsiveness in clinical transplantation.

2. Chimeric Proteins to Induce T-Cell Death: Cytokine-Toxin Conjugates

Another interesting strategy is to fuse a cytokine gene with a toxin gene to induce death of the T cells that bind the cytokine. Examples are fusion proteins in which the receptor binding domain of IL-2 is fused with the G-protein binding domain of diphtheria or tetanus toxin. Several studies in rodents have shown that these reagents can prevent rejection (59).

3. Antisense Nucleic Acids

Nucleic acids that are antisense to RNA encoding a protein essential to T-cell growth can, in theory, prevent rejection. Two strategies are used to get antisense nucleic acids into cells (60). A cumbersome strategy is to transfect cells with a DNA that encodes antisense RNA. The transfected cells transcribe the antisense RNA. This then binds to the normal (sense) RNA of the gene of interest and prevents its translation into protein. Besides being cumbersome, this approach has fallen into disrepute because experimental results have been variable.

A simpler strategy is to introduce antisense oligonucleotides into the cells. These oligos can bind to the RNA of interest and prevent its translation. Currently there is emphasis on developing modified oligonucleotides that are resistant to degradation by extracellular nucleases and are less toxic to cells (61). Most of these efforts are targeted toward inhibiting oncogenes and preventing growth of cancers (62), but the strategy would be applicable to prevention of rejection.

The versatility of in vitro molecular biological techniques is tremendous. Therefore, almost any combination of reagents can be made using these techniques. However, the challenge is to figure out a strategy that will be effective in clinical transplantation.

C. Gene Transfer to Prevent Rejection

1. Gene Transfection to Induce Donor-Specific Unresponsiveness

Historically, donor-specific transfusion (DST) is known to induce tolerance in experimental animals. With gene transfer technology, it became possible to test the hypothesis that histocompatibility genes or cells incapable of presenting antigens may induce tolerance. Wood and coworkers showed that transfusion of fibroblasts transfected with MHC of potential donors led to donor-specific unresponsiveness in recipients of mouse heart allografts (63). An interesting modification of this strategy is to introduce an allogeneic MHC class I gene into the bone marrow of the recipients of allografts. In experiments by Sykes and coworkers, reteroviral vectors were used to transduce the allogeneic MHC class I gene into T-cell-depleted bone marrow cells (64). Although only about 5% of bone marrow cells expressed the allogeneic MHC gene after reconstitution, prolonged survival of MHC-disparate allografts was achieved.

Knechtle and colleagues have utilized a novel method to achieve donor-specific unresponsiveness (65). Their approach is based on the observation that myoblasts take up injected DNA readily. Initially they demonstrated that plasmids containing MHC class I gene constructs injected directly into heart muscle expressed allogeneic MHC class I protein. This group then transfected myoblasts and myotubes with the allogeneic MHC gene and injected the myoblasts intrathymically into potential recipients of allografts. The intrathymic injections induced tolerance to fully disparate liver allografts and to subsequent heart allografts. It is interesting to note that expression of allogeneic MHC molecules in myoblasts in extrathymic locations accelerates rejection (65). These experiments demonstrate the antigen-presenting capacity of "nonprofessional" APCs and suggest a strategy to induce tolerance using gene therapy approaches.

2. Direct Gene Transfer in Organs and Tissues

a. Physical Methods. DNA can be introduced into mammalian cells with the help of several physical agents. A commonly used physical method for gene transfer is via liposome-mediated DNA transfection. In this technique, cationic liposomes act as carriers of negatively charged DNA molecules. Liposomes presumably fuse with the cell membranes and lead to DNA transfection by endocytosis. The efficiency of liposome mediated DNA transfection (transient) can approach 30 to 40% in vitro. The other advantages of the liposomes is that they are easy to use, have a capacity to carry large pieces of DNA, and can be used to transfect almost any type of cell (66). However, liposomes are frequently toxic to cells. Recent improvements in liposome fabrication have reduced this toxicity. It is possible to obtain systemic expression of a desired gene in several organs by intravenously injecting the gene complexed with liposomes (67).

As an alternative to liposomes, genes can be directly injected into tissues by suspending DNA in sucrose solutions. This method works optimally in muscles, because the injected DNA disseminates in the syncytia of myocytes. The tolerance induction experiments of Knechtle and coworkers, described above, have utilized this method to express alloMHC genes in cardiac and skeletal muscles.

b. Biological Methods (Adenovirus and Retroviruses). Biological methods of gene transfer involve employing viral vectors to carry the gene of interest. Retroviral and adenoviral vectors are most commonly used for gene therapy. Retroviruses infect dividing cells most efficiently. Therefore, gene transfer using these vectors is generally possible only in vitro. Genes introduced via retroviral vectors are stably integrated into the genome of the infected cells. The efficiency of retroviral vector-mediated gene transfer can approach 100%. A variety of reteroviral vectors have been created to accommodate foreign DNA. Vectors have been designed so that they cannot replicate independently. These vectors (and the genes inserted in them) are propagated and amplified with the help of helper viruses. This system is a safeguard against inadvertent spread of retroviruses containing foreign genes.

Adenoviruses (Adv) and adeno-associated viruses (Aav) hold the greatest promise as vectors of choice for gene therapy. Their advantages are that they transfer genes with high efficiency to almost all cell types, although their natural tropism is to respiratory cells. Also, in contrast to retroviruses, the Adv and AAv infect nondividing cells. However, as a general rule, these viruses do not integrate into the host genome but exist as episomal elements. The Aav integrate in the genome in certain cell types. Due to their advantages, the Adv and the Aav are increasingly being used in phase I and II clinical trials of gene therapy.

Although gene therapy is in its infancy, this approach holds the greatest promise in clinical allotransplantation. An important advantage of this approach is that it is potentially feasible in cadaveric donors. Organs can be perfused with foreign genes after recovery. The main objective now is to devise efficient and nontoxic techniques to deliver genes into solid organs. Finally, although technically very difficult, it is possible to express entire gene complexes by transfecting eukaryotic cells with YAC vectors.

3. *Gene Transfer During Embryonic Development*

An exciting and powerful approach to prevent rejection is to manipulate genes in vivo to produce donor organs that will escape immunosurveillance. In vivo manipulation can be used either to introduce new genes (transgenes) or delete a constituent gene (gene "knockouts"). Although, historically, transgenic animals have been utilized to dissect the alloresponse (68), currently transgenic large animals are being created to evade the immune response.

a. Transgenic Animals. Production of transgenic mice is now commonplace due to developments in microinjection techniques. Using micropipettes, the transgenes are injected as cDNA into pronuclei of one-cell eggs. These eggs are reimplanted into the oviducts of pseudopregnant females. Progeny are tested to determine if the transgene is expressed and founder mice are established. Although production of transgenic animals is performed with relative ease, propagation of mice expressing the transgene involves a considerable expenditure of time and energy. Nonetheless, valuable information has been gained regarding the mechanisms of tolerance by experiments with mice transgenic for MHC and TCR genes (69).

Pigs transgenic for the human complement inhibitor decay accelerating factor c"DAF" have been created and are currently being bred (70) to provide organs for xenotransplantation. DAF accelerates the decay of a key component in the complement pathway, and DAF genes are species-specific. Therefore, organs from pigs transgenic for human DAF are expected to express this molecule and thus to escape hyperacute rejection when transplanted to humans.

b. Gene "knockout" Animals. Gene "knockout" mice are created on the principle of homologous recombination (71). This is based on the observation that genes introduced in dividing embryonic stem (ES) cells tend to be integrated in the same place as the constituent homologous genes (and sometimes to replace the homologous genes by recombination). If the introduced genes are defective (mutated), they replace the constituent functional gene with a defective gene.

MHC knockout mice were created by mutating the β2 microglobulin gene. This gene was introduced into ES cells, which were then injected into blastocysts obtained from pregnant mice. As a result of mixing the introduced ES cells with the embryonic cells, the blastocyst and subsequent progeny were chimeras. The germinal cells in some of these mice were a mixture of cells containing either functional or defective β2 microglobulin genes. The F2 progeny of these mice consisted of either β2 microglobulin–expressing or –nonexpressing mice. The mice lacking β2 microglobulin do not express MHC class I molecules (72,73), since MHC class I molecules are not transported to the cell surface in the absence of β2 microglobulin.

MHC class II–deficient mice were produced similarly except that the β chain encoding gene I-E was knocked out in C57B16 mice. The C57B16 mice normally lack the other class II (I-a) molecules. Thus, knocking out the I-E gene led to mice that were completely deficient in class II expression. An alternate strategy consisted of knocking out the gene for the invariant chain which normally transports the MHC class II molecules to the cell surface (74,75). In the final step, the class I– and class II–deficient mice were mated to produce mice that lacked expression of either gene (76). The "double knockouts" lacked $CD4^+$ and $CD8^+$ T cells but had significant numbers (5 to 50% of wild type) of $CD4^-CD8^-TCR\alpha\beta^+$ T cells in the periphery. Interestingly, these mice rejected fully allogeneic skin grafts despite the lack of $CD4^+$ or $CD8^+$ T cells.

V. CONCLUSIONS AND FUTURE DIRECTIONS

Molecular biology is a relative newcomer to transplant biology. Therefore, definitive diagnosis of rejection is still based on clinical and histopathological criteria. Molecular biological approaches are now being employed in an attempt to facilitate the diagnosis by either providing clues for earlier diagnosis or providing increased sensitivity of diagnosis. For example, determining the cytokine profile in tissue obtained from a biopsy may provide clues for earlier diagnosis. Although much of this work is in its early stages, a combination of histopathological and molecular techniques is quite likely to provide a higher level of sophistication in diagnosing rejection and thus increasing graft survival.

The ultimate goal of transplantation is to achieve long-term tolerance. Although immunosuppression could achieve this goal, it is far more desirable to induce tolerance without immunosuppression. Molecular biology has started to provide the foundation for this goal. Organs from transgenic animals can be made to express tolerogenic genes. On the other hand, "knocking out" genes that are important in rejection by manipulating the genes at the embryonic level can provide organs in which the immunogenic genes are not expressed. In the adult, gene transfer (therapy) provides the exciting opportunity of inserting tolerance-inducing genes into organs during perfusion. As can be surmised, the development of these technologies depends heavily on understanding the mechanisms of rejection.

The "brave new world" is on the horizon. Clinical trials with organs from pigs transgenic for human soluble complement receptor (sCr) gene are expected to begin shortly. This is not to say that xenografts will provide organs and reduce the organ shortage in the immediate future, but these steps are major achievements of the fusion of molecular biology with transplant immunology. This fusion will pave the way for transplantation tolerance.

ACKNOWLEGMENTS

The authors gratefully acknowledge discussion with Mary S. Leffell, Ph.D., Co-Director, Immunogenetics Laboratory, The Johns Hopkins Hospital regarding DNA-based HLA typing, and the secretarial assistance of P. Morris. D.S.K. has been supported by NIH R29-25550.

REFERENCES

1. Kittur DS, Kittur SD, Adler W. Molecular biology of transplant rejection. In: Burdick JF, Racusen LC, Solez K, Williams GM, eds. Kidney Transplant Rejection: Diagnosis and Treatment. 2d ed. New York: Marcel Dekker, 1992:741–756.
2. Sambrook J, Fritsch EF, and Maniatis, T, eds. Molecular Cloning: A Laboratory Manual. Vol. 1. 2d ed. New York: Cold Spring Harbor Laboratory Press, 1989.
3. Sambrook J, Fritsch EF, and Maniatis, T, eds. Molecular Cloning: A Laboratory Manual. Vol. 2. 2d ed. New York: Cold Spring Harbor Laboratory Press, 1989.
4. Sambrook J, Fritsch EF, and Maniatis, T, eds. Molecular Cloning: A Laboratory Manual. Vol. 3. 2d ed. New York: Cold Spring Harbor Laboratory Press, 1989.
5. Colowick SP, Kaplan NO, Wu R, eds. Methods in Enzymology—Recombinant DNA. Vol. 68, New York: Academic Press, 1979.
6. Colowick SP, Kaplan NO, Wu R, Grossman L, Moldave K, eds. Methods in Enzymology—Recombinant DNA. Vol. 100, part B. New York: Academic Press, 1983.
7. Colowick SP, Kaplan NO, Wu R, Grossman L, Moldave K, eds. Methods in Enzymology—Recombinant DNA. Vol. 101, part C. New York: Academic Press, 1983.
8. Colowick SP, Kaplan NO, Grossman MM, eds. Methods in Enzymology—Molecular Genetics of Mammalian Cells. Vol. 151. New York: Academic Press, 1987.
9. Colowick SP, Kaplan NO, Wu R, Grossman L, eds. Methods in Enzymology—Recombinant DNA. Vol. 153, part D. New York: Academic Press, 1987.
10. Colowick SP, Kaplan NO, Grossman L, eds. Methods in Enzymology—Recombinant DNA. Vol. 154, part E. New York: Academic Press, 1987.
11. Colowick SP, Kaplan NO, Wu R, eds. Methods in Enzymology—Recombinant DNA Vol. 155, part F. New York: Academic Press, 1987.
12. Colowick SP, Kaplan NO, Goeddel DV, eds. Methods in Enzymology—Gene Expression Technology. Vol. 185. New York: Academic Press, 1990.
13. Ausubel FM, Brent R, Kingston RE, et al, eds. Current Protocols in Molecular Biology. Vol. 1. New York: John Wiley, 1989.
14. Riley E, Olerup O. HLA polymorphisms and evolution. Immunol Today 1992; 13:333–335.
15. Brown MG, Driscoll J, Monaco JJ. MHC-linked low-molecular mass polypeptide subunits define distinct subsets of proteasomes. J Immunol 1993; 151:1193–1204.
16. Monaco JJ. Major histocompatibility complex-linked transport proteins and antigen processing. Immunol Rev 1992; 11:125–132.
17. Erlich H, Bugawan T, Begovich A, Scharf S. Analysis of HLA class II polymorphism using polymerase chain reaction. Arch Pathol Lab Med 1993; 117:482–485.
18. Zemmour J, Praham P. HLA class I nucleotide sequences, 1992. Immunobiology 1993; 187 (1–2):70–101.
19. Bidwell J, Bidwell E. DNA-RFLP analysis and genotyping of HLA-DR and DQ antigens. Immunol Today 1988; 9:1.
20. Cros P, Allibert P, Mandrand B, et al. Oligonucleotide genotyping of HLA polymorphism on microtitre plates. Lancet 1992; 340:870–873.
21. Ota M, Seki T, Fukushima H, et al. HLA-DRB1 genotyping by modified PCR-RFLP method combined with group-specific primers. Tissue Antigens 1992; 39:187–202.

22. Zetterquist H, Olerup O. Identification of the HLA-DRB1*04, -DRB1*07, and -DRB1*09 alleles by PCR amplification with sequence-specific primers (PCR-SSP) in 2 hours. Hum Immunol 1992; 34:64–74.
23. Olerup O, Zetterquist H. HLA-DR typing by PCR amplification with sequence-specific primers (PCR-SSP) in 2 hours: An alternative to serological DR typing in clinical practice including donor-recipient matching in cadaveric transplantation. Tissue Antigens 1992; 39:225–235.
24. Olerup O, Zetterquist H. DR "low-resolution" PCR-SSP typing—A correction and an up-date. Tissue Antigens 1993; 41:55–56.
25. Mickelson E, Smith A, McKinney S, et al. A comparative study of HLA-DRB1 typing by standard serology and hybridization of non-radioactive sequence-specific oligonucleotide probes to PCR-amplified DNA. Tissue Antigens 1993; 41:86–93.
26. Doherty DG, Donaldson PT. HLA-DRB and DQB typing by a combination of serology, restriction fragment length polymorphism analysis and oligonucleotide probing. Eur Immunogenet 1991; 18:111–124.
27. Santamaria P, Lindstrom AL, Boyce-Jacino MT, et al. HLA class I sequence-based typing. Hum Immunol 1993; 37:39–50.
28. Mytilineos J, Scherer S, Dunckley H, et al. DNA HLA-DR typing results of 4000 kidney transplants. Transplantation 1993; 55:778–781.
29. Opelz G, Mytilineos J, Scherer S, Analysis of HLA-Dr matching in DNA-typed cadaver kidney transplants. Transplantation 1993; 55:782–785.
30. Strom TB, Waldmann H. Transplantation. Curr Opin Immunol 1994; 6:755–756.
31. Suthanthiran M, Strom TB. Renal transplantation. N Engl J Med 1994; 331:365–376.
32. Weiss A, Littman D. Signal transduction by lymphocyte antigen receptors. Cell 1994; 76: 263–274.
33. Sheng M, Greenberg ME. The regulation and function of c-fos and other immediate early genes in the nervous system. Neuron 1990; 4:477–485.
34. Angel P, Karin M. The role of Jun, Fos and the AP-1 complex in cell proliferation and transformation. Biochim Biophys Acta 1991; 1072:129–157.
35. Andersson G, Peterlin BM. NF-X2 that binds to the DRA X2-box is activator protein 1: Expression cloning of c-Jun. J Immunol 1990; 145:3456–3462.
36. Jain J, McCaffrey PG, Vale-Archer VE, Rao A. Nuclear factor of activated T cells contains Fos and Jun. Nature 1992; 356:810.
37. Dallman MJ, Wood KJ, Hamano K, et al. Cytokines and peripheral tolerance to alloantigen. Immunol Rev 1993; 133:5–18.
38. Fair JH, Mattei P, Guo YP, et al. Oligoclonal V beta usage in vitro after in vivo exposure to pig xenoantigen extracorporeal pig liver perfusion. Transplant Proc 1994; 26:1340–1341.
39. Hall BL, Finn OJ. PCR-based analysis of the T-cell receptor V beta multigene family: Experimental parameters affecting its validity. Biotechniques 1992; 13:248–257.
40. Kirk AD, Li RA, Kinch MS, et al. The human antiporcine cellular repertoire: In vitro studies of acquired and innate cellular responsiveness. Transplantation 1993; 55:924–931.
41. Hall BL, Finno OJ. T cell receptor V beta gene usage in allograft-derived cell lines analyzed by a polymerase chain reaction technique. Transplantation 1992; 53:1088–1099.
42. Starzl TE, Demetris AJ, Trucco M, et al. Systemic chimerism in human female recipients of male livers. Lancet 1992; 340:876–877.
43. Starzl TE, Demetris AJ, Murase N, et al. Donor cell chimerism permitted by immunosuppressive drugs: A new view of organ transplantation. Trends Pharmacol Sci 1993; 14:217–223.
44. Wilborn F, Schmidt CA, Siegert W. Demonstration of chimerism after allogeneic bone marrow transplantation by polymerase chain reaction of Y-chromosome-specific nucleotide sequences—Characterization of a new technical approach. Leukemia 1993; 7:140–143.
45. Saiki RK, Walsh PS, Levenson CH, Erlich HA. Genetic analysis of amplified DNA with immobilized sequence-specific oligonucleotide probes. Proc Natl Acad Sci USA 1989; 86:6230–6234.

46. Feuerbach D, Etteldorf S, Ebenau-Jehle C, et al. Identification of amino acids within the MHC molecule are important for the interaction with the adenovirus protein E3/19K. J Immunol 1994; 153:1626–1636.
47. Hadley GA, Linders B, Mohanakumar T. Immunogenicity of MHC class I alloantigens expressed on parenchymal cells in the human kidney. Transplantation 1992; 54:537–542.
48. Hadley GA, Linders B, Mohanakumar T. Kidney cell-restricted recognition of MHC class I alloantigens by human cytolytic T cell clones. Transplantation 1993; 55:400–404.
49. Platt JL, Holzknecht ZE, Lindman BJ. Porcine endothelial antigens recognized by human natural antibodies. Transplant Proc 1994; 26:1387.
50. Parimoo S, Patanjali SR, Shukla H, et al. cDNA selection: Efficient PCR approach for the selection of cDNAs encoded in large chromosomal DNA fragments. Proc Natl Acad Sci USA 1991; 88:9623–9627.
51. Geraghty DE, Pei J, Lipsky B, et al. Cloning and physical mapping of the HLA class I region spanning the HLA-E to HLA-F interval by using yeast artificial chromosomes. Proc Natl Acad Sci USA 1992; 89:2669–2673.
52. Denizol F, Mattei MG, Vernet C, et al. YAC-assisted cloning of a putative G-protein mapping to the MHC class I region. Genomics 1992; 14:857–862.
53. el Kahloun A, Chauvel B, Mauvieux V, et al. Localization of seven new genes around the HLA-A locus. Hum Molec Genet 1993; 2:55.
54. Hruban RH, Long PP, Perlman EJ, et al. Fluorescence in situ hybridization for the Y-chromosome can be used to detect cells of recipient origin in allografted hearts following cardiac transplantation. Am J Pathol 1993; 142:975–980.
55. Xia W, Fearon DT, Kirkman RL. Effect of repetitive doses of soluble human complement receptor type I on survival of discordant cardiac xenografts. Transplant Proc 1993; 25(1 pt 1): 410–411.
56. Pruitt SK, Kirk AD, Bollinger RR, et al. The effect of soluble complement receptor type I on hyperacute rejection of porcine xenografts. Transplantation 1994; 57:363–370.
57. Linsley P, Ledbetter J. The role of the CD28 receptor during T cell responses to antigen. Annu Rev Immunol 1993; 11:191–212.
58. Turka LA, Linsley PS, Lin H, et al. T-cell activation by the CD28 ligand B7 is required for cardiac allograft rejection in vivo. Proc Natl Acad Sci USA 1992; 89:11102–11105.
59. Shapiro ME, Kirkman RL, Kelley VR, et al. In vivo studies with chimeric toxins: Interleukin-2 fusion toxins as immunosuppressive agents. Targ Diagn Ther 1992; 7:383–393.
60. Zamecnik PC. Introduction: Oligonucleotide base hybridization as a modulator of genetic message readout. In: Prospects for Antisense Nucleic Acid Therapy of Cancer and AIDS. Wiley-Liss, 1991:1–6.
61. Vlassov VV, Yakubov LA. Oligonucleotides in cells and in organisms: Pharmacological considerations. In: Prospects for Antisense Nucleic Acid Therapy of Cancer and AIDS. Wiley-Liss, 1991:243–266.
62. Leserman L, Degols G, Machy P, et al. Targeting and intracellular delivery of antisense oligonucleotides interfering with oncogene expression. In: Prospects for Antisense Nucleic Acid Therapy of Cancer and AIDS. New York: Wiley-Liss, 1991:25–33.
63. Madsen JC, Sperina RA, Wood KJ, Morris PJ. Immunological unresponsiveness induced by recipient cells transfected with donor MHC genes. Nature 1988; 332:161–164.
64. Sykes M, Sachs DH, Nienhuis AW, et al. Specific prolongation of skin graft survival following retroviral transduction of bone marrow with an allogeneic major histocompatibility complex gene. Transplantation 1993; 55:197–202.
65. Knechtle SJ, Wang J, Jiao S, et al. Induction of specific tolerance by intrathymic injection of recipient muscle cells transfected with donor class I major histocompatibility complex. Transplantation 1994; 57:990–996.
66. Farhood H, Gao X, Son K, et al. Cationic liposomes for direct gene transfer in therapy of cancer and other diseases. Ann NY Acad Sci 1994; 716:23–35.

67. Zhu N, Liggitt D, Liu Y, Debs R. Systemic gene expression after intravenous DNA delivery into adult mice. Science 1993; 261:209–211.
68. Yeung RS, Penninger J, Mak TW. Genetically modified animals and immunodeficiency. Curr Opin Immunol 1993; 5:585–594.
69. Miller JFAP. Introduction: Use of transgenic mice in the investigation of self-tolerance and the repertoire of T and B lymphocytes. Semin Immunol 1989; 1:93–94.
70. Rosengard A, Cary NRB, Langford GA, et al. Tissue expression of human complement inhibitor, decay accelerating factor (DAF), in transgenic pigs—A potential approach for preventing xenograft rejection. Transplantation. In press.
71. Song K-Y, Schwartz F, Maeda N, et al. Accurate modification of a chromosomal plasmid by homologous recombination in human cells. Proc Natl Acad Sci USA 1987; 84:6820–6824.
72. Zijlstra M, Bix M, Simister NE, et al. β2-microglobulin deficient mice lack CD4-8+ cytolytic T cells. Nature 1990: 344:742–746.
73. Koller BH, Marrack P, Kappler JW, Smithies O. Normal development of mice deficient in the B_2M, MHC class I proteins, and CD8+ T cells. Science 1990; 248:1227–1230.
74. Grusby MJ, Johnson RS, Papaioannou VE, Glimcher LH. Depletion of CD4+ T cells in major histocompatibility complex class I deficient mice. Science 1991; 253:1417–1420.
75. Cosgrove D, Gray D, Dierich A, et al. Mice lacking MHC class II molecules. Cell 1991; 66: 1051–1066.
76. Grusby MJ, Auchincloss H Jr, Lee R, et al. Mice lacking major histocompatibility complex class I and class II molecules. Proc Natl Acad Sci USA 1993; 90:3913–3917.

23

New Immunosuppressive Agents

Bernhard Ryffel,* Qinjxiang Su, Hans-Pietro Eugster, and B. D. Car
Institute of Toxicology of the ETH and University of Zürich, Schwerzenbach-Zürich, Switzerland

I. INTRODUCTION: DRUG DISCOVERY, IMMUNOBIOLOGY OF TRANSPLANT REJECTION, AND IMMUNOLOGICAL INTERVENTION

A. Drug Discovery

The surgical success in vascular anastomoses at the beginning of our century was thwarted by loss of the kidney due to rejection. The immunological basis of events involved in graft rejection was unknown at that time; the notion of histocompatibility antigens and their differences between individuals emerged 60 years later. Successful allotransplantation was performed between identical twins as early as 1950. Irradiation and chemical immunosuppression were first attempted as adjunct therapies in the early 1960s. The milestones of renal transplantation are summarized in Table 1. The discovery of azathioprine and its combined use with glucocorticosteroids hailed the beginning of a new era in organ transplantation. Surgeons, encouraged by results with chemical immunosuppression, attempted the transplantation of several other organs, including the liver and heart. Rejection crises were treated with high doses of glucocorticosteroids and/or antilymphocyte serum. An important limitation of the treatment was the toxicity of the immunosuppressants: leukopenia induced by the purine analogue azathioprine and Cushing's syndrome by chronic glucocorticosteroid excess.

The discovery of cyclosporine (1) and its introduction into the clinic in 1978 (1,2) heralded a therapeutic breakthrough that enabled controlled immunosuppression to be employed in transplant patients. Cyclosporine proved to be much more selective for the immune system and devoid of adverse effects on the hematopoietic system. However, despite the excellent results achieved, clinicians retain reservations concerning the use of cyclosporine for at least two reasons: renal dysfunction as the major side effect and failure to induce lasting immunological tolerance with cyclosporine (1). The role of newer immunosuppressants emerging from microbiological research, such as the macrolide-structured

Present affiliation: Institute of Pathology, Basel, Switzerland.

Table 1 Milestones of Kidney Transplantation

1902	Experimental kidney transplantation (Ullmann)
1906	Xenotransplantation into humans (Jaboulay)
1954	Kidney transplantation between twins (Murray et al.)
1960	Azathioprine immunosuppression (Calne, Zukoski)
1967	Antilymphocyte globulin (Starzl)
1978	Cyclosporine (Calne)
1983	OKT-3 antibody (Cosimi)
1990	FK506 (Starzl)
1995–2000	Rapamycin, MPA, BQR, Leflunomide?

molecules FK506 and rapamycin, and a few novel chemicals mostly derived from cancer chemotherapy, are discussed in this chapter.

From this short introduction it is already evident that each immunosuppressant has its specific profile of adverse effects. The specific toxicities of novel immunosuppressive agents are the focus of the present chapter. Since side effects are tightly related to the pharmacological activity, the present knowledge of the mode of action of the immunosuppressants is reviewed and the possible relations to the mode of action are discussed. Understanding of molecular drug action may help to predict drug toxicity; this approach may be necessary for the novel immunosuppressants which have not yet reached the market.

B. Immunobiology of Transplant Rejection

A simplified scheme of cellular events occurring during the interaction between the grafted organ and its host is given in Fig. 1. Schematically, three phases may be distinguished: first, an afferent phase, which includes the recognition of the foreign tissue—i.e., the allograft; second, a central phase occurring within the immune system, comprising the differentiation of alloantigen-specific lymphocytic clones into effector cells; and the final efferent phase, characterized by cellular and humoral effector mechanisms, leading to the ultimate rejection of the allograft (reviewed in Ref. 3). Genetic differences between donor and host are defined by histocompatibility complex molecules expressed on the cell membrane. Donor cells with histocompatibility molecules differing from those of the host are recognized by the host's immune system. Continuous alloantigenic stimulation results in profound activation of helper T cells with the release of several cytokines leading ultimately to the maturation of effector immune cells, e.g., cytotoxic T cells, activated macrophages, natural killer cells, and plasma cells. These activated effector cells, acting in concert with several cytokines—e.g., interferon and interleukins, which increase the class II expression within the graft, and TNF, with its direct cytotoxic effect—and specific antibodies attack the graft and cause its rejection. The tremendous progress in the areas of allorecognition, cytokines, and the identification of their specific membrane receptors will allow a better understanding of the molecular events of the graft rejection (4,5).

C. Possible Sites of Immunological Intervention

The interaction of the antigen-presenting cell with the antigen receptor on helper T lymphocyte surface is the central event leading to the activation of the immune system

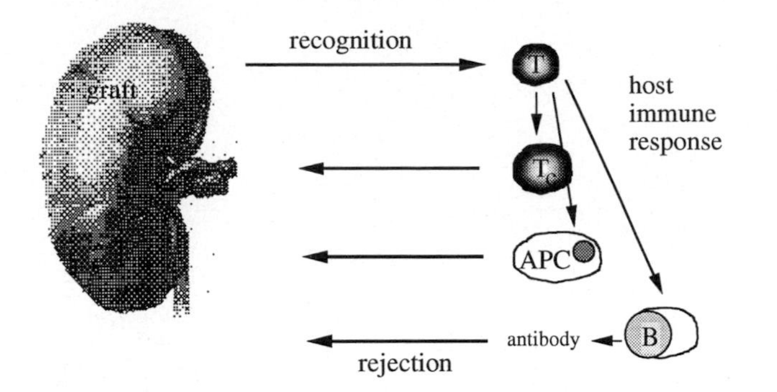

Figure 1 Cellular events leading to graft rejection. Afferent limb: Alloantigen from the graft is presented by dendritic cells (APC). Central part: Recognition of alloantigen by host immune system, activation of antigen presenting cells (APC), T cells, and B cells. Efferent limb: Activated lymphocytes, antibodies and complement, macrophages, and lymphokines destroy the graft.

(reviewed in Ref. 3) (Table 2). The activation of the T-helper cells (T_H) results in the synthesis and release of several cytokines, affecting the maturation of effector cells with cytotoxic function (Tc, NK) and of B-lymphocytes (Fig. 2). In the induction of immune suppression, the first potential site of intervention in the host immune system would be at the level of antigen uptake, followed by processing and final assembly into the host class II antigen of antigen presenting cells (APC). While such specificity of suppression is possible in vitro, it may be difficult to achieve in vivo. Agents that inhibit the activation of APC and their release of cytokines (e.g., IL-1, IL-6, or TNF), however, may have a profound effect on subsequent T-cell activation. The T-cell receptor (TcR), consisting of a heterodimeric antigen-recognition domain and several invariant associated chains (known as the CD3 complex), is another potential site of immunointervention, which would theoretically prevent recognition of the antigenic signal (6). Antibodies directed against TcR or CD3 may block the access of the processed antigen presented by the class II molecules. Instead of antibodies, irrelevant peptides may be utilized, which compete for the class II site, thereby preventing correct recognition by the TcR. The interaction of TcR with the specific antigenic peptide presented by class II molecules provides the specificity of the reaction

Table 2 Potential Sites of Immunosuppression: Macrophage/T-Helper Cell

Antigen presentation	Inhibition of antigen processing
	Presentation on MHC class II antigen
	Bioengineered xenotransplants
Signal recognition	Blocking antibodies against T-cell receptor, accessory molecules of T-cell activation, specific peptides
Signal transduction	Inhibition of specific kinases or phosphatases: fyn-, lck-kinase, CD45 phosphatase, calcineurin, PLCγ, MAP-kinase, G-proteins
Gene transcription	Inhibition of cytokine or receptor
	Modulation of regulatory gene (myc, myb, rb, p53, cyclins)
Cytokine action	Neutralizing antibodies against cytokine or cytokine receptor
	Soluble receptors
Inhibition of cell cycle	Antimetabolites

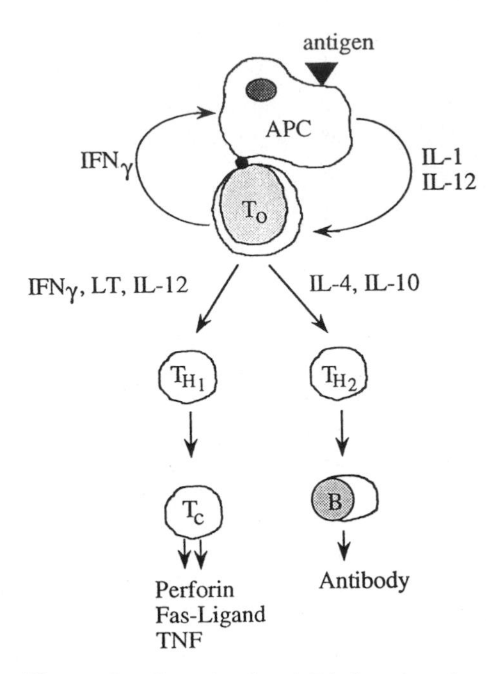

Figure 2 Central role of T-helper lymphocyte, cellular interactions. Antigen is processed by antigen-presenting cells (APC) and presented within the major histocompatibility molecules to the T-cell (T_O) receptor. Activated APC release IL-1, IL-12, and TNF, while activated T-helper cells (TH) synthesize several interleukins, which have multiple regulatory effects, shifting the immune response to a TH1-type response with the differentiation of cytotoxic T lymphocaters (Tc) or to a TH2 response, resulting in B-cell differentiation and antibody-secreting plasma cells (PC).

but is alone insufficient for T-cell activation. Other membrane molecules, such as CD4/8 and several adhesion molecules, are necessary to increase the affinity of the cellular interaction. Thus, prevention of these additional contact sites, predominantly by antibodies, is another potential avenue for inhibition of T-cell activation.

Upon recognition by the TcR, the antigenic signal is transduced through complex biochemical pathways, which include the activation of several enzymes—such as phospholipase C_γ, kinases (e.g., fyn, lck, and MAP kinase) and phosphatases, including CD45 and calcineurin. A key feature of this transduction is the release of inositol-3-phosphate, thus mobilizing intracellular calcium, which with diacylglycerol activates protein kinase C. Recent reports concerning CsA and FK506 have concluded that the phosphatase calcineurin plays an important role through dephosphorylation of the nuclear factor NFAT. Upon dephosphorylation, NFAT is translocated into the nucleus, where it binds to the interleukin-2 (IL-2) promotor, resulting in IL-2 gene transcription (see below). However, other factors (e.g., NFKB and AP-1) were shown to be necessary for IL-2 gene activation. The control of IL-2 gene activation/transcription is an active area of research.

The genetic program induced by antigen stimulation is complex and includes the active transcription of at least 70 genes. The inhibition of gene expression of molecules such as cytokine receptors, interferons, and TNF must also be considered for the induction of immunosuppression.

Pharmacological modulation of antigenic processing within the APC is also a potential avenue to immunosuppression that remains unexploited.

II. OVERVIEW OF IMMUNOSUPPRESSIVE AGENTS

This chapter provides a short overview of presently used immunosuppressants or drugs that are in phase II or III clinical trials (Table 3):

Azathioprine: Azathioprine is an imidazole derivative of 6-mercaptopurine, a purine analogue with antimetabolite properties, inhibiting primary immune responses. Since azathioprine immunosuppression is mediated by inhibition of cell proliferation, it is not surprising that other systems, especially the hemopoietic system, are also adversely affected. Leukopenia is the main dose-limiting side effect (7–10). Azathioprine is often combined with steroids and CsA as maintenance immunosuppressive therapy, but has no effect in antirejection therapy.

Antilymphocyte antibodies: Polyclonal antibodies raised against human lymphocytes in rabbit or horse are in clinical use for the treatment of transplant rejection. These antisera bind to circulating lymphocytes, causing a sequestration in the spleen and resulting in subsequent lympholysis. Monoclonal antibodies (anti-CD3) have the advantage of being a homogenous product, in contrast to the antisera. Although acting similarly to the polyclonal antibodies, an important difference is the mitogenic activity of anti-CD3 monoclonal antibodies on T cells, which leads to their activation, resulting in fever due to the release of cytokines (11–14).

Glucocorticosteroids: Steroids inhibit T-lymphocyte activation by blocking the release of IL-1 from macrophages and subsequent IL-2 synthesis. Furthermore, steroids cause the lysis of lymphocytes. The immunosuppressive properties of steroids can be used clinically for maintenance and antirejection therapy.

Steroids have pleiotropic effects on other systems in the body, e.g., inhibition of

Table 3 Overview of Immunosuppressant Agents: Chemical and Biological

Drug	Mode of Action	Side Effects
Azathioprine	Antimetabolite, inhibition of purine biosynthesis	Myelotoxicity
Cyclosporine	IL-2 gene transcription	Nephrotoxicity
Glucocorticosteroids	Inhibition of IL-1 synthesis	Cushing's syndrome
FK506	IL-2 gene transcription	Nephrotoxicity
Rapamycin	IL-2 signal transduction, inhibition of S6 kinase	?
Leflunomide	IL-2 signal transduction	?
Deoxyspergualin (DSG)	IL-2 signal transduction?	?
RS 61443 (MPA)	Inhibition of de novo purine synthesis	?
Brequinar (BQR)	Inhibition of de novo purine synthesis	?
OKT3	Activation and sequestration of T lymphocytes	Fever
Antibodies	MHC class II IL-2R ICAM-1, LFA-1, CD4, B7, CTLA4 IFNγ, TNF	?

inflammation, interference with several metabolic pathways causing hyperglycemia, etc. The adverse metabolic effects of chronic therapy, manifesting as Cushing's syndrome, are usually dose-limiting (15,16).
Cyclosporin A (CsA): Cyclosporin A is a fungal peptide, which inhibits IL-2 gene transcription. The immunosuppressive property of CsA is successfully used clinically for maintenance and antirejection therapy.
Recent investigations revealed that CsA confers immunosuppression by inhibiting the calcineurin phosphatase. It is assumed that deficient dephosphorylation of NFAT prevents its nuclear translocation and IL-2 gene transcription (1).
FK506, rapamycin: These molecules are two novel and potent immunosuppressants with macrolide structure. While FK506 has a similar mode of action to CsA (i.e., inhibition of IL-2 gene transcription by affecting calcineurin phosphatase), rapamycin is the prototype of a novel class of immunosuppressants. Rapamycin has no effect on IL-2 gene expression but potently blocks IL-2 signal transduction by inhibition of the S6 kinase as discussed below (2,17,18).

III. CYCLOSPORINE—NEW INSIGHTS INTO ITS MODE OF ACTION, RELATION TO TOXICITY

Cyclosporin A (CsA) is a member of the cyclic undecapeptides (Fig. 3), which have immunosuppressive properties (1). It has been successfully used to prevent allograft rejection and to treat several autoimmune diseases (2). Molecular studies on its mode of action have revealed that CsA prevents T-lymphocyte activation at the level of cytokine gene transcription (reviewed in Refs. 3,18,17). Recent investigations with macrolide immunosuppressants showed that FK506 has the same effect on cytokine gene transcription as CsA, thereby inhibiting T-lymphocyte activation (19–22). These findings provoked investigations at the molecular level designed to identify possible pathways common for both immunosuppressants. Such studies may provide important insights into the control of cytokine gene activation.

Cellular uptake of CsA, evidence of intracellular receptors: Specific, saturable, and reversible binding was shown for murine and human mononuclear blood leukocytes utilizing a ^{3}H-CsA derivative (23,24). Investigations over a broader concentration range in erythrocytes and in several nucleated cell types revealed two components of cell binding (3): a saturable cytosolic binding at low CsA concentrations and a nonsaturable, nonspecific partitioning into the membrane at higher CsA concentrations. These findings, together with evidence for CsA accumulation within the cell, suggest the existence of an intracellular binding protein (25).

The discovery of cyclophilin A (CPH-A), an 18-kDa protein that specifically binds CsA, was a seminal contribution to the understanding of CsA-mediated events (26), opening many avenues of further research. The amino acid sequence of CPH-A was apparently not related to any known protein (27); however, it was later established that CPH-A was homologous to a prolyl-peptidyl cis-trans-isomerase, also known as rotamase (28,29). Active cyclosporines were shown to bind to CPH-A (30) and inhibit its rotamase activity.

The specificity of cyclosporin-CPH-A binding was investigated by hydrophobic interactions using an LH-20 column (27), competitive solid phase enzyme-linked immunosorbant assay (31,32), and photoaffinity labeling (33). Binding to CPH-A correlated with the

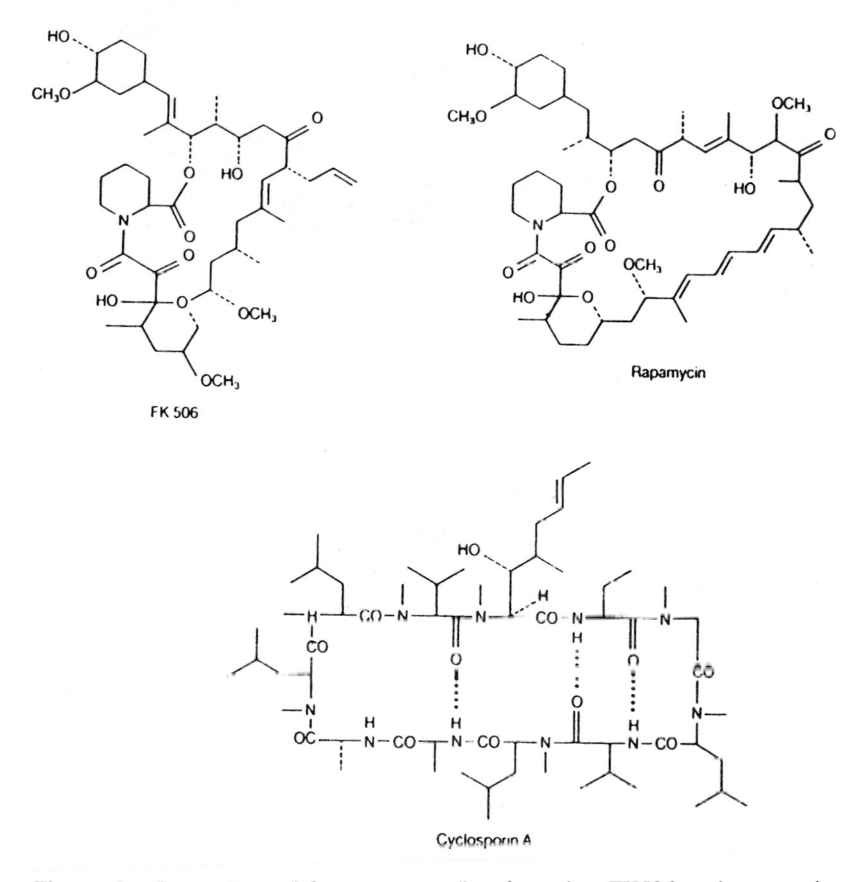

Figure 3 Comparison of the structures of cyclosporine, FK506, and rapamycin.

immunosuppressive activity of cyclosporine analogues. Amino acids 1, 2, 10, and 11 of the CsA molecule were found to be essential for cyclophilin binding. Subtle changes in these residues reduced both the affinity for CPH-A and in vitro immunosuppressive activity (32,34).

The synthesis of a photoaffinity-labeled cyclosporine analogue allowed the identification of several additional CsA binding proteins (33,35,36). In the T-cell line Jurkat, labeled proteins of 21, 25, 40, and 60-kDa were identified (37). The labeled proteins at 21 and 25-kDa were identical with CPH-A and CPH-B (Fig. 4). CPH-B is a second CsA binding protein, which has an endoplasmic reticulum retention signal (38–40). Two new members of this family were also identified (Table 4): CPH-C, which reportedly has a restricted tissue distribution (41), and CPH-D (42). These latter proteins are less abundant than CPH-A and have a molecular mass of approximately 22 kDa; thus, they were not distinguishable from CPH-B by photoaffinity labeling. Kieffer et al. (43) purified a 40-kDa protein (CPH-40) by affinity chromatography; the partial sequence analysis of this protein showed homology with CPH-A. CPH-40 antiserum did not cross-react with CPH-A in immunoblot analysis. Another 45-kDa CsA binding protein, which is phosphorylated, was reported but not further characterized (44).

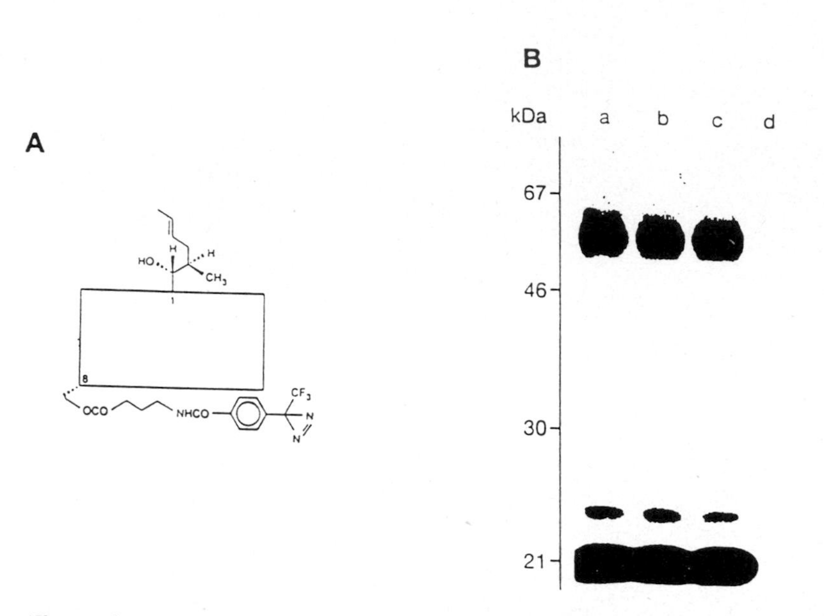

Figure 4 In vivo detection of CsA receptor proteins (A). Structure of photoaffinity-labeled derivative (B). The human T-cell line Jurkat is incubated with titrated photoaffinity label–probe. After UV cross-linking, the labeled cellular proteins are separated by SDS-PAGE and the proteins detected by fluoroautoradiography (a). The specificity of binding is defined by competition with 10× molar excess CsA (d) or by lack of competition by inactive CsH (b) or FK506 (c).

Table 4 Properties of CsA and FK506 Binding Proteins (Immunophilins)

	Molecular weight				
Name	(kDa)	(%)	Homology	Location[a]	Rotamase activity
Cyclophilins					
CPH-A	18		—	c	+
CPH-B	22		64	m	+
CPH-C	23		?	?	+
CPH-D	22		72	m	+
CPH-40	40		?	c	+
CPH-45	45		?		
FKBPs					
FKBP12	12			c	+
FKBP13	13		60	m	+
FKBP25	25		40	n	+
FKBP59	59			n?	+

[a]Cellular location: membrane (m), cytosol (c), nuclear (n).

Cyclophilin distribution and function: All the members of the CPH family have rotamase (prolyl-peptidyl cis-trans-isomerase) activity, which is inhibited by CsA (42,45). CPH-A exhibits the highest specific activity and is most sensitive to CsA inhibition. Macrolide-derived immunosuppressants, however, do not affect this CPH rotamase activity. All CPHs, with the possible exception of CPH-C, are highly abundant in both lymphoid and nonlymphoid tissues. The subcellular localization of CPH proteins has been investigated by biochemical cell fractionation studies and immunoelectron microscopy. Cyclophilin A and B are found in both cytosol and nucleus, and demonstrate no specific association with organellar structures (46–48). CPH-B and D possess a membrane localization signal and are found in the endoplasmic reticulum-membrane fraction.

The relative abundance and high conservation of cyclophilins suggest, however, an important role in normal cell function (26,46,49,50). The search for an endogenous ligand of CPH has been hitherto unsuccessful. The initial uptake and intracellular concentration of active cyclosporines at cytosolic and/or nuclear sites (25), followed by inhibition of rotamase activity are two potential roles for CPH-A in CsA-mediated immunosuppression. However, the role of rotamase inhibition has been questioned, since the IL-2 gene transcription is fully inhibited at just 1% occupancy of CPH-A.

The CsA-cyclophilin binding site: The CsA-cyclophilin complex has been investigated by x-ray and nuclear magnetic resonance (NMR) techniques (51–55). CPH-A exhibits a β barrel shape with a radius of 17 Å. The main structural elements are two perpendicular four-stranded β sheets and two well-defined α helices (Fig. 5A). Most of the hydrophobic side chains are packed in a hydrophobic core. Other hydrophobic residues occur in the contact region between the two helices, the β sheets, and in the CsA binding site. Replacement of the two cysteines (Cys 62 and 115) by alanine affected neither CsA binding nor rotamase activity. The sole tryptophane residue (Trp 121) is, however, necessary for binding (56). The macrolide binding protein, FKBP (see below), has no significant homology with CPH-A. Common three-dimensional surface structures that could preexist or be induced by CsA or FK506 on their respective immunophilins are presently an area of intense research.

Calcineurin as a target of the CsA-cyclophilin complex: As shown in Fig. 5, the photolabile cyclosporine derivative labeled not only cyclophilin but also a 60-kDa protein in Jurkat T cells, which is most likely calcineurin. It was recently demonstrated that the phosphatase calcineurin forms a complex with the drug and immunophilin (41,57). The complex was only formed in the presence of the CsA and cyclophilin together with calmodulin and calcium.

Calcineurin consists of catalytic (A) and regulatory subunits (B). Calcineurin B has a molecular weight of 19-kDa and high homology to calmodulin. Calcineurin A, the 61-kDa subunit, contains the catalytic domain of the serine-threonine phosphatase. Calcineurin occurs ubiquitously in the body and is a highly conserved protein. Two isozymes of calcineurin A (type I and II) are formed as the result of alternative splicing events (58). The C terminus contains an inhibitory domain and an adjacent calmodulin binding domain, which are rapidly removed by limited proteolysis. The central part of the protein, being resistant to proteolysis, harbors the catalytic domains and is identical for the two isozymes of calcineurin. This region shows extensive similarities to the catalytic subunits of protein phosphatases 1 and 2B, which define a distinct family of protein phosphatases. The 40 amino acid N-terminal fragment, which is specific for calcineurin, contains 11 successive prolines, possibly important for the binding to CPH-A/B or to FKBP. Preliminary results show that CsA binds to the catalytic domain of calcineurin A, thereby inhibiting its phosphatase activity.

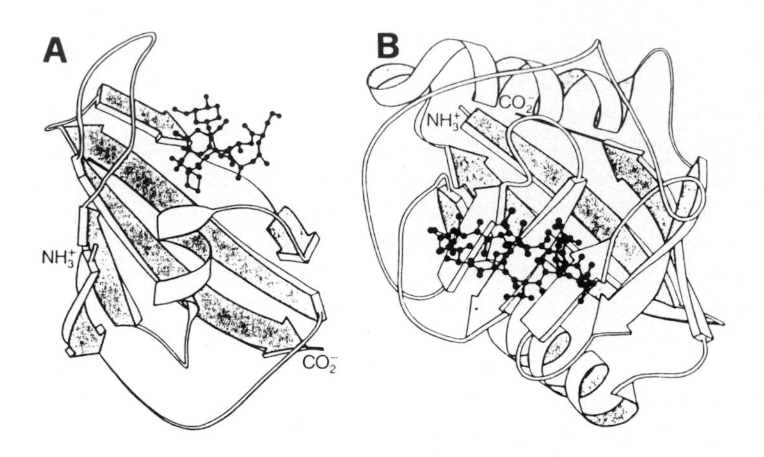

Figure 5 Three-dimensional structure of the complex of human FKBP (A) with FK506 and human CPH-A with CsA (B). The data were obtained by x-ray and NMR analyses (From Refs. 51 and 72.)

Role of calcineurin in IL-2 gene transcription: Calcineurin is abundant in lymphoid cells (59). Fruman et al. (60) demonstrated calcineurin phosphatase activity in lysates of Jurkat T cells. CsA inhibited cellular calcineurin activity at drug concentrations that inhibit IL-2 synthesis in activated T cells. These findings taken together suggest that calcineurin plays a role in T-cell activation. Another approach chosen to investigate the role of calcineurin T-cell activation was the cotransfection of an IL-2 promotor-linked reporter-gene construct together with murine calcineurin A into Jurkat cells. As expected, the overexpression of calcineurin caused relative resistance to the immunosuppressants, necessitating higher concentrations in order to achieve the same immunosuppressive effect (61,62). These results implicate calcineurin as a component of the T-cell receptor signal transduction pathway. The present understanding of the molecular events leading to the inhibition of IL-2 gene transcription is depicted in Fig. 6.

Molecular mechanisms leading to CsA nephrotoxicity: The mechanisms leading to nephrotoxicity are being examined. At immunosuppressive doses, CsA causes a reduction of the glomerular filtration rate (GFR) and slight arterial hypertension (63,64). The present knowledge of the pathogenesis of this renal dysfunction is summarized in Fig. 7: CsA may affect renal mesangial cells directly, resulting in reduction of the GFR. In addition, endothelial cells and smooth muscle cells, especially of the afferent arterioles, may respond directly to CsA and release further vasoactive mediators. At higher concentrations, the tubular epithelial cells themselves may develop degenerative changes. The toxicity of cyclosporine is discussed further in Chap. 24.

The abundance of CPH-A, B, and calcineurin, at least as determined by Western blot analysis, does not differ between drug-sensitive (lymphocytes and kidney) and drug-resistant organs. Friedman and Weissman (41) claimed that CYP-C occurs only in the immune system and the kidney. CPH-C could, therefore, explain the relative tissue-specificity of CsA action and perhaps account for the specificity of organ toxicity—i.e., nephrotoxicity. These findings have yet to be confirmed by other investigators. Attempts have been made by several groups to correlate the ability of several CsA derivatives to bind cyclophilin with their immunosuppressive and toxic activity in vivo (22). However, pres-

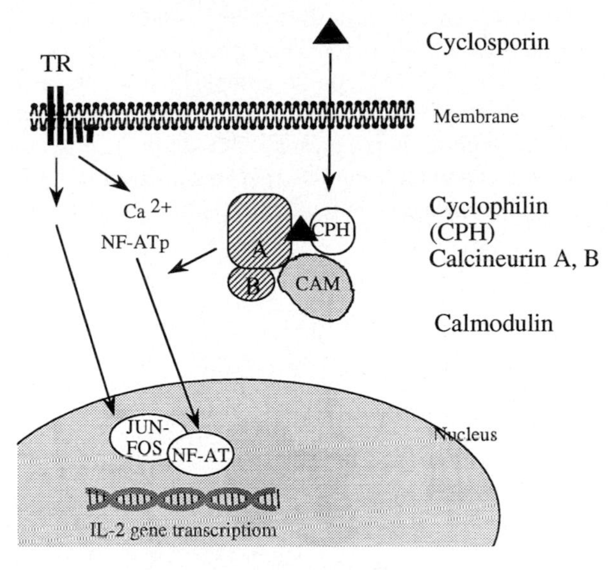

Figure 6 Schematic representation of the drug-immunophilin complex, binding and inhibition of the calcineurin phosphatase, thus inhibiting the translocation of the cytosolic subunit of the nuclear factor of T-cell activation (NF-ATc).

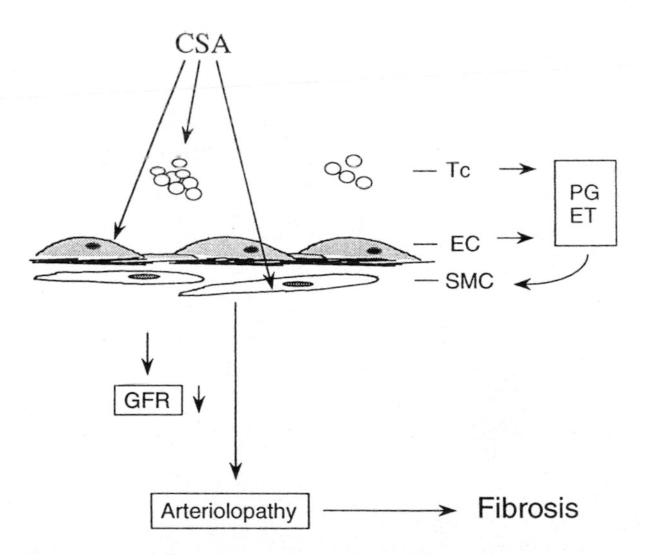

Figure 7 The cellular targets of cyclosporine comprise endothelial cells (EC); smooth muscle cells (SMC); and thrombocytes (Tc). CsA may cause adherence of platelets to the endothelium and synthesis and/or release of endothelin (ET) and prostaglandin (PG), which may be followed by endothelial and smooth muscle cell damage and regeneration. The direct or indirect contractile effect of CsA on the smooth muscle cell causes a reduction of glomerular filtration rate (GFR); the progressive arteriolar damage (arteriolopathy) results in focal interstitial fibrosis.

ently available in vitro data do not confirm such a relationship. The formation of drug-immunophilin complexes with calcineurin is very likely in renal target cells, since abundant calcineurin is present in the kidney (125). The CsA-cyclophilin complex associates with renal calcineurin and inhibits its phosphatase activity in vitro. Higher-molecular-weight complexes consisting of calcineurin and cyclophilin in the presence but not in the absence of CsA were found (Fig. 8). Thus, receptor-bound CsA inhibits renal calcineurin in vitro.

The next question is the identification of the substrate of renal calcineurin-immunophilin

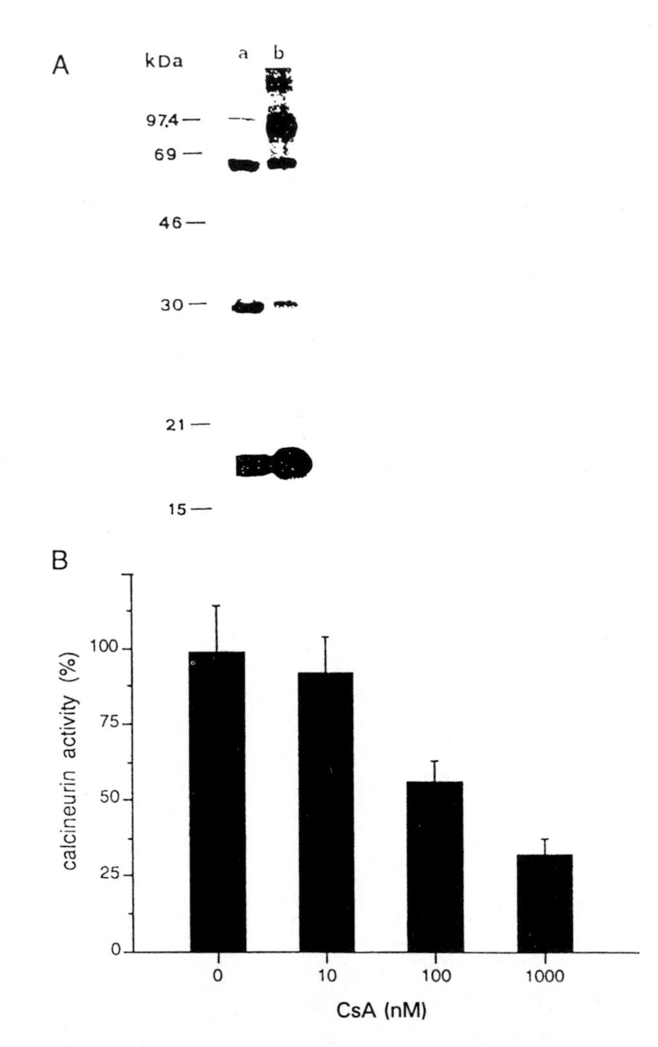

Figure 8 Evidence for immunophilin-drug-calcineurin complex and inhibition of calcineurin activity in rat kidney. (A) Ternary complex of calcineurin with cyclophilin and CsA in rat kidney. Renal tissue lysate was incubated in the absence (a) or presence of 1nM CsA (b) with the chemical cross-linker DST; the proteins were separated on a 7.5% SDS PAGE, transferred on nitrocellulose, and calcineurin complexes were detected with anticalcineurin A/B antiserum. (B) Inhibition of calcineurin phosphatase activity by CsA. Renal tissue lysate was incubated with several concentrations of CsA, and calcineurin activity was determined using a radiolabeled synthetic peptide (125).

complex. Possible candidate substrates include the effector peptides, leading to toxicity or factors upstream, leading to effector molecules of toxicity. Presently, candidate peptides considered as important for the development of nephrotoxicity are endothelin, renin, tissue factor, and TGFβ.

Despite initial enthusiastic reports, FK506 was shown to cause a similar form of nephrotoxicity to CsA in controlled clinical trials. The related macrolide rapamycin with its different mode of immunosuppression-induction is devoid of nephrotoxic side effects (Ryffel, unpublished). One possible explanation is that rapamycin neither binds to calcineurin nor inhibits calcineurin-phosphatase activation. These findings suggest that the immunophilin drug-calcineurin complex may indeed be involved in the development of the nephrotoxicity of both CsA and FK506.

IV. FK506 AND RAPAMYCIN—MACROLIDES INTERRUPTING DISTINCT PATHWAYS

Macrolide immunosuppressants are a structurally distinct family of immunosuppressants, composed of FK506 and rapamycin (Fig. 4). While FK506 inhibits cytokine gene transcription in a manner identical to that of CsA, rapamycin has a completely different mode of action (65,66).

Cellular receptors: Both FK506 and rapamycin bind to a 12-kDa cytosolic protein, FKBP12 (67–74). FKBP12 has no homology to any known protein but has rotamase activity comparable to that of the CPHs. The rotamase activity of FKBP12 is inhibited by FK506 and rapamycin but is not affected by CsA. Since both FK506 and rapamycin have similar inhibitory effects on FKBP12, inhibition of the rotamase fails to explain the different actions of the two drugs. Additional members of the family with binding specificity for the macrolide immunosuppressants were sought (Table 4). FKBP13, a membrane form like CPH-B, was reported by Jin (75). FKBP13 has similar properties to the cytosolic form, FKBP12, in that it binds to both FK506 and rapamycin.

The discovery of FKBP25 proved to be interesting in that it appears to selectively bind rapamycin (76). The N-terminal 101 amino acids of FKBP25 are unrelated to those of the FKBP proteins and consists of an α helix. The C-terminal 114 amino acids are homologous to FKBP12 except for a nuclear targeting sequence. The selective inhibition of the S6-kinase pathway by rapamycin (66) but not by FK506 or CsA, in lieu of the selectivity of rapamycin for FKBP25 and its special structural features, lead to the suggestion that FKBP25 may be important in the signaling of this pathway.

Finally, a FKBP59 binding both rapamycin and FK506 was identified and shown to be related to and associated with heat shock proteins and the corticosteroid receptor (77). It is important to note that there is no sequence homology between members of the cyclophilin and FKBP families.

The three-dimensional structure was investigated by NMR and x-ray crystallography (Fig. 5B). The main structural elements are a five-stranded antiparallel β sheet which wraps around a short helix without any similarity to CPH-A. FK506 binds in a shallow cavity between the α helix and the β sheet, half of the ligand being buried in the receptor protein. The binding site is composed of conserved aromatic residues (for review, see Ref. 18).

Calcineurin as a common target of drug-immunophilin complex: Since it was shown that the rotamase activity was also inhibitable by nonimmunosuppressant macrolides and that the rotamases have no absolute substrate specificity, it was suggested that the FKBPs and immunophilins in general may have a "dominant" function; binding of the drug to the cognate immunophilin may thus result in a gain of function (37). Proline binding by immunophilins might be an important property for the association with common target proteins. The demonstration that the phosphatase calcineurin forms a complex not only with CsA-cyclophilin but also with FK506-FKBP was an exciting observation, possibly explaining the identical mode of action (41,57). The complex forms only in the presence of the drug, its cognate immunophilin, calmodulin, and calcium. Rapamycin bound to FKBP does not form a complex with calcineurin. The immunosuppressants CsA and FK506 inhibit calcineurin phosphatase activity in the presence of their specific immunophilins and calcium.

FK506, but not rapamycin, blocks IL-2 gene transcription by inhibiting the calcineurin phosphatase: Fruman et al. (60) demonstrated that calcineurin phosphatase activity in lysates from Jurkat T cells was inhibited by CsA and FK506, with rapamycin having no effect. Cotransfection of an IL-2 promotor-linked reporter-gene construct together with murine calcineurin A into Jurkat cells caused relative resistance to the immunosuppressants CsA and FK506 (61,62). These results implicate calcineurin as a component of the T-cell receptor signal transduction pathway. A likely substrate of calcineurin is the nuclear factor of activated T cells (NFAT), a cytoplasmic phosphoprotein. It is hypothesized that upon T-cell activation, NFAT is dephosphorylated and translocated into the nucleus, where it binds to the IL-2 promotor region. Thus, it may be assumed that inhibition of the calcineurin phosphatase prevents this dephosphorylation and subsequent IL-2 gene transcription (Fig. 6).

Rapamycin inhibits signal transduction through S6 kinase activation: It is well established that rapamycin has no effect on calcineurin activity and does not inhibit IL-2 gene transcription. The discovery that rapamycin completely and rapidly inhibits IL-2–induced phosphorylation and activation of p70 S6 kinase was a major breakthrough in the understanding of the differing modes of action of the closely related molecules. The blockade of biochemical events proximal to p70 S6 kinase activation by rapamycin implicates this signaling pathway in the regulation of T-cell entry into the S phase. In addition, Chung et al. (78) showed that rapamycin blocked phosphorylation and activation of p70 S6 kinase in a variety of animal cells of nonlymphoid origin. These studies demonstrate that a growth factor–induced signaling event, not merely restricted to T cells, may be impinged upon by rapamycin through the induction of a blockade of entry into the S phase.

Rapamycin, which binds to the same immunophilin as FK506, FKBP12, neither associates nor inhibits calcineurin phosphatase. Importantly, rapamycin has no effect on IL-2 gene transcription. An interesting observation was the recent discovery of FKBP25 (Table 4), a rapamycin-specific receptor. It may be speculated that FKBP25 targets rapamycin to the rapamycin-sensitive S6 kinase. In contrast to CsA and FK506, rapamycin inhibits the activation process at a later stage—e.g., the IL-2 receptor-induced entry into S phase and subsequent T-cell proliferation (79–81). Kuo et al. (65) presented evidence that IL-2 selectively induces the phosphorylation and activation of the p70 S6 kinase.

V. AZATHIOPRINE, STEROIDS, AND ANTILYMPHOCYTE ANTIBODIES STILL USEFUL FOR MAINTENANCE IMMUNOSUPPRESSION AND REJECTION THERAPY

Azathioprine, an imidazole derivative of 6-mercaptopurine, was the first immunosuppressant that allowed successful renal transplantation to be performed. Azathioprine was synthesized by Hitching and Elion and was found to be more portent than 6-mercaptopurine (82). Both compounds are purine analogues and inhibit cell replication in general. The importance and relative specificity of the inhibited pathway of purine metabolism for lymphocytes is clearly demonstrated by the profound immune incompetence associated with adenosine deaminase deficiency. Azathioprine proved to be a potent immunosuppressant and is useful in preventing allograft rejection, but it has no therapeutic effect in acute rejection episodes. Azathioprine is usually combined with steroids for effective immunosuppression. In this combination, 1-year graft survival is on the order of 50%. The main limitation of azathioprine immunosuppression, referable to its general inhibitory effect on cell replication, is myelosuppression (7–10).

Glucocorticosteroids, which are normally produced by the adrenal cortex, have a broad spectrum of activity; they possess metabolic, anti-inflammatory, and immunosuppressive activities. Their anti-inflammatory and immunosuppressive properties are used to therapeutic advantage in several clinical conditions, including autoimmune diseases, allergic reactions, and allograft rejection. The effect of steroids on the immune system are fairly well established. Steroids inhibit the release of the macrophage-derived IL-1, thereby blocking the IL-1–dependent activation of T lymphocytes and synthesis of IL-2, the central T-cell growth factor. Steroids also result in the lysis of T lymphocytes, an effect that is more profound in murine than in human lymphocytes (15,16).

Steroids used at low doses are useful as adjunct immunosuppressants and are of prime importance in rejection therapy. For rejection therapy, high-dose IV bolus injections of methylprednisolone (up to 1 g) are given in combination with antilymphocyte serum or anti-CD3 antibody.

Adverse effects of steroids, especially of long-term therapy, are well known and include osteoporosis, diabetes, gastric ulcer, infections, and water and electrolyte retention, described as Cushings syndrome.

Antilymphocyte antibodies: Polyclonal antibodies raised against human lymphocytes in rabbit or horse are in clinical use for the treatment of transplant rejection. These antisera bind to circulating lymphocytes, causing a sequestration in the spleen and resulting in subsequent lympholysis. Monocloncal antibodies (anti-CD3) have the advantage of being a homogenous product, in contrast to the antisera. Although acting similarly to the polyclonal antibodies, an important difference is the mitogenic activity of anti-CD3 monoclonal antibodies on T cells, which leads to their activation, resulting in fever due to the release of cytokines (11–14).

Thus, the main side effect is the so-called cytokine release syndrome, which usually is manifest by fever and rarely by more severe signs such as rash or hypersensitivity reaction and very rarely by allergic shock, since the patients have a maintenance immunosuppressive therapy. A common fear with combinations of immunosuppressants is the higher risk of developing lymphoma, which has been reported with OKT3, but is a common concern for any drug combination.

VI. NOVEL EXPERIMENTAL IMMUNOSUPPRESSANTS: HOPE FOR THE FUTURE

A number of the newer experimental drugs are described below (Table 3; Fig. 9).

15-Deoxyspergualin (DSG): 15-Deoxyspergualin was isolated from *Bacillus laterosporous* and has an analogous structure to the antitumor drug spergualine. 15-Deoxyspergualin inhibits alloantigen- and mitogen-induced murine and human lymphocyte prolifera-

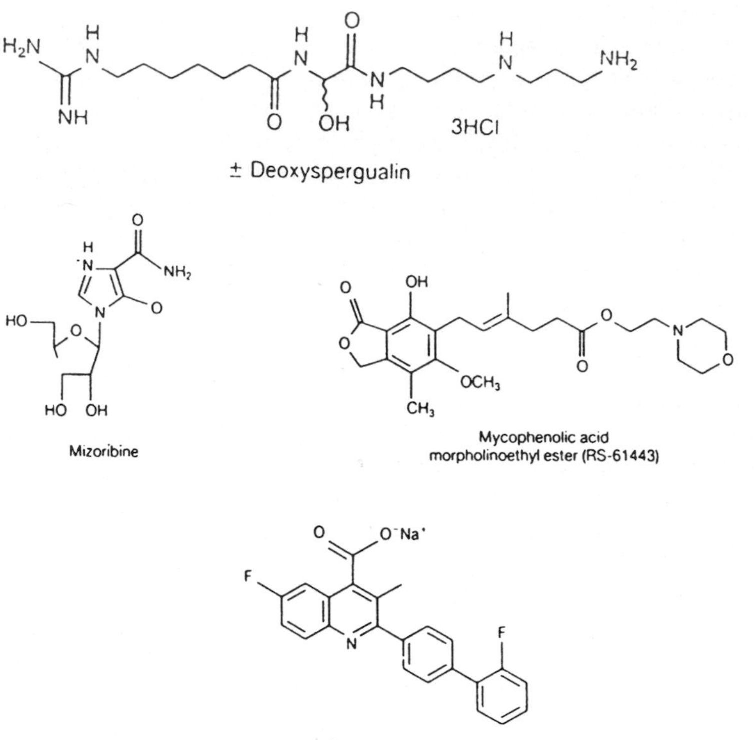

Figure 9 Chemical structure of newer immunosuppressants.

tion. It has no effect on IL-2 production but inhibits IL-2–dependent growth. It seems that DSG inhibits monocyte/macrophage functions—e.g., IL-1 and interferon γ synthesis, expression of MHC class II antigens, synthesis of lysosomal enzymes. 15-Deoxyspergualin binds to heat shock proteins and may interfere with a pathway common to that of steroids. 15-Deoxyspergualin prolongs the in vivo survival of different types of allografts in several species. Although preventing longer-term rejection, 15-deoxyspergualin does not inhibit an acute rejection reaction. The most promising area for this drug is xenotransplantation, where it is highly efficacious (83–93). Toxicity is presently unknown, but may be related to the inhibition of cell proliferation in general. Hence, the bone marrow might be a likely target of toxicity.

Mycophenolic acid (MPA, RS 61443): Mycophenolate mofetil is a prodrug of the antiproliferative agent mycophenolic acid (MPA) with antitumor, antiviral, and immunosuppressant activities. MPA inhibits two key enzymes of the de novo biosynthetic pathway of guanosine. Lymphocytes lack this salvage pathway for purine synthesis, which is present in most other cells, and depend on the de novo synthesis; they are therefore sensitive to MPA. Lack of GMP inhibits the cell cycle progression of lymphocytes but has no effect on interleukin synthesis. MPA inhibits allograft rejection but has low activity in mice due to rapid metabolism. A synergism with CsA has been reported.

MPA may be superior to azathioprine in preventing transplant rejection, since the therapeutic index is higher. Furthermore, MPA can reverse ongoing rejection which is steroid- and OKT3-resistant. Finally, experimental data suggest that MPA might be used for xenotransplantation (94–103).

The toxicity profile seems to be low, but insufficient information is presently available to exclude toxicity of MPA.

Brequinar (BQR): The sodium salt of brequinar is a novel antitumor agent that inhibits de novo pyrimdine biosynthesis by blocking dihydroorotate dihydrogenase in mitochondria. Lymphocyte proliferation is suppressed by its cytostatic activity. Brequinar is effective in the prevention of rat allograft rejection and in prolonging cardiac xenograft survival from hamsters in rats (104–108). Toxicity again may be related to the antiproliferative effect of BQR.

Mizoribin (Bredinin): Mizoribine is an imidazole nucleoside antimetabolite isolated from *Eupenicillium brefeldianum*, which inhibits the biosynthesis of purine. Phosphorylated mizoribin inhibits de novo purine biosynthesis at the level of GMP synthase and IMP dehydrogenase. Bredinin inhibits T-lymphocyte proliferation and prevents graft rejection in experimental models when given with CsA (109).

Mizoribine is presently used in combination with azathioprine or CsA: it has no effect in graft rejection therapy. The toxicity of mizoribine is probably of low order.

Leflunomide: Leflunomide is an isoxazol derivative which has common features with the mode of action of rapamycin—e.g., inhibition of antigen and mitogen as well as IL-2–induced lymphocyte proliferation, with no effect on synthesis of IL-2 or IL-2 receptor. The inhibitory effect, however, occurs at concentrations about 50-fold higher than those of rapamycin. In vivo leflunomide inhibits acute rejection of kidney, heart, and skin allografts. As for rapamycin there is probably a synergistic effect with CsA immunosuppression (110). No specific toxicity has been reported.

Antibodies: Several antibodies directed against the T-cell receptor (TcR) or associated membrane receptor molecules (MHC class II, ICAM-1, LFA-1, CD4, CD28, CTLA4) are presently being developed to block T-cell activation. The experimental results are very promising and clinical trials are ongoing (111–113).

In view of the central role of IL-2 in T-cell activation, the use of inhibitory antibodies to the IL-2R to block cell activation were considered for use in therapy early on. Interleukin-2 and several other cytokines are released during an immune response. The administration of neutralizing antibodies to, for example, TNF, IFNγ, etc., may, therefore, represent another way to block or mitigate an ongoing immune response (114–116).

Since several cytokines are synthesized and released during rejection response of the host, attempts are being made to neutralize circulating cytokines by antibodies or soluble receptors. Recombinant soluble receptors for interferon γ and TNF have been produced and are presently considered in allograft rejection. Clinical trials with antibody blocking the IL-2 receptor are ongoing and may have a role in acute rejection therapy (117,118).

VII. RISKS OF IMMUNOSUPPRESSION AND DRUG TOXICITY

Any form of immunosuppression bears the risk of infections and tumor development. The incidence of infection depends on the dose and the specificity of the immunosuppressant. Viral infections are presently the most frequent complication. With respect to tumor development, one may distinguish between direct genetic damage and indirect or epigenetic mechanisms (119,120). Although alkylating agents predominantly make up the first group, any type of immunosuppressant increases the risk of tumor development due to a weakening of immune surveillance. The tumor types found in immunosuppressed patients include lymphomas, skin tumors, and occasionally brain tumors (120). The risk of these complications may be reduced by minimal dose immunosuppressive therapies.

Specific toxicity associated with a given immunosuppressant is tentatively given in Fig. 10. For the experimental drugs, the clinical toxicity is merely speculative and is deduced from the biological activity of the drugs:

- Fever and malaise after OKT3 therapy (known as cytokine-release syndrome) commonly occur and are due to the systemic release of endogenous cytokines, including TNF, IL-1, and interferons. Therapy with antibodies against other cellular targets (e.g., IL-2 receptor antibody, adhesion molecules, etc.) likely will have some systemic adverse reactions, as outlined for OKT3 (118).
- The bone marrow is a common target of antiproliferative drugs. Bone marrow and leukopenia depression after azathioprine and several of the novel immunosuppressants, which have emerged from the area of tumor therapy and have general antiproliferative properties, are frequent and will be dose-limiting.
- Glucocorticosteroids used at high dose for the prevention of acute rejection are also a common component of maintenance immunosuppressive regimens in combination with CsA or azathioprine. However, the long-term administration of steroids is followed by the well-known Cushing's syndrome.
- Reduction of glomerular filtration rates occur commonly with CsA and FK506 immunosuppression. Dose-limiting of such a therapy is, however, renal arteriolar disease, resulting in interstitial fibrosis and occasionally in renal failure. This is a well-recognized complication and can be avoided by switching to an alternative immunosuppressive regimen.

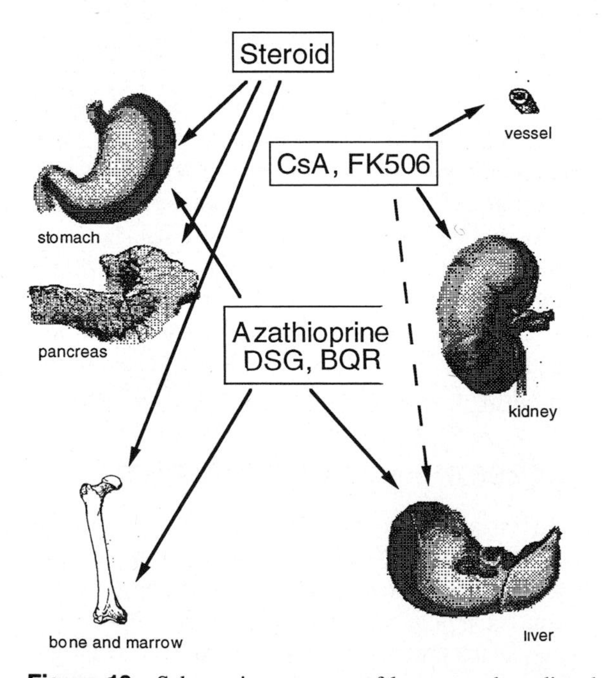

Figure 10 Schematic summary of known and predicted toxicity of immunosuppressants.

• Gastrointestinal erosions, bleeding, and ulcers are found with steroids and all the antiproliferative type of immunosuppressants.

• Chronic rejection is one of the major threats to long-term heart and kidney transplant function. Chronic graft rejection is characterized by progressive narrowing of the graft arteries and arterioles, interstitial cellular infiltration and fibrosis, glomerular changes, and tubular atrophy. The obliteration of the vascular lumen is due to infiltration of the intima by mononuclear cells, proliferation of vascular smooth muscle cells and fibroblasts of the media, and migration into the intima, with increased deposition of extracellular matrix proteins. Graft failure due to chronic rejection is an important cause of graft loss within 5 to 10 years following transplantation. The pathophysiology of chronic rejection is complex and involves a number of mechanisms, including endothelial cell damage, monocyte-macrophage activation, proliferation of smooth muscle cells and fibroblasts due to the release of several cytokines and oxygen radicals, and release of vasoactive peptides, including endothelin and nitric oxygen, as reviewed in Fellström and Larsson and Häyry et al. (121,122). Since the pathology is characterized by invasion of immunoreactive cells within the vessel wall, a key to the prevention of chronic vascular rejection might be the optimization of the immunosuppressive treatment. Presently there is no established means of preventing chronic vascular rejection and the proposed experimental strategies—such as interruption of prostaglandin metabolism, somatostatin inhibitors, and others—have to be tested in patients (121).

VIII. EFFECTIVE IMMUNOSUPPRESSION WITHOUT RISK—THE FUTURE?

A more philosophical topic is what we may achieve in the near future. Two lines of research will probably lead to the desired goal of long-term graft acceptance and maybe to tolerance; first, further developments in drug discovery, and, second, genetic modifications of the graft or host.

For drug discovery, the long list of novel immunosuppressants with only limited adverse effects is a source of hope. Most of the discoveries were made by an ever-increasing and more sophisticated screening of natural products. Mechanistic studies with the novel experimental immunosuppressants might provide new insights into pathways of gene activation, and we are curious to know what secrets of nature will be revealed in the near future. The identification of pivotal proteins such as regulatory phophatases and/or kinases may also represent the key for a rationale drug design.

The ultimate dream of the clinician and patient alike is the induction of transplant tolerance, a goal that is presently achievable only in rodent models. Since some of the novel agents have promise in the prevention of xenograft rejection, it is quite possible that these agents may help to unravel novel pathways.

With the advent of novel immunosuppressive agents and technical improvements in transplant surgery, xenotransplantation is being considered in light of the shortage of human kidneys, so that more patients might benefit from organ-replacement therapy. The rejection of discordant xenografts is very different from classic cell-mediated allograft rejection. It appears to involve the binding of naturally occurring host antibodies to xenograft antigens, followed by the activation of complement (123,124).

Genetic modifications of the graft or the host will be an area of intense research. These procedures must include the identification of the relevant target proteins for graft acceptance, of stable and safe vectors for gene transfer, and establishment of an ethical basis for such procedures in our society.

Xenotransplantation of healthy organs with tolerance induction is the ultimate goal of pharmaceutical or genetic intervention in the immune system. Although impressive theoretical and experimental advances in the area of tolerance have been achieved, the clinical application of this goal is still far away.

REFERENCES

1. Borel JF. Pharmacology of cyclosporin (Sandimmune). Pharmacol Rev 1989; 42:260–372.
2. Morris PJ. Cyclosporin, FK506 and other drugs in organ transplantation. Curr Opin Immunol 1991; 3:748–751.
3. Ryffel B. Pharmacology of cyclosporin, cellular activation: Regulation of intracellular events by cyclosporin. Pharmacol Rev 1989; 41:407–421.
4. Young PR. Protein hormones and their receptors. Biotechnology 1992; 3:408–421.
5. Akira S, Kishimoto T. Mechanisms of soluble mediators. Immunology 1992; 4:307–313.
6. Janeway CA. The T cell receptor as a multicomponent signalling machine: CD4/CD8 coreceptors and CD45 in T cell activation. Annu Rev Immunol 1992; 10:645–674.
7. Elion GB, Callahan S, Bieber S, et al. Cancer Chemother Rep 1961; 14:93–98.
8. Calne RY, Alexandre GPJ, Murray JE. Ann N Y Acad Sci 1962; 99:743–761.
9. Murray JE, Merrill JP, Dammin GJ, et al. Ann Surg 1962; 156:337–355.
10. Bach JF, ed. The Mode of Action of Immunosuppressive Agents. Amsterdam: North Holland, 1975.
11. Min DI, Monaco AP. Complications associated with immunosuppressive therapy and their management. Pharmacotherapy 1991; 11:119S–125S.
12. Walker RG, d'Apice AJF, Mathew TH, et al. Transplant Proc 1987; 19:2834–2836.
13. Mussche MM, Ringoir SGM, Lamiere NN. Nephron 1976; 16:289–291.
14. d'Apice AJ, Becker GJ, Kincaid-Smith P, et al. Transplantation 1984; 37(4):373–377.
15. Cupps TR, Fauci AS. Corticosteroid-mediated immunoregulation in man. Immunol Rev 1982; 65:133–155.
16. Claman HN. Corticosteroids and lymphoid cells. N Engl J Med 1972; 287:388–394.
17. Sigal N, Dumont FJ. Cyclosporin A, FK-506 and rapamycin: Pharmacological probes of lymphocyte signal transduction. Annu Rev Immunol 1992; 10:519–560.
18. Schreiber S, Crabtree G. The mechanism of action of cyclosporin A and FK506. Immunol Today 1992; 13:136–142.
19. Baumann G, Geisse S, Sullivan M. Cyclosporin A and FK-506 both affect DNA binding of regulatory nuclear proteins to the human interleukin-2 promotor. New Biol 1991; 3:270–278.
20. Granelli-Piperno A. Lymphokine gene expression in vivo is inhibited by cyclosporin A. J Exp Med 1990; 171:533–544.
21. Mattila P, Ullman K, Fiering S, et al. The actions of cyclosporin A and FK506 suggest a novel step in the activation of T lymphocytes. EMBO J 1990; 9:4425–4433.
22. Sigal N, Dumont F, Turette T, et al. Is cyclophilin involved in the immunosuppressive and nephrotoxic mechanism of action of cyclosporin A? J Exp Med 1991; 173:619–628.
23. Ryffel B, Goetz U, Heuberger B. Cyclosporin receptors on human lymphocytes. J Immunol 1982; 129:1978–1982.
24. Foxwell B, Frazer G, Winters M, et al. Identification of cyclophilin as the erythrocyte cyclosporin-binding protein. Biochem Biophys Acta 1988; 938:447–455.
25. Merker M, Handschumacher R. Uptake and nature of the intracellular binding of cyclosporin A in a A murine thymoma cell line BW5147. J Immunol 1984; 132:3064–3070.
26. Handschumacher R, Harding M, Rice J, Drugge R. Cyclophilin: A specific cytosolic binding protein for cyclosporin A. Science 1984; 226:544–547.

27. Harding M, Handschumacher R, Speicher D. Isolation and amino acid sequence of cyclophilin. J Biol Chem 1986; 261:8547–8555.
28. Fischer G, Wittmann-Liebold B, Lang K, et al. Cyclophilin and peptidyl-prolyl cistrans isomerase are probably identical proteins. Nature 1989; 337:476–473.
29. Takahashi N, Hayano T, Suzuki M. Peptidylprolyl cis-trans isomerase is the cyclosporin A-binding protein cyclophilin. Nature 1989; 337:473–475.
30. Quesniaux VFJ. Pharmacology of cyclosporin (Sandimmune): III. Immunochemistry and monitoring. Pharmacol Rev 1989; 41:249.
31. Quesniaux VFJ, Schreier MH, Wenger RM, et al. Cyclophilin binds to the region of cyclosporin involved in its immunosuppressive activity. Eur J Immunol 1987; 17:1359–1365.
32. Quesniaux VFJ, Schreier MH, Wenger RM, Van Regenmortel MHV. Molecular characteristics of cyclophilin-cyclosporin interaction. Transplantation 1988; 46:23S–27S.
33. Foxwell B, Woerly G, Husi H, et al. Identification of several cyclosporin binding proteins in lymphoid and non-lymphoid cells in vivo. Biochem Biophys Acta 1992; 1138:115–121.
34. Hsu V, Heald S, Harding M, et al. Structural elements pertinent to the interaction of cyclosporin A with its specific receptor protein, cyclophilin. Biochem Pharmacol 1990; 40:131–140.
35. Foxwell B, Mackie A, Ling V, Ryffel B. Identification of the multi-drug resistance related p-glycoprotein as a cyclosporin binding protein. Mol Pharmacol 1989; 36:543–546.
36. Wenger RM. Cyclosporin: Conformation and analogues as tools for studying its mechanisms of action. Transplant Proc 1988; 20:313–318.
37. Schreiber S. Chemistry and biology of the immunophilins and their immunosuppressive ligands. Science 1991; 251:283–287.
38. Caroni P, Rothenfluh A, McGlynn E, Schneider C. S-cyclophilin, new member of the cyclophilin family associated with the secretory pathway. J Biol Chem 1991; 266:10739–10742.
38. Danielson P, Forss-Petter S, Brown M, et al. p1B15: A cDNA clone of the rat mRNA encoding cyclophilin. DNA 1988; 7:261–267.
39. Hasel KW, Glass JR, Godbout M, Suthcliffe JG. An endoplasmatic reticulum-specific cyclophilin. Mol Cell Biol 1991; 11:3484–3491.
40. Price ER, Cldowski LD, Jin M, et al. Human cyclophilin B, a second cyclophilin gene encodes a peptidyl-prolyl isomerase with a signal sequence. Proc Natl Acad Sci USA 1991; 88:1903–1907.
41. Friedman J, Weissman I. Two cytoplasmic candidates for immunophilin action are revealed by affinity for a new cyclophilin: One in the presence and one in the absence of CsA. Cell 1991; 66:799–806.
42. Bergsma DJ, Eder C, Gross M, et al. The cyclophilin multigene family of peptidyl-prolyl isomerases. J Biol Chem 1991; 266:23204–23214.
43. Kieffer LJ, Thalhammer T, Handschumacher RE. Isolation and characterization of a 40-kDa cyclophilin-related protein. J Biol Chem 1992; 267:1–5.
44. Foxwell B, Hiestand P, Wenger R, Ryffel B. A comparison of cyclosporin binding by cyclophilin and calmodulin and the identification of a novel 45KD cyclosporin-binding phosphoprotein in Jurkat cells. Transplantation 1988; 46:35S–40S.
45. Schönbrunner ER, Mayer S, Tropschug M, et al. Catalysis of protein folding by cyclophilins from different species. J Biol Chem 1991; 266:3630–3635.
46. Marks WH, Harding MW, Handschumacher R, et al. The immunochemical distribution of cyclophilin in normal mammalian tissues. Transplantation 1991; 52:340–345.
47. McDonald ML, Ardito T, Marks WH, et al. The effect of cyclosporin administration on the cellular distribution and content of cyclophilin. Transplantation 1992; 53:460–466.
48. Ryffel B, Foxwell G, Gee A, et al. Cyclosporin-relationship of side effects to mode of action. Transplantation 1988; 46:90S–96S.
49. Koletsky A, Harding M, Handschumacher R. Cyclophilin: Distribution and variant properties in normal and neoplastic tissues. J Immunol 1986; 137:1054.
50. Ryffel B, Woerly G, Greiner B, et al. Distribution of the cyclosporin binding protein cyclophilin in human tissues. Immunology 1991; 72:399–404.

51. Fesik SW, Gampe RT Jr, Holzman, TF, et al. Isotope-edited NMR of cyclosporin A bound to cyclophilin: Evidence for a Trans 9,10 amide bond. Science 1990; 250:1406–1409.
52. Kallen J, Spitzfaden C, Zurini MG, et al. Structure of human cyclophilin and its binding site for cyclosporin A determined by x-ray crystallography and NMR spectroscopy. Nature 1991; 353: 276–279.
53. Ke H, Zydowsky L, Liu J, Walsh C. Crystal structure of recombinant human T-cell cyclophilin A at 2.5 A resolution. Proc Natl Acad Sci USA 1991; 88:9483–9487.
54. Spitzfaden C, Weber HP, Braun W, et al. Cyclosporin A-cyclophilin complex formation: A model based on x-ray and NMR data. FEBS Lett 1992; 300:291–300.
55. Wüthrich K, von Freyberg B, Weber Ch, et al. Receptor-induced confirmation, change of the immunosuppressant cyclosporin A. Science 1991; 254:953–955.
56. Liu J, Albers MW, Chen CM, et al. Cloning expression and purification of human cyclophilin in Escherichia coli and assessment of the catalytic role of cysteines by site-directed mutagenesis. Proc Natl Acad Sci USA 1990; 87:2304–2308.
57. Liu J, Farmer JD, Lane WS, et al. Calcineurin is a common target of cyclophilin-cyclosporin A and FKBP-FK506 complexes. Cell 1991; 66:807–815.
58. Guerini A, Klee CB. Cloning of human calcineurin A: Evidence for two isozymes and identification of a polyproline structural domain. Proc Natl Acad Sci USA 1989; 56:9183–9187.
59. Kincaid RL, Takayama H, Billingsley ML, Sitkovsky V. Differential expression of calmodulin-binding proteins in B, T lymphocytes and thymocytes. Nature 1987; 330:176–178.
60. Fruman DA, Klee CB, Bieber BA, Burakoff SJ. Calcineurin phosphatase activity in T lymphocytes is inhibited by FK 506 and cyclosporin A. Proc Natl Acad Sci USA 1992; 89:3686–3690.
61. Clipstone NA, Crabtree GR. Identification of calcineurin as a key signaling enzyme in T-lymphocyte activation. Nature 1992; 357:695.
62. O'Keefe St, Tamura J, Kincaid RL, et al. FK-506- and CsA-sensitive activation of the interleukin-2 promoter by calcineurin. Nature 1992; 357:692–694.
63. Mason J. Pathophysiology and toxicology of cyclosporin in humans and animals. Pharmacol Rev 1989; 41:423–434.
64. Mihatsch MJ, Thiel G, Ryffel B. Renal side-effects of cyclosporin A with special reference to autoimmune diseases. Br J Dermatol 1990; 36:101–115.
65. Kuo CJ, Chung J, Florentino DF, et al. Rapamycin selectively inhibits interleukin-2 activation of p70 S6 kinase. Nature 1992; 358:70–73.
66. Morris RE. Rapamycins: Antifungal, antitumor, antiproliferative, and immunosuppressive macrolides. Transplant Rev 1992; 6:39–87.
67. Van Duyne GD, Standaert RF, Karplus PA, et al. Atomic structure of FKBP-FK506, an immunophilin-immunosuppressant complex. Science 1991; 252:839–842.
68. Michnick SW, Rosen MK, Wandless TJ, et al. Solution structure of FKBP, a rotamase enzyme and receptor for FK 506 and rapamycin. Science 1991; 252:836–839.
69. Moore JM, Peattie DA, Fitzgibbon MJ, Thomson JA. Solution structure of the major binding protein for the immunosuppressant FK506. Nature 1991; 351:248–250.
70. Standaert RF, Galat A, Verdine GL, Schreiber SL. Molecular cloning and overexpression of the human FK506-binding protein FKBP. Nature 1990; 346:671–674.
71. Harding WM, Galat A, Uehling, DE, Speicher DW. A receptor for the immunosuppressant FK506 is a cris-trans peptidyl-prolyl-isomerase. Nature 1989; 341:758–760.
72. Lane WS, Galat A, Harding MW, Schreiber SL. Complete amino acid sequence of the FK506 and rapamycin binding protein, FKBP, isolated from calf thymus. J Protein Chem 1991; 10: 151–160.
73. Maki N, Sekiguchi F, Nishimaki J, et al. Complementary DNA encoding the human T-cell FK 506-binding protein, a peptidylprolyl cis-trans isomerase distinct from cyclophilin. Proc Natl Acad Sci USA 1990; 87:5440–5443.

74. Siekierka JJ, Hung SHY, Poe M, et al. A cytosolic binding protein for the immunosuppressant FK506 has peptidyl-prolyl isomerase activity but is distinct from cyclophilin. Nature 1989; 341:755–757.
75. Jin YJ, Albers MW, Lane WS, et al. Molecular cloning of a membrane-associated human FK 506- and rapamycin-binding protein, FKBP-13. Proc Natl Acad Sci USA 1991; 88:6677–6681.
76. Galat A, Lane WS, Standaert RF, Schreiber SL. A rapamycin-selective 25-kDa immunophilin. Biochemistry 1992; 31:2427–2434.
77. Tai PK, Albers MW, Chang H, et al. Association of a 59-kilodalton immunophilin with the gluco-corticoid receptor complex. Science 1992; 256:1315.
78. Chung J, Kuo CJ, Crabtree GR, Blenis J. Rapamycin-FKBP specifically blocks growth-dependent activation of and signaling by the 70 kd S6 protein kinases. Cell 1992; 69:1227–1236.
79. Bierer BE, Mattila P, Standaert R, et al. Two distinct signal transmission pathways in T lymphocytes are inhibited by complexes formed between an immunophilin and either FK506 or rapamycin. Proc Natl Acad Sci USA 1990; 87:9231–9235.
80. Bierer BE, Somers P, Wandless T, et al. Probing immunosuppressant action with a nonnatural immunophilin ligand. Science 1990; 250:556–559.
81. Staruch M, Sigal N, Dumont F. Differential effects of the immunosuppressive macrolides FK-506 and rapamycin on activation-induced T-cell apoptosis. Int J Immunopharmacol 1991; 13:677–685.
82. Hamilton D. Kidney transplantation: A history. In: Morris PJ, ed. Kidney Transplantation: Principles and Practice. Philadelphia: Saunders, 1989
83. Okubo M, Amemiya K, Kamata K, et al. Toxicological and immunological evaluation of the immunosuppressant 15-deoxyspergualin in BALB/c mice: An in vivo and in vitro study. Immunopharmacology 1991; 21:99–107.
84. Krzymanski M, Waaga AM, Ulrichs K, Muller-Ruchholtz W. Long standing rat kidney graft survival by a combination of organ perfusion with MHC class II monoclonal antibody and immunosuppression with reduced doses of 15-deoxyspergualin. Immunol Invest 1991; 20:253–256.
85. Takasu S, Sakagami K, Morisaki F, et al. Immunosuppressive mechanism of 15-deoxyspergualin on sinusoidal lining cells in swine liver transplantation: Suppression of MHC class II antigens and interleukin-1 production. J Surg Res 1991; 51:165–169.
86. DeMasi R, Araneda D, Gross U, et al. Improved xenograft survival with continuous infusion deoxyspergualin and RATG. J Invest Surg 1991; 4:59–67.
87. Okubo M, Umetani N, Inoue K, et al. Reversal of established nephropathy in New Zealand B/W F1 mice by 15-deoxyspergualin. Nephron 1991; 57:99–105.
88. Nemoto K, Hayashi M, Ito J, et al. Deoxyspergualin in lethal murine graft versus host disease. Transplantation 1991; 51:712–715.
89. Fukao K, Iwasaki H, Yuzawa K, et al. Immunosuppressive effect and toxicity of 15-deoxyspergualin in cynomologus monkey. Transplant Proc 1991; 23:556–558.
90. Hibasami H, Tsukada T, Suzuki R, et al. 15-deoxyspergualin: An antiproliferative agent for human and mouse leukemia cells shows inhibitory effects on the synthetic pathway of polyamines. Anticancer Res 1991; 11:325–330.
91. Yabuuchi H, Nakajima Y, Segawa M, et al. Prominent prolongation of islet xenograft survival in combination therapy with FK 506 and 15-deoxyspergualin. Transplant Proc 1991; 23:859–861.
92. Carobbi A, Araneda D, Patselas T, et al. Effect of splenectomy in combination with FK 506 and 15-deoxyspergualin on cardiac xenograft survival. Transplant Proc 1991; 23:549–550.
93. Nadler StG, Tepper MA, Schacter B, Mazzucco ChE. Interaction of the immunosuppressant deoxyspergualin with a member of the Hsp70 family of heat shock proteins. Science 1992; 258:484–486.

94. Platz KP, Eckhoff DE, Hullett DA, Sollinger HW. RS-61443 studies: Review and proposal. Transplant Proc 1991; 23:33–35.
95. Simmons RL, Wang SC. New horizons in immunosuppression. Transplant Proc 1991; 23: 2152–2156.
96. Morris RE, Wang J, Blum JR, et al. Immunosuppressive effects of the morpholinoethyl ester of mycophenolic acid (RS-61443) in rat and nonhuman primate recipients of heart allografts. Transplant Proc 1991; 23:19–25.
97. Allison AC, Almquist SJ, Muller CD, Eugui EM. In vitro immunosuppressive effects of mycophenolic acid and an ester pro-drug, RS-61443. Transplant Proc 1991; 23:10–14.
98. Allison AC, Eugui EM. Immunosuppressive and long acting anti-inflammatory activity of mycophenolic acid and derivative, RS-61443. Br J Rheumatol 1991; 30:57–61.
99. Platz KP, Bechstein WO, Eckhoff DE, et al. RS-61443 reverses acute allograft rejection in dogs. Surgery 1991; 110:736–741.
100. Hao L, Calcinaro F, Lafferty KJ, et al. Tolerance induction in adult mice: Cyclosporin inhibits RS-61443 induced tolerance. Transplant Proc 1991; 23:733–734.
101. Platz KP, Sollinger HW, Hullett DA, et al. RS-61443 a new, potent immunosuppressive agent. Transplantation 1991; 51:27–31.
102. Eugui EM, Mirkovich A, Allison ACC. Lymphocyte-selective antiproliferative and immunosuppressive activity of mycophenolic acid and its morpholinoethyl ester (RS-61443). Transplant Proc 1991; 23:15–18.
103. Burlingham WEJ, Grailer AP, Hullett DA, Sollinger HW. Inhibition of both MLC and in vitro IgG memory response to tetanus toxoid by RS-61443. Transplantation 1991; 51:545–547.
104. Cramer DV, Chapman FA, Jaffee BD, et al. The effect of a new immunosuppressive drug, brequinar sodium, on concordant hamster to rat cardiac xenografts. Transplant Proc 1992; 24:720–721.
105. Cramer DV, Chapman FA, Jaffee BD, et al. The effect of a new immunosuppressive drug, brequinar sodium, on heart, liver and kidney allograft rejection in the rat. Transplantation 1992; 53:303–308.
106. Lakaschus G, Loffler M. Differential susceptibility of dihydroorotate dehydrogenase/oxidase to brequinar sodium (NSC 368 390) in vitro. Biochem Pharmacol 1992; 43:1025–1030.
107. Chen SF, Perrella FW, Behrens DL, Papp LM. Inhibition of dihydroorotate dehydrogenase activity by brequinar sodium. Cancer Res 1992; 52:3521–3527.
108. Loffler M. The "anti-pyrimidine effect" of hypoxia and brequinar sodium (NSC 368390) is of consequence for tumor cell growth. Biochem Pharmacol 1992; 43:2281–2287.
109. Dayton JS, Turka LA, Thompson CB, Mitchell BS. Comparison of the effects of mizoribine with those of azathioprine, 6-mercaptopurine, and mycophenolic acid on T lymphocyte proliferation and purine ribonucleotide metabolism. Mol Pharmacol 1992; 41:671.
110. Amemiya H, Itoh H. Mizoribin (Bredenin). Mode of action and effects on graft rejection. In: Thomson, AW, Starzl TE, eds. Immunosuppressive Drugs: Developments in Anti-Rejection Therapy. London: Edward Arnold, 1992.
111. Chong AS-F, Finnegan A, Jian XL, et al. Leflunomide: A novel immunosuppressive agent. Transplantation 1993; 55:1361.
112. Shizuru JA, Alters SE, Fathman CG. Anti CD4 monoclonal antibodies in therapy: Creation of nonclassical tolerance in the adult. Immunol Rev 1992; 129:105–130.
113. Cobbold SP, Qin S, Leong LYW, et al. Reprogramming the immune system for peripheral tolerance with CD4 and CD8 monoclonal antibodies. Immunol Rev 1992; 129:165–201.
114. Waldmann TA. Immune receptors: Targets for therapy of leukemia/lymphoma, autoimmune diseases and for the prevention of allograft rejection. Annu Rev Immunol 1992; 10:675–704.
115. Ozmen L, Gribaudo G, Fountoulakis M, et al. Mouse soluble IFN-γ receptor as IFN-γ inhibitor. J Immunol 150:32698–2705.
116. Vassalli P. The pathophysiology of tumor necrosis factors. Annu Rev Immunol 1992; 10: 411–452.

117. Cantarovich D, Le Mauff B, Hourmant M, et al. Prevention of acute rejection episodes with an anti-interleukin 2 receptor monoclonal antibody. Transplantation 1994; 57:198–203.
118. Chatenoud L. Safety and efficacy of the therapeutic monoclonal antibodies in clinical therapy. Immunol Today 1993; 14:421–425.
119. Ryffel B. The carcinogenicity of ciclosporin. Toxicology 1992; 73:1–22.
120. Penn I. The price of immunotherapy. Curr Probl Surg 1981; 18:681.
121. Fellström BC, Larsson E. Pathogenesis and treatment perspectives of chronic graft rejection (CVR). Immunol Rev 1993; 134:83–98.
122. Häyry P, Isoniemi H, Yilmaz S, et al. Chronic allograft rejection. Immunol Rev 1993; 134: 33–81.
123. Lo D. T Cell tolerance. Current Opinion Immunol 1992; 4:711–715.
124. Platt JL, Vercellotti GM, Dalmasso AP, et al. Transplantation of discordant xenografts: A review of progress. Immunol Today 1990; 11:450–456.
125. Su Q, Weber L, Lettir M, Engster HP, Ryffel B. Nephrotoxicity of Cyclosporin A and FK506: Inhibition of calcineurin phosphatase. Renal Physiol Biochem 1995; 18:128–139.

24

Nephrotoxicity of Cyclosporine and Newer Immunosuppressive Agents

Kim Solez
University of Alberta, Edmonton, Alberta, Canada

Lorraine C. Racusen
Johns Hopkins University School of Medicine, Baltimore, Maryland

Michael Mihatsch
Institut für Pathologie der Universität Basel, Basel, Switzerland

I. INTRODUCTION

At the beginning of this decade it had been predicted that the development of new immunosuppressive drugs would soon end the problem of renal failure brought about by antirejection agents. However, two of the new agents that were clearly nonnephrotoxic—brequinar and anti-CD45—have recently proven ineffective in renal transplantation trials. Meanwhile, the new agents that *have* proven effective in clinical trials or are still in active development either have potential for nephrotoxicity themselves (FK506, rapamycin, and anti-T-cell monoclonal antibodies) or are commonly used with the potentially nephrotoxic agent cyclosporine (mycophenolate mofetil and 15-deoxyspergualin). Thus it appears that nephrotoxicity will be a possible complication of successful antirejection drug regimens for some time to come.

In this chapter, we review the nephrotoxicity of cyclosporine, with brief mention of the differential diagnosis of thrombotic microangiopathy in renal transplants and the nephrotoxic potential of FK506, rapamycin, and OKT3. Before commencing, it is worth reflecting on the relationship between immunosuppressive action and nephrotoxicity in cyclosporine and FK506. Both agents are believed to owe their immunosuppressive effects in part to inhibition of calcineurin (1–4). The two agents are structurally quite dissimilar and have differing extrarenal side effects. However, both agents have similar toxic effects in the kidney (5–16). This suggests that calcineurin may be necessary for normal renal function and that it will not be possible to dissociate calcineurin inhibition from nephrotoxicity. Nevertheless, with the potent antirejection agents available, it is possible to find treatment regimes that minimize nephrotoxic effects.

II. CYCLOSPORINE NEPHROTOXICITY

A. Introduction

Cyclosporine has a number of nonrenal side effects including excess hair growth, gum hypertrophy, hypertension, tremor, and seizures (17,18). However, its ability to impair renal function and to produce structural changes in the kidney remained the principal toxic effect that limited its wider use until physicians became familiar with strategies to deal with this effect.

There have been detailed descriptions of cyclosporine nephrotoxicity for over 12 years (3–9), and a standard approach to biopsy diagnosis has been suggested (19). Discussions of nephrotoxicity constitute a substantial portion of the more than 14,000 articles have been written on cyclosporine (Fig. 1). Therefore the authors of any new review have a special responsibility to provide new concepts that improve practical understanding of this important subject. Our aim has been to provide the reader with a useful approach to this topic.

Most reviews of medical conditions emphasize that the pathogenesis of the disorder being described is incompletely understood. However there is a level of phenomenology below pathogenesis where much is known, and a summary of existing knowledge at this level can be of considerable practical value. Certainly there can be a firm grasp on those features necessary for diagnosis without full knowledge of pathogenesis. In this section we have attempted to provide a clear description of the relationship between the lesions observed in cyclosporine nephrotoxicity and to set forward a conceptual framework that uses morphological findings to establish diagnosis and prognosis.

If toxicity is defined as an influence that impairs organ function, then cyclosporine is capable of exerting a number of toxic effects, running the gamut from purely functional, possibly short-lived changes to extensive structural changes that are longer-lasting (Fig. 2).

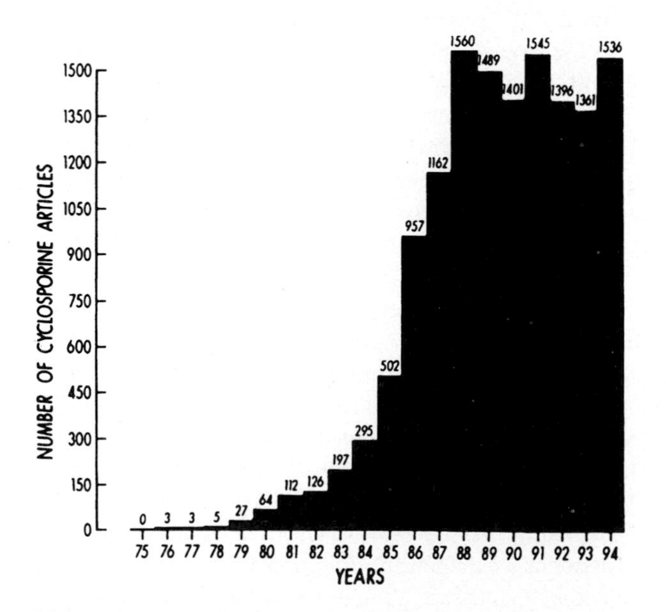

Figure 1 Histogram showing number of articles on cyclosporine published per year. The rapid rise in interest in the years 1979–1987 and the sustained high interest since then is apparent. The number of published articles on cyclosporine now exceeds 14,000.

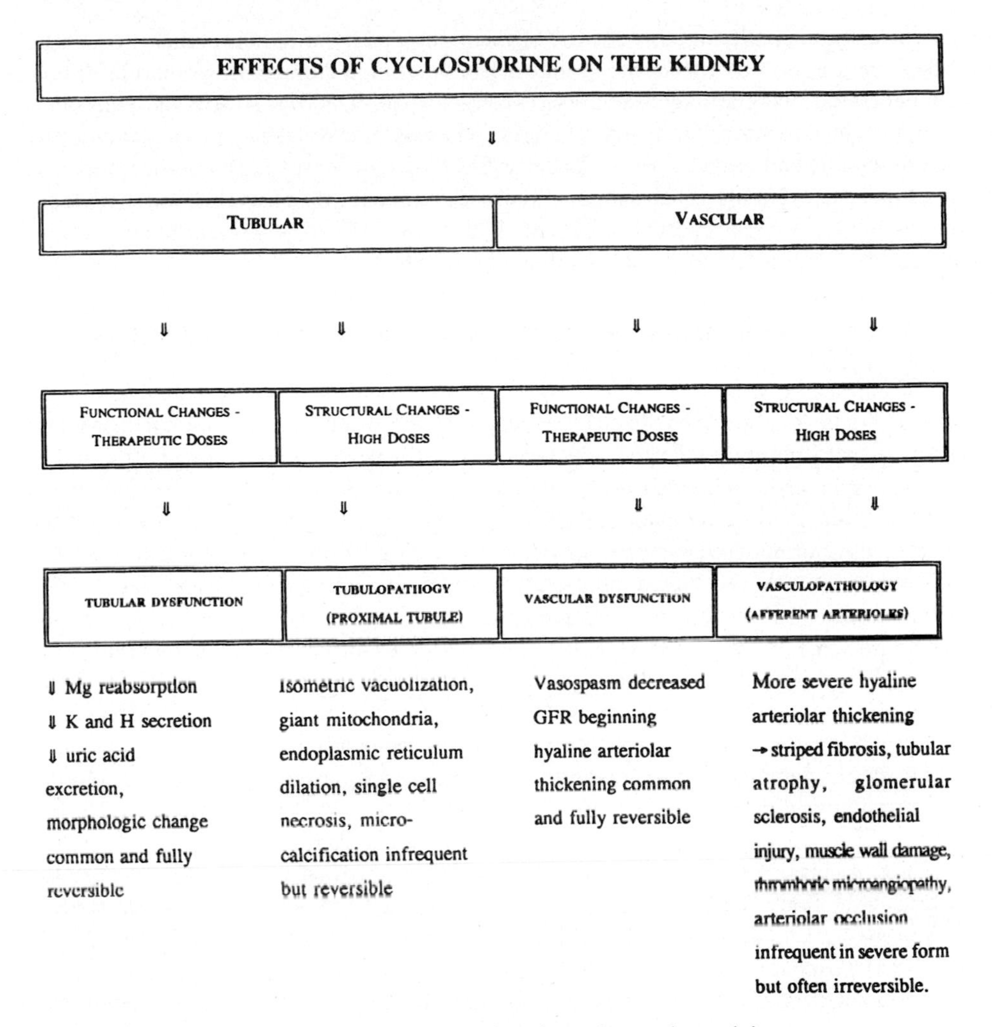

Figure 2 Diagram showing various types of cyclosporine nephrotoxicity.

B. Relationship of Toxicity to Dose

Different sensitivities and various risk factors determine the severity of cyclosporine nephrotoxicity in individual patients (20–22). Functional changes due to cyclosporine include renal side effects that are not associated with distinct morphological renal lesions and that may already be present at therapeutic trough levels and doses. Most patients develop functional changes at therapeutic dose levels above 5 mg/kg, corresponding to cyclosporine trough levels (whole blood) of more than 200 to 500 ng/mL or 20 to 60 ng/mL (serum), respectively. Functional changes are characterized by a slight increase in the serum creatinine concentration, reflecting a decreased glomerular filtration rate and variable signs of tubular dysfunction. Acute renal failure with oligoanuria immediately after kidney grafting is considered to be a special form of functional toxicity due to cyclosporine, which develops only in this specific situation. At high dose and trough levels, structural toxicity (i.e., tubulopathy, arteriolopathy, or microangiopathy and their clinical sequelae) may be superimposed on functional changes. The functional damage in glomerular filtration is believed to be due largely to arteriolar vasospasm, which, if severe and persistent enough, may lead to arteriolar hyaline changes. Whereas functional changes and tubulopathy are reversible and arteriolopathy can be reversed in some cases (23), microangiopathy may result in irreversible renal damage. These different forms of cyclosporine toxicity in the kidney have been reported in patients with kidney, liver, heart, and bone marrow transplants as well as in those with autoimmune diseases.

C. Frequency and Time of Presentation of Cyclosporine-Related Lesions

No precise data can be given on the frequency of the different morphological lesions induced by cyclosporine. In the 1981–1990 series of Mihatsch et al. (12), about 50% of the 1000 biopsy specimens obtained from renal transplant patients showed lesions thought to be induced by cyclosporine. In about half of the specimens in which rejection was evident, signs of cyclosporine toxicity were also found (24,25). Despite the complexity of the lesions observed, allograft biopsy influences therapeutic decisions in 83% of cases (26).

The frequency of cyclosporine-related lesions in kidney transplant biopsy specimens varies significantly in various transplant centers owing to differences in therapeutic regimens and the indications for performing renal biopsies. In four different transplant centers, the frequency of acute renal failure with diffuse interstitial fibrosis varied between 0 and 19%, tubular toxicity occurred with a prevalence of 9 to 37%, the frequency of the striped form of interstitial fibrosis was 5 to 50%, and cyclosporine-associated arteriolopathy occurred with a prevalence of 5 to 30% (24,25).

An analysis of the 1000 transplant biopsy specimens examined at the University of Basel showed signs of tubular toxicity in 43% of those obtained within the first 2 weeks after transplantation, decreasing to 5% in those obtained more than 3 years later (8). Cyclosporine-associated arteriolopathy was found in 12% of specimens taken within 2 weeks after transplantation and increased to 38% in specimens obtained more than 3 years after transplantation. Cyclosporine-associated arteriolopathy may be observed within the first week after transplantation (25,27–29). The corresponding prevalences of the striped form of interstitial fibrosis were 9% within 2 weeks and 77% after 3 years, respectively. Comparison of two intervals (1981–1985 vs. 1986–1990) showed no significant differences with respect to the overall frequency of cyclosporine-associated lesions in biopsy specimens (27,30). However, in the biopsy specimens from Basel, a center that has engaged in strict low-dose therapy since 1985, the prevalence of cyclosporine-associated arteriolopathy 4 years after transplantation decreased from 40 to 20%. The number of diagnostic biopsies also decreased over this period despite a continuous increase in the number of transplants, indicating that fewer patients developed clinical problems related to cyclosporine toxicity. At the University of Basel, the frequency of vascular and interstitial toxicity decreased from about 30 to 15% with the use of lower doses of cyclosporine in the first year after transplantation (31).

The severity of cyclosporine-related lesions has dramatically decreased in patients with autoimmune diseases. Whereas early reports described a prevalence of cyclosporine-related lesions in about 50% of the patients (32–34), the frequency in a recent large series was found to be 21% (21).

D. Functional Toxicity

1. *Clinical Findings*

When cyclosporine is given in a daily oral dose of 10 mg/kg, which is below the previously recommended initial dose for organ transplantation, a decrease in renal function can be observed in almost all patients. Soon after commencement of therapy, a slight increase in the serum creatinine concentration is observed. This increase is reversible if the dose of cyclosporine is reduced. There is a parallel decrease in glomerular filtration rate and renal plasma flow, keeping the filtration fraction within the normal range. When well-functioning kidney grafts in patients receiving cyclosporine treatment are compared with similar successful grafts in patients treated with azathioprine, the creatinine clearance is about 20% lower in the cyclosporine group (35). Similar functional changes are seen in the native kidneys of patients treated with cyclosporine for nonrenal organ transplants or for autoimmune diseases (36–40).

Hypertension is observed in about 40% of patients undergoing kidney transplantation. In patients receiving heart transplants, hypertension occurs even more frequently. Hyperkalemia, mild metabolic acidosis, hypomagnesemia, and hyperuricemia secondary to reduced uric acid clearance occur only rarely as complications of cyclosporine therapy (41–48).

2. *Morphology*

Systematic biopsy studies of cases with functional toxicity are lacking. The morphological findings can only be inferred from occasional biopsies performed in patients with kidney transplants and poor renal function as well as from a few systematic biopsies in patients with autoimmune disease (45–48). Except for preexisting damage, the renal tissue is either essentially normal (6,8,24) or is affected by peritubular capillary congestion (49) (Fig. 3). The number of Tamm-Horsfall protein casts may be increased. Peritubular capillary congestion differs from normal renal tissue only by the presence of dilated peritubular

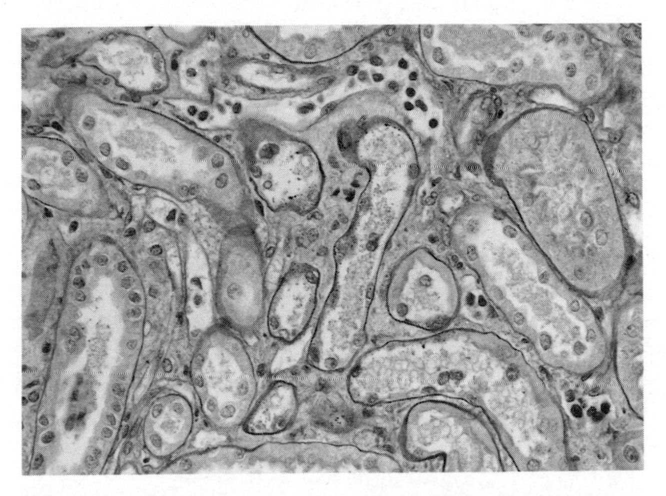

Figure 3 Congestion of peritubular capillaries containing aggregates of mononuclear cells. Slight interstitial edema is also present. (Hematoxylin and eosin, ×300.)

capillaries containing mononuclear cells, which disappear after increased corticosteroid therapy (8). Peritubular capillary congestion is seen only in patients with kidney transplants. It is often associated with tubular toxicity (24–25) and in the medulla is a nonspecific finding that is often observed in acute renal failure of any etiology in patients not treated with cyclosporine (24,50). The juxtaglomerular apparatus in functional toxicity was believed to be enlarged (36). Some quantitative studies in larger series, however, showed no difference in comparison with zero hour biopsies (Ström and Mihatsch, unpublished).

E. Acute Renal Failure with Oligoanuria

1. Clinical Findings

Acute renal failure with oligoanuria—either the primary form resulting from delayed kidney graft function or the secondary form—was found more frequently with the administration of cyclosporine than with conventional treatment. The incidence of delayed kidney graft function increased to as high as 23% in some transplant centers. Furthermore, the duration of oligoanuria was usually longer (up to 13 days) than with conventional immunosuppression. Cold ischemia lasting more than 36 to 48 hr was associated with an increased incidence of primary nonfunctioning kidneys and significantly poorer graft survival (51–55). Today, with the use of low doses, the prevalence of acute renal failure in cyclosporine-treated patients is similar to those treated with conventional immunosuppression. Patients with other solid-organ transplants may also experience acute renal failure following cyclosporine therapy (40,55–57).

2. Morphology

Acute tubular necrosis (ATN) occurring in patients treated with cyclosporine has no characteristic morphology but is characterized by more frequent necrosis of entire tubular cross sections than transplant ATN in patients treated with steroid-azathioprine immunosuppression (58).

In cases of prolonged oligoanuria of more than 2 to 3 weeks' duration, slight diffuse interstitial fibrosis may develop (12,59–62). The tubules are separated from each other by an excess of collagen fibers and edema (Fig. 4). The tubules do not show gross atrophy. Signs of preceding acute tubular necrosis may still be present, however. Vascular lesions are absent. After recovery of renal function, interstitial fibrosis disappears completely or fibrotic foci may remain (60,63). Biopsies of transplants with a prolonged ischemia time of more than 24 hr have been found to exhibit a greater degree of fibrosis than those with a shorter duration of cold ischemia (8).

Long-lasting oligoanuria is responsible for diffuse interstitial fibrosis, often with little tubular atrophy (64,65). This is distinguished from the striped interstitial fibrosis described below. After 2 to 3 weeks of oligoanuria secondary to hemolysis and after other causes of acute renal failure in the native kidney, interstitial fibrosis may also develop in patients who have not been treated with cyclosporine. Thus, this type of diffuse interstitial fibrosis is not the result of cyclosporine toxicity but is rather secondary to prolonged oligoanuria (64,65). An animal model of diffuse fibrosis following acute renal failure has not been established.

F. Tubulopathy

1. Clinical Findings

The clinical findings do not differ qualitatively from those previously described under functional toxicity. However, the rise of serum creatinine concentration may be greater than

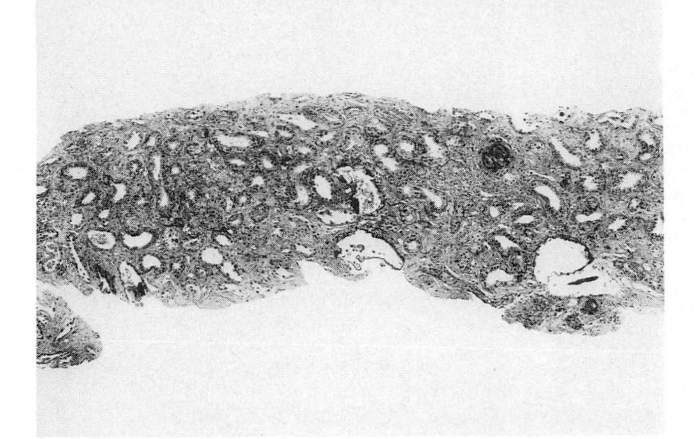

Figure 4 Diffuse interstitial fibrosis with widening of the interstitial space. (Chromotrope aniline blue, ×80.)

100%. Interestingly enough, there is little evidence of proximal tubular dysfunction. Features of proximal tubular effects, such as in the Fanconi syndrome, have not been described in tubulopathy (66). Hyperuricemia, rather than hypouricemia, is present. Lysozymuria and N-acetyl glucosaminidase excretion are within normal limits (67–71). Gluthatione transferase, in contrast, is increased (72). Beta$_2$-microglobulin may be a good indicator as well (73,74). Proximal tubular cell antigens in the urine are also indicators of proximal tubular dysfunction and are not increased (75). Thus, the morphological lesions do not appear to correlate with tubular dysfunction.

2. Morphology

Low-power magnification often shows more or less normal renal tissue. The morphological changes seen in tubulopathology (24,76) include inclusion bodies in tubular epithelial cells that correspond to giant mitochondria, isometric tubular vacuolization, and microcalcification. The different lesions of tubulopathy are most often found in a single biopsy (24). They may, however, occur in any combination, and giant mitochondria, isometric vacuolization, or microcalcifications may be found alone. Vascular and glomerular lesions are usually absent, as are interstitial lesions such as edema. Tubulopathy is found in kidney transplants as well as in bone marrow and heart transplant recipients and in patients treated for autoimmune diseases (20,33,77–79).

Giant mitochondria occur predominantly in the convoluted part (S_1 and S_2 segments) of the proximal tubule, usually one per cell (Fig. 5). Multiple tubular inclusion bodies must be considered to be phagolysosomes. Giant mitochondria are distributed inhomogeneously and are rare, even in cases of severe toxicity. Whereas some tubular cross sections may contain many giant mitochondria, adjacent ones may contain none. Giant mitochondria reach about half the size of a nucleus, are mostly round or oval, rarely cigar-shaped, and lie adjacent to the nuclei. The morphology of giant mitochondria lacks any specificity. They usually have few cristae and frequently contain paracrystalline inclusions, large matrix granules, and lipid droplets. Because of the rarity of cristae and their polymorphism, they are easily mistaken for lysosomes. The other mitochondria vary slightly in size

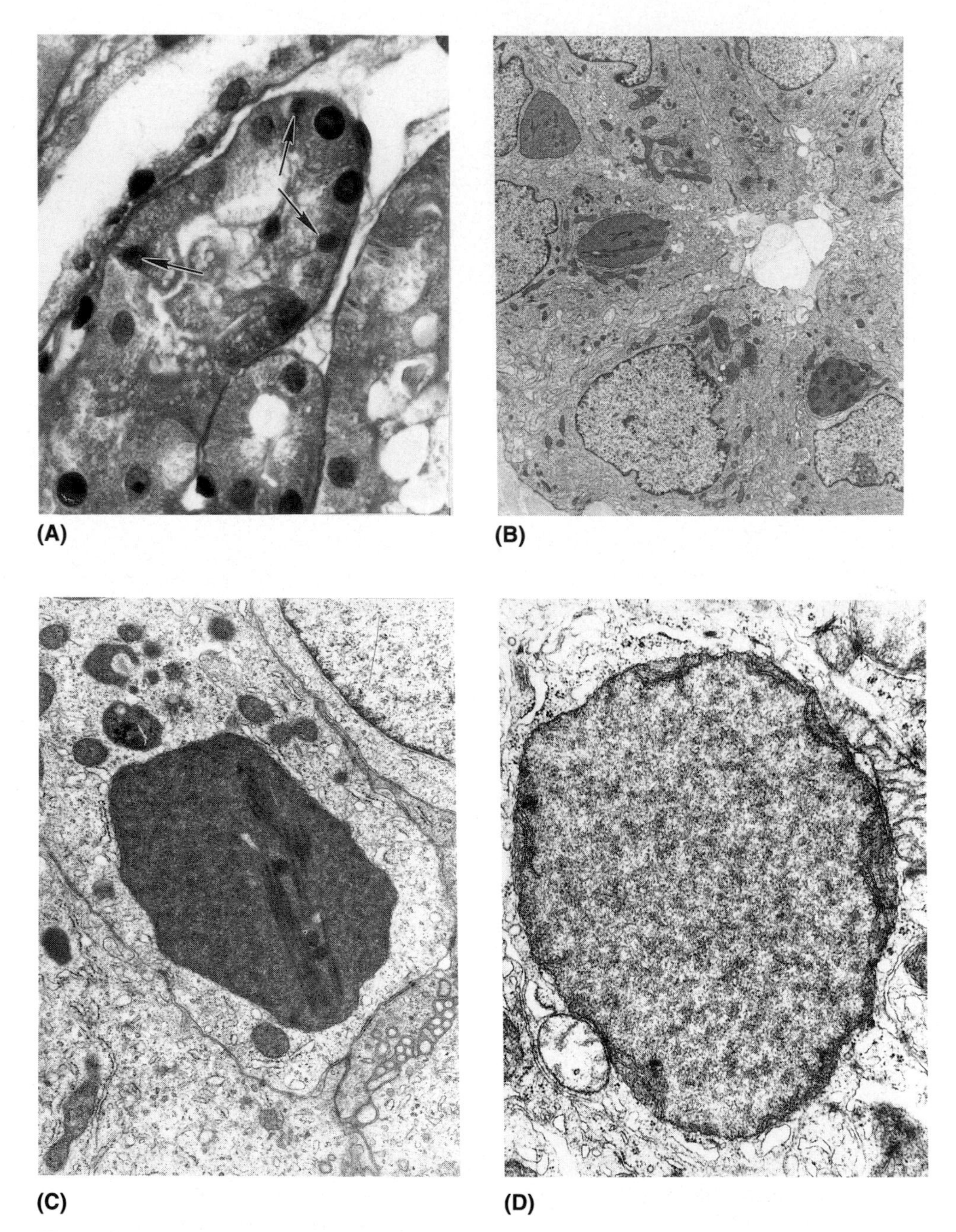

Figure 5 Giant mitochondria. A. Light microscopy (arrows). (Chromotrope aniline blue, × 950.) B. Two giant mitochondria adjacent to nuclei. Note the absence of lysosomes. (×3300.) C and D. Two giant mitochondria with paracrystalline inclusions and scarcity of cristae. (×23000.) (From Ref. 12.)

and shape. In rare cases, autophagolysosomes contain fragments of mitochondria. Giant mitochondria are often found in the tubule lumen.

Isometric vacuolization is found almost exclusively in the straight part of the proximal tubule, or S_3 segment of some nephrons. The light microscopic picture is identical to that of osmotic nephrosis (Fig. 6). Most of the tubular cells in a cross section contain densely packed vacuoles of equal size that are free of lipids. Vacuolization is at least partly the result of dilatation of the smooth endoplasmic reticulum. Giant mitochondria and isometric vacuolization are never observed in the same cell. Sometimes the nuclei look pyknotic, and the brush border of the affected cells may be missing.

Microcalcifications of single tubular cells or proximal tubular groups of them are found in various parts of the nephron. They are round, crescentic, or polycyclic. Microcalcifications are the result of calcification of Tamm-Horsfall protein casts and possibly also of necrotic tubular cells. They are an infrequent finding by light or electron microscopy.

The morphological features of tubulopathy can be found not only in core biopsy specimens but also in fine-needle aspiration biopsies (80–86) and cytologic smears of the urine (77,86–89). The diagnosis of tubulopathy is difficult by light microscopy. The quality and type of histological technique are important (8,24). For light microscopic identification of tubular lesions, the following points should be considered (1) 4% buffered formalin seems to be superior to any other fixative; (2) sections 2 to 3 μm thick are needed; (3) special stains such as chromotrope aniline blue (90) for the identification of giant mitochondria and von Kossa's stain for microcalcifications are most helpful; (4) serial sections must be evaluated at a final magnification of at least 400×; and (5) unequivocal demonstration of giant mitochondria is possible only by the use of electron microscopy, although this is impractical for routine diagnosis.

3. *Specificity of Lesions*

There has been much debate about the specificity of giant mitochondria and somatic vacuolization of the tubules (59,79,91). These morphological lesions are nonspecific although highly characteristic, especially when giant mitochondria, isometric vacuolization, and microcalcification are present in the same biopsy. Giant mitochondria may be found in a variety of conditions (92–94), including glomerulonephritis, systemic lupus erythematosus, minimal change nephrotic syndrome, and hereditary and metabolic renal diseases as well as following kidney transplantation and conventional immunosuppressive therapy. They were shown to occur with significantly greater frequency, however, after treatment with cyclosporine than after conventional immunosuppressive regimens, an observation that has been confirmed by others (52,94). The isolated occurrence of giant mitochondria in kidney transplants may be interpreted as suggestive of cyclosporine toxicity. In autoimmune disease with renal involvement, in which giant mitochondria may occur spontaneously in the absence of cyclosporine therapy, their presence must be interpreted with caution.

Isometric vacuolization must be differentiated from coarse and irregular vacuolization seen in ischemic renal damage, as in acute tubular necrosis or at the periphery of infarcts. In patients receiving other agents which can cause vacuolization, such as mannitol, dextran, sucrose, or contrast media (95–98), isometric vacuolization must not be interpreted as indicative of cyclosporine toxicity. In patients receiving cyclosporine and one of these other agents, however, widespread vacuolization may be found, even after low doses of mannitol or similar infusion solutions and with low cyclosporine trough levels. By light microscopy,

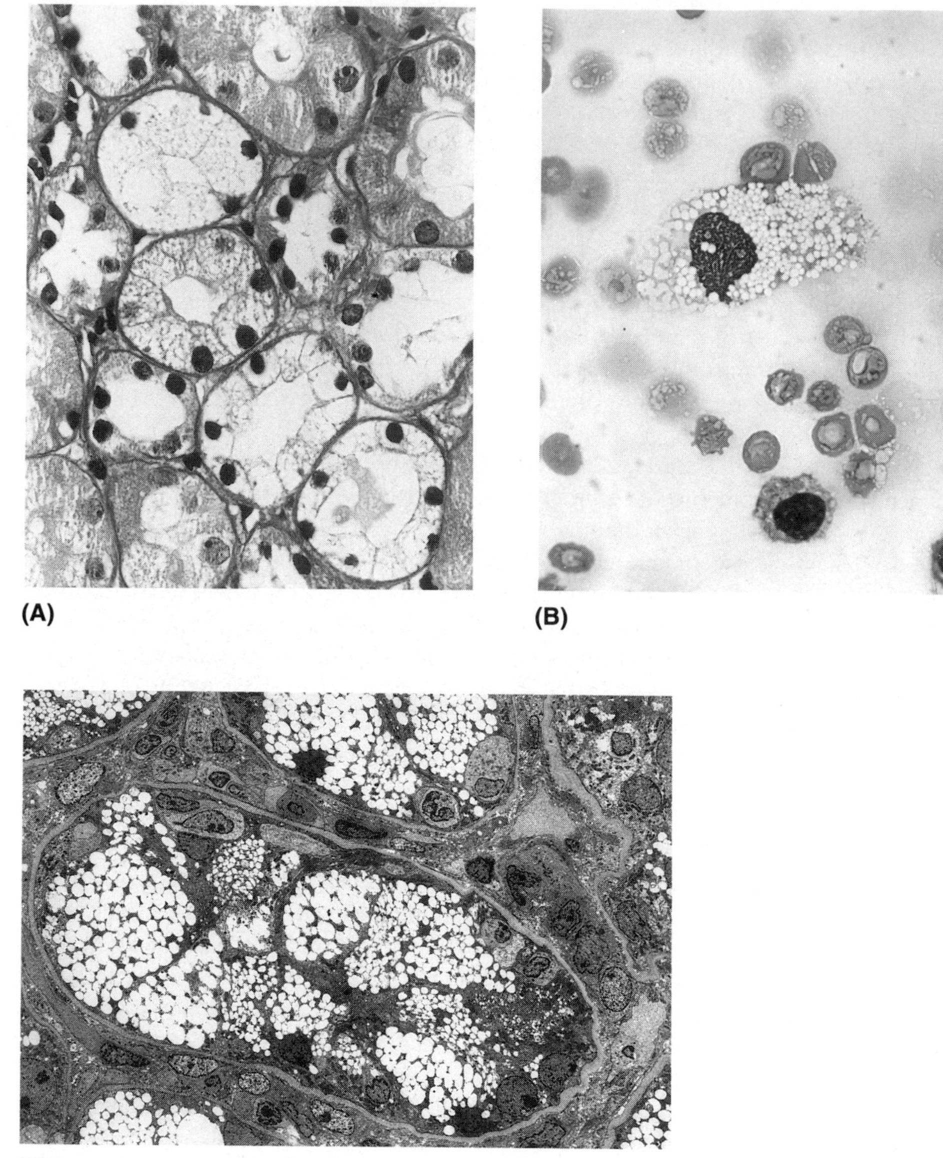

Figure 6 Isometric vacuolization. A. Tubular cells with fine vacuolization of the cytoplasm. (Chromotrope aniline blue, ×320.) B. Vacuolated tubular cell as seen in a fine-needle aspirate. (Giemsa, ×980.) C. Most tubular cells have empty vacuoles. The nuclei are pyknotic and the brush border is lacking in most cells. (×4900.) (From Ref. 12.)

isometric vacuolization in patients treated with cyclosporine is similar but not identical to osmotic nephrosis. In the former, dilatation of endoplasmic reticulum as well as formation of pinocytotic vacuoles and phagolysosomes occur, whereas in the latter dilatation of the endoplasmic reticulum is noted (96,96,98). In patients with autoimmune disorders, tubular vacuolization is found mostly in patients with type I diabetes. Microcalcification, in contrast, is seen mostly in patients with minimal change disease associated with the nephrotic syndrome (100). Microcalcifications seen after acute tubular necrosis are usually much larger than those attributable to cyclosporine. If microcalcifications are present alone, they must not be interpreted as a sign of toxic tubulopathy. Extensive tubular necrosis, as seen in gentamicin toxicity, is not found after treatment with cyclosporine alone (101,102).

4. *Etiology and Pathogenesis*

The essential etiological factor in the development of tubulopathy is a toxic cyclosporine trough level. Toxic tubulopathy is an expected finding in patients with cyclosporine trough levels exceeding 1000 ng/mL in whole blood, which corresponds to 200 ng/mL in serum (6,24). In the rat, a highly significant correlation exists between trough level and morphology (103). No tubulopathy can be found in the rat with cyclosporine doses of less than 10 mg/kg/day. In the presence of additional renal damage, especially ischemia and rejection, tubulopathy may be found at cyclosporine trough levels that are usually nontoxic (6,24). Giant mitochondria in tubules develop quickly. After a mean exposure time of 12 min, an increased number of giant mitochondria was found in zero-hour biopsy specimens of human renal allografts at whole blood concentrations of cyclosporine of 300 to 600 ng/mL (104). Increased individual sensitivity to cyclosporine may account for the occurrence of tubular lesions at low cyclosporine trough levels even in the absence of additional risk factors.

The pathogenesis of toxic tubulopathy is not clear. It must be considered a result of direct tubular damage. The toxicity is attributable to the parent compound rather than its metabolites (105,106).

G. Microangiopathy and Tubulointerstitial Lesions

1. *Clinical Findings*

Clinical findings that are the consequence of microangiopathy and tubulointerstitial lesions are often superimposed on the symptoms of cyclosporine-induced functional changes. These can have both an acute and a chronic component. The clinical signs are similar in patients with kidney, heart, bone marrow, and liver transplants as well as in patients with autoimmune disease (34,35,37,39,40,107–114). Slowly progressive deterioration of renal function and, eventually, hypertension are the most important signs. Initially, glomerular filtration rate and renal plasma flow decrease (37,115) and vascular resistance increases (111). Creatinine clearance and even inulin clearance are not sensitive enough to detect early nephron loss, which is compensated for by the intrinsic reserve capacity [i.e., hyperfiltration in less affected nephrons (38)]. Thus, the increase in serum creatinine concentration is not an early sign, but ultimately the creatinine concentration always increases with significant renal damage. Proteinuria is mild or absent. After discontinuation of cyclosporine therapy, an improvement in renal function will occur in some but by no means all patients (35,110–115). The residual renal dysfunction after cessation of cyclosporine therapy may be the result of irreversible structural lesions.

An indicator of vascular damage is the finding of increased levels of factor VIII and antithrombin III, both of which are of endothelial origin (116–118). Furthermore, platelet aggregation (119,120) and platelet deposition are found in kidney grafts with microangiopathy, with or without other clinical signs of hemolytic-uremic syndrome (29). Several examples of these lesions resembling hemolytic-uremic syndrome have been reported in patients with kidney (118–127), liver (128), and bone marrow transplants (124–138) as well as in patients with autoimmune disease (139).

2. *Morphology*

Vascular-interstitial lesions caused by cyclosporine may affect the small vessels (arterioles, eventually together with the glomeruli), the tubulointerstitial space alone, or both (6,24). Vascular-interstitial lesions may be classified as follows:

1. Cyclosporine-associated microangiopathy:
   a. Cyclosporine-associated arteriolopathy: early lesions, thrombotic lesion, typical lesion (cyclosporine-associated arteriolopathy) (6,24,140–142)
   b. Cyclosporine-associated glomerulopathy: thrombotic lesion, typical hemolytic-uremic syndrome–like lesion, focal segmental glomerular sclerosis
2. Tubular atrophy with concomitant interstitial fibrosis (striped form)

Vascular-interstitial lesions are found not only in kidney transplant recipients but also in patients with bone marrow (112,129–138,143), liver (144), and heart transplants (55) and in those with autoimmune diseases (33,37,48,145,146).

Cyclosporine-associated microangiopathy predominates in the peripheral vascular tree, including the arterioles (afferent vessels) and arteries with up to two layers of smooth muscle cells. The vascular lesions sometimes extend downstream into the glomerulus and upstream into arteries, close to where they branch into arterioles. Proliferative arteriolopathy of interlobular or arcuate arteries (147) or intimal mononuclear cell infiltrates are not a feature of cyclosporine toxicity in our experience (140). Intimal fibrosis in arteries, however, is common in patients with severe and long-standing cyclosporine-associated arteriolopathy.

a. Cyclosporine-Associated Microangiopathy. The description of this lesion follows concepts derived from biopsy specimens of bone marrow, heart, and kidney transplant recipients (Fig. 7) (12,143).

i. *Early (Minor) Lesions.* Early minor lesions (Fig. 7) include vacuolization (at least partly attributable to a dilatation of endoplasmic reticulum), inclusion bodies resembling giant mitochondria or giant lysosomes (20), single-cell necrosis of endothelial or smooth muscle cells, and, most often, a clear cell transformation of smooth muscle cells. Except for giant vacuoles in smooth muscle cells and the clear cell transformation, the early minor lesions are hardly ever seen by light microscopy.

ii. *Thrombotic Lesions.* Arteriolar or glomerular (see later) fibrin or platelet thrombi or both (28,29,140) usually affect only a few arterioles or glomeruli (Fig. 8). In rare cases all glomeruli and arterioles may be involved. We found fibrin thrombi in about 3% of diagnostic kidney transplant biopsy specimens from patients treated with cyclosporine (8,25,140).

In routine biopsy specimens, thrombi were found in about 26% of the patients 1 and 4 weeks after transplantation. In 25 to 50% of the patients with thrombi, cyclosporine-associated arteriolopathy was also present (25,28,29,140). In one study of recipients of bone marrow transplants, glomerular or arteriolar thrombi or both were found in three of the autopsies performed (129). Thrombi in arterioles, glomeruli, or both were present in 40% of bone marrow transplant recipients and in 10% of heart transplant recipients in another autopsy series (143). In 75% of the cases, thrombi were seen in association with cyclosporine-associated arteriolopathy. We are not aware of any report concerning thrombi in patients with autoimmune diseases except for those with overt hemolytic uremic syndrome (139).

iii. *Typical Cyclosporine-Associated Arteriolopathy.* Cyclosporine-associated arteriolopathy occurs in two forms, which may coexist (6,24,141,142) (Figs. 9 and 10). In the

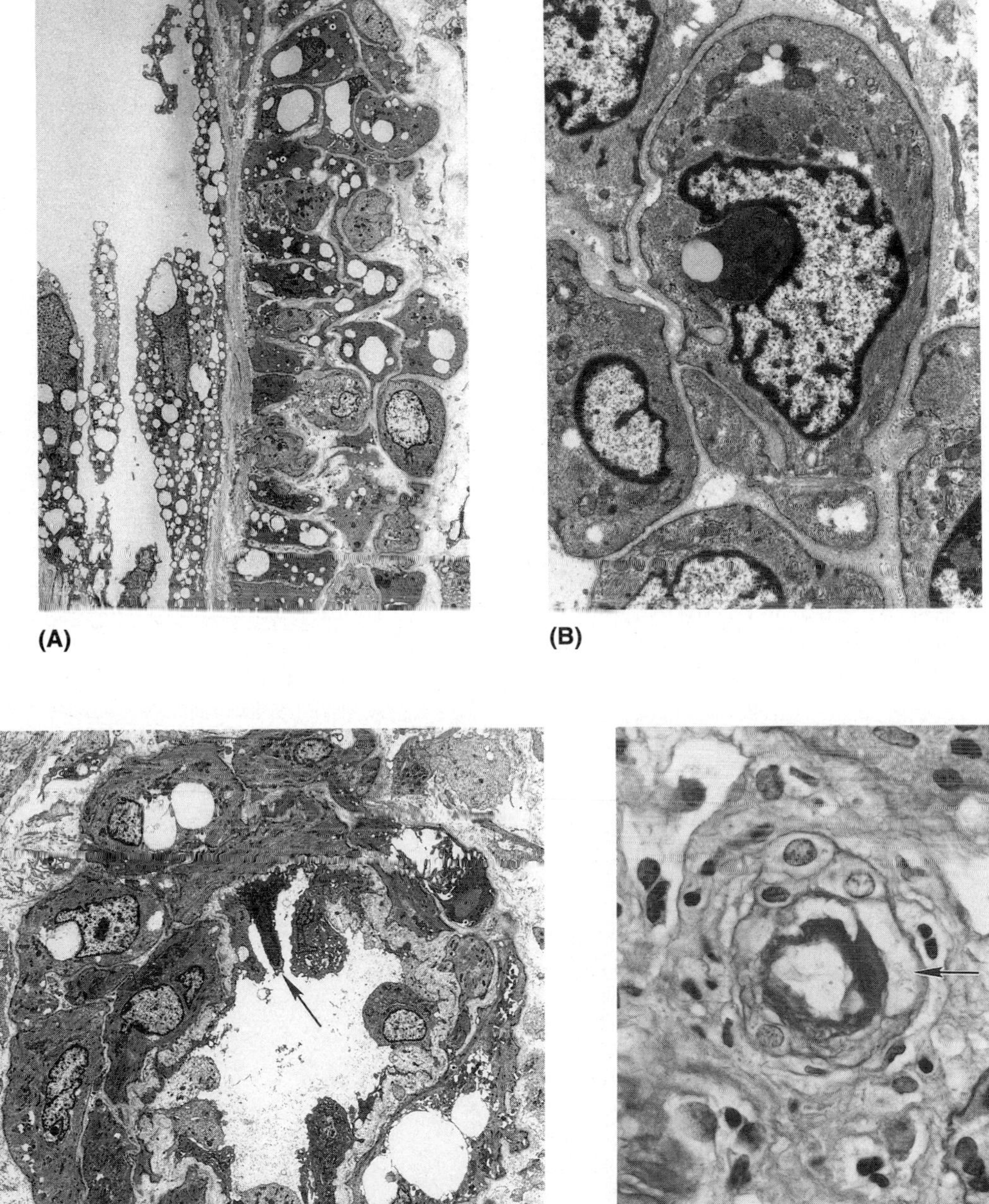

Figure 7 Minor vascular lesions. A. Marked vacuolization of smooth muscle and endothelial cells. (×1900.) B. Smooth muscle cell with large inclusion body (lysosome or giant mitochondrion). (×9400.) C. Arteriolar cross section with vacuolization of smooth muscle cells and necrosis of individual endothelial and smooth muscle cells. (×2400.) D. Early light microscopic findings in arterioles. Note clear cell transformation of the cytoplasm and loss of individual cell (arrow). (Periodic acid-Schiff, ×1500.) (From Ref. 12.)

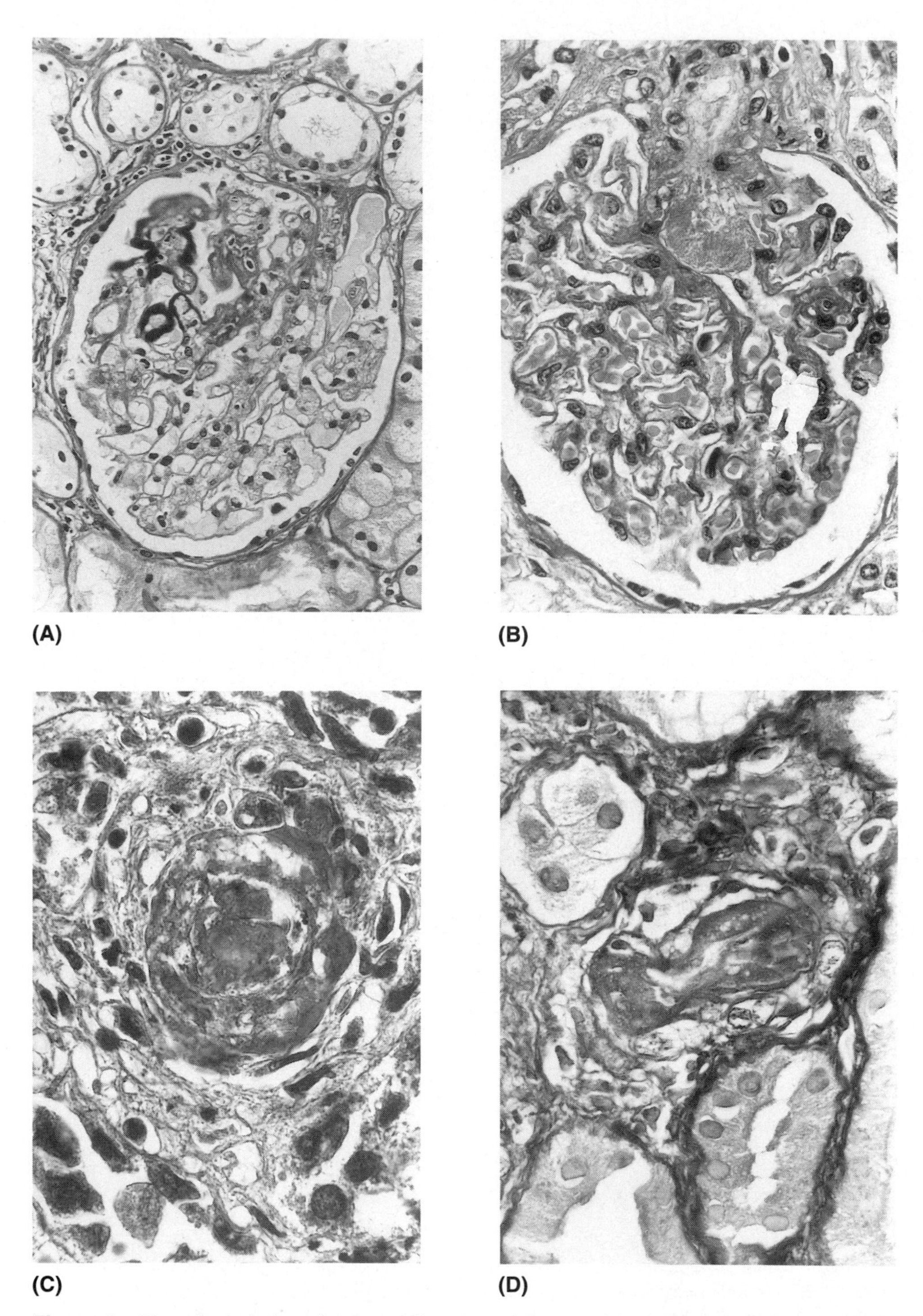

Figure 8 Thrombotic lesions in glomeruli and arterioles. A. Glomerulus with fibrin thrombi in renal transplant. (Acid fuchsin orange G, ×340.) B. Glomerular microthrombus at the vascular pole in a heart transplant recipient (periodic acid-Schiff, ×450.) C. Fibrin thrombus in an arteriole with complete necrosis of the vascular wall in a bone marrow transplant recipient. Periodic acid-Schiff, ×920.) D. Fibrin thrombus in a degenerated arteriole in a patient with renal transplant. (Periodic acid-Schiff, ×795.) (From Ref. 12.)

first form, circular nodular protein deposits may permeate the arteriolar wall and may narrow or even occlude the vascular lumen. Often, the protein deposits are arranged in a pattern resembling a pearl necklace or cloverleaf. Electron microscopy reveals that the protein deposits replace necrotic myocytes. The protein deposits contain IgM and/or complement (C3, Clq, C5B-9) by immunofluorescence (6,24). Fibrin is present in up to 20% of affected patients as well (25). This lesion may have the character of severe arteriolar hyalinosis or fibrinoid necrosis by light microscopy. The second form of arteriolopathy, which is rare, consists of a mucoid thickening of the intima that results in narrowing of the vascular lumen. Electron microscopy reveals thickening of the intimal layer by a loose, amorphous material. Necrotic myocytes are also present as indicated by positive immunofluorescence (6,24).

The more common form of arteriolopathy can develop within a week posttransplantation (30). Repeat biopsies in patients with cyclosporine-associated arteriolopathy have shown that, after the dose of cyclosporine is reduced or stopped, the arteriolopathy may either progress to complete vascular occlusion or remodeling of the vascular lesion may take place. If complete severe circular involvement of the arteriole is present, the arteriole may either become completely scarred or eventually merge and finally vanish with the interstitial fibrosis. In the case of incomplete involvement of the arteriole, remodeling of the vascular wall may develop with progressive decrease of protein deposits, so that in the end patent arterioles are found with an increase in basement membrane material throughout the vessel wall (24,148) (Fig. 11).

b. Cyclosporine-Associated Glomerulopathy. In general, at least subtle glomerular lesions are probably always associated with cyclosporine-associated arteriolopathy, as found in bone marrow (143), heart (37,143), and renal transplant recipients (149) and in patients with autoimmune diseases (32,139). Thus, cyclosporine-associated glomerulopathy may be interpreted as the extension of arteriolopathy into the glomerulus. The frequency of cyclosporine-associated glomerulopathy decreases in parallel with the severity of arteriolopathy: 65% in cases of severe cyclosporine-associated arteriolopathy, 45% and 25% in medium severe and slight forms, respectively; and none in cases without arteriolopathy (149). In bone marrow and heart transplant recipients, the overall frequency of cyclosporine-associated glomerulopathy was similar to that of renal transplant recipients (143).

The morphological pattern of cyclosporine-associated glomerulopathy is variable (149) (Fig. 12). The changes include (1) fibrin or platelet thrombi, (2) the pouch lesion (i.e., thrombotic and proliferative lesion at the vascular pole of the glomerulus), (3) changes resembling those of the hemolytic-uremic syndrome, (4) mesangiolysis, and (5) segmental focal glomerular sclerosis. These lesions of cyclosporine-associated glomerulopathy may be accompanied by other nonspecific changes, including glomerular collapse, glomerular obsolescence, and thickening and multilayering of the basement membrane of Bowman's capsule.

The glomerular lesions are usually focal. In some cases, only a single glomerulus may be affected. The involved glomerulus is usually supplied by an arteriole showing cyclosporine-associated arteriolopathy. This finding may be helpful in the distinction of cyclosporine-associated glomerulopathy from similar glomerular lesions observed in transplant glomerulopathy or recurrent segmental focal glomerular sclerosis.

c. Tubular Atrophy and Interstitial Fibrosis (Striped Form). Irregular foci or stripes of tubular atrophy accompanied by fibrosis are observed in the renal cortex (Fig. 13) (6,24). The atrophic tubules exhibit mostly basement membrane thickening, but basement membrane thinning may also be present. Tubules in other areas appear to be essentially normal. A sparse mononuclear cell infiltrate is often seen in the fibrotic area, not only in

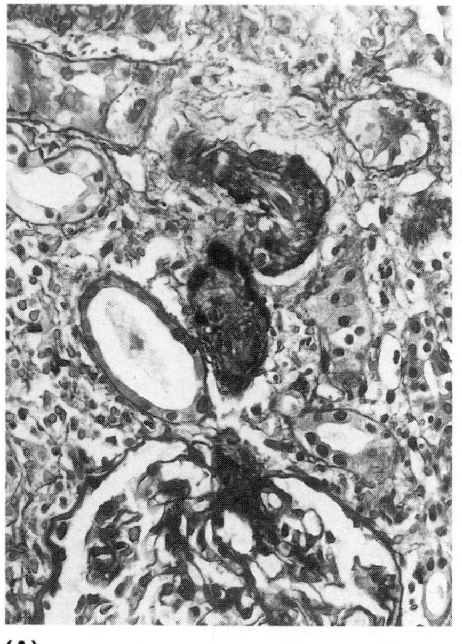

(A)

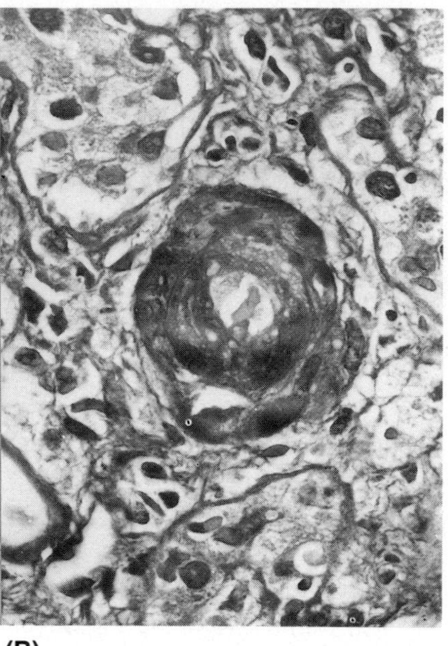

(B)

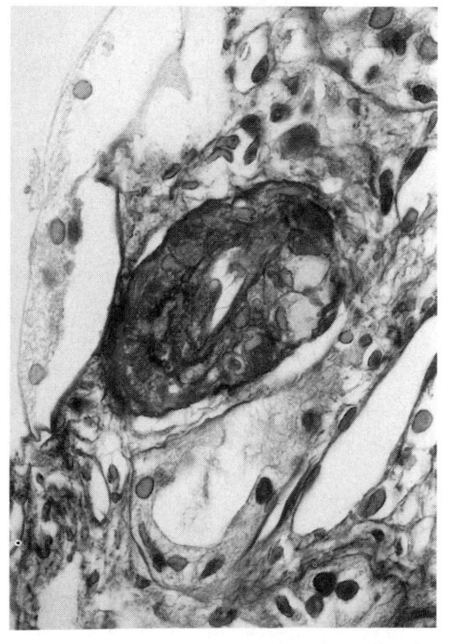

(C)

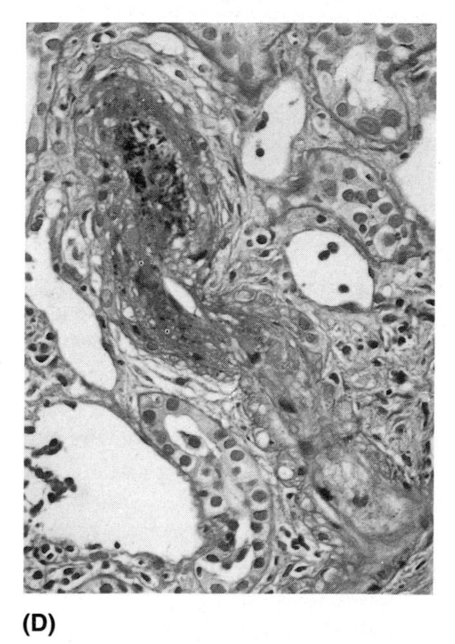

(D)

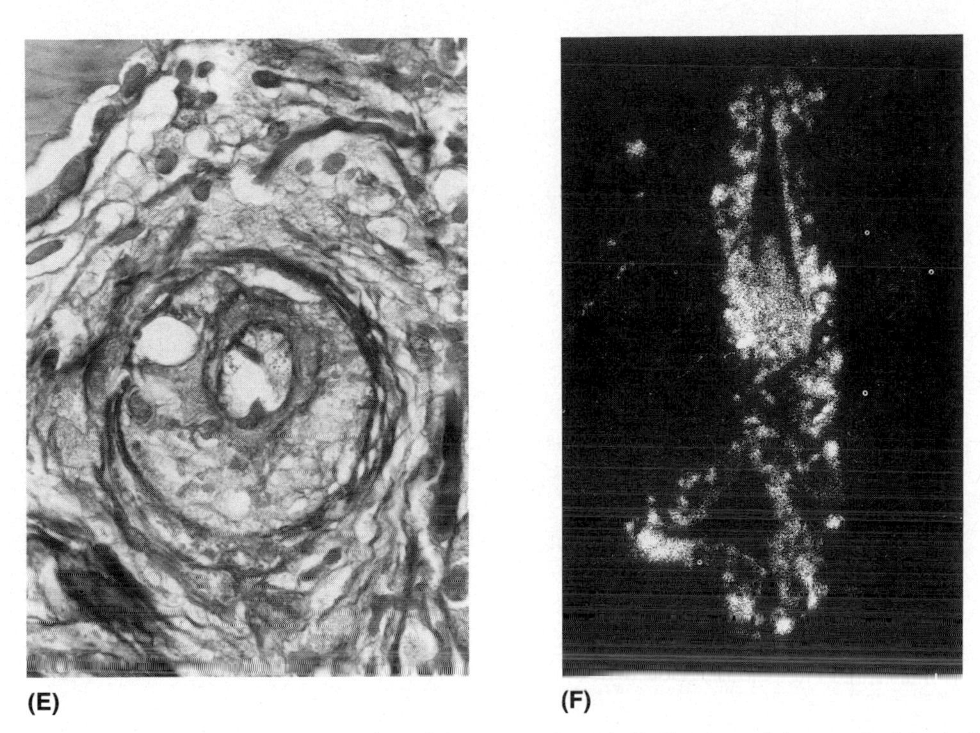

Figure 9 Cyclosporine-associated arteriolopathy. A through C. Circular nodular protein deposits in place of necrotic smooth muscle cells. (Acid fuchsin orange G, ×340–380.) D. Arteriolopathy with wall necrosis and fibrin/protein plugging of the lumen transgressing into the mucoid type of arteriolopathy (bottom). (Acid fuchsin orange G, ×380.) E. Arteriolopathy with mucoid thickening of the intima and necrosis of smooth muscle cells. (Acid fuchsin orange G, ×370.) F. Nodular complement (C3) deposits in the arteriolar wall. (Immunofluorescence microscopy, ×340.) (From Ref. 12.)

patients with kidney transplants but also in those with autoimmune disease without primary renal involvement. Tubular atrophy and interstitial fibrosis may be associated with any of the morphological lesions described earlier or may be found alone, which is most often the case in patients with autoimmune diseases. Intimal fibrosis may be seen in the arteries. Glomerular changes, mainly completely obsolescent glomeruli, are usually not prominent but become more common in patients with advanced interstitial fibrosis and tubular atrophy (110). An increase in the glomerular cross-sectional area of the remaining patent glomeruli is found with progressive glomerular obsolescence (150). Completely scarred arterioles or noncharacteristic arteriolar lesions may also be present.

3. Specificity of Lesions

The morphological lesions seen in vessels, glomeruli, and the tubulointerstitial space are nonspecific. The changes of cyclosporine-associated arteriolopathy are similar to those that may be found in advanced cases of thrombotic microangiopathy, independent of cyclosporine treatment. The differentiation of early cyclosporine-associated arteriolopathy from hypertensive or diabetic arteriolar hyalinosis is usually easy, owing to the presence of focal nodular deposits that are situated inside the intact smooth muscle cells in the latter (141), in comparison to the deposits in cyclosporine-associated arteriolopathy, which are circular and replace necrotic smooth muscle cells. In advanced cases of hypertensive or diabetic

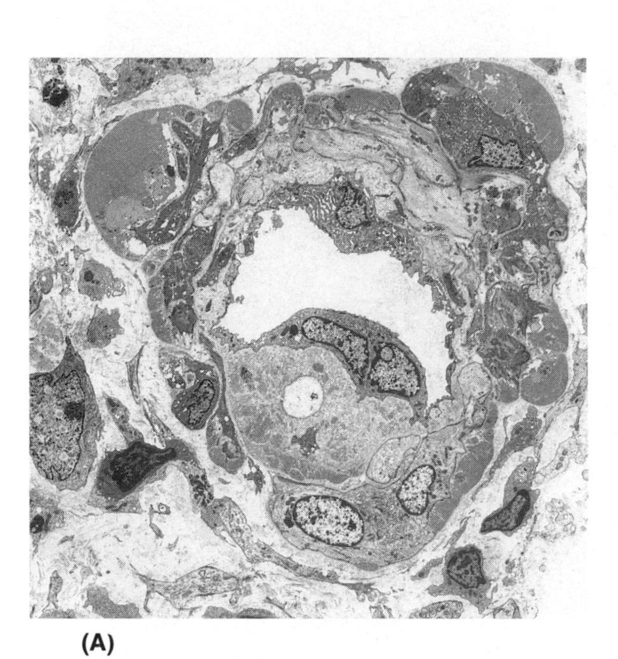

(A)

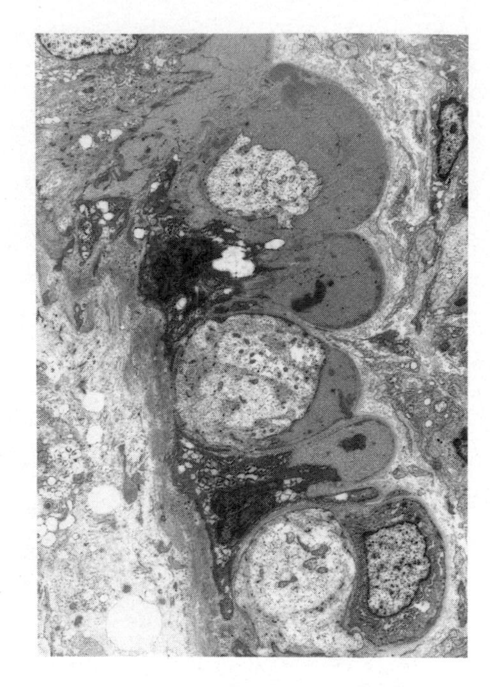

(B)

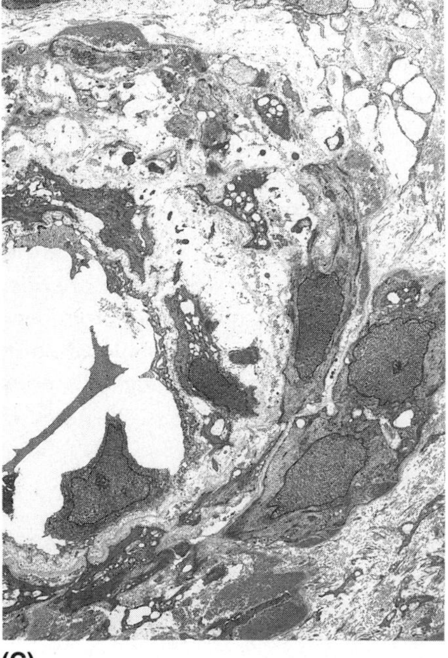

(C)

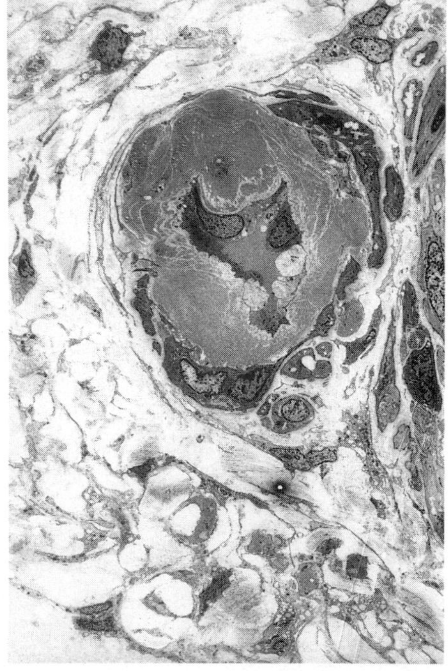

(D)

arteriolopathy or in the late stages of cyclosporine-associated arteriolopathy, differentiation by light microscopy may be difficult or even impossible. Because of the rarity of cyclosporine-associated arteriolopathy in patients with autoimmune diseases and the increased frequency of nonspecific arteriolar hyalinosis, the latter may be considered a forme fruste of the more typical cyclosporine-associated lesions.

Identification of cyclosporine-associated glomerulopathy is usually easy because of the consistent correlation with cyclosporine-associated arteriolopathy. In questionable cases, serial sections may be helpful to show the concurrence of cyclosporine-associated arteriolopathy in individual glomeruli. In cases in which the primary renal disease is a hemolytic-uremic syndrome or segmental focal glomerular sclerosis, correct interpretation of the glomerular lesions may be difficult or even impossible

Differentiation of cyclosporine-induced vascular-interstitial lesions from vascular lesions seen in transplant rejection may be extremely difficult (12,152). Depending on the stage of rejection, intravascular coagulation, proliferative or sclerosing vascular changes, or both may be present. Arterial lesions with arteritis predominate in acute rejection; if arteriolar lesions occur, they are always associated with lesions in the arteries. We have never observed acute rejection limited to the arterioles in transplant recipients receiving conventional treatment (151). Kidney transplant biopsy specimens showing fibrin thrombi limited to the arterioles, glomeruli, or both without any arterial lesions pose a special problem. In the case of concomitant arterial involvement or interstitial rejection, the thrombi are interpreted as most likely due to rejection. In the absence of arterial involvement, cyclosporine toxicity is considered to be the most likely diagnosis. However, many other factors are capable of causing similar changes (see "Differential Diagnosis," below). As a rule, predominant involvement of the arteries in patients with kidney transplants is usually attributable to rejection, whereas predominant involvement of the arterioles is more likely the result of cyclosporine toxicity. The determination of human leukocyte antigen class II expression on tubular epithelium is helpful in the differentiation between toxicity and rejection. In the former it is entirely negative; in the latter it is diffusely positive (152).

Interstitial fibrosis with tubular atrophy is also a nonspecific renal lesion. Numerous pathogenic causes result in this type of interstitial fibrosis. It should not be attributed to cyclosporine therapy unless other pathogenetic factors are excluded.

H. Prognosis of Cyclosporine Nephrotoxicity

It is clear that cyclosporine is capable of causing fixed morphological changes in the kidney and some degree of permanent renal functional impairment. Just as previous episodes of acute rejection are a risk factor for chronic rejection, so are previous episodes of acute cyclosporine nephrotoxicity a risk factor for chronic changes (153).

The key question in this area is whether cyclosporine leads to a progressive decline in

---

Figure 10 Cyclosporine-associated arteriolopathy in comparison with common arteriolar hyalinosis. A. Cyclosporine-associated arteriolopathy with circular nodular protein deposits replacing degenerated or necrotic smooth muscle cells. (×1400.) B. Part of the arteriolar wall: nodular protein deposits replace necrotic and pyknotic smooth muscle cells. (×2725.) C. Mucoid form of arteriolopathy with extensive necrosis of smooth muscle cells and small protein deposits along the periphery of the vessel wall. (×2160.) D. Severe arteriolar hyalinosis in hypertension. Subendothelial deposits are evident, but no smooth muscle cell necrosis is noted. (×2160.) (From Ref. 24.)

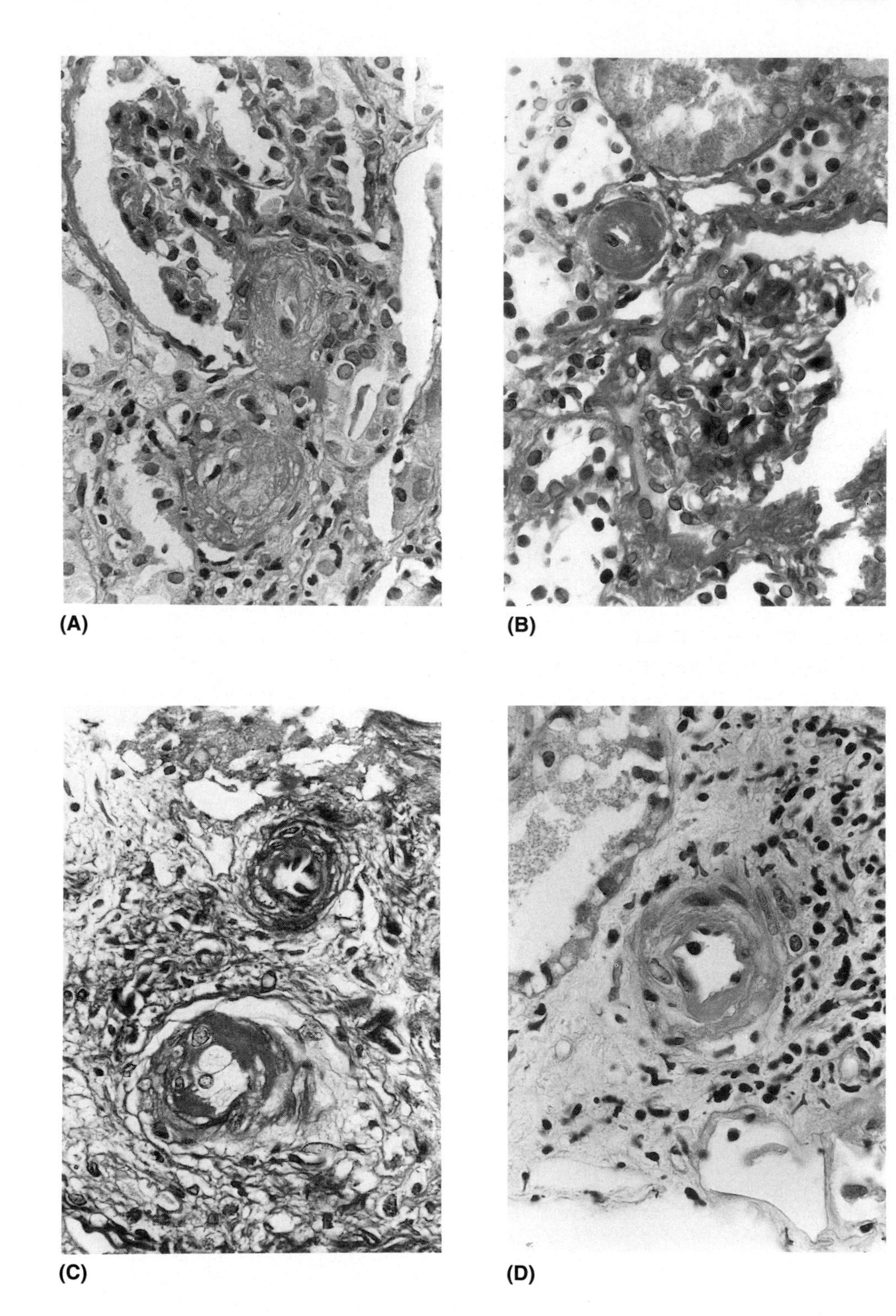
(A)
(B)
(C)
(D)

renal function culminating in end-stage renal failure, and, if it does, how frequently this occurs. Recent studies indicate that chronic renal insufficiency caused by cyclosporine is in most cases not progressive (153–157). Late rejection due to noncompliance or too low a dose of cyclosporine is a significantly greater risk factor for graft failure than is cyclosporine nephrotoxicity (153). In patients treated with cyclosporine for nonrenal transplants or autoimmune disease, there is usually an initial decline in renal function followed by stabilization after 6 months (154,155). In the personal series of Mihatsch et al., reviewing more than 100 nephrectomy specimens of renal grafts, only a single case of terminal renal failure that could be attributed entirely to cyclosporine toxicity was found. In none of 50 autopsy cases had cyclosporine toxicity caused terminal renal failure. Stopping the drug in transplant recipients is more harmful than continuing with the lowest possible dose. Of 20 kidney transplant recipients in the series of Mihatsch et al., 8 lost their grafts to rejection that developed after stopping the drug (148).

In summary, cyclosporine-associated arteriolopathy is a relatively benign lesion that is acceptable in patients with life-threatening diseases. The use of the lowest possible dose of cyclosporine will prevent the development of terminal renal insufficiency in most patients. In patients with non-life-threatening autoimmune diseases, it is hoped that strict adherence to the recommended doses and laboratory monitoring will prevent the development of serious renal insufficiency (158).

III. DIFFERENTIAL DIAGNOSIS: OTHER CAUSES OF THROMBOTIC MICROANGIOPATHY IN TRANSPLANTS

Many cases of thrombotic microangiopathy (TMA) in allograft recipients are not caused by cyclosporine at all or involve another etiological factor that is partially responsible. As a topic closely related to the discussion above, it is worth considering the other factors that can be responsible for thrombotic microangiopathy in transplant patients. These include cytomegalovirus (CMV) infection (159–160), AIDS (161), OKT3 treatment (162–164), recurrence of hemolytic uremic syndrome (164–166), malignant hypertension (167–168), antibody-mediated rejection (169–171), presence of lupus anticoagulant (172), sepsis (173), treatment with radiation (173–174), mitomycin C and other cancer chemotherapeutic agents (173–179), and FK506 (180–181).

Cytomegalovirus infection has been implicated as a factor predisposing the kidney to endothelial injury, leading to thrombotic microangiopathy (159–160). Hmiel et al. found that 60% of renal allograft recipients with thrombotic microangiopathy had evidence of simultaneous acute CMV infection (159). This association was stronger than the association with clinical cyclosporine toxicity. Symptomatic CMV infection was significantly more frequent in patients who subsequently developed thrombotic microangiopathy (160).

Figure 11 Chronologic changes of cyclosporine-associated arteriolopathy in repeat biopsy specimens in a patient with a renal transplant. A. Severe thrombotic necrotizing cyclosporine-associated arteriolopathy (second biopsy). B. Severe circular necrotizing cyclosporine-associated arteriolopathy (third biopsy). C. Irregular thickening of the vascular wall with hyalinosis 4 years after stopping cyclosporine (fourth biopsy). D. Remodeling of the vascular wall with minimal subendothelial protein deposits (fifth biopsy) more than 4 years after stopping cyclosporine. (Periodic acid-Schiff, ×300–450.) (From Ref. 23.)

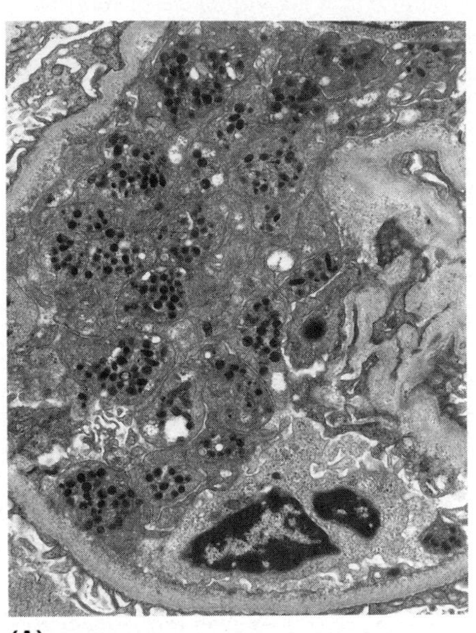

(A)

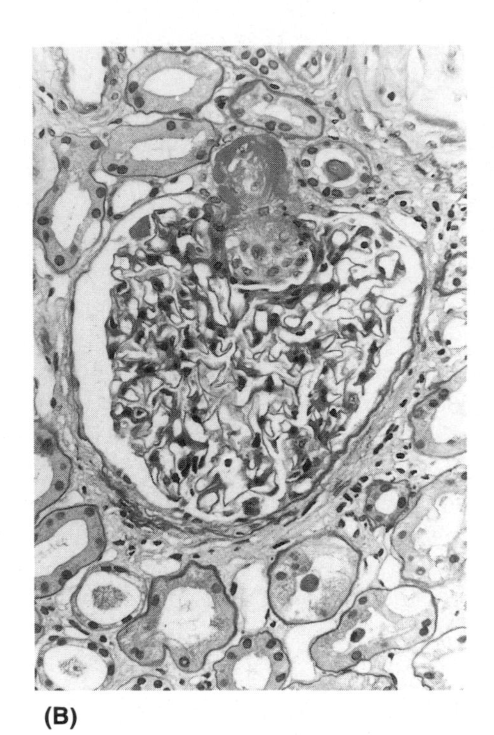

(B)

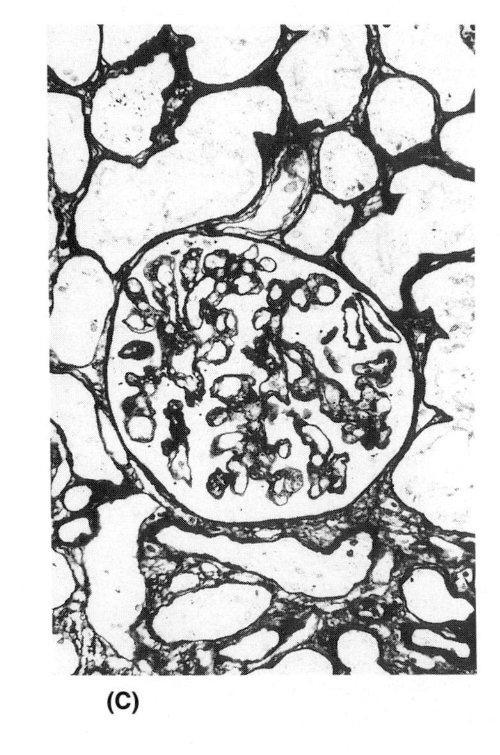

(C)

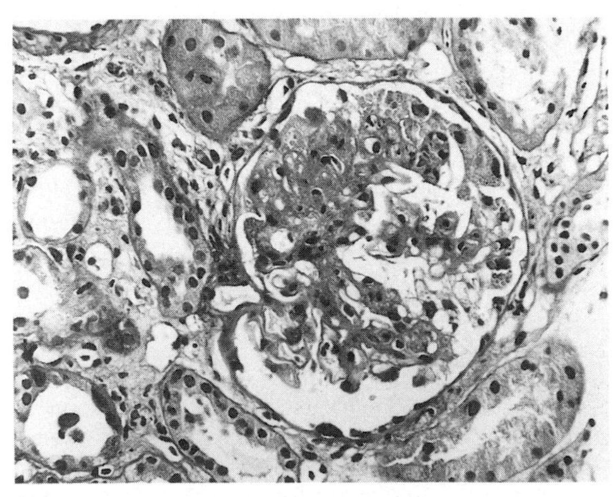

(D)

There is a single case report of thrombotic microangiopathy in a patient with subclinical AIDS infection (161).

Thrombotic microangiopathy has also been described as a side effect of OKT3 administration (162–164). Abramowicz et al. (162) reported that among 93 consecutive kidney transplant patients who received prophylactic OKT3 10 mg/day for 2 weeks, 9 had intragraft thromboses within 2 weeks of transplantation. The thromboses were in renal artery in 1 patient and in veins in 3. The remaining 5 patients had thromboses of glomerular capillaries and thrombotic microangiopathy similar to that seen in the hemolytic-uremic syndrome. All treatments failed, and the 9 grafts had to be removed. Plasma concentrations of prothrombin fragment 1 and 2 were higher 4 hr after the first OKT3 dose in OKT3 recipients than in transplant patients who received other prophylaxis, confirming that OKT3 has procoagulant effects in vivo. In another study, fibrin degradation products (FDP) and von Willebrand factor (VWF) antigen, a molecule released by activated or damaged endothelial cells, were also significantly increased after injection of OKT3. Tumor necrosis factor has been implicated in these procoagulant effects of OKT3 (163).

In patients whose original disease was hemolytic uremic syndrome, fulminant recurrence of the syndrome has been reported within 2 days of transplantation (164–165). Often there are several etiological factors all promoting the disorder, such as cyclosporine, OKT3, and recurrence (164,166). Malignant or accelerated hypertension as a complication of the underlying renal disease can lead to similar morphological changes in the renal allograft (167,168).

Rejection due to the late appearance of anti–class I antibody also frequently shows an appearance of thrombotic microangiopathy, with accumulation of polymorphs in peritubular capillaries and the presence of severe arteritis with fibrinoid change (169–171). Thrombotic microangiopathy and renal failure occur in a large proportion of bone marrow transplant recipients. Often the inciting factors are a combination of radiation damage, sepsis, and treatment with cytotoxic agents that injure the endothelium (173–179). The chemotherapeutic agent mitomycin C has a special propensity to cause thrombotic microangiopathy, which has been successfully treated with plasmapheresis (175–176). The new immunosuppressive agent FK506 has been reported to cause a thrombotic state resembling microangiopathy, similar to that seen with cyclosporine (see below) (180–182).

IV. FK-506 (TACROLIMUS) NEPHROTOXICITY

As discussed in the introduction to this chapter, the common mechanism of action of FK-506 and cyclosporine probably leads inevitably to similar nephrotoxicity (1–16, 183). Studies in liver transplant recipients suggest that FK506 is at least as nephrotoxic as cyclosporine (184–188). In a study comparing the hemodynamic responses to FK-506 and cyclosporine at 4 weeks (184), it was found that FK-506 produced as much or more renal

---

Figure 12 Different types of glomerular lesions. A. Platelet thrombus in a glomerular loop. (×6500.) B. So-called pouchlike lesion; complete necrosis of the afferent arteriole with fibrin deposits and slight proliferation at the vascular pole of undefined cells. (Periodic acid-Schiff, ×240.) C. Hemolytic-uremic syndrome–like glomerular lesion with extensive basement membrane doubling and thickening. (Periodic acid-Schiff-silver methenamine, ×240.) D. Early segmental glomerular sclerosis. (Periodic acid-Schiff, ×240.) (From Ref. 12.)

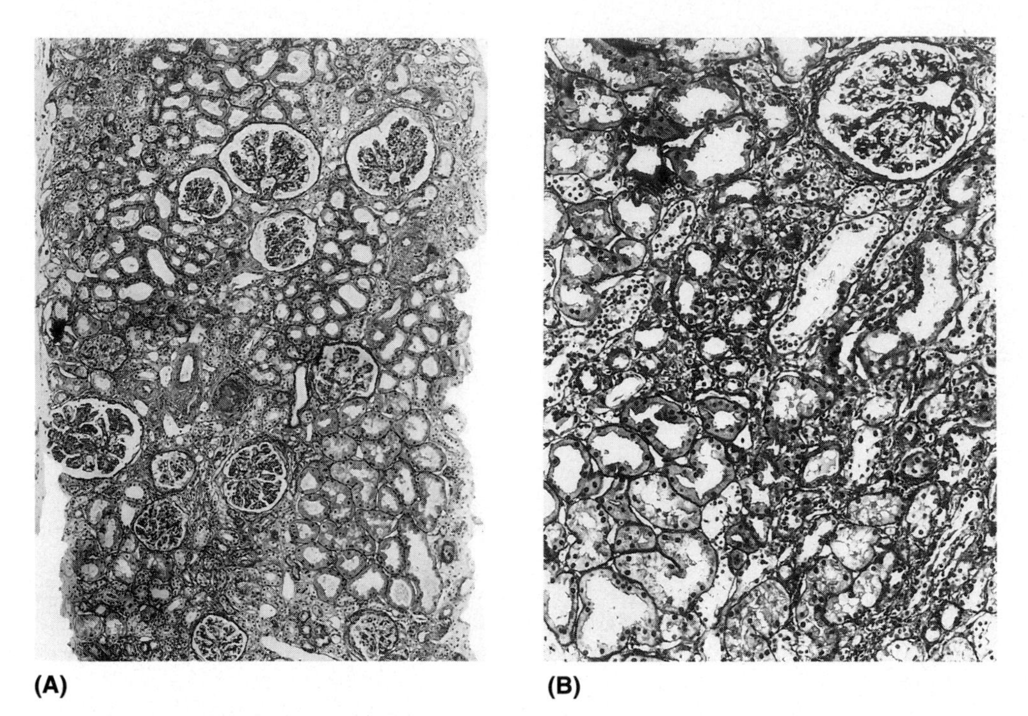

Figure 13 Striped form of interstitial fibrosis with tubular atrophy. Atrophic tubules with thickened basement membranes embedded in a fibrotic interstitium are adjacent to areas exhibiting normal tubules. A: acid fuchsin orange G, ×80; B: acid fuchsin orange G, ×150. (From Ref. 12.)

vasoconstriction as cyclosporine but was associated with less systemic vasoconstriction and less hypertension.

Morphological changes brought about by the two compounds are also quite parallel. Randhawa et al. (181) described tubular vacuolization, striped fibrosis, and arteriolar hyaline thickening as typical lesions in patients treated with FK-506. Focal glomerular sclerosis was observed in some patients, but it is not clear that this was a direct effect of the drug. Thrombotic microangiopathy and focal arteriolar fibrinoid change are also sometimes observed (see previous discussion) (180–182). Vascular smooth muscle cell vacuolization similar to that seen after administration of amphotericin or chemotherapeutic agents has also been described, along with peritubular calcification (181).

V. RAPAMYCIN NEPHROTOXICITY

It is not clear that rapamycin is nephrotoxic in human beings. In the rabbits treated for 60 days, hyaline arteriolar thickening, interstitial fibrosis, and tubular atrophy similar to that observed after cyclosporine treatment were found (189). The range of serum creatinine and the glomerular filtration rate (GFR) reported suggest that mild renal functional impairment may have occurred in occasional animals, but overall no significant effect on renal function could be documented. It is possible that in rodent models the diabetogenic effect of the drug causes glomerular hyperperfusion, thus obscuring any GFR-lowering effect (190). In Sprague-Dawley rats, rapamycin given for 14 days in a dose of 1.5 mg/kg/day produced a slight rise in serum creatinine on its own and significantly worsened the renal functional impairment brought about by cyclosporine 15 mg/kg/day (191). These effects in rats are strain- and dose-dependent (192,193). The current clinical trials in renal allograft patients will reveal whether these effects in animals have any relevance for humans (189).

VI. OKT3 NEPHROTOXICITY

Although OKT3 has no direct toxic effect on the kidney, it can induce renal failure by causing thrombotic microangiopathy through its procoagulant effect (162–164) (see above) or by producing a systemic capillary leak syndrome with consequent renal hypoperfusion (194–199). Both of these effects are probably due to release of tumor necrosis factor alpha and other cytokines (163,194–201).

The capillary leak syndrome is a particular feature of the reaction to the first dose of OKT3 and may be attenuated by concomitant administration of steroids, indomethacin, or pentoxifylline (196–199). There is a transient rise of creatinine averaging 57% during these reactions, accompanied by increased shedding of tubular cells in the urine (195). In addition to tumor necrosis factor, interleukin-2, and gamma-interferon release, complement activation is also believed to play a role (201). The renal morphology has not been well studied, but one would expect to see changes of prerenal azotemia with juxtaglomerular apparatus hyperplasia but few other morphologic changes. However, it is now known how often these first-dose reactions are accompanied by subtle microthrombotic changes, representing a form fruste of the more overt thrombotic microangiopathy changes sometimes seen later in the course of OKT3 treatment (162–164).

The higher peak serum creatinine during renal allograft rejection episodes treated with OKT3 is attributed to the combined effects of the microthrombotic and first-dose effects of OKT3 (202–203). The availability of humanized, more specific anti-T-cell monoclonal antibodies (204–205) should, in the future, eliminate the side effects currently experienced with OKT3.

REFERENCES

1. Flanagan WM, Corthesy B, Bram RJ, Crabtree GR. Nuclear association of a T-cell transcription factor blocked by FK506 and cyclosporin A. Nature 1991; 352:803–806.
2. Liu J, Farmer JD, Lane WS, et al. Calcineurin is a common target of cyclophilin-cyclosporin A and FKBP-FK506 complexes. Cell 1991; 66:807–815.
3. Fruman D, Klee C, Brierer B, Burakoff S. Calcineurin phosphatase activity in T lymphocytes is inhibited by FK506 and cyclosporin A. Proc Natl Acad Sci USA 1992; 89:3686–3690.
4. Lyson T, Ermel LD, Belshaw PJ, et al. Cyclosporine- and FK506-induced sympathetic activation correlates with calcineurin-mediated inhibition of T-cell signalling. Circ Res 1993; 73:596–602.
5. McDiarmid SV, Colonna JO II, Shakad A, et al. A comparison of renal function in cyclosporine- and FK506-treated patients after primary orthotopic liver transplantation. Transplantation 1993; 56:847–853.
6. Mihatsch MJ, Thiel G, Spichtin HP, et al. Morphological findings in kidney transplants after treatment with cyclosporine. Transplant Proc 1983; 15:2821–2835.
7. Racusen LC, Solez K. Cyclosporine nephrotoxicity. In: GW Richter, K Solez, eds. International Review of Experimental Pathology, Vol 30. San Diego: Academic Press, 1988:107.
8. Bergstrand A, Bohman SO, Farnsworth A, et al. Renal histopathology in kidney transplant recipients immunosuppressed with cyclosporin A. Clin Nephrol 1995; 24:107–119.

9. Kahan BD. Cyclosporine: the agent and its actions. Transplant Proc 1985; 17:5–18.
10. Remuzzi G, Bertani T. Renal vascular and thrombotic effects of cyclosporine. Am J Kidney Dis 1989; 13:261–272.
11. Zachariae H, Hansen HE, Kragballe K, Olsen S. Morphologic renal changes during cyclosporine treatment of psoriasis: studies on pretreatment and posttreatment kidney biopsy specimens. J Am Acad Dermatol 1992; 26(3 pt 2):415–419.
12. Mihatsch MJ, Ryffel B, Gudat F, Thiel G. Cyclosporine nephropathology. In: CC Tisher, BM Brenner, eds. Renal Pathology: With Clinical and Functional Correlations, 2d ed. Philadelphia: Lippincott, 1994:1641–1681.
13. Demetris AJ, Banner B, Fung J, et al. Histopathology of human renal allograft rejection under FK506: a comparison with cyclosporine. Transplant Proc 1991; 23:944–946.
14. Alessiani M, Cillo U, Fung JJ, et al. Adverse effects of FK506 overdosage after liver transplantation. Transplant Proc 1993; 25:628–634.
15. Textor SC, Wiesner R, Wilson DJ, et al. Systemic and renal hemodynamic differences between FK506 and cyclosporine in liver transplant recipients. Transplantation (US) 1993; 55:1332–1339.
16. Andoh TF, Burdmann EA, Lindsley J, et al. Enhancement of FK506 nephrotoxicity by sodium depletion in an experimental rat model. Transplantation (US) 1994; 57:483–489.
17. Krupp P, Gulich A, Timoren P. Side effects and safety of Sandimmune in long-term treatment of renal transplant. Transplant Proc 1986; 18:991.
18. Rossi SJ, Schroeder TJ, Hariharan S, First MR. Prevention and management of the adverse effects associated with immunosuppressive therapy (review). Drug Safety 1993; 9:104–131.
19. Mihatsch MJ, Antonovych T, Bohman SO, et al. Cyclosporin A nephropathy: standardization of the evaluation of kidney biopsies. Clin Nephrol (Germany) 1994; 41:23–32.
20. Mihatsch MJ, Thiel G, Ryffel B. Morphology of cyclosporin nephropathy. Prog Allergy 1986; 38:447–465.
21. Feutren G, Mihatsch MJ. Risk factors for development of cyclosporine-associated nephropathy in patients with autoimmune or inflammatory diseases. N Engl J Med 1992; 326:1654–1660.
22. Mihatsch MJ, Steiner K, Abegwickrama KH, et al. Risk factors for the development of vascular interstitial nephrotoxicity after cyclosporin. Clin Nephrol 1988; 29:165–175.
23. Morozumi K, Thiel G, Albert FW, et al. Studies on morphological outcome of cyclosporine-associated arteriolopathy after discontinuation of cyclosporine in renal allografts. Clin Nephrol (Germany) 1992; 38:1–8.
24. Mihatsch MJ, Thiel G, Basler V, et al. Morphologic patterns in cyclosporin A treated renal transplant recipients. Transplant Proc 1985; 17(suppl 1):101–116.
25. Ulrich W. Morphologiw von Nierentransplantaten. Wien, Springer-Verlag, 1986.
26. Kiss D, Landmann J, Mihatsch M, et al. Risks and benefits of graft biopsy in renal transplantation under cyclosporin-A. Clin Nephrol 1992; 38:132–134.
27. Mihatsch MJ. Selectivity has still its price: personal experiences with cyclosporine (Sandimmune) over the last 10 years. Transplant Proc 1992; 24(4 suppl 2):67–70.
28. Neild GH, Reuben R, Hartley RB, Cameron JS. Glomerular thrombi in renal allografts associated with cyclosporin treatment. J Clin Pathol 1985; 38:253–258.
29. Leithner C, Schwarz M, Sinzinger H, Ulrich W. Limited value of 111-indium platelet scintigraphy in renal transplant patients receiving cyclosporin. Clin Nephrol 1986; 25:141–148.
30. Strøm EH, Thiel G, Mihatsch MJ. Prevalence of cyclosporine-associated arteriolopathy in renal transplant biopsies from 1981 to 1992. Transplant Proc 1994; 26:2585–2587.
31. Thiel G. The use of cyclosporin blood level measurements in renal transplantation. In: Cyclosporin, Proceedings of a Workshop, Oxford, Medical Education Services, 1986:12–19.
32. Palestine AG, Austin HA III, Balow JE, et al. Renal histopathologic alterations in patients treated with cyclosporin for uveitis. N Engl J Med 1986; 314:1293–1298.

33. Svenson K, Bohman SO. Cyclosporin-associated nephropathy in patients with autoimmune diseases. Klin Wochenschr 1988; 66:43–47.
34. Mihatsch MJ, Helmchen U, Casanova P, et al. Kidney biopsy findings in Cyclosporine-treated patients with insulin-dependent diabetes mellitus. Klin Wochenschr 1991; 69:354–359.
35. Feutren G. Functional consequences and risk factors of chronic cyclosporin nephrotoxicity in type I diabetes trials. In: Kahan BD, ed. Cyclosporin. Vol 4. Orlando, FL: Grune & Stratton, 1988:356–365.
37. Myers BD, Ross J, Newton L, et al. Cyclosporin associated chronic nephropathy. N Engl J Med 1984; 311:699–705.
38. Myers BD. Cyclosporine nephrotoxicity. Kidney Int. 1986; 30:964–974.
39. Yee GC, Kennedy MS, Deeg HJ, et al. Cyclosporine-associated renal dysfunction in marrow transplant recipients. Transplant Proc 1985; 17(suppl 1):196.
40. Iwatsuki S, Esquivel CO, Klintmalm GBG, et al. Nephrotoxicity of cyclosporin in liver transplantation. Transplant Proc 1985; 17:191.
41. Stahl RAK, Kanz I, Maier B, Schollmeyer P. Hyperchloremic metabolic acidosis with high serum potassium in renal transplant recipients: a cyclosporine A associated side effect. Clin Nephrol 1986; 25:245–248.
42. Adu D, Turney J, Michael J, McMaster P. Hyperkalaemia in cyclosporin-treated renal allograft recipients. Lancet 1983; 2:370–372.
43. Foley RJ, Hamner RW, Weinmann EJ. Serum potassium concentrations in cyclosporine- and azathioprine-treated renal transplant patients. Nephron 1985; 40:280–295.
44. June CH, Thompson CB, Kennedy MS, et al. Profound hypomagnesemia and renal magnesium wasting associated with the use of cyclosporine for marrow transplantation. Transplantation 1985; 39:620–624.
45. June CH, Thompson CB, Kennedy MS, Loughran TP. Correlation of hypomagnesemia with the onset of cyclosporine-associated hypertension in marrow transplant patients. Transplantation 1986; 41:47–51.
46. Thompson CB, June CH, Sullivan KM, Thomas ED. Association between cyclosporin neurotoxicity and hypomagnesaemia. Lancet 1984; 2:1116–1120.
47. Cohen SL, Boner G, Rosenfeld JB, et al. Hyperuricaemia in cyclosporin treated renal transplant recipients. Transplant Proc 1982; 19:1829–1830.
48. Siamopoulos KC, Drosos AA, Moutsopoulos HN, Mihatsch MJ. Renal pathology after low dose cyclosporin (CyA) in patients with primary Sjögren's syndrome. In: Andreucci VE, Dal Canton A, eds. Current Therapy in Nephrology. Boston, Kluwer, 1989:551–553.
49. Sibley RK, Rynasiewicz J, Ferguson RM, et al. Morphology of cyclosporine nephrotoxicity and acute rejection in patients immunosuppressed with cyclosporin and prednisone. Surgery 1983; 94:225–235.
50. Solez K, Kramer EC, Fox JA, Heptinstall RH. Medullary plasma flow and intravascular leukocyte accumulation in acute renal failure. Kidney Int. 1974; 6:24–37.
51. Opelz G. Multicenter impact of cyclosporin on cadaver kidney graft survival. Prog Allergy 1986; 38:329–345.
52. Keown PA, Stiller CR, Wallace AC. Nephrotoxicity of cyclosporin A. In: Williams GM, Burdick JF, Solez K, eds. Kidney Transplant Rejection. New York; Marcel Dekker, 1986: 423–457.
53. Landmann J, Thiel G, Harder F. Einfluss der Ischämiezeiten auf die Funktion von Leichennierentransplantaten. Helv Chir Acta 1985; 52:91–95.
54. Belitski P (for the Canadian Transplant Study Group). Initial non-function of cyclosporine treated cadaver renal allografts preserved by simple cold storage. Transplant Proc 1985; 17:1485–1488.
55. Goldstein J, Thoua Y, Wellens F, et al. Cyclosporine nephropathy after heart and heart-lung transplantation. In Davison AM, Guillou PJ, eds. Proceedings, European Dialysis and Trans-

plant Association—European Renal Association. Vol. 21. London: Pitman Press, 1985: 973–981.
56. Novick AC, Ho-Shieh H, Steinmuller D, et al. Detrimental effect of cyclosporine on initial function of cadaver renal allografts following extended preservation. Transplantation 1986; 42:154–158.
57. Greenberg A, Egel JW, Thompson ME, et al. Early and late forms of cyclosporin nephrotoxicity: studies in cardiac transplant recipients. Am J Kidney Dis 1987; 9:12–22.
58. Solez K, Racusen LC, Marcussen N, et al. Morphology of ischemic acute renal failure, normal function, and cyclosporine toxicity in cyclosporine-treated renal allograft recipients. Kidney Int. 1993; 43:1058–1067.
59. Farnsworth A, Hall BM, Kirwan P, et al. Pathology in renal transplant patients treated with cyclosporin. Transplant Proc 1983; 15:636–638.
60. Farnsworth A, Hall BM, Ng ABP, et al. Renal biopsy morphology in renal transplantation: A comparative study of the light microscopic appearances of biopsies from patients treated with cyclosporin A or azathioprine, predisone and antilymphocyte globulin. Am J Surg Pathol 1984; 8:243–252.
61. Klintmalm GBG, Ivatsuki S, Starzl TE. Nephrotoxicity of cyclosporin A in liver and kidney transplant. Lancet 1981; 1:470–471.
62. Hall BM, Tiller DJ, Duggin GG, et al. Post-transplant acute renal failure in cadaver renal recipients treated with cyclosporine. Kidney Int. 1985; 28:178–186.
63. Farnsworth A, Hall BM, Duggin GG, et al. Interstitial fibrosis in renal allografts in patients treated with cyclosporin. Lancet 1984; 2:1470–1471.
64. Zollinger HU. Anurie bei Chromoproteinurie. Stuttgart: Thieme, 1952.
65. Bohle A, Jahnecke J, Meyer D, Schubert GE. Morphology of acute renal failure: comparative data from biopsy and autopsy. Kidney Inst. 1976; 10:9–16.
66. Hoyer PF, Brodehl J, Byrd DJ, et al. Effect of cyclosporin on the renal tubular amino acid handling after kidney transplantation. Transplant 1988; 46:73–78.
67. Palestine AG, Austin HA III, Nussenblatt RB. Renal tubular function in cyclosporine treated patients. Am J Med 1986; 81:419–424.
68. Cantarovich F, Lardet G, Monti I, et al. Diagnostic role of urinary enzymes in renal transplant monitoring. Transplant Proc 1986; 18:1042–1044.
69. Loerstcher R, Scholer A, Brunner F, et al. Klinische Relevanz der N-Acetyl-Glukosaminidase-Bestimmung im Urine bei Nierentransplantatempfängem mit und ohne Cyclosporin A. Schwiez Med Wochenschr 1982; 112:1658–1664.
70. Shen SY, Weir MR, Litkowski I, et al. Enzyme-linked immunosorbent assay for serum renal tubular antigen in kidney transplant patients. Transplantation 1985; 40:642–647.
71. Wurster U, Patzold U, Ehrich JHH. Assessment of enzymuria in multiple sclerosis patients treated with cyclosporin A. In: Bach PH, Lock Ea, eds. Proceedings of the 2nd International Symposium on Nephrotoxicity. Chichester, England: Wiley, 1985:457–460.
72. Bäckman L, Appelkvist EL, Ringdén O, Dallner G. Glutathione transferase in the urine: a marker for post-transplant tubular lesions. Kidney Int 1988; 33:571–577.
73. Berg KJ, Førre Ø, Bjerkhoel F, et al. Side effects of cyclosporin A treatment in patients with rheumatoid arthritis. Kidney Int. 1986; 29:1180–1187.
74. Berg KJ, Førre Ø, Djøseland Ø, et al. Renal side effects of high and low cyclosporine A doses in patients with rheumatoid arthritis. Clin Nephrol 1989; 31:232–238.
75. Tolkoff-Rubin NE, Cosimi AB, Delmonico FI, et al. Monitoring of renal proximal tubular injury in transplantation with a monoclonal antibody-based assay for the adenosine deaminase binding protein. Transplant Proc 1986; 18:716–718.
76. Keown PA, Stiller CR, Wallace AC. Nephrotoxicity of cycloporin A. In: Burdick JF, Racusen LC, Solez K, Williams GM, eds. Kidney Transplant Rejection: Diagnosis and Treatment, 2d ed. New York: Marcel Dekker, 1992.

77. Marbet UA, Graf U, Mihatsch MJ, et al. Renale Nebenwirkungen der Therapie mit Cyclosporin-A bei der chronischen Polyarthritis und nach Knochenmarktransplantation. Schweiz Med Wochenschr 1980; 110:2017–2020.
78. Chomette G, Auriol M, Beaufils H, et al. Les lésions renales provoquées par la cyclosporine. Ann Pathol 1986; 6:29–36.
79. Mihatsch MJ, Olivieri V, Marbet U, et al. Giant mitochondria in renal tubular cells and cyclosporin-A. Lancet 1982; 1:1162.
80. Willebrand VE, Häyry P, Ahonen J. Differential diagnosis of cyclosporin nephrotoxicity versus rejection on fine needle aspiration biopsy. Kidney Int. 1983; 24:418.
81. O'Brien JP, Horsburgh T, Veitch P, Bell PRF. Experience with fine needle aspiration biopsies from renal transplant patients on different immunosuppressive regimens. Transplant Proc 1985; 17:2089–2090.
82. Santelli G, Ouziala M, Charpentier B, Fries D. Predictive value of fine needle aspiration biopsy for cyclosporine nephrotoxicity. Transplant Proc 1985; 17:2094–2095.
83. Egidi F, de Vecchi A, Pagliari B, et al. Lack of relationship between blood cyclosporine levels and nephrotoxicity as assessed by fine needle aspiration biopsy of renal allografts. Transplant Proc 1985; 17:2096–2097.
84. Baumgartner D, Burger HR, Binswanger U, Largiader F. Routine fine needle aspiration biopsy adds clinically relevant information for evaluation and treatment of renal transplant recipients with primary oliguria. Transplant Proc 1985; 17(suppl 5):2080–2082.
85. Jarck HU, Block T, Hammer C, Bernheim C. Immunosuppressive and nephrotoxic effect of cyclosporin A and ALG in renal allotransplantation. Langenbecks Arch Chir 1983; 359: 189–193.
86. Stella F, Troccoli R, Stella C, et al. Urinary cytologic abnormalities in bone marrow transplant recipients of cyclosporin. Acta Cytol 1987; 31:615–619.
87. Klima G, Spielberger M, Konig P, Margreiter R. Fine needle aspiration biopsy and urinary sediment cytology in renal allograft recipients. Transplant Proc 1985; 17(suppl 5):2083–2084.
88. Winkelmann M, Bürig KF, Koldowsky U, et al. Cyclosporin-A altered renal tubular cells in urinary cytology. Lancet 1985; 2:667.
89. Cortesini R, Stella F, Renna Molajoni E, et al. Urinary exfoliative cytology in kidney allografts under cyclosporin therapy. Transplant Proc 1984; 16:1200–1201.
90. Scheuer PJ. Liver Biopsy Interpretation, 3d ed. London, Baillière Tindall, 1978.
91. Verani RR, Fletcher SM, Van Buren CT, Kahan BD. Acute cellular rejection or cyclosporin A nephrotoxicity? A review of transplant renal biopsies. Am J Kidney Dis 1984; 4:185–191.
92. Suzuki T, Furusato M, Takasaki S, Ishikava E. Giant mitochondria in the epithelial cells of the proximal convoluted tubules of diseased human kidneys. Lab Invest 1975; 33:578–590.
93. Chedid A, Jao W, Port J. Megamitochondria in hepatic and renal disease. Am J Gastroenterol 1980; 73:319–324.
94. Kirwan PD. Giant mitochondria and multiple cilia in proximal convoluted tubules of renal transplant patients receiving cyclosporin-A immunosuppression. Micron 1982; 13:353–354.
95. Diomi P, Ericsson JLE, Matheson NA, Shearer JR. Studies on renal tubular morphology and toxicity after large doses of dextran 40 in the rabbit. Lab Invest 1970; 22:355–360.
96. Rohr HP, Zollinger HU. Die sogennnante Zuckerspeicherniere unter besonderer Berücksichtigung elektronenoptisch-autoradiographischer Untersuchungen mit ^{14}C-Saccharose. Virchows Arch (a) 1966; 341:115–122.
97. Moreau JF, Droz D, Subato J, et al. Osmotic nephroses induced by water soluble tri-iodinated contrast media in man. Radiology 1975; 115:329–336.
98. Schwartz SL, Johnson CB. Pinocytosis as the cause of sucrose nephrosis. Nephron 1971; 8:246–254.
99. Brunner FP, Hermle M, Mihatsch MJ, Thiel G. Mannitol potentiates cyclosporin nephrotoxicity. Clin Nephrol 1986; 25:130–136.

100. Mihatsch MJ, Thiel G, Ryffel B. Hazards of cyclosporine A therapy and recommendations for its use. J Autoimmun 1988; 1:533–543.
101. Ryffel B, Müller AM, Mihatsch MJ. Experimental cyclosporine nephrotoxicity: Risk of concomitant chemotherapy. Clin Nephrol 1986; 25:121–125.
102. Bennett WM. Comparison of cyclosporine nephrotoxicity with aminoglycoside nephrotoxicity. Clin Nephrol 1986; 25:126–129.
103. Mihatsch MJ, Ryffel B, Hemle M, et al. Morphology of cyclosporine nephrotoxicity in the rat. Clin Nephrol 1986; 25:2–8.
104. Thiel G, Mihatsch MJ. Morphologic findings in "zero-hour" biopsies of renal transplants. Clin Nephrol 1991; 36:215–222.
105. Burke MD, Whiting PH. The role of drug metabolism in cyclosporin A nephrotoxicity. Clin Nephrol 1986; 25:111–116.
106. Ryffel B, Porter G. Nephrotoxicity versus benefit to mankind: lessons from the history of development of cyclosporine. In: Solez K, Racusen L, Dekker M, eds. Acute Renal Failure. New York: Marcel Dekker, 1991:227–231.
107. Svenson K, Bohman SO, Hällgren R. Clinical effects and renal side effects in patients with autoimmune disease treated with cyclosporin A. In: Schindler LR, ed. Cyclosporin in Autoimmune Disease: First International Symposium. Berlin: Springer-Verlag, 1985.
108. Svenson K, Bohman SO, Hällgren R. Renal interstitial fibrosis and vascular changes. Arch Intern Med 1986; 146:2007–2010.
109. Kabalan S, Dische FE, Neild GH, et al. Cyclosporin A nephrotoxicity: comparison of biopsy histological findings in renal transplant patients treated with cyclosporin A or azathioprine. In: Davison AM, Guillou PJ, eds. Proceedings, European Dialysis and Transplant Association—European Renal Association, 22nd Congress, Brussels, June 25–29, 1985. London: Baillière Tindall, 1985:540–545.
110. Myers BD, Newton L. Cyclosporin-induced chronic nephropathy: an obliterative microvascular renal injury. J Am Soc Nephrol 1991; 2(2 suppl 1):S45–S52.
111. Myers BD, Newton L, Boshkos CH, et al. Chronic injury of human renal microvessels with low-dose cyclosporin therapy. Transplantation 1988; 46:694–703.
112. Dieterle A, Gratwohl A, Nizze H, et al. Chronic cyclosporin-associated nephrotoxicity in bone marrow transplant patients. Transplantation 1990; 49:1093–1100.
113. Clasen W, Kindler J, Mihatsch MJ, Sieberth HG. Long-term treatment of minimal change nephrotic syndrome with cyclosporine: a control biopsy study. Nephrol Dial Transplant 1988; 3:733–737.
114. Hors J, Mihatsch MJ, Paillard M, et al. Factors associated with early remission of type 1 diabetes in children treated with cyclosporin. N Engl J Med 1988; 318:663–670.
115. Thiel G, Mihatsch MJ, Landmann J, et al. Is cyclosporin A induced nephrotoxicity in recipients of renal allografts progressive? Transplant Proc 1985; 17(suppl 1):169–175.
116. Huser B, Lämmle B, Tran TH, et al. Blutungsneigung von Nierentransplantatträgem unter Cyclosporin A? Schwiez Med Wochenschr 1984; 114:1397.
117. Varenterghem Y, Roels L, Lerut T, et al. Thromboembolic complications and haemostatic changes in cyclosporin-treated cadaveric kidney allograft recipients. Lancet 1985; 1:999–1002.
118. Brown Z, Neild GH, Willoughby JJ, et al. Increased factor VIII as an index of vascular injury in cyclosporine nephrotoxicity. Transplantation 1986; 42:150–153.
119. Cohen H, Neild GH, Patel R, et al. Evidence for chronic platelet hyperaggregability and in vivo activation in cyclosporin-treated renal allograft recipients. Thromb Res 1988; 49:91–101.
120. Grace AA, Barradas MA, Mikhailidis DP, et al. Cyclosporin A enhances platelet aggregation. Kidney Int 1987; 32:889–895.
121. Nyberg G, Sandberd L, Rydberg L. ABO autoimmune hemolytic anemia in a renal transplant patient treated with cyclosporin A: case report. Transplantation 1984; 37:529–530.
122. Leithner C, Sinzinger H, Pohanka E, et al. Occurrence of haemolytic uremic syndrome under

cyclosporin treatment: Accident or possible side effect mediated by a lack of prostacylin-stimulating plasma factor? Transplant Proc 1983; 15:2787–2789.
123. Wolfe JA, McCann RL, Sanfilippo F. Cyclosporine-associated microangiopathy in renal transplantation: a severe but potentially reversible form of early graft injury. Transplantation 1986; 41:541–544.
124. Berden JHM, Netten P, van Liessum PA, et al. Hemolytic-uremic syndrome during cyclosporine immunosuppression in renal allograft recipients. Clin Transplant 1987; 1:246–252.
125. Buturovic J, Kandus A, Malovrh M, et al. Cyclosporin-associated hemolytic-uremic syndrome in four renal allograft recipients: resolution without specific therapy. Transplant Proc 1990; 22:1726–1727.
126. Fago A, Hakim RC, Sagiura M, et al. Severe endothelial injury in a renal transplant patient receiving cyclosporin. Transplantation 1990; 49:1190–1192.
127. Yoshimura N, Oka T, Ohmori Y, et al. Cyclosporin-associated microangiopathic bemolytic anemia in a renal transplant recipient. Jpn J Surg 1989; 19:223–228.
128. Bonser RS, Adu D, Franklin L, McMaster P. Cyclosporin induced haemolytic uraemic syndrome in liver allograft recipient. Lancet 1984; 2:1337.
129. Shulman H, Striker G, Deeg HJ, Kennedy M, Storb R, Thomas ED. Nephrotoxicity of cyclosporin A after allogeneic marrow transplantation. N Engl J Med 1981; 305:1392–1395.
130. Gluckman E, Arcese W, Devergie A, Boiron M. Cyclosporin-A prophylactic treatment of graft-versus-host disease in human allogeneic bone marrow transplantation: preliminary results. Transplant Proc 1981; 13:368–370.
131. Biggs JC, Atkinson K, Hayes J, et al. After allogeneic bone marrow transplantation cyclosporin A is associated with faster engraftment, less mucositis and three distinct syndromes of nephrotoxicity when compared to methotrexate. Transplant Proc 1983; 15:1487–1489.
132. Atkinson K, Biggs JC, Hayes J, et al. Cyclosporin A–associated nephrotoxicity in the first 100 days after allogenic bone marrow transplantation: three distinct syndromes. Br J Haematol 1983; 54:59–67.
133. Hows JM, Chipping PM, Fairhead S, et al. Nephrotoxicity in bone marrow transplant recipients treated with cyclosporin-A. Br J Haematol 1983; 5:69–78.
134. Mackenzie JC, Lumley HS, Hughes RG, et al. Haemolytic uraemic syndrome in bone marrow transplantation. Exp Haematol 1983; 11:18.
135. Powles RL, Kay HEM, Clink HM, et al. Mismatched family donors for bone marrow transplantation as treatment of acute leukaemia. Lancet 1983; 1:612–615.
136. Powles RL, Evans B, Poole C, et al. Cyclosporin for the prevention of graft-versus-host disease in 72 patients with acute myeloblastic leukaemia in first remission receiving matched sibling bone marrow transplants. Transplant Proc 1983; 15:2624–2627.
137. Cohen H, Bull HA, Seddon A, et al. Vascular endothelial cell function and ultrastructure in thrombotic microangiopathy following allogenic bone marrow transplantation. Eur J Haematol 1989; 43:207–214.
138. Chappell ME, Keeling DM, Prentice HG, Sweny P. Haemolytic uraemic syndrome after bone marrow transplantation: an adverse effect of total body irradiation? Bone Marrow Transplant 1988; 3:339–347.
139. Beaufils H, de Groc F, Gubler MC, et al. Hemolytic uremic syndrome in patients with Behçet's disease treated with cyclosporine A: report of 2 cases. Clin Nephrol 1990; 34:157–162.
140. Landmann J, Mihatsch MJ, Ratschek M, Thiel G. Cyclosporin A and intravascular coagulation. Transplant Proc 1987; 19:1817–1819.
141. Banfi G, Tarantino A, Fogazzi GB, et al. Significance of vascular lesions in cyclosporine treated renal transplants. Kidney Int. 1985; 28:392.
142. Stoffner D, Castro LA, Hillebrand G, et al. Über die chronische Nephrotoxizität von Cyclosporin nach Nierentransplantation (lanzeituntersuchung im Vergleich mit Azaothioprin-behandelten Patienten). Nieren Hockdruckkrankeit 1986; 15:145–148.

143. Nizze H, Mihatsch MJ, Zollinger HU, et al. Cyclosporin-associated nephropathy in patients with heart and bone marrow transplants. Clin Nephrol 1988; 30:248–260.
144. Dische FE, Neuberger J, Keating J, et al. Kidney pathology in liver allograft recipients after long-term treatment with cyclosporine A. Lab Invest 1988; 58:395–402.
145. Austin HA III, Palestine AG, Sabnis SG, et al. Evolution of cyclosporin nephrotoxicity in patients treated for autoimmune uveitis. Am J Nephrol 1989; 9:392–402.
146. Mihatsch MJ, Beghiti D, Bohman SO, et al. Kidney biopsies in control or cyclosporin A-induced psoriatic patients. Br J Dermatol 1990; 122(suppl 36):95–100.
147. Sommer BG, Jeffrey TT, Whitehurst RM, et al. Cyclosporine-associated renal arteriolopathy results in loss of allograft function. Am J Surg 1985; 149:756–764.
148. Morozumi K, Thiel G, Albert FW, et al. Studies on morphological outcome of cyclosporine associated arteriolopathy after discontinuation of cyclosporine in renal allograft. Clin Nephrol 1992; 38:1–8.
149. Morozumi K, Gudat F, Thiel G, Mihatsch MJ. Is cyclosporin associated glomerulopathy a new glomerular lesion in renal allografts using CSA? Presented before the 14th International Congress of the Transplantation Society, Paris, France, August 6–21, 1992.
150. Myers B, Sibley R, Newton L, et al. The long-term course of cyclosporin-associated chronic nephropathy. Kidney Int. 1988; 33:590–600.
151. Zollinger HU, Mihatsch MJ. Renal Pathology in Biopsy. Berlin, Springer-Verlag, 1978.
152. Alexopoulos E, Leontsini M, Daniilidis M, et al. Differentiation between renal allograft rejection and cyclosporin toxicity: a clinicopathological study. Am J Kidney Dis 1991; 18:108–115.
153. Burke JF Jr, Pirsch JD, Ramos EL, et al. Long-term efficacy and safety of cyclosporine in renal transplant recipients. N Engl J Med 1994; 331:358–363.
154. Van Buren DH, Burker JF, Lewis RM. Renal function in patients receiving long-term cyclosporine therapy. J Am Soc Nephrol 1994; 4:S17–22.
155. Pei Y, Scholey JW, Katz A, et al. Chronic nephrotoxicity in psoriatic patients treated with low-dose cyclosporine. Am J Kidney Dis 1994; 23:528–536.
156. Salomon D, Brunson M, Vansickler J, et al. A retrospective analysis of late renal graft function: correlation with mean cyclosporine levels and lack of evidence for chronic cyclosporine toxicity. Transplant Proc 1991; 23(1 Pt 2):1018–1019.
157. Almond PS, Gillingham KJ, Sibley R, et al. Renal transplant function after ten years of cyclosporine. Transplantation 1992; 53:316–323.
158. Consensus conference on cyclosporin A for psoriasis. Br J Dermatol 1992; 126:621–623.
159. Hmiel SP, Brennan DC, Shenoy S, et al. Cytomegalovirus association with episodes of thrombotic microangiopathy in cyclosporine treated renal allograft patients. Abstracts of the 14th Annual Meeting of the American Society of Transplant Physicians May 14–17, 1995, p. 105.
160. Hochstetler LA, Flanigan MJ, Lager DJ. Transplant associated thrombotic microangiopathy: the role of IgG administration as initial therapy. Am J Kidney Dis 1994; 23:444–450.
161. Frem GJ, Rennke HG, Sayegh MH. Late renal allograft failure secondary to thrombotic microangiopathy—human immunodeficiency virus nephropathy. J Am Soc Nephrol 1994; 4:1643–1648.
162. Abramowicz D, Pradier O, Marchant A, et al. Induction of thromboses within renal grafts by high dose prophylactic OKT3. Lancet 1992; 339:777–778.
163. Pradier O, Marchant A, Abramoxicz D, et al. Procoagulant effect of the OKT3 monoclonal antibody: involvement of tumor necrosis factor. Kidney Int 1992; 42:1124–1129.
164. Doutrelepont JM, Abramowicz D, Florquin S, et al. Early recurrence of hemolytic uremic syndrome in a renal transplant recipient during prophylactic OKT3 therapy. Transplantation 1992; 53:1378–1379.
165. Mochon M, Kaiser BA, de Chadarevian JP, et al. Cerebral infarct with recurrence of hemolytic-uremic syndrome in a child following renal transplantation. Pediatr Nephrol 1992; 6:550–552.

166. Gagnadoux MF, Habib R, Broyer M. Outcome of renal transplantation in 34 cases of childhood hemolytic-uremic syndrome and the role of cyclosporine. Transplant Proc 1994; 26:269–270.
167. Fournier A, el Esper N, Makdassi R, et al. Hypertension and progression of renal insufficiency. Nephrol Dial Transplant 1994; 9(suppl 3):28–34.
168. McEnery PT, Nathan J, Bates SR, Daniels SR. Convulsions in children undergoing renal transplantation. J Pediatr 1989; 115:532–536.
169. Halloran PF, Wadgymar A, Ritchie S, et al. The significance of the anti-class I antibody response: I. Clinical and pathologic features of anti-class I-mediated rejection. Transplantation 1990; 49:85–91.
170. Halloran PF, Schlaut J, Solez K, Srinivasa NS. The significance of the anti-class I response: II. Clinical and pathologic features of renal transplants with anti-class I-like antibody. Transplantation 1992; 53:550–555.
171. Trpkov K, Campbell P, Pazderka F, et al. Pathology of anti-class I antibody-induced rejection. Abstracts of the 14th Annual Meeting of the American Society of Transplant Physicians May 14–17, 1995, p 110.
172. Kincaid-Smith P, Nicholls K. Renal thrombotic microvascular disease associated with lupus anticoagulant. Nephron 1990; 54:285–288.
173. Zager RA. Acute renal failure in the setting of bone marrow transplantation. Kidney Int 1994; 46:1443–1458.
174. Antignac C, Gubler MC, Leverger G, et al. Delayed renal failure with extensive mesangiolysis following bone marrow transplantation. Kidney Int. 1989; 35:1336–1344.
175. Garibotto G, Acquarone N, Saffioti S, et al. Successful treatment of mitomycin C–associated hemolytic uremic syndrome by plasmapheresis. Nephron 1989; 51:409–412.
176. Poch E, Gonzalez-Clemente JM, Torras A, et al. Silent renal microangiography after mitomycin C therapy. Am J Nephrol 1990; 10:514–517.
177. Oursler DP, Holley KE, Wagoner RD. Hemolytic uremic syndrome after bone marrow transplantation without total body irradiation. Am J Nephrol 1993; 13:167–170.
178. Loomis LJ, Aronson AJ, Rudinsky R, Spargo BH. Hemolytic uremic syndrome following bone marrow transplantation: a case report and review of the literature. Am J Kidney Dis 1989; 14:324–328.
179. Cohen EP, Lawton CA, Moulder JE, et al. Clinical course of late-onset bone marrow transplant nephropathy. Nephron 1993; 64:626–635.
180. Schmidt RJ, Venkat KK, Dumler F. Hemolytic-uremic syndrome in a renal transplant recipient on FK 506 immunosuppression. Transplant Proc 1991; 23:3156–3157.
181. Randhawa PS, Shapiro R, Jordan ML, et al. The histopathological changes associated with allograft rejection and drug toxicity in renal transplant recipients maintained on FK506. Am J Surg Pathol 1993; 17:60–68.
182. Holman MJ, Gonwa TA, Cooper B, et al. FK506-associated thrombotic thrombocytopenic purpura. Transplantation 1993; 55:205.
183. Lea JP, Sands JM, McMahon SJ, Tumlin JA. Evidence that inhibition of NA+/K+-ATPase activity by FK506 involves calcineurin. Kidney Int 1994; 46:647.
184. Textor SC, Weisner R, Wilson DJ, et al. Systemic and renal hemodynamic differences between FK506 and cyclosporine in liver transplant recipients. Transplantation 1993; 55:1332.
185. European FK506 Multicentre Liver Study Group. Randomised trial comparing tacrolimus (FK506) and cyclosporin in prevention of liver allograft rejection. Lancet 1994; 344:423.
186. The U.S. Multicenter Liver FK506 Liver Study Group. A comparison of tacrolimus (FK506) and cyclosporine for immunosuppression in liver transplantation. N Engl J Med 1994; 331:1110.
187. Porayko MK, Textor SC, Krom RA, et al. Nephrotoxic effects of primary immunosuppression with FK-506 and cyclosporine regimens after liver transplantation. Mayo Clin Proc 1994; 69:105.
188. Platz KP, Mueller AR, Blumhardt G, et al. Nephrotoxicity following othotopic liver trans-

plantation: a comparison between cyclosporine and FK506. Transplantation 1994; 58: 170–178.
189. Thliveris JA, Yatscoff RW. Effect of rapamycin on morphological and functional parameters in the kidney of the rabbit. Transplantation 1995; 59:427–4239.
190. Bennett WM. The nephrotoxicity of immunosuppressive drugs. Clin Nephrol 1995; 43(suppl 1):S3–S7.
191. Whiting PH, Woo J, Adam BJ, et al. Toxicity of rapamycin-a comparative and combination study with cyclosporine at immunotherapeutic dosage in the rat. Transplantation 1991; 52:203–208.
192. Di Joseph JF, Sharma RN, Chang JY. The effect of rapamycin on kidney function in the Sprague-Dawley rat. Transplantation 1992; 53:507–513.
193. Di Joseph JF, Mihatsch MJ, Sehgal SN. Influence of rat strain on rapamycin's kidney effects. Transplant Proc 1993; 25(1 pt 1):714–715.
194. Gaston RS, Deierhoi MH, Patterson T, et al. OKT3 first-dose reaction: association with T cell subsets and cytokine release. Kidney Int. 1991; 39:141–148.
195. Simpson MA, Madras PN, Cornaby AJ, et al. Sequential determinations of urinary cytology and plasma and urinary lymphokines in the management of renal allograft recipients. Transplantation 1989; 47:218–223.
196. Chatenoud L, Legendre C, Ferran C, et al. Corticosteroid inhibition of the OKT3-induced cytokine-related syndrome—dosage and kinetics prerequisites. Transplantation 1991; 51: 334–338.
197. Gaughan WJ, Francos BB, Dunn SR, et al. A retrospective analysis of the effect of indomethacin on adverse reactions to orthoclone OKT3 in the therapy of acute renal allograft rejection. Am J Kidney Dis 1994; 24:486–490.
198. Chatenoud L, Ferran C, Legendre C, et al. In vivo cell activation following OKT3 administration. Systemic cytokine release and modulation by corticosteroids. Transplantation 1990; 49:697–702.
199. De Vault GA Jr, Kohan DE, Nelson EW, Holman JM Jr. The effects of oral pentoxifylline on the cytokine release syndrome during inductive OKT3. Transplantation 1994; 57:532–540.
200. Abramowicz D, Schandene L, Goldman M, et al. Release of tumor necrosis factor, interleukin-2, and gamma-interferon in serum after injection of OKT3 monoclonal antibody in kidney transplant recipients. Transplantation 1989; 47:606–608.
201. Raasveld MH, Bemelman FJ, Schellekens PT, et al. Complement activation during OKT3 treatment: a possible explanation for respiratory side effects. Kidney Int 1993; 43:1140–1149.
202. Goldman M, Van Laethem JL, Abramowicz D, et al. Evolution of renal function during treatment of kidney graft rejection with OKT3 monoclonal antibody. Transplantation 1990; 50:158–159.
203. Toussaint C, De Pauw L, Vereerstraeten P, et al. Possible nephrotoxicity of the prophylactic use of OKT3 monoclonal antibody after cadaveric renal transplantation. Transplantation 1989; 48:524–526.
204. Brown PS Jr, Parenteau GL, Dirbas FM, et al. Anti-Tac-H, a humanized antibody to the interleukin 2 receptor, prolongs primate cardiac allograft survival. Proc Natl Acad Sci USA 1991; 88:2663–2667.
205. Tinubu SA, Hakimi J, Kondas JA, et al. Humanized antibody directed to the IL-2 receptor betachain prolongs primate cardiac allograft survival. J Immunol 1994; 153:4330–4338.

Index

About the Editors

KIM SOLEZ is Professor of Pathology at the University of Alberta, Edmonton, Alberta, Canada. The recipient of the Borden Award, the Schwentker Award, and a Research Career Development Award from the National Institutes of Health, Dr. Solez is the author or coauthor of over 200 publications concerning acute renal failure, renal pathology, and vascular disease. He serves on the editorial boards of *Renal Failure* and *Laboratory Investigation*, and is the editor or coauthor of several books, including (with Lorraine C. Racusen) *Acute Renal Failure: Diagnosis, Treatment, and Prevention*, (with James F. Burdick, Lorraine C. Racusen, and G. Melville Williams) *Kidney Transplant Rejection: Diagnosis and Treatment, Second Edition*, and (with Leendert C. Paul) *Organ Transplantation* (all titles except *Laboratory Investigation*, Marcel Dekker, Inc.). Dr. Solez is a member of numerous professional societies, including the American Society of Nephrology, the American Society for Investigative Pathology, the International Society of Nephrology, the U.S./Canadian Academy of Pathology, the Alberta Society of Laboratory Physicians, the Canadian Medical Association, the Canadian Association of Pathologists, and the Royal College of Physicians and Surgeons of Canada. He is Chairman of the International Society of Nephrology Commission on Acute Renal Failure and Chair of the Nephrology Informatics Committee. He is the owner of the NEPHROL Internet discussion group. Dr. Solez received the M.D. degree (1972) from the University of Rochester School of Medicine and Dentistry, Rochester, New York.

LORRAINE C. RACUSEN is Associate Professor of Pathology at The Johns Hopkins University School of Medicine, Baltimore, Maryland. Her research interests include the pathophysiology of toxic injury in the kidney, GI tract, and central nervous system, as well as animal models and in vitro cell culture studies of renal tubular injury and acute renal failure. The author of over 60 publications, Dr. Racusen serves on the editorial board of *Renal Failure*, is a reviewer for the *American Journal of Pathology*, and is coeditor (with Kim Solez) of *Acute Renal Failure: Diagnosis, Treatment, and Prevention* and (with James F. Burdick, Kim Solez, and G. Melville Williams) of *Kidney Transplant Rejection: Diagnosis and Treatment, Second Edition* (all titles except *American Journal of Pathology*, Marcel Dekker, Inc.). She is a member of the U.S./Canadian Academy of Pathology, the Kidney Council of the American Heart Association, the American Society of Nephrology, the American Association for the Advancement of Science, the International Academy of Pathology, the International Society of Nephrology, and the New York Academy of Sciences. The recipient of the American Heart Association and Stetler Research Foundation Fellowships and a Mellon Clinician Scientist Award, Dr. Racusen received the M.D. degree (1975) from the University of Vermont, Burlington.

MARGARET E. BILLINGHAM is Professor of Pathology Emeritus (active) in the Department of Cardiothoracic Surgery at Stanford University School of Medicine, Stanford California. Dr. Billingham is the author or coauthor of over 300 professional publications on heart and lung transplantation, endomyocardial biopsy, cardiac pathology, and cardiac toxicities. A Fellow of the Royal College of Pathologists, the American College of Cardiology, the American College of Chest Physicians, and the American College of Pathologists, she is a founding member of the International Society for Heart Transplantation and the International Association for Cardiac Biological Implants, Past-President of the Society for Cardiovascular Pathology, and a member of the International Academy of Pathology and the Pathological Society of Great Britain and Ireland, among others. Dr. Billingham received the M.B.B.S. degree (1954) from the Royal Free Hospital School of Medicine, London University, United Kingdom.